RESEARCH FOR NURSES:
METHODS AND INTERPRETATION

RESEARCH FOR NURSES: METHODS AND INTERPRETATION

Angela Gillis, BSN, PhD
Professor and Chair
Department of Nursing
St. Francis Xavier University
Antigonish, Nova Scotia

Winston Jackson, PhD
Professor of Sociology
St. Francis Xavier University
Antigonish, Nova Scotia

F.A. DAVIS COMPANY • PHILADELPHIA

F. A. Davis Company
1915 Arch Street
Philadelphia, PA 19103
www. fadavis.com

Printed in the United States of America

Last digit indicates print number: 10 9 8 7 6 5 4 3 2 1

Acquisitions Editor: Melanie Freely
Developmental Editor: Laura Bonazzoli
Production Editor: Nwakaego Fletcher-Perry
Cover Designer: Louis Forgione

As new scientific information becomes available through basic and clinical research, recommended treatments and drug therapies undergo changes. The author(s) and publisher have done everything possible to make this book accurate, up to date, and in accord with accepted standards at the time of publication. The author(s), editors, and publisher are not responsible for errors or omissions or for consequences from application of the book, and make no warranty, expressed or implied, in regard to the contents of the book. Any practice described in this book should be applied by the reader in accordance with professional standards of care used in regard to the unique circumstances that may apply in each situation. The reader is advised always to check product information (package inserts) for changes and new information regarding dose and contraindications before administering any drug. Caution is especially urged when using new or infrequently ordered drugs.

Library of Congress Cataloging-in-Publication Data

Gillis, Angela, 1953–
    Research for nurses : methods and interpretation / Angela Gillis,
Winston Jackson.—1 st ed.
    p. cm.
    Includes bibliographical references and index.
    ISBN 0-8036-0896-9 (pbk.)
    1. Nursing—Research. 2. Nursing—Research—Methodology. I.
Jackson, Winston. II. Title.
    RT81.5 .G53 2001
    610.73′07′2—dc21

To my mother, father, and sisters, Liza and Catherine, who taught me love. To my husband, Phonse, and daughters, Rita and Catherine, who tolerated my absence when they would have preferred my presence, and who continually remind me that love is what is really important. — AG

. . . and to all the nursing students, past and present, for their commitment and enthusiasm…thanks for the memories and all your wonderful projects. — WJ

Preface

The authors of this text set out with one major goal—to write a book that would demystify the research process as much as possible and to present the material in an exciting, fresh, and innovative manner. The book examines both qualitative and quantitative approaches available to the nurse researcher because no single theory, research design, data collection method, measurement procedure, or statistical approach can provide a satisfactory answer to all research questions.

The text prepares students to be both knowledgeable *users* and *doers* of research. We believe students learn most by active involvement. Where possible, the book presents rules and steps for understanding each stage in evaluating and conducting research. In order to empower and encourage the student, the book provides many ideas for feasible projects that have been undertaken by graduate and undergraduate nursing students. In short, the book is student-friendly, useful, and relevant to contemporary nursing.

Research for Nurses: Methods and Interpretation does not assume that the student has prior knowledge of statistics or of research design. Indeed the strength of the text is that it is comprehensive enough to be used as a graduate text, yet written in a simple and straightforward manner with numerous examples so that the senior un-

dergraduate student with no research experience can grasp the concepts discussed. It is also appropriate for post-registered nurse degree students returning to pursue a baccalaureate degree.

Part 1 focuses on basic concepts of research, the fundamental importance of research to nursing, and the process of identifying important researchable problems.

Part 2 presents five chapters that address the most popular quantitative and qualitative designs in contemporary usage.

Part 3 examines bias and ethical issues in research.

Part 4 discusses basic statistical concepts. This material provides the foundation for the next part.

Part 5 discusses the actual planning and implementation of a research project.

Part 6 deals with analyzing the findings of a study.

Part 7 focuses on reporting and disseminating the findings, critiquing research, and utilizing the findings to enhance practice.

Part 8, a section not typically featured in other nursing research methods texts, explains how to process data using Statistical Package for the Social Sciences (SPSS). This section walks the first-time user through the various steps in analyzing research data and in reading SPSS output.

Other features are:

- Easy-to-follow guidelines for reading and critically appraising quantitative and qualitative research projects.
- A section devoted to new-wave applied designs such as action research, health promotion studies, feminist, and evaluation research.
- Down-to-earth steps to guide the student through a project. This feature helps the student to realize that he or she can engage in rigorous research to answer questions that emerge in the practice setting.
- Case studies and sample projects presented in "Nursing Researchers at Work" boxes to illustrate key approaches, methods, and findings. This is an important feature that helps ground nursing research in the "real" world of nursing.
- Step-by-step instructions for questionnaire design and administration and for sample size determination.

- A chapter devoted to the problem of bias in nursing research. This is a unique feature of the text on a topic that is not sufficiently discussed in most nursing research texts, yet it is a problem that plagues every aspect of the research process.
- A two-chapter statistics primer covering basic statistical material. Advanced techniques such as regression analysis, discriminant analysis, multivariate analysis of variance, and factor analysis are presented in Chapter 18.
- An overview of what NUD*IST means, and a discussion of how it can be used to analyze qualitative data.
- A series of 10 laboratory assignments to train students in the use of SPSS (SPSS^x, SPSS PC+, and SPSS for Windows version 10.0) are included in the instructor's manual along with a sample data on attitudes toward euthanasia.
- Numerous Web site addresses, including the authors' Web site, which includes 160 sample questionnaires designed by student researchers. Other sites will be identified to assist students.

Acknowledgements

Many individuals have freely given their advice on different aspects of this text as it was being developed. We would especially like to thank the many students at St. Francis Xavier University who challenged us with interesting research problems and who taught us so much. To the chapter reviewers at F. A. Davis: thank you for your expertise, promptness, and many suggestions. We hope you can recognize the places where your suggestions improved the text, and perhaps not notice where we did not follow your counsel. To the F. A. Davis staff: thank you for your professionalism, and your editorial and production work. In particular, we would like to thank our acquisitions editor, Melanie Freely, for her enthusiasm, encouragement, creative ideas, and belief in this project; our development editor, Laura Bonazzoli, for her clarity of thought, spirited advise, patience, and skilled editing; our production editor, Nwaka Fletcher-Perry, for her constructive suggestions and attention to last-minute details. To our friends and colleagues: thank you for the insightful comments and the welcomed coffee breaks—without which we could not have written the text as well as we have. We also give our thanks and our gratitude to Donna Beiswanger, Gary Brooks, Lisa Keeping, Tanya Greencorn, Marlies Jackson, Shirley Laffrey, Ellen MacFarlane, Jean MacInnis, Jason Ryan MacLean, Debbie Murphy, Dorothy Payne, Barbara Phillips, Maria Sangster, Judith Shaw, and Saru Sony.

We wish to acknowledge the contribution of St. Francis Xavier University in providing the sabbatical leave that gave us the opportunity to work on the manuscript. The support of Hugh Gillis, Ron Johnson, and Ed McAlduff is most appreciated.

We are also indebted to SPSS Inc. for permission to present the commands for SPSS. As always, SPSS personnel have been most helpful. In particular, we would like to thank Marcus Hearne of SPSS Inc., Chicago, Illinois, who was most generous in providing a copy of version 10.0 of SPSS for Windows to help in the development of Appendix A.

Finally we wish to acknowledge our families for their love, patience, understanding, and support throughout this intensive but exciting endeavor.

Angela Gillis
Winston Jackson
February, 2001

Consultants

Elizabeth Black, MSN, BSN
Assistant Professor
Director ASN Program
Gwynedd-Mercy College
Gwynedd Valley, Pennsylvania

E. Joyce Black, RN, EdD
Education Consultant
Registered Nurses Association of British
  Columbia
Vancouver, British Columbia

Dr. Janet Brookman, DSN, RN
Clinical Associate Professor
The University of Alabama in Huntsville
Huntsville, Alabama

Elizabeth S. Carlson, PhD, RNC
Assistant Professor
School of Nursing
Loyola University-Chicago
Maywood, Illinois

Ann M. Dollins, AD, BSN, MPH, MSN, PhD
Director BSN Program
Northern Kentucky University
Highland Heights, Kentucky

Karen Fernengel, PhD, FNP, CS
Chair Graduate Nursing Program
Graceland University
Leavenworth, Kansas

Rebecca L. Hartman, EdD, RN
Coordinator, Allied Health Professions
Assistant Professor, Nursing
Indiana University of Pennsylvania
Indiana, Pennsylvania

Catherine Blackwell Holland, BS, MS, PhD
Assistant Professor
Southeastern Louisiana University
Baton Rouge Campus
Baton Rouge, Louisiana

Mary Taylor Martof, RN, EdD
Associate Professor
Louisiana State University Health Sciences
  Center
New Orleans, Louisiana

Martha MacLeod, RN, PhD
Associate Professor
University of British Columbia,
British Columbia, Canada

Sharon Moore, RN, PhD
College Research Officer
Faculty of Health and Community Studies
Mount Royal College
Calgary, Alberta

Mary Jo Gorney-Moreno, PhD, RN
School of Nursing
San Jose State University
San Jose, California

Carla Mueller, PhD, RN
Associate Professor
University of St. Francis
Fort Wayne, Indiana

Kathleen Poindexter, RN, DNSc
Assistant Professor
College of Allied Health
Temple University
Philadelphia, Pennsylvania

Rosalee J. Seymour BSN, MSN, EdD
Associate Professor
School of Nursing
East Tennessee University
Johnson City, Tennessee

Teresa Shellenbarger, DNSc, MSN, BS
Professor of Nursing
Indiana University of Pennsylvania
Indiana, Pennsylvania

Maria A. Smith, DSN, RUN, CCRN
Professor
School of Nursing
Middle Tennessee State University
Chattanooga, Tennessee

Susan Urbanski, MSN, RN
President /Executive Director
CIGNA Behavioral Health of California
Glendale, California

Contents

Part 1

GETTING STARTED

C hapter 1 introduces students to a variety of nursing research approaches. In addition to describing research and its utilization as a key to the progress of nursing science, the chapter outlines the major methodological approaches in nursing scholarship. Chapter 2 describes the role of theory in understanding human behavior. Various nursing theoretical frameworks are discussed, along with approaches to testing them. Chapter 3 begins our exploration of how research projects are designed.

Chapter 1

Introduction to Nursing Research

CHAPTER OUTLINE

KEY TERMS

Aesthetics

Applied research

Conceptual hypothesis

Conceptual level

Conceptual variable

Contemporary applied research

Critical perspective

Descriptive research

Empirical knowledge

Epistemology

Ethical knowing

Evidence-based practice

Explanatory research

Field studies

Hypotheses

Interpretive perspective

Macrovariables

Mechanistic model

Methodological triangulation

Microvariables

NUD*IST

Operational level

Operationalization

Participatory action research

Personal knowledge

Positivist perspective

Predictive research

Pure research

Quantitative research

Qualitative research

Reliability

Research

Research process

Scientific method

SPSS

Theoretical level

Validity

Research has been given a bad rap. Many people would have you think of it as dull, intimidating, and even immobilizing, when in reality, conducting research can be fun and exciting as well as crucial to the development of nursing as a profession and the achievement of excellence in practice. For those who approach research with trepidation, this text will help you to realize that the essence of research is reflected in nurses' everyday practice. It is not an obstacle to be avoided but an essential tool that we hope you will come first to understand, then to use, and finally, to embrace.

Nurses have a responsibility to ensure that their clients are the recipients of care that reflects the most current and relevant knowledge available. Thus, research has become a highly valued activity for nurses. As you yourself are experiencing, baccalaureate and graduate-level nursing programs now prepare students with courses in research methods. You also probably have noticed that content in nursing textbooks reflects current research findings as an evidence base for practice. On the professional level, nursing leaders for decades have been challenging nurses to use research findings to improve care. Research utilization has long been a priority in the nursing literature (Lindeman, 1975) and remains a priority today (Moore, 1995; Robinson, 1997). Finally, hospitals, clinics, agencies, and clients expect nurses to engage in **evidence-based practice**—that is, nursing practice should be informed and modified in the light of systematic research that evaluates the effectiveness of alternative interventions.

The authors of this text believe every nurse can develop the skills needed to become actively engaged in the research process. We therefore invite you to take up the challenge of nursing research, and to do so with confidence! In return, we promise that you will soon come to respect the power of nursing research to enhance the quality of your care, further your career goals, and advance the status of the entire nursing profession.

Nursing research includes both qualitative and quantitative approaches. There are fundamental differences between these approaches on virtually every aspect of research. Throughout this text, we will attempt to alert the reader to such differences and to point out how both approaches are legitimate in their own right and both will make significant contributions to nursing research in the years ahead. Later in this chapter, we explore some of the differences between the two approaches. Chapters 6, 7, and 8 are devoted to exploring qualitative research strategies. We will begin our journey on familiar ground, with a comparative view of the nursing process.

A. RESEARCH AND NURSING: PARALLEL PROCESSES

The steps of the **research process** should not be totally new to you because you perform similar activities every day when you engage in critical thinking, reflect on your practice, and apply the nursing process. For example, you engage in *data collection* about your client when you read the client's chart; receive reports; and engage in dialogue with colleagues, the client, and the family. Based on this information and your observations, you formulate a diagnosis of the client's health needs. This stage is similar to *naming, taxonomy,* or *problem identification.* Next, you develop a plan of care specific to the client's identified needs. This is similar to the *methodology plan* that the researcher develops after the problem statement is clearly defined. Your plan is based on an expectation that certain interventions produce intended outcomes for the client. This is similar to *prediction* in the quantitative research process. Finally, you evaluate the effect of the interventions on the client's outcomes and recommend modifications to the plan as new evidence becomes available. This is similar to *interpretation of findings* and the *recommendation stage* of the research process.

Table 1.1 compares the steps of the nursing process with those of the research process, which will be described in detail later in this chapter and throughout this text. For now, it is important to remember that both the nursing process and the research process are simply series of actions taken by the nurse to achieve a specific goal. Ultimately, the general goal of both processes is to improve the quality of care provided to our clients and their families, although specific differences do exist in the means that each process uses to achieve this end.

In effective application of the nursing process, the staff nurse is concerned with similar issues as the researcher. In both processes, the nurse uses problem solving, critical thinking, and complex reasoning to guide logical decisions. Issues of concern to both include:

- Are data about the client valid and reliable?
- Have the relevant problems (diagnoses) been accurately identified?
- Is the client's perspective truly represented in the diagnosis and plan of care?
- What relationships, among which variables, are responsible for the client's outcomes?
- What other variables need to be considered by the nurse?
- What other alternative explanations could account for the intervention results?

As we have stated, although the nursing process and the research process contain parallel elements, their intended purposes are quite different. Quantitative research is conducted to produce findings that are generalizable and meaningful to others. Findings of the nursing

Table 1.1 Comparison of Steps of Nursing Process and Stages of Nursing Research

Nursing Process	Qualitative Research Process	Quantitative Research Process
Assessment and interpretation of data	Selection of a social context	Problem identification Literature review Selection of conceptual framework or theory
Diagnosis of problem	Formulation of research question Explication of researcher's beliefs	Formulation of research question or hypothesis
Development and implementation of plan of care	Development and implementation of methodology plan Cyclical process of data collection, analysis, and concept formation and modification	Development and implementation of methodology plan
Evaluation of plan of care	Interpretation of findings May involve review of the literature at this stage Validation of findings with participants	Interpretation of the findings
Revision of plan based on evaluation	Communication of the findings Implications and recommendations	Communication of the findings, implications, and recommendations

process and of qualitative research, in contrast, are specific to a particular client and setting and are not necessarily generalizable to others. Also, in applying the nursing process and in qualitative research, the nurse may not necessarily have reviewed the literature about a client problem or situated the problem within a theoretical framework. The nurse also may not describe the various factors in a client situation precisely enough that any other nurse could take the same intervention and effectively demonstrate the same results. There is no attempt in the nursing process or in qualitative research to control all of the variables in the environment to the extent that the nurse can be sure that the action taken really accounts for the results.

In addition, the research process is quite simply more complex than the nursing process. It requires that the nurse learn a new vocabulary and a specific set of rules and methods that must be rigorously applied. Without this new knowledge, you will not be able to perform nursing research effectively.

As a nursing student, you apply the nursing process on a consistent basis with ease and confidence. Through working with this text, you will learn to apply the research process with the same ease and to build a body of scientific knowledge that will enhance your practice and increase the accountability of your profession to the public you serve.

B. CONCEPTUALIZING RESEARCH IN NURSING

The term *research* generally implies a systematic inquiry into a subject to discover new knowledge or to validate or refine existing knowledge. Such evidence-based knowledge is the foundation of professional nursing practice. As an inquisitive student of nursing, you may already have asked yourself some fundamental ques-

tions about the type and nature of knowledge you need to practice nursing. These questions may include:

- What is nursing knowledge?
- What knowledge do nurses need to practice nursing?
- How is nursing knowledge created?
- Is nursing knowledge different from that required by other health-care professionals?
- What is nursing research?
- What are the important questions to be researched in nursing?
- When should research results be used to change practice?

The world of nursing research you are about to explore will help you reflect on responses to these questions, spark your curiosity for research possibilities, and challenge your intellectual creativity. Let us begin our exploration by reflecting on the nature of research itself.

1. What Is Research?

Researchers frequently attach different meanings to the term **research;** however, there is consensus that research implies a formal, rigorous, and precise process. These characteristics require research to be a planned and systematic activity. A second point on which there is consensus in the literature is that the aim of research is to discover new knowledge and relationships and find solutions to problems or questions. Box 1.1 provides common definitions of research with varied meanings.

You will notice that whereas some definitions call for a single approach to development of knowledge, requiring objectivity of the researcher, others allow more diversity in the method. The authors of this text believe a broad definition inclusive of both quantitative and qualitative approaches is most useful to advancing the development of nursing knowledge.

BOX 1.1 *Definitions of Research*

Research is a systematic, controlled, empirical, and critical investigation of hypothetical propositions about the presumed relations among natural phenomena (Kerlinger, 1973, p. 11).

Research is a systematic, formal, rigorous, and precise process used to gain solutions to problems or discover and interpret new facts and relationships (Waltz & Bausell, 1981, p. 1).

Research is a process in which observable, verifiable data are systematically collected from the empirical world (i.e., the world we know through our senses) to describe, explain, predict, or control events (Seaman, 1987, p. 3).

Research is an attempt to increase the sum of what is known, usually referred to as a "body of knowledge," by the discovery of new facts or relationships through a process of systematic scientific enquiry (Macleod & Hockey, 1989).

Research is application of formalized methods of obtaining reliable and valid knowledge about empirical experience (Chinn & Kramer, 1995, p. 75).

2. What Is Nursing Research?

Nursing research is similar to research conducted by other professional groups or disciplines in that the same rigorous steps must be followed and the research design and method of investigation must be appropriate to the problem or question studied. What, then, distinguishes research in nursing from research conducted by other health-care disciplines? The past decade has witnessed a lively debate in the literature in response to this question. The diversity of the human experience and the nature of nursing practice require flexibility in our definition, which must make provision for the variations that occur across professional practice settings. This is particularly true today as globalization of our world community highlights the differences in nursing practice and contexts across first-world, second-world, and developing countries. The American Nurses Association provides a definition that is broad enough to include this variety within nursing practice:

> *Nursing research is investigation into the area of knowledge in which the physical and behavioral sciences meet and influence one another in an effort to study how health problems relate to human behavior and how behavior relates to health and illness. It addresses the human and behavioral questions that arise in the treatment of disease, in the prevention of illness, and in the promotion and maintenance of health (ANA, 1976, p.1).*

Defining nursing research requires determining the relevant knowledge for nursing. Since Florence Nightingale's era, nurses have been expanding their professional practice foundation through research efforts designed to develop and test knowledge. This text defines nursing research as research into phenomena that are predominantly and appropriately the responsibility of nurses in their professional practice. This definition implies that we as nurse researchers need to analyze the work that nurses do as a basis for determining what needs to be known and what gaps exist in nursing's knowledge base. Nursing is a professional as well as an academic discipline; hence, it incorporates a clinical practice component as an integral part of its activities. Nurses are responsible for provision of client care, administration of nursing and health-care services, and education of practitioners. Therefore, research in nursing encompasses systematic investigation into each of these areas. We believe that this comprehensive view has considerable potential to contribute to advancing the professional identity of nursing and promoting excellence in practice through knowledge development.

3. What Are the Goals of Nursing Research?

A *goal* is something toward which one's efforts are directed. The goals of nursing research reflect its importance to the discipline. Although they may vary somewhat from researcher to researcher, most would agree on the following five goals:

1. To produce an understanding of human responses across the life span to health and illness states in ever-changing environments. In relation to this goal, we ask, Why do we find regularities, or patterns, in human responses? Which patterns are unique to partic-ular health or illness states and environments, and which are common across settings? We want not only to document these regularities but also to understand the complexity of human responses to therapeutic measures to promote health and minimize the negative impact of illness states.
2. To improve the quality of nursing care and promote health through the application of research methods. To do this, nurses must ask questions about their practice and seek systematic answers.
3. To enhance the recognition of nursing as a science. This recognition is important in attracting to nursing the brightest and best minds and in increasing the respectability of nursing in the research community.
4. To enable nursing, as a practice discipline, to control the provision of its services. To do so, research on those services and the knowledge research can yield are essential. Knowledge provides a basis for professional power and autonomy.
5. To empower nurses. Research efforts help to empower nurses and distinguish nursing's body of knowledge from those of other sciences. On an individual level, the use of knowledge generated through research to change practice empowers the nurse. At the level of the profession, research knowledge justifies nursing services by establishing their validity to clients and other important stakeholders.

To do research in nursing requires intellectual integrity, curiosity, knowledge of the scientific method, and a belief that nursing is important enough to warrant investigation. If we want to argue that nursing makes a difference, that our interventions are cost effective and efficacious and our services socially relevant, then we need to produce evidence to support our claims. The research process and scientific knowledge generated through research are important tools to help us accomplish these goals.

C. THE VARIETIES OF NURSING KNOWLEDGE

1. Sources of Nonresearch-Based Nursing Knowledge

A great deal of our nursing knowledge is not generated through research. Rather, nurses typically draw on knowledge from a variety of sources, each offering something unique to holistic nursing practice. These include tradition, authority, trial and error, personal experience, intuition, and logical reasoning. The difficulty with non–research-based knowledge is that it has limited scientific predictability and cannot be used to justify nursing actions or provide new scientific information to direct practice. The following discussion of alternative sources of nursing knowledge highlights the strengths and limitations of acquiring knowledge in this manner, creating the context for discussing the process of acquiring knowledge through research.

a. Tradition

Folklore and tradition abound in nursing practice and are powerful sources of knowledge. Many established customs and methods of procedure in nursing are embedded in our culture and passed down from one generation of nurses to the next through verbal and written communication. The advantage of this source of knowledge is that it is usually grounded in past experiences that were successful and effective; therefore, it is usually an efficient way of solving a nursing problem.

Many traditions, however, have not been tested for accuracy or effectiveness. For example, the tradition of restricted visiting hours on children's units was thought useful in helping children deal with the separation from home and family. Research into separation anxiety and coping in hospitalized children revealed, however, that children benefit greatly from the presence of a parent, family-centered care approaches, and unrestricted visiting privileges. Although tradition may offer useful solutions to practice problems, nurses need to be aware that such knowledge has not withstood the test of empirical validation. Nurses should be cognizant that new research information may invalidate knowledge and practices derived from tradition.

b. Authority

Authority becomes a source of nursing knowledge when one accepts something an authoritative person says as truth. Historically, nursing has accepted an organizational hierarchy in health care that gave a great deal of authority to those who had the highest level of education or experience. For example, expert nurses who passed on their knowledge and skills to student nurses were considered authorities, as were physicians. Indeed, until the latter half of the 20th century, physicians were often the instructors of nursing students, and they selected topics that perpetuated nurses' role as their "handmaidens." In that era, nurses did not question the knowledge that was passed down

to them. Conformity was expected and rewarded. Today, nursing authorities more often include nursing professors, instructors, clinical associates, and nurse managers. Although these individuals often possess useful information, it is nevertheless important to question and challenge their knowledge through empirical testing. Many times the information is of value; however, prudent nurses will be aware that knowledge from authority sources is not infallible.

c. Trial and Error

The trial and error approach to nursing knowledge usually involves multiple attempts to solve a particular problem until a satisfactory solution is found. For example, a pediatric nurse who is consoling an immobilized child in the hospital may try a number of different play techniques based on the child's developmental stage until finding one that is effective. This method of knowing is inefficient because a number of attempts are usually required before a solution is found. Depending on the situation, trial and error could be hazardous to client safety, and it is often fallible. Additionally, the solution that is found may be specific to a particular client and setting and not generalizable to a broad population. A more structured approach similar to the scientific process would be more practical, efficacious, and frugal in terms of human and financial resources.

d. Personal Experience

Personal experience is a rich source of knowing in nursing. Extensive clinical experience provides nurses with opportunities to recognize patterns of responses in practice and then make predictions about future responses based on observations of the practice. This important source of knowledge allows nurses to transfer learning from one situation to a similar situation with another client.

The work of Benner (1984) has been revolutionary in highlighting the important relationship between clinical experience and nursing knowledge. Benner identified five levels of clinical expertise: novice, advanced beginner, competent, proficient, and expert practitioner. Although personal experience is a functional source of knowledge, it can be limiting if the field of experience is not sufficiently diverse to allow an adequate breadth of rich experiences. Also, the values and beliefs of the knower can bias it.

e. Intuition

Intuitive knowing is the ability to understand a situation or phenomenon as a whole without reasoning or previous study. It has been described as a "gut feeling" or "hunch" that causes a nurse to respond appropriately in unfamiliar situations. Nurses often seem to possess a tacit knowledge within themselves that is deeply rooted in the subconscious until it is required in a practice situation (Meerabeau, 1992). Intuition plays a critical role in the reflective process and, therefore, is central to nursing practice. It has been cited as the exclusive gift of expert practitioners, but others see it as a universal human experience (Mitchell, 1994). However, controversy exists regarding its validity because it does not conform to the recent requirements for evidence-based practice in health care—that is, intuitive knowing is not predictable, measurable, and generalizable. At the same time, it has unquestionably enabled nurses to make significant decisions in client care.

f. Common Sense Reasoning

Reasoning is the ability to understand phenomena and draw conclusions through logical thinking. Reasoning enables nurses to develop an argument to support their conclusions about a particular clinical situation. Two types of reasoning exist, deductive and inductive.

Common sense deductive reasoning is that by which a nurse reaches a conclusion by moving from the general to the specific. It is the approach used to test predictions and validate existing relationships. For example, an obstetrics nurse has noticed over many years of practice that women who have no support person with them while giving birth require more supportive nursing care than those accompanied by a partner, mother, friend, or professional labor coach. When this nurse then admits a 22-year-old woman who is in labor who arrives at the hospital alone by cab, the nurse anticipates that additional care measures will be appropriate for this client.

Common sense inductive reasoning, by contrast, moves from the specific to the general. Specific situations are observed and then combined into a larger, more general statement that can be tested through research. The obstetrics nurse described observed hundreds of individual clients in labor over many years. From these observations of individual clients, the nurse was able to propose a general theory about women who are in labor that could then be tested through formal research.

The validity of nursing knowledge generated through reasoning depends on the accuracy of the information or premises with which one is working. The conclusions are valid only if the premises (statements) on which they are based are valid. Research is used to confirm or refute premises so nurses in practice may use them.

2. Four Ways of Knowing

Epistemology is the study of the nature of knowledge. It seeks to determine how we know what we know. A number of authors have studied ways of knowing in nursing.

A seminal piece of work by Carper (1978) suggested that there are four fundamental ways of knowing in nursing:

a. Aesthetics or the Art of Nursing

Aesthetics is the study of the nature of beauty or art. In nursing, aesthetic knowledge allows nurses to perceive the beauty underlying each encounter with each client. The art of nursing is best expressed through the virtue of empathy, which is the capacity to vicariously experience the feelings of another. The more skilled a nurse becomes in empathizing with clients, the greater the knowledge and understanding that will be gained of alternate modes of reality. Orem (1995) speaks of the art of nursing as the individual nurse's creativity and style in designing nursing care that is effective and satisfying. Aesthetic knowledge involves perception, understanding, empathy, and intuition, and acknowledges the value of everyday experiences lived by individuals. In this respect, it is associated with the interpretive research perspective that will be discussed later in this chapter.

b. Ethics or the Moral Component of Nursing Knowledge

Ethical knowing in nursing focuses on obligation, on what should be done. This pattern of knowing in nursing requires an understanding of different philosophical positions regarding what is good, what is right, and what is desired. The ethical component involves more than knowledge of morality and ethical codes; it involves judgment of moral value in relation to nursing actions and intentions. Nursing involves carrying out deliberate actions that are subject to interpretation and judgment. The moral component of knowledge influences difficult decisions that nurses must make in the context of increasingly complex health care services.

c. Personal Knowledge as a Pattern of Knowing

Personal knowledge involves the interpersonal interactions and relationships between a nurse and a client. It is concerned with the knowing and encountering of the individual self. Through the component of personal knowledge, a nurse using "therapeutic use of self" rejects approaching the client as an object and strives to establish an authentic personal relationship. This requires an acceptance that each client is not a fixed entity but someone constantly engaged in the process of becoming. In therapeutic encounters, nurses develop authentic personal relationships with others, a process possible only because they have learned about themselves. Personal knowledge is of extreme importance to all areas of nursing practice. It is difficult to imagine the development of practice without this essential element that is implicit in everything a nurse does for a client. It is the personal knowledge and opportunity to reflect on personal feelings that enables nurses to recognize the most personal aspects of a situation and respond to the needs of the particular client (Barragan, 1998).

d. Empirics or the Science of Nursing

Empirical knowledge refers to knowledge of the experienced or empirical world. This type of knowledge is generated through scientific methods and is usually organized into laws and theories that help to describe, predict, and explain phenomena. This knowledge is embedded within the positivist perspective that is discussed later in this chapter. In recent years, much emphasis has been placed on developing scientific knowledge for nursing practice.

Although the focus of this text is an exploration of the methods that create the science of nursing, it is important to keep

BOX 1.2 *Nurse Researchers at Work*

SEXUAL HARASSMENT: EVERYDAY VIOLENCE IN THE LIVES OF GIRLS AND WOMEN

Violence is a significant public health issue with consequences for individuals, families, and communities. The emergence of a rapidly growing international organization, the Nurses' Network on Violence against Women International, speaks to the critical interest of nurses in this complex problem. An insidious form of violence that particularly affects girls and young women is sexual harassment. Growing evidence suggests that sexual harassment is a common occurrence in their everyday lives. This project explored how violence becomes "normalized" in the lives of girls and young women.

The objectives of the project were twofold: (1) to explicate the diverse ways in which girls and young women are socialized to expect violence in their lives, and (2) to examine how social policies, legislation, and institutions alleviate or perpetuate the problem in this population.

The study used a *participatory action research* approach and was guided by the principles of *feminist research*. Implicit in the assumptions of the research was the assertion that traditional notions of "girls at risk" may not be useful when addressing the topic of violence. Rather, given the insidious and pervasive nature of many forms of violence, including sexual harassment, all girls must be considered "at risk."

Focus group interviews were conducted in five national centers with ethnically and geographically diverse groups of girls. Questions explored the girls' thoughts about a range of issues such as growing up female, likes and dislikes about being a girl, the most significant joys and challenges of "girlhood," and how they learned about what being a girl is "supposed to be." Although no specific questions about violence or harassment were asked in the focus group interviews, the theme of subtle and explicit forms of violence emerged in all of the sessions. The girls described experiences that evoked fear, intimidation, feelings of belittlement, and a diminished sense of self. When speculating on factors that may have contributed to such experiences, the girls mentioned media, religious dogma, and educational factors. Notably absent from their discussion was the role of gender, including male power and control within a patriarchal society.

The study suggests that nurses have numerous opportunities to empower adolescent girls to deal with sexual harassment. Teaching girls a process of resistance—including behaviors such as adopting a range of healthful habits, speaking out against sexism, and maintaining relationships with which they are able to speak freely and hear their own voices—may help girls minimize the impact of such violence on their lives.

Nurses are in an ideal position to develop health education programs for girls that incorporate a gender-based analysis of the challenges girls face. In addition to empowerment program development, the study challenges nurses to "simultaneously, actively, and loudly join in the larger political struggle against male dominance and one of its primary weapons, sexual harassment."

SOURCE: Summarized from Berman, H., McKenna, K., Arnold, C., et al (2000). Sexual harassment: Everyday violence in the lives of girls and women. *Advances in Nursing Science*, 22(4), 32–46.

such as Ethnograph, Superfile, Framework, and TEXTAN are popular programs that perform content analysis. In addition, most word processing programs can perform sort operations and search a text file for selected words or a string of words. **NUD*IST** (non-numerical unstructured data indexing searching and theorizing) is a software program developed specifically for qualitative data analysis. It is designed to aid researchers in handling non-numerical and unstructured data in qualitative analysis, by supporting processes of coding data in an index system, searching text, or searching patterns of coding and theorizing about the data. Chapter 7 explains NUD*IST commands that are used in computer analysis of qualitative data.

The **SPSS** (Statistical Package for the Social Sciences) is a collection of procedures for processing social science and nursing data. Versions of SPSS date back to the 1960s. Most universities and many research organizations have SPSS. Although many statistical packages are available, few can match the scope of SPSS. Appendix A of this book explains SPSS commands (SPSS for Windows version 10.0) that are used in computer analysis. Readers who have access to earlier versions of SPSS will find that, with a few modifications, the commands presented in this book will work. In addition, a special SPSS supplement is available to instructors using this text, which contains a series of computer assignments designed to familiarize students with SPSS.

E. KEY METHODOLOGICAL PERSPECTIVES IN NURSING SCIENCE

Among the research literature, we identify three important perspectives in the development of nursing science: the *positivist perspective,* the *interpretive perspective,* and the *critical perspective.* Let us investigate the assumptions that these perspectives make about science, human behavior, and values as well as their preferred methodologies and possible weaknesses.

1. The Positivist Perspective

Most people have some familiarity with the **positivist perspective** because it is the one used in the physical sciences. It emerged from a branch of philosophy known as logical positivism, which operates on strict rules of logic, truth, axioms

(general principles), and predictions. Early nurse researchers modeled knowledge development on the physical sciences using the positivist perspective. Many labels, such as behaviorist, empiricist, and scientist, are attached to its practitioners, along, of course, with some less-flattering labels, such as *abstracted empiricist* or *number cruncher.* Some critics of the positivist perspective claim that positivist researchers have become overly impressed with the numbers and the tools used to process them and have lost sight of the goal of trying to understand human behavior and responses. In any case, positivism is the predominant approach that nursing science has taken to develop knowledge. But, as we shall see, the past decade has witnessed an interest in the interpretive and the critical perspective in nursing.

Most positivists would agree with Carlo Lastrucci's definition of science as ". . . an objective, logical, and systematic method of analysis of phenomena, devised to permit the accumulation of reliable knowledge" (1967, p. 6). An *objective* approach is designed to minimize bias, is impersonal, and seeks its authority in fact, not opinion. A *logical* approach uses deductive rules, and a *systematic* approach is consistently organized and makes use of such techniques as statistical analysis. Finally, *reliable knowledge* refers to knowledge one can count on, knowledge that allows one to predict outcomes accurately: ". . . reliable knowledge is that which is both objectively and empirically verifiable" (Lastrucci, 1967). Predictions are empirically verifiable if they can be tested for accuracy by making systematic observations.

a. Positivist Assumptions about Science and Human Behavior

There are a number of basic postulates, or working assumptions, that positivist nurse scientists make in approaching their research. Again, following Lastrucci, we can summarize seven of the major postulates as follows (1967, p. 37–46):

1. *All behavior is naturally determined.* To understand human behavioral responses, we should look for causes in the natural world. This postulate emphasizes a mechanistic view of the world: each outcome is produced by one or more external causes.

2. *Humans are part of the natural world.* Human responses can therefore be studied using the methods used to study the behavior of other species, although the study of human behavior is made far more complex by the need to take language into account.

3. *Nature is orderly and regular.* The natural world is orderly, predictable, and therefore knowable. The patterns of nature may be identified and observed. Events that appear to be random may simply reflect our inability to fully comprehend the natural forces at work.

4. *All objective phenomena are eventually knowable.* There are no intellectual limits on what we may eventually know about nature or about human behavioral responses.

5. *Nothing is self-evident.* Our knowledge of human responses should be demonstrated objectively. And although we may wish to use folk wisdom or "common sense" as a starting point, ultimately we must test ideas systematically.

6. *Truth is relative.* What is regarded as a scientific truth today may be disproved or modified tomorrow. There is a dynamic element to what we know. Our knowledge is always on the road to some ultimate truth, but never quite reaches it.

7. *Knowledge comes from experience.* The belief that we need to test our understanding of the world systematically with knowledge gained through our senses is a fundamental principle of science.

Positivists are interested in understanding the patterns of human response. An emphasis is placed on identifying, measuring, and expressing the relations among variables with mathematical precision. And because cause-and-effect relationships are of central concern to the positivist, it is no surprise that emphasis is placed on prediction.

Positivists search out ways of testing theories of human behavior. For positivists, this implies using the traditional research process or quantitative research. Typically, this is accomplished by establishing *hypotheses* (predictions) about relationships, measuring the variables, and then analyzing the relationships to see if evidence can support or refute the prediction. Efforts are then made to replicate (repeat) the study to see if similar findings result when studying a different population. According to this process, information gained from one study is never sufficient to include in the body of science. A study must be replicated several times with similar results produced each time before the information can be considered a "fact." Facts from studies are then related to each other using abstract thought processes, in a way that seems to best explain the abstract world.

A key indicator of an adequate explanation for positivists is the ability to predict outcomes. Thus, positivists wish to identify the key causes in the variation of some variable. For example, positivists may be interested in identifying the factors that contribute to health-promoting lifestyles in adolescent girls, or compliance with medication schedule in asthmatic children, or job satisfaction of staff nurses working in nurse-run clinics, or the choice of nontraditional comfort measures for women in labor. In each case, the researcher is interested in understanding which factors best predict the phenomenon under investigation. Thus, one measure of the success of a study is when most of the variation is accounted for, and when the causes can be linked to some general theory useful to nursing practice.

Unfortunately, the reputation of nursing science that deals with human responses and natural systems is not impressive when it comes to accurate predictions. Generally, it is thought that only the physical sciences are sufficiently well developed to predict with mathematical accuracy. Indeed, most of the highly predictable outcomes in science are based not on natural, unaltered systems, but rather on engineered systems—systems designed to take into account various influencing factors.

For example, you can predict that no matter what the weather, the bridge you drive over every day to work will be there for you tomorrow. It will be there because it is designed to withstand weather and traffic conditions well beyond its normal loads. So unless something catastrophic happens, the bridge will be there. In contrast, the leaf that blew off the tree in your yard may or may not have moved since yesterday. To estimate its current location would be foolhardy because so many factors could influence where it has moved to since yesterday. Similarly, a huge challenge confronts a nurse who wishes to predict the amount and type of social support required by adolescents to resist smoking. So many factors may influence the adolescent's decision to smoke or not to smoke in a given context. Prediction for a positivist nurse scientist is akin to estimating the whereabouts of the leaf. Natural systems pose a tough challenge for researchers keen on prediction.

b. Positivist View of the Role of Values in Research

Positivists argue that research should be value free. Researchers should put their personal values aside to avoid influencing the outcomes of studies. Positivists maintain that science progresses when researchers systematically test alternative explanations of behavior (attempting to rule them out) without trying to support some pet theory or favored project.

c. Research Designs Associated with Positivism

The positivist perspective relies mainly (but by no means exclusively) on *experiments, surveys,* and *secondary data analysis* (information collected by persons other than the researcher). Typically, positivist perspectives rely on some form of numerical analysis rather than on verbal descriptions.

d. Criticisms of Positivism

Many criticisms have been leveled against the positivist perspective to knowledge. Some of the major criticisms are:

- Some critics argue that value-free research is an unattainable goal. Some studies have shown that despite the best intentions, it is extremely difficult for a researcher to prevent his or her biases or expectations from exerting some influence on the results of a study (see Chapter 9).
- Some critics argue that the so-called *value neutrality* of positivism is itself a value.
- Other critics argue that some areas within nursing do not lend themselves to scientific measurement. For example, it is difficult to quantify the experience of meaning in life in the elderly, the phenomenon of courage in the face of terminal illness, or resilience in victims of sexual abuse.
- Some scholars argue that the positivistic view ignores a crucial aspect of social reality—namely, that different people may experience and perceive the same events differently. The sub-

jective experience of a client's world is an alternate social *reality* that may be explored by a nurse scientist; it is the one emphasized particularly by those who use the interpretive perspective.

- Qualitative researchers believe that the whole is greater than the sum of the parts and that in their treatment of data, positivists treat only the isolated "parts"—therefore, positivists seem to be defining the whole as a sum of the parts.

2. The Interpretive Perspective

The German scholar Max Weber (1864–1920) was particularly influential in developing methodological approaches that stressed the importance of the interpretation *individuals* put on their actions and on the actions and reactions of others. He emphasized *Verstehen,* the empathetic understanding of behavior. The researcher should try to imagine how a particular individual perceives social actions. How does the individual feel? What are the individual's motivations? What meaning does the individual attach to a particular event?

The interpretive perspective and methodologies were further developed by others outside of nursing, such as Mead (1934), Goffman (1962), Glaser and Strauss (1967), Lincoln and Guba (1985), Denzin and Lincoln (1994), and Strauss and Corbin (1997). However, within the past two decades, this perspective has gained increasing popularity as an appropriate approach for exploring the depth, richness, and complexity of nursing phenomena. The works of Chenitz and Swanson (1986), Leininger (1985, 1990), Morse (1991, 1998), Parse (1987), Sandelowski (1995), Streubert and Carpenter (1999), and Stern (1998) have brought this perspective to the forefront of knowledge development in nursing. The interpretive perspective will no doubt undergo evolu-

tionary changes within the field of nursing as more researchers use it to develop the field's knowledge base.

a. Interpretive Assumptions about Science and Human Behavior

Rather than confining itself to behavior alone, the **interpretive perspective** examines how people make sense of their lives, how they define their situation, and how their sense of self develops in interaction with others. In this perspective, humans act and interact on the basis of symbols that have meaning for them. Humans are always in a process of *becoming;* they are influenced by how they see themselves, by how others see them, and by what they want to become. Symbolic interactionists, for example, stress the idea of *role modeling*—that is, the extent to which an individual chooses to emulate someone else's attitudes and behaviors. Note that in this view, the individual is actively choosing to be similar to someone else. In contrast, most theories that use the positivist or critical perspectives emphasize the extent to which individuals are *shaped,* or molded, by the institutions in their society.

The interpretive perspective believes a single reality does not exist. Rather, reality is based on perceptions, so it can be different for each person and can change with time. Interpretive scientists believe that what we know has meaning only within a given context. Meaning is produced by perceptually putting pieces together to make wholes. Because perception varies with the individual, many different meanings to a situation or event can exist.

The philosophical underpinnings of the interpretive perspective are very much in keeping with the nursing field's own understanding of the world. Its focus on a context-related and holistic approach to knowledge development that underpins practice is consistent with many of the field's central values (Masterson, 1996). This perspective encourages us to work with clients in their own environment to enhance our understanding of the emotions and perceptions involved in a given situation. As an example, Finfgeld (1998) explored courage among middle-aged adults with long-term health concerns. This study described the process of being courageous and the role that nurses can play in bolstering clients' courageous desires and behaviors. It provided specific examples of skills that nurses should use in their practice with chronically ill clients. Therefore, this study is an example of how knowledge gained from the interpretive perspective can be used to improve nursing practice.

b. Interpretive Views of the Role of Values in Research

Interpretive nurse scientists argue that values are relative—that is, they would argue that definitions of what constitutes appropriate or inappropriate behavior depend on the socialization that one has received from one's society. These definitions shift over time and across societies. Researchers should try to understand (empathetically) and to explain the values of the people being studied (i.e., the "actors").

c. Research Designs Associated with the Interpretive Perspective

The interpretive perspective relies mainly on field studies and emphasizes using participant observation and in-depth interviewing techniques. Some of the most frequently used qualitative methodologies in nursing include phenomenology, grounded theory, ethnography, and ethnomethodology. Interpretive field studies typically involve a few individuals who are described in detail because there is a desire to provide in-depth understanding of the social world from the participant's view. A key question for these researchers is, "Does the explanation offered make sense to the people whose behavior is being explained?" Communication of the results of such studies usually emphasizes rich textual descriptions rather than numerical analyses.

d. Criticisms of the Interpretive Perspective

As we have seen, the interpretive perspective differs markedly from the positivist perspective. Any proponent of the existence of general abstract laws would criticize the interpretive perspective for its subjectivity. Moreover, some critics reject the interpretive theorists' assessment that all values are equally valid and point out that this assessment is itself a value. Other critics argue that, with its emphasis on field studies, the interpretive perspective does not enable the researcher to make clear generalizations. We cannot easily determine whether the findings of a case study are particular to it or more generally applicable. The difficulty is even more acute when studies cannot be replicated—an ethnomethodological study of individual understandings of events would be a good example. The emphasis on the single case gets us into an old dilemma of knowing more and more about less and less, but in fairness, this criticism can be leveled in varying degrees against all types of systematic inquiry. Finally, if emphasis is placed on the individual level of analysis, it seems to be difficult to understand social patterns: to what extent can we understand interrelations among client groups by studying interactions among individual clients? But the response to this criticism may be that no nursing or related theory can hope to explain all client behavior.

3. The Critical Perspective

Numerous schools are included under the **critical perspective,** but the theorists generally credited with developing this perspective are Karl Marx (1818–1883) and George Simmel (1858–1918). Variants of critical theory abound in all social science disciplines. In brief, the essential themes that a critical researcher might explore include the scientific study of social institutions and the meanings of social life; the historical problems of domination, alienation, and social struggles; and a critique of society and the visioning of new possibilities (Creswell, 1998). The philosophy of critical social theory guides the researcher in seeking to understand how people communicate and how they develop symbolic meanings in a society. Many of the meanings in society have been taken for granted rather than discussed and debated. Nurses need to be aware of this because a number of meanings impede free and equal participation of nurses and clients in society. A nurse researcher using this perspective tries to uncover constraints that limit full participation by all members in society. Understandably, then, in many ways, *feminist theory* fits well with the critical perspective and could be considered a subset of critical social theory even though, methodologically, feminism draws much of its inspiration from the interpretive perspective. Proponents of the critical perspective share a common desire to improve the condition of humanity.

Participatory action research uses critical social theory methods. It is research for the purpose of taking action and creating change. The focus is on learning about how people actually experience a specific issue or problem. This knowledge is key to knowing what actions will make a practical difference in people's lives and why. Through action research, challenges can be made to current nursing practice and, on some occasions, even result in the transformation of practice (Stevens and Hall, 1992). The critical paradigm can help nurses to see the world through a different lens. It can be viewed from a global perspective in terms of the world of nursing and its development. Also, it can be seen from a practical perspective in terms of multidisciplinary relationships in which issues such as gender, relationships with medicine, and the perceived role in society have caused nurses to feel oppressed (Barragan, 1998). Research in this tradition can lead to emancipation for nurses and a valuing of their contributions to health care.

a. Critical Assumptions about Science and Human Behavior

According to the critical perspective, human behavior consists of different groups who are attempting to enhance their interests at the expense of less powerful groups. Whether it is physicians exerting influence over members of the health-care team or men exercising dominance over women, this perspective stresses that conflicting interests characterize human relations. Proponents of the critical perspective argue that scientists have an obligation to act as advocates working for changes in society, changes needed to bring social justice to all. Researchers help bring about such changes by making us more sensitive to social problems. In turn, this knowledge empowers citizens, helping them to become agents of social transformation (Fay, 1987, p. 27). The fundamental goal of the critical perspective is to bring about a truly egalitarian society—one with an *equality of opportunity* as well as an *equality of result.*

b. Critical View of the Role of Values in Research

Critical scientists forthrightly declare that whereas certain values are correct, others are not. In short, the critical perspective takes an absolutist view of values. Researchers working in the critical tradition would argue that the relativist position of mainstream social science has had the consequence of supporting the established order in society, and has had, therefore, little impact on reducing social inequities. Scientists in the critical tradition favor imposing moral absolutes in order to deal with inequalities.

c. Research Designs Associated with Critical Perspectives

The research designs associated with the critical perspective span a broad range. But, given the interest in understanding the relations between groups in society and in understanding how social change occurs, it is no surprise that critical social scientists tend to work with historical materials and thus pay particular attention to the analyses of secondary data. This focus tends to emphasize **macrovariables** (i.e., properties of societies) rather than **microvariables** (i.e., properties of individuals).

Research and explanations are judged to be valid if they lead to an improvement in the social condition of humanity. The critical perspective thus has a strong practical orientation. Social science analysis is seen as a means of achieving greater social justice for all.

d. Criticisms of the Critical Perspective

Similar to the positivist perspective, the critical perspective relies on general theories. But positivists, as well as interpretive researchers, would reject the imposition of absolute values. Positivist critics would argue that the difficulty with adopting a value position in any scholarly discipline is that it enhances the likelihood of distorting research to promote one's personal values. Critical researchers may be too selective, reporting only findings that are compatible with their values and

ignoring all others. Critics maintain that critical researchers are unlikely to make a rigorous attempt to exclude competing explanations of behavior or to find support for competing value systems. In fairness, however, this criticism could be leveled at all perspectives.

Table 1.2 summarizes the main ideas of the three major contemporary methodological perspectives. Each perspective can increase our understanding of human responses to health and illness situations across the life span. Rather than rejecting any one of them outright, we would do well to regard each perspective as potentially valuable in our quest for nursing knowledge.

F. TYPES OF RESEARCH: SOME IMPORTANT DISTINCTIONS

Before you can begin to conduct research, you need to become familiar with a variety of choices of techniques, types, and populations. These distinctions are described in this section and are summarized in Table 1.3.

I. Quantitative Versus Qualitative Approaches

Research approaches can be classified as either *quantitative* or *qualitative*. The distinction is based on the degree to which the analysis is done by converting observations to numbers or using narrative text to describe human experiences. The distinction also reflects differences in the types of questions asked, the kinds of evidence considered appropriate for answering a question, and the methods used to process this evidence. It is probably best to think of the quantitative–qualitative distinction as a continuum.

a. Quantitative Research

Quantitative research seeks to quantify, or reflect with numbers, observations

Table 1.2 Summary of Three Key Methodological Perspectives in Nursing Research

Criterion	Positivist	Interpretive	Critical
View of science	A tool for uncovering general laws of cause and effect in social behavior	A tool for understanding the reality experienced by people	A tool that should be used to improve the condition of the oppressed
View of human behavior	Caused by forces acting on the individual Characterized by regularity and order	Determined by context and individual perception of meaning	Consists of groups attempting to exploit others for their own advantage
Goals of research	To predict behavior; to test general theories of behavior by testing of hypotheses	To provide an adequate reflection of peoples' experience of the social world Testing grounded theory	To improve the social conditions of the oppressed To achieve a just society Advocacy
Role of values in research	Research should be value free; relativistic	Research should be value free; relativistic	Absolutist; research should impose moral absolutes derived from theory
Research designs associated with	Surveys, experiments, quasi-experiments, secondary data, historical analysis (tends toward quantitative orientation)	In-depth interviews, participant observations, field studies, document analyses (tends toward qualitative orientation)	Historical, comparative, interviews, advocacy research (uses both qualitative and quantitative approaches)

about human behavior. It emphasizes precise measurement, the testing of hypotheses based on a sample of observations, and a statistical analysis of the data. Quantitative researchers attempt to describe relationships among variables mathematically and to apply some form of numerical analysis to the relationships being examined. Quantitative researchers, like physical scientists, treat their subject matter like an object. Quantitative research is characteristic of the positivist perspective. It is also used (together with qualitative research) in the critical perspective. Box 1.3 provides an example of quantitative research.

Quantitative research can be conceived of as having three levels: the theoretical, the conceptual, and the operational.

(i) Theoretical Level

The **theoretical level** in a project is the most abstract, general conceptualization of the research problem. Theories propose explanations of phenomena—how things work, how parts are interconnected, and how things influence each other. Theories provide explanations to account for social patterns or for relationships. Many theories are required to account for the multitude of experiences encountered by human beings. The more general the theory, the greater the number of predictions that can be derived from it. Indeed, the number of predictions that can be derived from a theory is also a measure of the theory's power. Theories may be viewed as lying on a continuum of explicitness. At one end of this continuum, we would place a theory in which there are detailed statements of the relationships between the concepts of the theory and a specification of its underlying assumptions (in Chapter 2 we refer to these as *grand theories*); at the other end, we would place the theories

Table 1.3   Summary of Key Distinctions in Types of Research

	Unit of Analysis			
	Individual		**Aggregation**	
Dimension	One or few	Several or many	One or few	Several or many
Tendency in orientation	Qualitative	Quantitative	Qualitative	Quantitative
Types of study	Case study Phenomenology Grounded theory Ethnomethodology	Survey Experiment Quasi-experiment	Case study Participant observation	Comparative
Disciplines	Psychiatry Sociology Nursing	Psychology Sociology Political science History Education Nursing	Anthropology Sociology Political science Archaeology Nursing	Anthropology Sociology Political science Archaeology Nursing
Example	Describing the birthing experience	Variations in desired family size by gender and age	Describing changes in birth rates over time in one community	Comparing birth rates by community
Types of analysis	Thematic analysis; verbatim quotations	Statistical	Content analysis of interview; verbatim quotations	Statistical

that offer explanations of particular relationships (these are identified as *practice theories*).

Nurse scientists use theories to describe, explain, or predict limited properties of reality. An important role of methodologists is to try to refine them to see if they hold true under all conditions. It is through efforts to *disconfirm* theories that we extend our general knowledge of human behavior. One way to test a theory is to derive a prediction (or hypothesis) from it and then test that hypothesis. Chapter 2 discusses the nature of theories and ways of testing them in greater detail.

(ii) Conceptual Level

The **conceptual level** defines the variables that are to be used in the research. A **conceptual variable** is an idea that has a dimension that can vary. Conceptual variables can be relatively simple or quite complex. Examples include gender, weight, intelligence, peer pressure, social support, and anxiety. Derivations made at the theoretical level may be formed into conceptual hypotheses. A **conceptual hypothesis** is a statement of the relationship between two or more conceptual variables. Ordinarily, a hypothesis will take the form of *the greater X, the greater Y.* For example, "the higher one's socioeconomic status, the higher one's perceived health status."

The conceptual definitions of variables serve two important purposes. First, they should provide a clear statement of what is meant by the variables. Second, they should help us decide how each variable should be measured. For example, if we define the concept *socioeconomic status* as "differences in access to scarce resources," then we would try to measure the variable with *indicators* that reflect this definition as precisely as possible. This brings us to the operational level, which we will consider next.

BOX 1.3 *Nurse Researchers at Work*

THE EFFECTS OF RELAXATION THERAPY ON PRETERM LABOR OUTCOMES

The purpose of this experimental study was to determine the effect of relaxation therapy on preterm labor outcomes in a sample of 84 pregnant women. Participants were recruited from private physician offices and a hospital-based maternity triage unit. A total of 44 participants were assigned to the experimental group and 40 were assigned to the control group.

The experimental treatment consisted of in-home audiotaped instructions on strategies for conscious release of tension. Subjects were instructed to do the exercises daily. Progress was monitored weekly through telephone contact by the researcher. Subjects in the control group were also contacted by telephone weekly and asked how they were progressing. This was meant to protect against the possibility that the telephone contact would contribute to the treatment effect. After several weeks in the study, 23 subjects in the experimental group reported that they had ceased doing the exercises. Data from this group of subjects were retained but analyzed as a third group.

Results suggest that women who remained loyal to the experimental protocol of daily relaxation exercises had significantly longer gestation periods, delivered larger newborns, and had higher rates of pregnancy prolongation than either the control group or the nonadherent group. These findings suggest that teaching daily relaxation strategies to pregnant mothers can reduce the incidence of premature labor and the complex problems that result from it. The use of such therapy warrants further investigation.

SOURCE: Summarized from Janke, J. (1999). The effects of relaxation therapy on preterm labor outcomes. *Journal of Obstetric, Gynecologic and Neonatal Nursing, 28,* 255–263.

(iii) Operational Level

Operationalization refers to the selection of indicators (measures) to reflect conceptual variables and to the implementation of a research project. If socioeconomic status is defined as "differences in access to scarce resources," any measurement should attempt to reflect this definition. In this case, a measure of annual income might appropriately reflect the conceptual variable, as defined. And, in the study of perceived health status, the classification of health status into excellent, very good, fair, and poor would constitute a measure of the concept. The **operational level** consists of the measurement of variables as well as the collection and analysis of data. Later chapters provide a number of suggestions for the measurement of variables and a variety of procedures for collecting and analyzing data.

(iv) Linkages between Levels: Validity and Reliability

The theoretical, conceptual, and operational levels of a research study do not exist in isolation from one another. Important linkages connect them: testing a theory properly entails documenting explicitly the connections between the theoretical and the conceptual levels and between the conceptual and the operational levels.

Quantitative nurse researchers use two terms, *validity* and *reliability,* to refer to the connection between the conceptual and the operational levels. **Validity** refers to the extent to which a measure reflects a concept, reflecting neither more nor less than what is implied by the definition of the concept. It is not unusual for researchers to use markedly different "indicators" for similar conceptual variables. Although one might define socioeconomic status as "differential access to scarce resources," another might define it as a "hierarchy of respect and prestige." Measures are valid to the extent that the chosen indicators reflect the concepts as defined.

Reliability refers to the extent to which, on repeated measures, an indicator will yield similar readings. One can think of reliability as the extent to which a measurement will produce similar readings for similar phenomena. A tire gauge that indicates 26 lb of pressure now, but 29 lb a moment earlier, suggests an unreliable gauge—either that or a bad leak in the tire. In survey research, we sometimes repeat a question to test for reliability. Both responses to the question should be the same if the item is generating reliable responses. (The concepts of validity and reliability are discussed in greater detail in Chapter 13.)

(v) Types of Questions Asked

The types of statements or questions asked in quantitative research often describe variables, examine relationships among variables, and determine cause-and-effect interactions between variables. Typical questions would include:

- What are Hispanic-American mothers' beliefs when their children have physical disabilities?
- What support factors in the work environment are most important in determining the level of job satisfaction experienced by nurses in critical care units?
- What is the relationship between use and need of nursing services in rural areas serviced by independent nurse practitioners?
- Is a school-based, health-promotion intervention program effective in increasing the rate of healthy lifestyle choices by adolescents?

(vi) Types of Analysis

In quantitative research, findings are typically expressed in terms of relationships that are presented in tables and graphs. Variables are sometimes *cross-classified* to show how one variable changes as another variable changes. A table might show, for example, how average levels of job satisfaction of nurses vary by degree of perceived autonomy in the workplace. This same finding could also be presented in the form of a graph. A great variety of statistical procedures are available to quantitative researchers. It is important to learn which procedures are appropriate for a given research problem.

b. Qualitative Research

Qualitative research emphasizes verbal descriptions and explanations of human behavior. Rather than concerning itself primarily with representative samples, qualitative research emphasizes careful and detailed descriptions of life experiences in an attempt to understand how the participants experience and explain their own world and give meaning to it. The tools for gaining information include participant observation, in-depth interviews, or an in-depth analysis of a single case. At the macro level, qualitative researchers tend to look at whole institutions or organizations; at the micro level, qualitative researchers focus on individual behaviors and responses. Qualitative research is characteristic of the interpretive perspective. It is also used (together with quantitative research) in the critical perspective. Box 1.4 provides an example of a qualitative research project.

We should note that the stages of a qualitative research project include most of those described earlier, but the sequence is typically cyclical rather than linear. This is because qualitative methods are concerned with gaining a deeper understanding of phenomena from the participant's perspective, which is ever evolving. Thus, inductive approaches to inquiry are used, in which the researcher moves back and forth between the data

BOX 1.4 Nurse Researchers at Work

A NURSE PRACTITIONER MODEL OF PRACTICE

The purpose of this qualitative investigation was to describe the nurse practitioner role in a neonatal intensive care unit (NICU) so that an advanced practice nursing model unique to the role of the nurse practitioner in the NICU could be developed. An ethnographic case study approach was used. The practices of seven NICU nurses were studied through participant observation and interview procedures.

The researcher, as ethnographer, operated in the participant-as-observer role and therefore had access to a wide range of information. Shadowing the NPs, the researcher took extensive notes and used a tape recorder to record observations. Unstructured, open-ended interviews were conducted with each NP at the conclusion of the observation period.

Data collection occurred over a 15-month interval. Data were analyzed for the presence of themes and patterns. The findings were reviewed with each participant for confirmation. Results suggest that NPs practice within a model of care that incorporates "medical and nursing role functions and emphasizes holism, caring, and a health perspective for critically ill neonates and their families." They function in a highly technological environment with a high level of responsibility and accountability. As one NP stated:

I think that advanced practice allows you to practice with a combination of the nursing and medical model. I think that not only do I make medical diagnoses and perform diagnostic procedures and order the therapeutic regimens or prescriptions but I think my role is different from, say, a physician in that I also look at the nursing piece of it and that is the effect that illness has on the infant and the family.

This study clearly delineates the role of the NP in NICU as one that blends nursing and medicine within a holistic approach to promoting health in critically ill neonates. Future research should address the outcomes of the NPs' holistic focus on the health of neonates and their families in NICUs.

SOURCE: Summarized from Beal, J. (2000). A nurse practitioner model of practice. *The American Journal of Maternal Child Nursing*, 25(1), 18–24.

---

collection and analysis stages to derive a dynamic truth that reflects human interaction in social settings.

(i) Types of Questions Asked

The types of questions asked in qualitative research often concern how social systems operate, how individuals relate to one another, how individuals perceive one another, and how they interpret their own and others' behavior. Questions such as these are typical:

- What is the meaning of the experience of participating in public health education sessions for mental health clients?
- What is the experience of men who are primary caregivers for spouses with Alzheimer's disease?

- How do nurses handle patients who refuse to follow instructions?
- What is it like to be diagnosed with a terminal illness?

(ii) Types of Analysis

In qualitative research, findings are typically expressed by quoting interviews or relating experiences the researcher has had in the field. The findings are compared with the literature to see if similar results have occurred in other studies. Most final reports have few, if any, tables or graphs. Because much qualitative research is based on a small number of participants or on an in-depth examination of one group, it is often inappropriate to even attempt to quantify the results.

Various sections of Chapters 6 and 7 elaborate on the procedures that may be used to conduct different types of qualitative studies and present an alternative view to that of quantitative researchers on such issues as the meaning of validity and the goals of research.

c. Choice of Strategy

Although considerable debate exists over the relative merits of quantitative and qualitative research strategies, the issue is a false one, to a large degree. It is false because both approaches have their legitimate place in nursing research. The choice of strategy is influenced by the following factors:

- **The nature of the question asked.** If the question has to do with the nature of a human experience, a small number of observations, or a single case, then the use of quantitative techniques would be inappropriate. If the question has to do with patterns of human responses or descriptions of whole populations or a test of relationships among variables or differences, the approach will be quantitative.
- **The predisposition of the researcher.** If the researcher has a preference for qualitative research strategies, he or she will tend to ask questions that are best answered by using such methods.
- **The philosophy and nursing paradigm (worldview) of the researcher.** If the researcher reflects beliefs about person, health, and environment (the phenomena of concern to nursing), from the *totality paradigm,* the researcher will tend to pose questions and study problems best answered by quantitative methods. The totality paradigm has been the primary operating belief system in nursing. It posits the person as a total organism with bio-psycho-social-spiritual features that interact with the environment to maintain balance

and achieve goals. The field of nursing's emergence alongside medicine has crystallized this view. If the researcher reflects beliefs about person, health, nursing, and the environment from the *simultaneity paradigm* (alternate worldview), he or she will tend to pose problems that are best suited to a qualitative approach. The simultaneity paradigm views person as a unitary being in continuous mutual interrelationship with the environment, co-creating health through mutual interchange with the environment (Parse, 1987). The emergence of different philosophies and nursing paradigms provides grounding for research and is necessary to advance the boundaries of the discipline.

Sometimes the author of a research report will use a qualitative reporting style in order to communicate effectively. Qualitative research uses language and presentations familiar to all educated members of a society.

It is also important to note that there are qualitative dimensions in quantitative research. In the process of turning observations into numbers, there are typically a number of judgment calls, a number of qualitative decisions that must be made. So, whether the researcher wishes to decide how to design a question to find out how much self-esteem someone has, or how to classify educational programs as promoting health, or what determines a healthy lifestyle choice, a number of subjective judgments must be made. And although these may be defined numerically, there is nonetheless a qualitative dimension to the research decision. Virtually all studies that claim to be quantitative have important qualitative dimensions to them.

d. Methodological Triangulation

Methodological triangulation is the application of diverse methods to generate and collect data about one phenomenon (Kimchi, Polivka, and Stevenson, 1991; Creswell, 1994). The methods may be drawn from "within-methods" approaches, such as different types of quantitative data collection strategies in the same study (e.g., a survey and experiment), or it may involve "between-methods" approaches drawing on quantitative and qualitative data collection procedures (e.g., ethnography and survey research) in the same study. *Triangulation* is a term borrowed from the navigational tradition and refers to the use of multiple referents to draw conclusions about what constitutes truth. It is based on the assumption that any bias inherent in particular data sources, investigators, and methods would be neutralized when used in conjunction with other data sources, investigators, and methods.

Nurse researchers are using methodological triangulation with increasing frequency as a means of achieving a more complete understanding of nursing phenomena. The complex nature of nursing lends itself well to study using multiple methods.

(i) Perspectives on Methodological Triangulation

Some researchers believe triangulation is a method for linking quantitative and qualitative methods in a single study. In 1959, Campbell and Fisk sought to use more than one method to study a psychological trait to ensure that the variance was reflected in the trait and not in the method. Hence, the triangulation method is not new to social scientists. It is, however, a new method for nursing science.

Rossman and Wilson (1985) identify three perspectives on triangulation: purist, situationalist, and pragmatist. *Purists* believe that quantitative and qualitative approaches are derived from different, mutually exclusive understandings and beliefs about the nature of research, and hence, the paradigms and methods should not be mixed. *Situationalists* believe that both quantitative and qualitative approaches have value for specific situations. They use both methods but usually in a parallel manner in a study with little integration of the procedures or the findings. The situation dictates the methods a situationalist will use. *Pragmatists* attempt to integrate quantitative and qualitative methods in a single study. They argue that a false dichotomy exists between the two approaches and that researchers should make the best available use of techniques to answer questions of substantive importance. This perspective views triangulation as a means to richer and more insightful analysis of complex phenomena rather than an end in itself. The increasing number of triangulated studies in the literature suggests that nursing is moving in the direction of the situationalist and pragmatist perspectives.

(ii) Models of Combined Designs

Creswell (1994) has advanced three models of combined design as a means of adding scope and breadth to a study. These include:

- **The two-phase design.** Here quantitative and qualitative studies are presented and discussed in two distinct phases. This enables the researcher to clearly separate the two paradigms and respective assumptions behind each phase. The disadvantage is that it becomes difficult for the reader to see the connection between the two phases.
- **The dominant/less-dominant design.** Here one paradigm, either quantitative or qualitative, dominates the study, and a small component of the study (typically, the data collection stage) is drawn from the alternate paradigm. A classic example of this approach is a quantitative study with a small qualitative interview component in the data collection phase. Gillis (1993) conducted a triangulated study following this classic approach. Determinants of

health-promoting lifestyles were explored in 184 adolescent girls and their mothers and fathers using self-administered questionnaires to measure the study variables. Triangulation was accomplished by analysis of data from semi-structured interviews with a subset of eight adolescent participants. Another example is qualitative observations with a limited number of informants followed by a quantitative survey of a sample from a population. This approach presents a consistent paradigm picture in the study and still gathers limited information to probe in detail one aspect of the study. The disadvantage is that purists from both the quantitative and qualitative worldviews claim that central assumptions of each method do not match the data collection procedures.

- **The mixed-methodology design.** Here the quantitative and qualitative paradigms are combined at many methodological steps in the design such as the purpose statement, literature review, and research questions. This approach enjoys the advantages of both the quantitative and qualitative paradigms but adds considerable complexity to the design. Inductive and deductive reasoning are required in the same study. A sophisticated knowledge of both paradigms is required by the researcher to link the diverse methods together appropriately in the mixed-method approach.

(iii) Benefits of Triangulation

The main benefits of methodological triangulation are convergence on truth and a deeper understanding of the phenomena under investigation. Additional benefits include the emerging of overlapping and different facets of a phenomenon, a developmental informing of the second method by the first method used sequentially, and increased credibility and validity of results owing to corroboration of data. Finally,

mixed methods may contribute to new dimensions, contradictions, and fresh perspectives that may lead to new research questions and significant areas of inquiry.

(iv) Challenges of Triangulation

Methodological triangulation presents unique challenges to researchers. Connelly, Bott, Goffart, and Taunton (1997) outline the major problems created by this approach. Combining quantitative and qualitative methods is resource intensive in terms of investigator knowledge, skill, time, and finances. On the other hand, if two or more researchers with skill and expertise in each paradigm work together, the best of both worlds can emerge. The interpretation of inconsistent and contradictory numerical and textual findings must be considered. When this happens, the researcher needs to explore possible explanations and reconcile differences in meaning. Furthermore, replication of combined design studies is difficult and time consuming. This may limit the number of investigations that would enable validation of known findings. Finally, the investigator must decide how to weigh data sources and determine whether each method is equally sensitive.

2. Descriptive versus Explanatory versus Predictive Research

In addition to determining whether your study should be purely quantitative, purely qualitative, or triangulated, you must also consider the goal, or the main concern, of your work: specifically, do you wish to describe, explain, or predict?

Descriptive research (also called *exploratory research*) emphasizes the accurate portrayal of nursing phenomena. A study that is primarily descriptive is mainly concerned with the accurate description of some aspect of society. A researcher may wish to assess specific dimensions or characteristics of individuals, groups, situations, or events by summarizing the commonalties found in discrete observations. Descriptive studies state "what is." For example, a nurse scientist may wish to assess the support among citizens for implementation of a national no-smoking policy in public areas. With the goal of gauging the general sentiments in a society toward the policy, the researcher tries to describe as precisely as possible what proportion of the population supports the policy.

Fundamentally, the descriptive study is about *what* and *how many* of *what.* It is directed toward answering questions such as, *What is this?* Descriptive research using the empirical method involves observation of a phenomenon in its natural setting. It uses case studies, surveys, grounded theory, ethnographies, and phenomenological approaches, all of which are explained in detail later in this text.

Because the goal of descriptive research is to describe, researchers frequently draw a sample to make estimations about a particular population. As used by researchers, the term *population* refers to the collection of individuals, communities, or nations about which one wishes to make a general statement. To save money and time, the researcher draws from the population a *sample* that will be representative of the population as a whole. Although including the whole population would prove to be more accurate (as in a census), the costs may be prohibitive. Public opinion pollsters, market researchers, and census takers typically emphasize descriptive accuracy in their research. All explanatory studies have descriptive dimensions, and some descriptive studies have explanatory dimensions.

To explore the differences between female students who initiate smoking in their teen years and female students who do not smoke, a researcher would want to describe the characteristics of the two sets of students. Are rural students more likely to be nonsmokers in their teen years? Are young women from higher so-cioeconomic levels more likely to initiate smoking during adolescence?

By contrast, the primary goal of **explanatory research** is to understand or to explain relationships. They engage correlational designs to study relationships between dimensions or characteristics of individuals, groups, situations, or events. They explain how the parts of a phenomenon are related to one another (Fawcett and Downs, 1986). For example, why is it that young women who initiate smoking behavior during their teen years are more likely to be from higher socioeconomic backgrounds than those who do not start smoking? Here the issue is twofold. First, what is the relationship between socioeconomic background and initiation of smoking behavior? Second, if there is a relationship, why does it exist? Explanatory studies ask *why* questions.

Predictive research moves beyond explanation to the prediction of precise relationships between dimensions or characteristics of a phenomenon or differences between groups. Predictive research typically engages the empirical method of experimentation. This involves the manipulation of some phenomenon to determine its effect on some aspect of another phenomenon. The area of health promotion provides a rich source for predictive studies on the impact of such interventions on health outcomes and longevity in various populations. Through prediction, one can estimate the likelihood of a particular outcome in a given context (Chinn and Kramer, 1991), although it does not necessarily enable one to control the outcome. A key objective of nursing research is to design studies that yield the necessary knowledge to enable nurses to control or manipulate the practice situation to produce the desired outcomes for clients.

3. Pure versus Applied Research

Intent is yet another distinction to consider when choosing a type of research.

Nurse scientists who accumulate information in order to further our understanding of relationships or to formulate or refine theory are engaging in **pure research;** those who are interested in figuring out how to bring about specific changes in nursing practice, education, or administration are engaging in **applied research.** Simply stated, whereas pure researchers value knowledge for its own sake, applied researchers wish to have an impact on some specific nursing problem.

a. Pure Research

A nurse scientist engaged in pure research tries to explain the patterns of human responses to health and illness states across the life cycle. However, it is usually possible to devise many different explanations to account for any particular response. A challenge of nursing science is to determine which, if any, of the possible explanations accounts for any given pattern. Patterns may be understood through a variety of qualitative and quantitative techniques. But whatever the approach, the ultimate goal is to offer better descriptions and better explanations of human responses to health and illness states.

Frequently nurse scientists are confronted with "interesting" findings that cry out for an explanation. Suppose, for example, that a project is being done that measures high school students' socioeconomic status (SES) and their intentions to follow a healthy diet. And suppose, during data analysis, that a relatively strong relationship emerges indicating that the higher an individual's SES, the greater the likelihood that the individual will consume a healthy diet. At this stage, a pure researcher may wonder what explains the pattern that has emerged. In this example, pure research means doing research to identify which of the following explains variation in healthy diets:

- Peers of high SES students have healthy nutritional practices and the students influence one another in selecting food choices.
- Parents of high SES students have greater expectations concerning the nutritional diet choices of their children.
- High SES students know that they have the financial resources to select nutritional food choices and therefore plan on it.
- High SES students have been more exposed to role models who select healthy food choices and are more likely to model themselves on such individuals.

We can identify three important goals of pure research:

- To test existing theories of human behavior
- To explain observed patterns of behavior
- To document our knowledge of the emergence, modification, and persistence of patterned human behavior

b. Applied Research

Again, applied research focuses on variables that can be changed by intervention to achieve desired goals. For example, an applied researcher may want to increase attendance at weekly prenatal classes for adolescent mothers, and thus would test the effectiveness of an intervention such as phoning class participants the night before the class meets to remind them to attend. Or, the researcher may want to increase people's use of seat belts and therefore studies the effect of watching a crash simulation with unrestrained drivers. Applied research includes feminist, action, evaluation, and health promotion research. These are discussed in Chapter 8.

4. Units of Analysis: Individuals versus Aggregations

Nurse scientists study communities, groups, institutions, and individuals. Moreover, an institution such as the family may be studied either across cultures or within a culture. In doing research, it is difficult to deal simultaneously with more than one level of analysis. At the outset of a project, we should ask ourselves, "Am I studying individuals or aggregations?"

a. The Individual as the Unit of Analysis

If we are studying individuals, then we should pose questions that concern individual properties only. All of the data collected should measure variations between individuals on a variety of subjects. And any analyses of the data will have individuals as the basic unit. Most surveys and experiments use the individual as the unit of analysis, although it is possible to have individuals report on data for other levels of analysis such as communities, companies, or groups. Furthermore, individuals may be counted and used to produce a measure for some aggregation: the proportion of college graduates in a community is an example of such a variable.

b. An Aggregation as the Unit of Analysis

Alternatively, if we are studying aggregations, then we should pose questions that concern properties of groups, institutions, communities, or nations. Individual characteristics, such as income, educational level, or ethnic background have to be expressed as averages or proportions. If we begin a study using an individual level of analysis, then it is difficult, without careful advance planning, to switch to a different level, such as the community level. By using computers, it is easy to compute average scores, but it is unlikely that we will have sufficient cases to produce meaningful averages for all of the communities. For example, if you studied 300 people from 25 different communities and then wanted to move from the individual to the community level, you would have only 12 people from each community on which to base the average for the community.

It is important, therefore, when you start designing a study to be absolutely clear about the units of analysis that you plan to use. Again, Table 1.3 summarizes the relationships between the many factors discussed in this section.

G. RESEARCH AS A PROFESSIONAL MANDATE

Because knowledge is the foundation of professional practice, all nurses can and should develop and apply research skills in practice. This means that, although not all nurses conduct research, every nurse should become an intelligent consumer of research, at the very least. This requires an understanding of the research process and the ability to critically read and evaluate research studies, determine their credibility, and assess the appropriateness of research findings for use in practice. Prudent evaluation and use of findings are critical to the development of a scientific knowledge base for practice.

Now that you understand the importance of nursing research to the provision of quality care and to the development of nursing as a scientific discipline, what role will you play in the research process? This is an important question for you to reflect on as you achieve full professional status as a registered nurse. As a professional nurse, the role you will play in research will be influenced by your level of educational preparation. The trend is toward an expanded researcher role with advanced education and expertise. However, as we have stated, nurses at all levels of educational preparation have roles and responsibilities to assume when it comes to nursing research. The following list delineates the research mandate appropriate to various educational backgrounds.

- **Associate degree education.** Graduates of associate degree programs have several important roles to play in the world of nursing research. They need to develop an appreciation of the significance of research to nursing practice. They can assist with the identification of clinical practice research problems, data collection, and appropriate use of research findings in practice in consultation with professional nurses (ANA, 1989).
- **Baccalaureate education.** Graduates of baccalaureate programs have an important role to play as consumers of research. This assumes they have an intimate understanding of the research process; an ability to critically read, analyze, and critique research studies; and the judgment to interpret and evaluate research findings and determine their appropriateness for use in the practice setting. Baccalaureate graduates may be active members of research teams, participating in various phases of a study under the direction of experienced researchers. In this capacity, these nurses may help generate clinical research questions to be investigated, participate in the collection and recording of data, administer research protocols to clients, and always act ethically to protect clients' rights.
- **Master's education.** Graduates of master's programs also play important roles in nursing research. They have a rich understanding of clinical practice and usually an in-depth perspective on nursing problems specific to various practice settings. This enables these nurses to identify clinically relevant problems and provide expert clinical advise on ways that services should be delivered and projects conducted. Graduate education enables these nurses to assist others in the use of research findings. According to the ANA (1989), nurses with master's degrees are clinical experts who collaborate with experienced researchers in proposal development, data collection, analyses, and interpretation.
- **Doctoral education.** The main goal of nurses at the doctoral and postdoctoral level is the development of research and scholarly ability. Doctoral programs focus on advanced research training, with emphasis on the process of building theory and advancing nursing knowledge. Graduates of doctoral programs are best prepared to appraise, design, and conduct research (LoBiondo-Wood and Haber, 1998). According to the ANA (1989), they develop nursing knowledge through original research and theory development. They also conduct funded independent research projects.

The purpose of nursing research is to generate a scientific knowledge base for practice. If the field of nursing is to be accountable to the clients it serves, it must develop an empirically grounded body of scientific knowledge on which to base clinical decisions and actions. The scientific approach as reflected in research provides a means to do this. In today's world of health-care restructuring and reform, nurses are increasingly required to be accountable for the quality of care they provide and demonstrate that they are engaging in evidence-based practice.

E X E R C I S E S

1. Examine one issue of a nursing research journal. For each article do the following:
   (a) Copy the title of each article.

   (b) Classify each article by whether it is predominantly quantitative or qualitative in orientation.

   (c) Classify each by whether it is predominantly descriptive, explanatory, or predictive.

   (d) Classify each by whether its intent seems to be pure or applied.

   (e) Classify each by whether it falls most into a positivist, interpretive, or critical perspective.

2. Identify five examples of research that fall predominantly into each of the positivist, interpretive, and critical perspectives. Did you encounter difficulties in coming up with examples for each perspective? Do you think there is a trend in nursing toward one of these perspectives? From your examination of various journals and books, estimate the percentage of research in nursing that would fall into each of the perspectives.

RECOMMENDED READINGS

Chow, J.D. (1999). Interruption to research design: Substance driven research. *Advances in Nursing Science, 22*(2), 39–47. The feminist and critical theory approaches guided this investigation of adolescent's perceptions of health messages in magazines geared toward teens. The article demonstrates how interpretive inquiry (hermeneutics) transformed the study to one that became substantively driven and contributes to the qualitative approaches in the human sciences.

Crookes, P., and Davies, S. (1998). *Research into Practice.* Edinburgh, Scotland: Balliere Tindall. This is a comprehensive text with an excellent discussion of essential skills for reading and applying research in nursing and health care.

Fain, J.A. (1999). *Reading, Understanding, and Applying Nursing Research.* Philadelphia: F.A. Davis. This book provides a compre-hensive introduction into the major methods used in nursing research.

Hilton, B., Thompson, R., and Moore-Dempsey, L. (2000). Evaluation of the AIDS Prevention Street Nurse Program: One step at a time. *Canadian Journal of Nursing Research, 32*(1), 17–38. This is a clear example of new wave research using both qualitative and quantitative methods in the area of participatory research.

Mitchell, M., and Jolley J. (1997). *Research Design Explained* (3rd ed). Orlando: Harcourt Brace Jovanovitch College Publishers. This is one of the most approachable methods texts in psychology. It contains numerous examples and helpful suggestions for students.

Streubert, H.J., and Carpenter, D. R. (1999). *Qualitative Research in Nursing* (2nd ed). Philadelphia: J.B. Lippincott. This clearly written text presents the essentials of qualitative research as it relates to nursing.

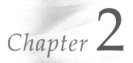
Understanding Theory

CHAPTER OUTLINE

KEY TERMS

Alternative explanations

Anecdotal evidence

Axiomatic derivation

Borrowed theories

Conceptual framework

Conceptual map

Concepts

Conditional variable

Confounding variable

Constructs

Controlled observations

Control variable

Dependent variable

Empathetic explanations

False dilemma

Grand theories

Hypotheses

Illegitimate appeal to authority

Independent variable

Intervening variable

Middle-range theories

Missing evidence

Objective

Practice theories

Precise communication

Propositions

Provincialism

Replacement of terms

Selected evidence

Situation-specific theory

Source of spuriousness variable

Structural equation modeling

Theory

Theoretical framework

Theoretical triangulation

Treatment variables

Unwarranted conclusion

Variables

Verifiable

As nurses, we want to further our understanding of human responses to health and illness in a constantly changing environment. But we lack well-confirmed and widely accepted theoretical explanations for client behavior. For this reason, the work of nurse researchers is vital. In their quest for understanding, they may challenge commonly accepted explanations for human behavior, gather new evidence to support existing theories, or generate new theories to guide nursing practice.

This chapter introduces beginning researchers to the role of theory in understanding the world of nursing. The basic elements of theory are described and the purpose of theoretical frameworks in research is explored. The chapter also summarizes three theoretical frameworks commonly used to guide nursing research. Finally, we present some simple theory-testing techniques that may be applied by beginning researchers to help them understand the elusive patterns found in the nursing world. We begin by examining the role of explanation in nursing knowledge and nursing research.

A. EXPLANATION

We probably could not survive in nursing without being able to anticipate, at least to some extent, the behavior of our colleagues and clients. For example, in greeting your nursing colleague, Nancy, you anticipate that you will get an upbeat, positive response rather than a hostile one. You have generalized from your previous experiences with her when you conclude that you will be greeted warmly. We rely on such generalizations to guide much of our interaction. In addition, all cultures have phrases that attempt to offer general explanations of human behavior. These are variously referred to as adages, old wives' tales, maxims, proverbs, sayings, aphorisms, clichés, folk

wisdom, and truisms. Indeed, it is sometimes difficult to find an outcome that is *not* covered by some cultural maxim.

There are problems, however, with nonscientific explanations. First, numerous pairs of contradictory explanations can be found: the first explains one result, and a parallel one explains the opposite outcome. No matter what happens, a ready explanation is available. This poses a tremendous threat to the advancement of nursing knowledge because scientific inquiry into client responses is snuffed out with pat answers: "Of course he won't practice his breathing exercises! You can't teach an old dog new tricks!" Box 2.1 lists a few contradictory proverbs to illustrate the prevalence of conflicting explanations in our world. Can you think of other conflicting ones?

Second, it is often true that the most compelling predictions that the nurse scientist can make will be those that run counter to "common sense." If you are able to make a prediction that goes startlingly against common understanding and it turns out to be true, you will have a powerfully convincing study.

I. Types of Explanations

We can ask whether there are different kinds of explanations that are more or less useful in understanding observations of the nursing world. In order to explain the occurrence and meaning of nursing phenomena, nurse researchers may use the following categories of explanation.

a. Deductive Explanation

When nurse scientists use deductive explanations, they try to show that the phenomenon to be explained is a logically necessary consequence of the explanatory premises. For example: if $A = B$ and $B = C$, then $A = C$. As a variant on Emile Durkheim's (1897) analysis of suicide, we

---

BOX 2.1 *A Few Contradictory Sayings*

Absence makes the heart grow fonder./Out of sight, out of mind.
Beauty is as good as ready money./ Beauty buys no beef.
Nothing ventured nothing gained./Better safe than sorry.
A farthing saved is twice earned./A penny saved is a penny earned.
Birds of a feather flock together./Opposites attract.
Judge not a book by its cover./Fine feathers make fine birds.
He will shoot higher who shoots at the sun than he who aims at a tree./Hew not too high lest the chips fall in thine eye.
Two heads are better than one./Too many cooks spoil the broth.
You can't teach an old dog new tricks./It's never too late to learn.
Haste makes waste./A stitch in time saves nine.
Better to have loved and lost than never to have loved at all./Better safe than sorry

---

might propose the following set of inter-related propositions:

(i) In any social grouping, the suicide rate (SR) varies inversely with the degree of social support (SS).

<SS $\longrightarrow$ SR (the less the social support, the higher the suicide rate)

(ii) The degree of social support (SS) varies with the degree of ruralness (RURAL)

>RURAL $\longrightarrow$ >S (the more rural the community, the greater the social support)

(iii) If the previous two statements are correct, we can deduce that:

>RURAL $\longrightarrow$ <SR (the more rural the community, the lower the suicide rate)

In the below example, we have a deductive model of the form:

>RURAL $\longrightarrow$ >Social support

<Social support $\longrightarrow$ >Suicide rate

<RURAL $\longrightarrow$ >Suicide rate

In this illustration, by combining a theoretical proposition (i) with an untested assumption (ii) and then using deductive

reasoning, we get a testable hypothesis (iii). If, indeed, the data are consistent with the prediction, this would constitute one piece of evidence that is supportive of the theory of suicide—namely, that "social support" explains the connection between "ruralness" and suicide rates. We could not claim to have *proven* the theory to be correct because alternative theories may also make the prediction that suicide rates will be comparatively low in rural communities. In this illustration, note that "social support" is a common term that links size of community (RURAL) to "suicide rate." The deductively derived hypothesis is easily tested by examining the relationship between suicide rate and community size.

b. Probabilistic Explanation

Probabilistic explanation rests on linking a particular case to its general category. When asked to explain why Mary, a nursing student, spends excessive hours in the library, if you respond by saying, "There are many nursing students in the library these days doing reserve readings," you have given a probabilistic explanation. Mary spends a lot of time in the library because she is a member of a category of individuals who are required to do reserve readings. The explanation suggests that an individual tends to be like others in the same category.

Another example is the explanation commonly offered in response to complaints that, "I've been buying lottery tickets for years, but I never win the big prize." The probabilistic explanation is that the chances of winning the jackpot are about one in 14 million. In other words, the odds are against any one individual.

c. Functional Explanation

Functional explanations explain the presence of some phenomenon in terms of the role it plays in maintaining some system. For example, if the presence of the family unit in all cultures is explained in terms of its role in producing new members for each society, this would be a functional explanation: the family exists to propagate to maintain the social system.

d. Causal Explanation

Causal explanations dominate the thinking of many researchers. In a causal explanation, an event is explained by making reference to preceding influencing events. The explanation traces the sequence of steps, each influencing the next, that has led to some event. Think of a line of dominoes falling in sequence after one has been knocked over, or consider all the factors that may influence choosing a healthful lifestyle.

e. Empathetic Explanation

Empathetic explanations are those that stress the experience of coming to see or to understand an imagined possibility. The individual feels, "Ah-ha, I've got it—I can see that I would do the same thing in similar circumstances." Everyday life is full of empathetic explanations and understandings. In the nursing world, where nurses and clients share intimate experiences such as birth, death, diagnosis of terminal illness, and so on, empathetic explanations take on increasing importance. Qualitative nurse researchers pay much attention to empathetic explanations because, to nurse scientists working in this tradition, they are the key to adequate explanations. An explanation or a description of a behavior that rings true to both the researcher and the client whose behavior is being revealed is key to judging the adequacy of an empathetic explanation.

2. The Nature of Nursing Science Explanations

Nursing science explanations serve the same function as proverbs, adages, and anecdotes: in all cases, they attempt to account for human behavior or to explain human responses to various health and illness states. Does a generalization made by a nurse scientist substantially differ from one made by a nonscientist? To begin to come to grips with this question, let's examine quantitative and qualitative evidence and argument.

a. Quantitative Evidence

For the quantitative nurse scientist, an important goal is to arrive at general statements, statements that can be applied to a variety of situations. A generalization depicts the typical. The following statements constitute generalizations:

- Among high school students, females experience more mental health problems than males.
- Males are more likely to be involved in motor vehicle accidents than females.
- Students who sit in the front or middle of the classroom get higher grades than those who sit in the back or to the sides of the classroom.

In contrast to nonscientists, the evidence a quantitative nurse scientist would look for would be based on objective, verifiable, controlled observations and would be communicated in a precise manner (Browne and Keeley, 1990). By **objective,** we mean observations that are free from bias; by **verifiable,** we mean information that could be confirmed by tests conducted by others; by **controlled observations,** we mean those in which other confounding factors are minimized or taken into account; and by **precise communication,** we mean that the information is unambiguous. In nursing science, many of our generalizations are probabilistic; this means that in most cases (but not all), the statement will be true. Certainly not all high school girls have more mental health problems than their male counterparts; and certainly not all students in the back row get lower grades than those sitting in the middle of the room. Because nurse scientists' arguments must be based on evidence, information must be collected and then appropriately analyzed. The resulting conclusion is then an informed opinion—that is, an opinion based on evidence that has been collected under controlled circumstances.

In making probabilistic generalizations, the nurse scientist has to indicate precisely how the information was collected, what kind of sampling procedures were used, and how the data were analyzed. A probabilistic generalization (e.g., students who choose nursing as a career are more likely to have altruistic vs. materialistic values) should indicate the population about whom the generalization is being made (e.g., all nursing students in the world; students in a particular country, region, community, or in the nursing program at the University of Texas). The researcher should also indicate the size and the method of selecting the sample on which the generalization is based (e.g., a convenience sample of 125 students in nursing and 125 students in non-nursing programs of study); and, finally, the researcher should indicate the procedures used to measure the variables and to process the resulting data.

b. Qualitative Evidence

For qualitative nurse scientists, more emphasis is placed on the extent to which explanations and descriptions ring true to both the researcher and to the people who are being described. The evidence itself may be based on a painstaking analysis of documents, on in-depth or focus group interviews, or on lengthy participation in a group (see Chapter 7). But in all cases, the evidence itself and the interpretations placed on it are judged in terms of how well they are perceived to deal with the matter at issue.

3. Flaws in Explanations

Nurse scientists design studies, make observations and analyze them, and then prepare a report on the results. During each stage, one must be careful not to fall prey to errors in thinking or in argument. The following section highlights common errors of particular relevance to nurse scientists.

a. Illegitimate Appeal to Authority

As researchers, sometimes we may be tempted to argue that something is bad (e.g., euthanasia) by using an **illegitimate appeal to an authority.** For example, in this case, we could state that euthanasia is bad because Nobel Prize winner in physics, Dr. X., claims that it is. In this case, the status of the person expressing the view should not influence our judgment. Legitimate authority, in contrast, is to be found in the peer-reviewed and scholarly literature of nursing and related disciplines. Does the preponderance of evidence in the research literature point to one conclusion? Are the exceptional findings to be explained by quirks in methodology or in the samples studied? In any case, nursing science proceeds by testing and retesting old ideas under new conditions.

b. Provincialism

As researchers, we carry with us the baggage of our culture. This makes us vulnerable to the danger of **provincialism,** of tending to see things as our culture sees them. Thus, if it is "politically correct" to view men and women as equally skilled at child rearing, then this may blind us from looking at areas in child rearing in which this may not be true. Kahane argues provincialism "tends to make us concentrate on our own society—to the exclusion of other cultures—and via loyalty, to influence our acceptance or rejection of alleged facts or theories, whatever the nature of the evidence" (1988, p. 47).

c. False Dilemma

A **false dilemma** is set up when a researcher argues that something is caused by either A or by B. Then, having provided some evidence that B is not responsible, the researcher falsely concludes that A must be the cause. The problem here is that there may be several other possibilities that have not been considered. For example, one may argue that either diet or a sedentary lifestyle explains the incidence of osteoporosis in women. Now suppose that the data from a small sample of women indicated that sedentary lifestyle was not related to osteoporosis in these women. Because other possible explanations have been omitted, this finding paves the way for an inappropriate conclusion that diet explains osteoporosis in women.

d. Missing Evidence

When the reports of researchers are examined, read carefully to make a judgment as to the adequacy of the evidence for each point made. Although it would be unrealistic to expect all assumptions to be identified and all statements to be demonstrated, watch out for signs of important **missing evidence** and be certain that evidence for key arguments is provided.

Frequently a nurse scientist is confronted with "interesting" findings for which an explanation should be offered. Suppose, for example, that a project is being done that measures high school students' scores in a health promotion course focusing on health behavior decision making and relates this variable to the age of their first experiencing sexual intercourse. And suppose, during data analysis, that a strong relationship emerges indicating that the higher one's score in the course, the older the average age of first sexual intercourse. At this stage, the researcher may wonder what explains the pattern that has emerged. Possibilities such as the following might come to mind:

- Peers of students with high course scores avoid early initiation into sex and influence their friends to do likewise.
- Among students with high course scores, parental supervision is such that the opportunities to engage in premarital sex are more limited.
- Students with high course scores have higher educational aspirations and avoid early initiation into sex because they think that to do so would impede their chances of going to college.

Unfortunately, the study may not have been designed to test, and possibly to rule out, competing explanations. Therefore, there may be no empirical evidence for the conclusion presented by the researcher. The problem here is that although much data may be presented documenting a variety of relationships, the reader of such a report may be convinced, inappropriately, that the researcher's numerous data, tables, and figures support the particular explanation being offered. Such explanations may sound good and appear reasonable, but they lack evidence.

e. Anecdotal Evidence

Suppose an incident of a person on a day pass from a mental health facility who commits an assault is cited in an attempt to justify the conclusion that the mental health care system is under-resourced. What do you conclude? Although this type of **anecdotal evidence** is commonly used, it is hardly sufficient to warrant the conclusion drawn. What are the overall rates of assault being committed by such persons? What are the social and human costs of more restrictive day passes? Are denials of day passes to mental health clients more likely to lead to rehabilitation, lead to decreases in assault rates, or provide greater protection, in the long run, to society? Be wary of anecdotal evidence.

Anecdotal evidence is the layperson's equivalent of arguments based on unrepresentative samples. When nurse scientists attempt to describe something (e.g., the effectiveness of a specific nursing intervention with breast cancer clients), they typically do so by working with samples. The conclusions should not go beyond the adequacy of the sample. A very small sample (e.g., an anecdote involving just one case) should not be used to generalize about all of humankind. You can imagine how inappropriate it would be to generalize about oncology clients' attitudes toward an alternative pain control procedure based on a sample of 10 breast cancer clients. Such a sample—likely one

of convenience (clients who were present at the oncology clinic the day when the questionnaire was administered)—is not only small but because the clients were not selected using a strict sampling procedure, it cannot be taken to represent even the oncology clients at that clinic. Avoid conclusions that state generalizations that go beyond those justified by the sampling procedure. (Details on sampling procedures are discussed in Chapter 15.)

f. Selected or Suppressed Evidence

In citing evidence, researchers should attempt to fairly represent the findings in the research literature and their own data. We are all familiar with public debates that have gone on in recent years on such issues as environmental illnesses, the dangers of smoking, abortion, and mercy killing. In each case, expert researchers who claim to have special knowledge on these matters and claim also to represent the consensus in their discipline have been called on to testify. The trouble is that each side seems to be able to produce an expert who supports its point of view. These experts are probably presenting **selected evidence,** choosing to report only studies that support a particular point of view, and ignoring the evidence that runs counter to what they are attempting to demonstrate. Advocacy is not science: both are legitimate enterprises, but they are not the same thing.

A similar situation exists with respect to researchers who report their own data. Given the need to keep reports short, some information is not reported; therefore, it is possible that researchers do not represent their own data fairly. Some information may be considered unreportable or insufficiently interesting to merit inclusion. Readers cannot tell how much information has been omitted.

g. *Unwarranted Conclusions*

Sometimes in analyzing data, a researcher will come to an **unwarranted conclusion.** Confusing correlation and cause is an example of this type of error in reasoning. Researchers take pains to measure variables and to investigate how they are related to one another. However, to show that *as A increases, so does B* does not demonstrate that A causes B. Although this issue is explored in greater detail in Chapter 17, let us look at one example here. Some theorists argue that there is a connection between engagement in health behaviors and health value. Let us assume that such a correlation, in fact, exists (some would disagree): are we justified in concluding that the valuing of health led to the engagement in health behaviors? What are the possibilities when we have a correlation between any two variables?

Health Value has influenced
engaging in Health Behaviors HV→HB

Engaging in Health Behaviors
influences Health Value   HB→HV

They influenced each other   HB↔HV

Other factor(s) influenced   both of them ?
                                 ↰HV HB↱

In drawing conclusions, it is important to sufficiently explore alternate possibilities. Be careful not to confuse association with cause.

B. THEORY

The term *theory,* similar to the term *research,* has many different meanings in nursing literature. The first step in understanding theory is to be clear on its meaning. This can prevent much confusion and frustration on the part of beginning researchers. Box 2.2 provides popular definitions of theory in the research literature. The term *theory* has different uses in the world of health care. Nurses use the term in everyday conversation to refer to a hunch or idea about some phenomena or event that is related. Scientists use the term in a precise manner. This text views **theory** as a systematic vision of reality that describes, explains, or predicts something. It is derived from the Greek word *theoria,* which means vision. Theories consist of words or symbols that represent something in the real world. Theories are not facts but simply ways of perceiving aspects of reality. Theories are dynamic and change with subsequent testing as scientists examine theory through research. Similar to theory in all sciences, nursing theory changes and is modified as new knowledge becomes available through research.

> **BOX 2.2** *Definitions of Theory*
>
> Theory is a statement that accounts for or characterizes some phenomena (Stevens, 1984).
>
> Theory is a general statement that explains the interrelationships among observed facts and propositions (Seaman, 1987).
>
> Theory consists of a set of concepts and propositions stating the relations between them. The set of propositions must be interrelated so that one can derive new propositions by combining them deductively, and furthermore, the propositions must be amenable to empirical testing (Homans, 1964).
>
> Theory is defined as a set of interrelated concepts, definitions, and propositions that present a systematic view of phenomena for the purpose of explaining and predicting phenomena (Chinn & Kramer, 1995; LoBionda-Wood, 1998).

I. Purpose of Theory

In order to survive in society, all of us need a shared understanding of human behavior. We learn what a frown means, what a jaunty wave of the hand means, and we come to a common understanding of what a vast array of words and symbols mean in our culture. We learn about appropriate and inappropriate behavior. As children, we might learn, for example, that it is okay to swear in front of our same-gender peers but that it is not acceptable to use the same words in front of our parents or in mixed company. We speculate on why others behave as they do and we think about our own behavior. Theory provides a structure for the interpretation of individuals' behavior and of events. Many theories are required to account for the multitude of experiences encountered by human beings. They state what something is, how something happens, or why it happens. Their function, therefore, is to describe, explain, or predict specific aspects of reality.

Theory serves a multitude of functions in nursing, but its *primary goal* is to provide a framework that links research and practice and contributes to making scientific findings meaningful and generalizable. Theory also functions to provide:

- A structure for interpreting observed behaviors, situations, and events
- A means of imposing order on unordered experiences
- An efficient means for summarizing and explaining observations from a number of isolated research studies. A theory enables a researcher to contribute the findings of even a small study to the larger theoretical perspective that uses the same theory.
- A source to generate hypotheses that predict what will be found when data are collected and analyzed
- A framework for guiding research. When a problem or research question is placed within the context of theory, the findings have greater potential for contributing to knowledge development in the discipline than isolated research that is not linked to a particular theory. This is because theories are abstract constructions of the mind and hence transcend the limits of specific circumstances such as time and place that apply in studies of a particular problem.
- A guide in selecting the appropriate method to answer the research question and in interpreting the results
- A source of professional autonomy. Theory guides the nurses' thinking and actions and provides a basis to describe, explain, or predict factors that influence nursing care. It enables nurses to explain nursing actions and their outcomes.

What do we gain by connecting research to new or existing theoretical perspectives? The answer has to do with *power*. Research that limits itself to the particular or to the unique will not contribute to our general understanding of the human condition. General explanations allow research to have implications for our overall understanding of human responses, as well as increase our knowledge of the particular variables involved in a nursing research project.

Unfortunately, in many journal articles, the research problem is not linked to a theory or conceptual framework. Silva (1986) suggests this may be caused in part by a lack of commitment to theory testing by the discipline. Silva conducted a study to identify the nursing theories that were tested in nursing research. She found 62 articles that reported "using" a nursing theory. Of the 62 articles, only nine actually tested a theoretical proposition. Deets (1990) reviewed 300 articles published in a 12-month period to identify studies that tested one or more of the field of nursing's metaparadigm concepts (nursing, person, health, and environment). Only six articles addressed one or more of the central concepts. Betz and Beal (1996) conducted a systematic analysis of 302 published pediatric nursing studies to evaluate use of nursing theories. Their review found that only 17 investigations used nursing theories as frameworks. If one accepts the assumption that one of the purposes of research is to test and generate theory and thus advance the science of nursing, then one must question doing nursing research that does not adequately address the theoretical elements in a study.

2. Relationship of Research, Theory, and Practice

Theory, research, and nursing practice are intimately related processes. As previously stated, the function of theory is to describe, explain, or predict the occurrence of nursing phenomenon. The function of research is to generate or test a theory (Fawcett, 1999; Chinn and Kramer, 1995) that will influence practice either directly or indirectly. Hence, we see the cyclical nature of the relationship. Research designed to test theory requires

you to collect data about relationships (with propositions or hypotheses) derived from the theory. The findings of the research can be woven into a program of research to build theory that will direct subsequent theory development. When the theory has been tested and validated through research and subsequently used to direct nursing practice, the cyclical relationship of theory–research–practice is complete. Research that generates theory requires the researcher to identify and describe nursing phenomena observed in practice and articulate the relationships between the phenomena. The existing knowledge about a nursing phenomenon guides the researcher in asking the appropriate question for a given study and guides him or her in selecting the design, method, and analysis to answer the research question.

3. Classification of Theory

The authors of this text believe there is some advantage to viewing theory along a continuum of abstractness that reflects the breadth of the concepts and relationship statements in the theory. Figure 2.1

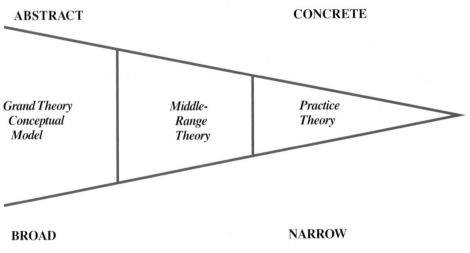

ABSTRACT   CONCRETE

Grand Theory *Conceptual Model*   *Middle-Range Theory*   *Practice Theory*

BROAD   NARROW

Figure 2.1   Theory continuum.

illustrates the theory continuum that runs from the most abstract grand theories to middle-range theories to practice-level theories. The major theories reported in the nursing literature can be classified along this continuum.

a. Grand Theories

Grand theories (or *conceptual models*) are the most abstract type of theories. They embody the beliefs, traditions, goals, and values of the discipline. They take into account the phenomena of central concern to nursing: person, health, nursing, and environment. They broadly define these concepts and link them together through relationship statements reflective of the theorist's view of the discipline. They explain universal relationships that describe what the discipline of nursing is all about. They remain broad, abstract representations of reality. Although grand theories are not directly tested through research, they serve as frameworks to guide the selection of concepts and phenomena important to nursing concerns. In this instance, grand theories highlight the importance of the phenomena for investigation (Fitzpatrick and Whall, 1996). Examples include Roy's adaptation model and Roger's science of unitary man model.

Researchers may examine relationships that are derived from grand theories. For example, most people are familiar with the simple deductive statement that if A=B and B=C, then A=C. In a similar manner, one may derive a relational statement from a grand theory to be tested in a research study. For example, in her Self-Care Model, Orem (1995) postulates that basic conditioning factors (i.e., age, health state, available resources, patterns of living) influence one's self-care agency (i.e., ability to engage in behaviors to keep one's self healthy). A researcher may deduce from this relationship that adolescents with adequate financial resources will engage in more health behaviors than adolescents with fewer financial resources. Use of grand theories in this way to derive statements to guide research is important in moving discussion of grand theory (conceptual models) down the continuum of abstractness to a more specific level. The deductive method is particularly useful in developing middle-range theory in substantive areas that are consistent with a given grand theory.

b. Middle-Range Theories

Middle-range theories are located on the continuum midway between the most abstract ideas and the most concrete. They deal with limited aspects of nursing phenomena and are more testable and generalizable than grand theories. They contain well-defined concepts and propositions. Common examples include the health promotion theory (Pender), stress and coping theory, and theories of social support. Lenz and associates (1995, 1997) suggest that nursing as a discipline must move from focusing on the current grand theories to middle-range theories if continued development is to occur. The lack of theory-testing studies in the nursing literature, discussed earlier, can be used as evidence to support the position of Lenz and associates.

c. Practice Theories

Practice theories are narrower in scope and more specific than middle-range theories. Concepts are specifically and narrowly defined and readily measured. Practice theory propositions produce clear directives for application in practice. Much of what nurses follow today in hospital procedure manuals is actually practice theory that has been developed inductively by expert nurses who have observed and described ways of practicing based on trial and error. Common examples include theory on mouth care, taking patients' oral temperature, decubitus ulcer therapy, and use of restraints. Practice theory is designed for immediate application to practice when appropriate.

A new level of theory known as *situation-specific theory* is emerging in nursing to incorporate diversities and complexities in nursing phenomena. It incorporates sociopolitical, cultural, and historic contexts of nursing encounters (Im and Meleis, 1999). According to these authors, **situation-specific theory** answers a set of coherent questions about situations that are limited in scope and focus. They characterize this level of theory as one that focuses on specific clinical practice phenomena, reflects a specific field of practice, is confined to developing and understanding of a specific population, and provides a blueprint for action. An example of an emerging situation-specific theory is the work of Im and Meleis (in press) on menopausal transition of Korean immigrant women. The situation-specific theory is developed from transitions theory, a middle-range theory. Although transition theory explains human beings during any kind of transition, the situation-specific theory is narrowly focused to explain the menopausal experience of a specific Korean immigrant population. As such, the concepts in the theory are grounded in Korean culture and the menopausal experience of immigrant women.

A criticism of some practice theory is that it may be so narrow in scope that it is not useful for the development of nursing theory beyond providing ideas for further theory development. If the practice theory deals with only one situation at one point in time, it is too narrow to be useful in many nursing situations.

4. Levels of Theory

Dickoff and associates (1968) produced a seminal piece of work that identified four levels of theory classified according to what the theory does. This work has been instrumental in guiding the development of theoretical research in nursing. The levels include:

- **Level 1,** referred to as *factor-isolating theory*. It is descriptive in nature, used when little is known about the phenomenon. It asks the question, "What is this?" Given the level of development of nursing as a scientific discipline, it is appropriate that many of our investigations are at this level.
- **Level 2** is *factor-relating theory*. It requires correlating factors in such a way that they create a meaningful situation. It concerns the relationship among concepts and asks the question, "What is happening here?"
- **Level 3** is *situation-relating theory*. It explains and predicts how situations are related. It focuses on the question, "What will happen if?"
- **Level 4** is *situation-producing theory*. It is prescriptive theory and it answers the question, "How can I make X happen?" Level 4 is the most powerful in terms of being able to prescribe nursing activity. It moves beyond description, explanation, and prediction to control.

Diverse views exist on what constitutes the appropriate level of theory in nursing. Given its complexity, we believe all levels are needed: theories of varying scope and specificity are required to account for the multitude of human responses to health and illness states.

C. CONCEPTS AND STATEMENTS: BUILDING BLOCKS OF THEORY

Nursing students often struggle with introductory chapters on research and theory because they do not understand the language used by scientists and researchers, who share a unique vocabulary. It is important that students and nurses interested in reading and applying research findings in their practice learn this new language so they can approach the research literature intelligently. The following terms are used frequently by members of the research community.

1. Concepts

Concepts are the building blocks of theory. They are abstract entities that represent broad general ideas that are not directly observable in the real world. However, they are formed from real-world observations of objects or events. For example, love is a concept. If asked to observe love in a population, most people would experience some confusion because the word can be defined in a number of ways. For research purposes, *love* would need to be defined in observable terms. Figure 2.2 illustrates the possible meanings of the concept of love.

a. Constructs

Constructs are concepts specified in such a way that they are observable in

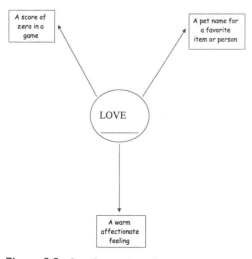

Figure 2.2   Specific meaning of concept.

the real world. Making a concept potentially observable facilitates testing of the idea. For love to be considered a construct, the researcher would have to list all of the aspects of love that could be observed in the real world. Some authors distinguish construct from concept by stating that constructs are "constructed or invented" by the researcher.

b. Variables

Variables are concepts that are observable, measurable, and have a dimension that can vary. For example, temperature is a variable that is observable, measurable, and varies from high to low.

Variables usually are so specific that they capture only a portion of the general meaning conveyed at the conceptual level. Concepts, constructs, and variables can be viewed along a continuum of specificity, similar to theory. At one end, we have concepts that are general, vague, and abstract, and at the other end we have variables that are narrow in meaning, observable, and measurable. For example, if the researcher takes the concept of love and defines it as a variable, the definition would be so explicit that it would clearly identify how the variable *love* is to be measured. Although the reader may not agree with this definition of the variable, the meaning and method of measurement or observation would be clearly understood. Figure 2.3 illustrates how the *concept* of love might be described, viewed as a *construct,* and defined as a *variable.*

c. Types of Variables

In designing, implementing, and evaluating studies to test theory, researchers distinguish various types of variables. The following discussion relates to variables as used in research studies. It is included in this chapter on theory to help

ABSTRACT

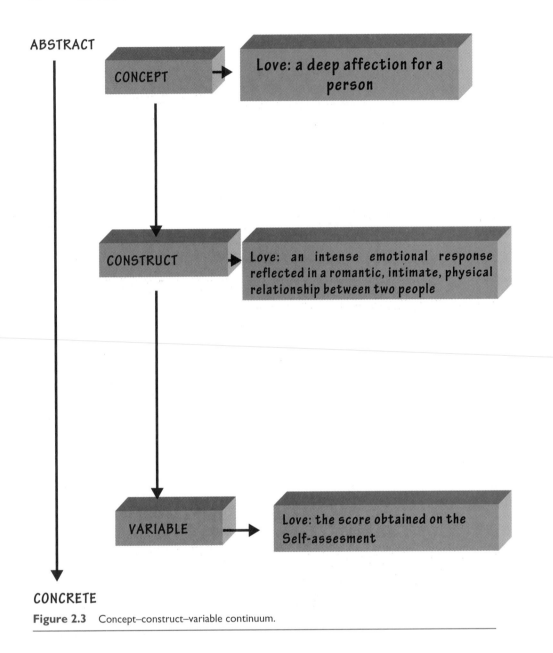

CONCEPT → Love: a deep affection for a person

CONSTRUCT → Love: an intense emotional response reflected in a romantic, intimate, physical relationship between two people

VARIABLE → Love: the score obtained on the Self-assesment

CONCRETE

Figure 2.3   Concept–construct–variable continuum.

students see the link between concepts as the basic building blocks of theory and variables as the basic unit of scientific research.

(i) Dependent Variables

A **dependent variable** is a variable thought to be influenced by other variables. It is the effect in a cause-and-effect relationship. As its name suggests, its variation depends on other variables. For example, in an investigation of the factors that influence women's decisions to choose home birthing rather than hospital birthing programs, birthing program choice would be treated as the dependent variable. However, this would not preclude exploring the possibility that, in turn, variations in birthing choice have an impact on a variable such as recovery rate. In such a case, recovery rate would be treated as the dependent variable.

(ii) Independent Variables

An **independent variable** is a cause in a cause-and-effect relationship. It is a variable that has been selected as a possible influence on variations in a dependent variable. Typically, one finds a number of independent variables in a study. Once again, it is how the variable is treated—that is, how it is thought of—that determines whether it is an independent or a dependent variable, not the nature of the variable itself.

In our example of birthing program choices, many different factors may be treated as independent variables. We might well include such factors as rural or urban home community, number of previous deliveries, types of family support available, socioeconomic status, mother's participation in the labor force, and the presence of role models who have opted for home birthing programs.

In experimental designs, **treatment variables** are those whose effect on some dependent variable is being assessed. For example, in an experiment to test the effectiveness of a structured exercise program on the perceived level of well being in middle-aged women, two groups of subjects would be assigned to either the exercise program group or to the group that did their standard routine of activities. In this study, exercise would be the treatment variable and well being would be the dependent variable. There may be several treatments used simultaneously, and their individual and joint effects would be assessed.

In general, we should be careful to ensure that the variables we treat as independent are indeed different variables. For instance, if we measured the weight of premature infants in pounds and then repeated the measurements, but this time using kilograms, our two sets of measures would lack independence. In short, they would simply represent different measures of the same variable. The researcher must be careful not to fall into the trap of thinking that there is a powerful causal connection between two variables when the measures lack independence and thus represent two different measures of the same thing.

(iii) Control Variables

A **control variable** is a variable that is taken into account in exploring the relation between an independent variable and a dependent variable. There are three basic types of control variables: the intervening variable, the conditional variable, and the source of spuriousness (or confounding) variable.

- Intervening variable. An **intervening variable** (I) is a variable that links an independent variable (X) to a dependent one (Y). An intervening variable represents an explanation of how the independent variable influences the dependent variable. It may be diagrammed as:

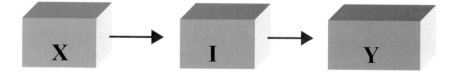

Suppose we are investigating the relation between socioeconomic status (SES) and preference for home birthing programs. A possible explanation of how SES influences the type of birthing program preferred would be that mothers with a high SES are more likely to be exposed to other mothers in home birthing programs. In other words, exposure to people in home birthing programs *intervenes* to account for the program preferred.

- Conditional variable. A **conditional variable** (C) is a variable that accounts for a change in the relationship between an independent variable (X) and a dependent variable (Y) when the general conditions change. Suppose we are investigating the relationship between SES and attitudes toward early discharge from the hospital: we might want to find out whether that relationship is fundamentally altered (or is entirely different) for each gender. Accordingly, we might test men and women separately for a relationship between SES and attitudes. Here gender would be the conditional variable, as in:

Males

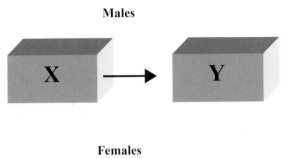

Females

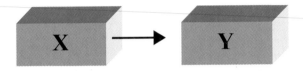

- Source of spuriousness variable. A **source of spuriousness variable** (S/S) is a variable that is viewed as a possible influence on both the independent variable (X) and the dependent variable (Y), in such a way that it accounts for the relationship between them. In other words, the relationship between X and Y is spurious because it is produced by the influence of S/S on both X and Y.

If we were exploring the relation between socioeconomic background and choice of a birthing program by pregnant women, we might consider the possibility that rural or urban background is a source of spuriousness. Here the idea is that it may be the type of community that the women come from that influences family socioeconomic achievement as well as influencing birthing program preferences. The relationship between SES and birthing program choice might therefore be spurious. As in:

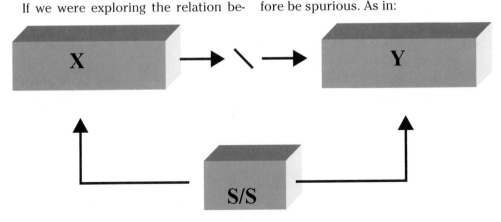

In experimental research, a source of spuriousness variable is typically referred to as a **confounding variable.** A confounding variable is one that may be influencing the outcome of an experiment systematically and that, after it is recognized, is treated in the design and controlled.

2. Propositions and Hypotheses

Propositions and hypotheses are elements of theories, and they represent different levels of abstraction.

a. Propositions

Propositions are statements of proposed relationships between two or more concepts in a theory. Propositions link concepts of a theory together so something can be described, explained, or predicted. The concepts in a proposition are not always measurable, rendering the proposition untestable. Propositions are also referred to as axioms or theorems. An example of a proposition would be the statement that "in any social grouping, the greater the social support, the lower the suicide rate."

b. Hypotheses

Hypotheses are statements of predicted relationship between two or more variables. Hypotheses are generally used in the context of a research study. They form a bridge between the abstract world of theory and the concrete reality of nursing's practice world. In this sense, they unify the two domains. Hypotheses may be directional (specifying a direction for the relationship, e.g., the greater X, the greater Y), or nondirectional (simply stating that there will be a difference between groups or variables, e.g., as X varies, Y varies). In the suicide example, the hypothesis derived might be "the more rural the place of residence, the lower the suicide rate." Hypotheses advance nursing knowledge by confirming or refuting the theoretical propositions from which they are derived.

D. THEORETICAL FRAMEWORKS

Theoretical frameworks are brief descriptions of a theory, or portions of a theory, to be tested in a research project. A theoretical framework describes the basic structure of ideas (i.e., theories, concepts, propositions) within which the study is to be conducted and the results interpreted (Diers, 1979). It is a verbal description of existing theory relevant to the phenomena under investigation, based on a review of the literature.

Nursing research studies that are guided by a theoretical framework usually make this fact known by explicitly describing the framework early in the research report. Typically a section titled *Theoretical Framework* briefly describes the major features of the theory or framework so readers will be able to understand the theoretical basis for the study.

I. Use of Nursing and Non-Nursing Frameworks

A well-developed study should have an explicitly stated framework—that is, the hypotheses should emerge from a theoretical framework that is explicitly stated in the article. Unfortunately, the frameworks in nursing studies are often implicit—leaving it to the reader to ponder the literature review to determine the relationships among variables from previous investigations. This may present a challenge for the beginning research student.

The theoretical framework for a nursing investigation depends, to a large extent, on the researcher's creativity in formulating what the particular problem, propositions, or hypotheses are an example of in the nursing world. For example, a pediatric problem related to appropriate preparation of toddlers for hospital admission may be conceptualized within the context of child development theory, social cognitive theory, or operant conditioning theory. However, it may also be thought about within the context of preparation for any new experience. When viewed in this manner, theories on preparation and information giving, theories on teaching or learning, and stress and adaptation theories may become part of the theoretical framework for the study of hospital preparation of toddlers.

Nursing research studies are often capable of being conceptualized in a number of ways because of the complex nature of nursing practice. Which theory to select as a framework is a choice made by the researcher. It is not a matter of choosing a correct theory or an incorrect theory to guide the investigation. Rather, it is important to be able to clearly see the logical links between the theoretical framework described and the research proposition or hypotheses to be tested.

As a young science, nursing often deals with phenomena that are not unique to nursing. As a consequence, a significant number of theories used as frameworks in nursing research are based on theoretical work from other disciplines, such as sociology (e.g., the sick role theory), psychology (e.g., social–cognitive theory) or physiology (e.g., theory of pain perception), to name a few. These are **borrowed theories**—that is, theories taken from other disciplines and applied to nursing questions and research problems. Borrowing is generally viewed as acceptable as long as the relevance of the theory to nursing is explained. Given the stage of development of nursing science, this trend toward multidisciplinary and multitheoretical perspectives is likely to be witnessed for some time in the nursing literature.

As we have seen, many nurse researchers who use a theoretical framework to guide their studies use one that has been previously developed and published elsewhere. But occasionally, nurse researchers may link their research project to theory by synthesizing the findings from previous studies to create a new theory. Unfortunately, some nursing studies claim a theoretical linkage after the fact. Even though this may enhance the meaningfulness of the findings, artificially linking a problem to a theory is not a desirable way to build knowledge in a discipline.

When a theory is retrospectively linked to a research problem, the researcher often fails to consider nuances of the theory in the study design. Ideally, a theoretical perspective is used to *direct* a study; then, the design of the study, the measurement of key constructs, the analysis of data, and the interpretation of findings will be influenced by that theory.

In reading research articles published in the nursing literature, you may encounter the term *conceptual framework*. Some authors make the distinction that the framework of a research study is called a **conceptual framework** when it does not contain a specific theory that explains the expected relationship between variables but rather synthesizes relevant literature about the proposed hypotheses. In most cases, the terms *theoretical* and *conceptual framework* are used interchangeably.

2. Conceptual Maps

A **conceptual map** is simply a diagram of the concepts and relationships expressed in a theoretical framework. A conceptual map is an efficient way to communicate what is known about a phenomenon more clearly than a verbal description. Conceptual maps contain all the concepts of a theory. Arrows indicate the proposed direction of the relationships among the concepts. Conceptual maps should be supported with references from the literature. Figures 2.4 through 2.6 are conceptual maps that illustrate the three theories described next.

3. Examples of Frameworks Guiding Nursing Research

A number of nursing theories appear in the literature today. Box 2.3 highlights some of the best-known theories used by nurse researchers to guide research investigations. For a detailed description of these theories, see the Recommended Readings at the end of this chapter. We encourage you to read these theories and speculate about them as possible sources of testable hypotheses or research questions.

This section briefly describes two popular nursing theories and one borrowed theory that have been used by nurse researchers to derive predictions that are tested through research. Also provided are summaries of published research studies that were conceptualized within the respective theoretical frameworks.

a. Orem's Theory of Self-Care

Orem's theory of self-care (1995) is an example of a nursing theory that has gained increasing popularity as a framework to guide research. Orem's theory describes the practice of nursing from the perspective of self-care. It focuses on the ability of an individual to take care of him- or herself (*self-care agency*). *Self-care* is the ability to initiate and perform activities on one's own behalf in order to maintain life, health, and well-being. A special type of self-care called *therapeutic self-care* is required when a person is ill or requires special skills or knowledge to perform self-care. If one is dependent in some way (e.g., physically challenged, frail, or on complete bedrest), then family members or support caregivers may assume the care role. This is referred to as *dependent care.*

The goal of nursing in Orem's theory is to help people meet their own therapeutic self-care demands. Nursing care is provided only when there is a deficit in the self-care or dependent care ability of the individual or the caregiver. When this occurs, the nurse operates within one of three nursing systems to meet the self-care needs of the client. The three nursing systems are *wholly compensatory, partly compensatory,* and *supportive–educative.* Figure 2.4 illustrates a model of Orem's theory, and Box 2.4 describes a nursing research study whose theoretical framework included Orem's theory as well as self-efficacy theory. As you read the summary of this nursing study, note

---

BOX 2.3 *Examples of Frameworks to Guide Nursing Research*

Grand Theories (Conceptual Models)

Roy's adaptation model
Roger's model: science of unitary man
Neuman's systems model

Middle-Range Theories

Pender's theory of health promotion
Jessor's problem behavior theory
Anderson's stress and nursing support systems theory

Practice Theories

Theory of interpersonal relations
Theory of clinical reasoning
Theory of non-nutritional infant sucking

Non-Nursing Theories (Borrowed Theories)

PRECEDE model of health behavior
Theory of reasoned action
The health belief model
Social learning theory

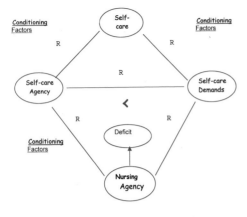

Note: R = relationship; < = deficit relationship

Figure 2.4   Model of Orem's theory of self-care. Note: R = relationship; < = deficit relationship. When the self-care demand of client is greater than his or her self-care agency (the ability of the client to engage in self-care), nursing agency (intervention by the nurse) is necessary to address the deficit (gap between self-care demand and self-care agency). (Adapted from Orem, D. [1995]. *Nursing Concepts of Practice* [5th ed]. St. Louis: Mosby.)

how the theoretical framework guided development of the study hypotheses and interpretation of results. For a complete description of the study, refer to the original source.

b. Peplau's Interpersonal Relations Theory

Peplau's interpersonal relations theory (1998) is a nursing theory that has been widely cited by nurses, particularly psychiatric nurses, as a framework that guides practice. This theory describes the nurse–client relationship as the crux of nursing. The theory states that this relationship evolves through four interconnected phases: orientation, identification, exploitation, and resolution. Figure 2.5 illustrates a model of Peplau's theory. The central components of the theory include interpersonal process, nurse, client, and anxiety. The interpersonal process is the primary component and includes the in-

teraction between the nurse in his or her professional role and the client in his or her state of anxiety manifested in illness. Through investigative interviewing, the nurse works with the client to uncover unused competencies and dormant powers. Through interpersonal interaction with the client, the nurse facilitates the client's ability to transform symptom-bound energy into problem-solving energy. Latent capacities become realized competencies by the client. The resultant transformation of anxiety moves the client toward health and outside the boundary of the nurse–client relationship. The theory has been used extensively to direct practice, but only limited empirical testing has been done through research.

Forchuk (1994) conducted a nursing investigation to test Peplau's theory by determining if variables she identified within her theory as significant were related to the development of the nurse–client relationship during the orientation phase of the process. Box 2.5 presents the highlights of this investigation.

c. Theory of Planned Behavior

The theory of planned behavior (Ajzen 1985, 1991) is a theory borrowed from the discipline of psychology. The theory can be used to explain virtually any behavior over which an individual has control. It is designed to predict behavior and to enhance understanding of the psychological determinants of that behavior (Fig. 2.6).

According to the theory, intention to perform or not perform a behavior is the immediate determinant of that behavior. Intention, in turn, is a direct function of three independent variables: attitude, subjective norms, and perceived behavioral control. The theory of planned behavior has been used by nurse investigators to study a multitude of health behaviors. Examples include sexual decision making, birth planning intentions, Lamaze childbirth intentions, contracep-

BOX 2.4 *Nurse Researchers at Work*

EFFECTS OF OREM-BASED NURSING INTERVENTION ON NUTRITIONAL SELF-CARE

The purpose of this study was to test the effectiveness of an intervention based on Orem's theory of nursing on the nutritional self-care of 104 patients who suffered from myocardial infarctions (MIs). Orem posited eight universal self-care requisites for maintenance of health. One of these, food, was the focus of this study. The theory of self-efficacy was also included in the theoretical framework. Self-efficacy is a person's belief in his or her own ability to perform a certain behavior and be motivated to persist in that behavior. It was expected that if the nursing interventions were effective in assisting patients to eat a healthful diet, then patients would be more confident in this ability and more motivated to eat a healthful diet because of their increased self-efficacy.

Nutritional self-care was measured with a 24-hour diet recall for 3 days and completion of the food habits questionnaire. Self-care agency (SCA) was measured with the SCA scale. Self-efficacy for healthful eating was measured by the eating habits confidence scale. Baseline data were collected from both groups in the hospital. Treatment group subjects were then visited in their homes 1 week after discharge to begin the treatment intervention, which included observation and questioning on dietary behavior, meal preparation, and encouragement in nutritional self-care. During the next 6 weeks, all subjects received three follow-up phone calls.

The control group did not receive the home visit nor were diet issues dealt with in the three follow-up phone calls unless the patient introduced the subject. Data were collected from both groups 7 weeks after discharge.

Results indicated significant differences between groups on their intake of total fat and saturated fat, and food habits questionnaire scores, with the treatment group scoring better on these measures at time 2. Significant changes over time on SCA and self-efficacy for healthful eating were noted for the treatment group between time 1 and 2. The control group increased only their self-efficacy during this period. At time 2, there were no significant differences between the group means on measures of either SCA or self-efficacy.

The nature of the relationship between SCA and nutritional self-care was expected to be positive and moderate because nutrition is only one of the eight aspects of self-care addressed in the instrument. Study findings were consistent with this expectation. The finding that self-care increased in the treatment group but not the control group suggested that the effect of the nursing action was related to SCA. Concepts from the psychological theory of self-efficacy were less useful in this study. In conclusion, Orem's theory proved useful in guiding strategies for effective care and in providing an explanation of how the intervention worked.

SOURCE: Summarized from Aish, A.E., and Isenberg, M. (1996). Effects of Orem-based nursing intervention on nutritional self-care of myocardial infarction patients. *International Journal of Nursing Studies, 33,* 259–270.

tive decision making, intention to engage in leisure activities, problem drinking, losing weight, and exercising. Box 2.6 presents the summary of a study by Hanson (1997), which applied the theory of planned behavior to cigarette smoking in teenage girls. The theory was tested using the path analysis method discussed later in this text. As you read the summary of this study, pay particular attention to the hypotheses statement and the results of the study, which lend some support to the theory of planned behavior. The study is an example of how research can lead to theory refinement and how theory can direct future research. For a complete description of the study, refer to the referenced source.

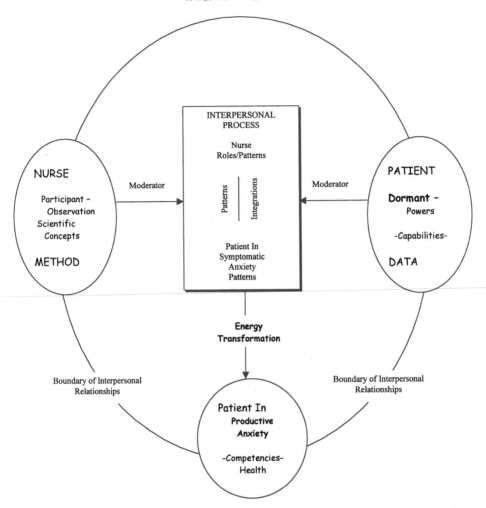

Figure 2.5 Model of Peplau's theory. (From Fitzpatrick, J., and Whail, A. [1996]. *Conceptual Models of Nursing: Analysis and Application* [3rd ed]. Stanford, CT: Appleton & Lange. Cited with permission.)

E. TESTING AND USING THEORY IN RESEARCH

As we have seen, the function of theory is to describe, explain, and predict—that is, to offer satisfactory, *testable* explanations for relationships. A testable explanation is one that can be disconfirmed (i.e., one that may turn out to be true or false). A satisfactory explanation is one that follows tough rules of evidence and is free from the flaws in explanation discussed at the beginning of this chapter.

As you know, a theory may be thought of as a cluster of tentative ideas put forward to explain something; research is then conducted to test the adequacy of these ideas. Considerable debate exists in nursing science about the proper relationship between theory and methods. Most seem to agree that they are best viewed as partners in our attempts to extend our understanding of human behavior. In that way, both theory and methods may be regarded as tools. Refinements in our theories are neither more nor less im-

BOX 2.5 *Nurse Researchers at Work*

THE ORIENTATION PHASE OF THE NURSE–CLIENT RELATIONSHIP: TESTING PEPLAU'S THEORY

This investigation used a correlational design to test Peplau's theory regarding influences during the orientation phase of the nurse–client relationship. The orientation phase is a clinically significant yet difficult phase with clients with a chronic mental illness. The study tested eight hypotheses that focused on the independent variables of preconceptions, interpersonal relationships, and anxiety, measured at the beginning of the nurse–client relationship. These were expected to predict later results for the dependent variable, the development of the therapeutic relationship as proposed by the theory. The hypotheses tested were:

i. Clients' more positive preconceptions of the nurse will be related to greater progress in the development of therapeutic relationships.
ii. Nurses' more positive preconceptions of the client will be related to greater progress in the development of therapeutic relationships.
iii. Clients' more positive interpersonal relationships will be related to greater progress in the development of therapeutic relationships.
iv. Nurses' more positive interpersonal relationships will be related to greater progress in the development of therapeutic relationships.
v. Higher levels of anxiety in the client will be related to less progress in the development of therapeutic relationships.
vi. Higher levels of anxiety in the nurse will be related to less progress in the development of therapeutic relationships.
vii. Taken together, the clients' preconceptions of the nurse, level of anxiety, and interpersonal relationships will be a better predictor of progress in the development of therapeutic relationships than any one client variable alone.

viii. Taken together, the nurses' preconceptions of the client, level of anxiety, and interpersonal relationships will be a better predictor of progress in the development of therapeutic relationships than any one nurse variable alone.

Purposive sampling was used to select subjects from a long-term care program serving mentally ill clients. The sample included 124 newly formed nurse–client dyads. Two instruments measured the dependent variable, development of the therapeutic relationship: The Relationship Form and the Working Alliance Inventory (WAI). The Personal Resource Questionnaire, the Beck Anxiety Inventory, and the Preconceptions Semantic Differential Scale measured the independent variables of interpersonal relations, anxiety, and preconceptions, respectively.

Results indicate that the preconceptions of both the nurse and client were most strongly related to the development of the therapeutic relationship (hypotheses i and ii supported). Clients' other relationships were significant on the WAI only (hypothesis iii partially supported), and nurses' other interpersonal relationships were not significant (hypothesis iv not supported). Anxiety, of nurses and clients, was not significantly related to progress in the relationship (hypotheses v and vi not supported). Hypothesis vii was partially supported, and hypothesis viii was not supported.

In conclusion, this study supports some of the tenets of Peplau's theory, but not others. It gives direction for further theory refinement and for future research. Specifically, anxiety and other relationships may be less important than the theory currently suggests. Continued testing of this theory will guide future theory refinement and the application of theory in practice.

SOURCE: Summarized from Forchuk, C. (1994). The orientation phase of the nurse-client relationship: Testing Peplau's theory. *Journal of Advanced Nursing, 20,* 532–537.

]

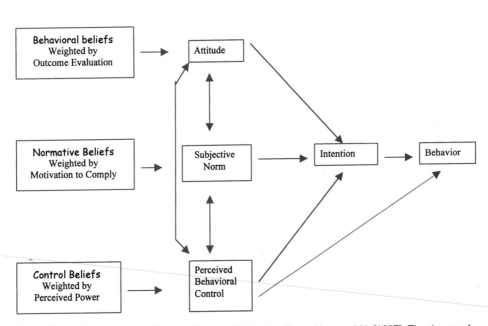

Figure 2.6 Conceptual map: Theory of planned behavior. (From Hanson, M.J. [1997]. The theory of planned behavior applied to cigarette smoking in African-American, Puerto Rican, and non-Hispanic white teenage females. *Nursing Research, 46*[3], 155–162. Cited with permission.)

portant than refinements in our methods. They are equal partners in the knowledge enterprise.

Hypothesis testing is a part of theory testing but, by itself, does not necessarily constitute a test of theory. The fundamental issue in theoretical research is to demonstrate the link between a set of theoretical propositions and the conceptual hypothesis that has been selected for examination. Only to the extent that this connection has been articulated successfully can we claim our research has bearing on theory. This section considers methods of testing theories.

I. Testing Middle-Range Theory

As the discipline of nursing matures, the emphasis on knowledge development is moving from grand theories to middle-range theories. It is likely that, as middle-range theory becomes the norm, new nursing research methods will be developed. Middle-range theories involve a number of formally stated, interconnected propositions; contain clearly defined variables; and indicate the nature (direct or inverse) and the direction (what is causing what) of the relationships among the variables. The propositions normally take the form of *the greater the A, the greater the B.* Not all the concepts in the propositions need to be directly measurable; however, at some point, a connection to measurable variables must be made. It is this link that must be specified for one's research to have bearing on a theoretical formulation. We will examine two methods used to demonstrate such connections: these are axiomatic derivations and replacement of terms.

BOX 2.6 *Nurse Researchers at Work*

THE THEORY OF PLANNED BEHAVIOR APPLIED TO CIGARETTE SMOKING

The purpose of this study was to evaluate the adequacy of Ajzen's Theory of Planned Behavior to predict cigarette smoking intention in three groups of teenage girls. Participants were 141 African-Americans, 146 Puerto Ricans, and 143 non-Hispanic whites, age 13 to 19 years.

The hypothesis tested was derived from the theory and tested all the predictor variables in the theory. It stated: "The belief-based measures of attitude, subjective norm, and perceived behavioral control have an indirect effect on cigarette-smoking intention and a direct effect on attitude, subjective norm, and perceived behavioral control, respectively. These, in turn, have direct effects on cigarette smoking intention in African-American, Puerto Rican, and non-Hispanic white teenage females." These represent the six essential paths diagrammed in Figure 2.6, the conceptual map of the theory.

The Fisbein/Ajzen-Hanson Questionnaire (FAHQ) was constructed in accordance with the Theory of Planned Behavior to measure the study variables. This instrument was administered to subjects attending family planning clinics.

Separate path analyses were used to test the study hypothesis for each group. To summarize, all six paths of the model were statistically significant for African-Americans. Hence, the hypothesis was supported for African-American teenage girls. For Puerto Rican and non-Hispanic whites, only the relationships among attitude, perceived behavioral control, and smoking intention were supported. Hence, the hypothesis was not supported for these two groups. This study suggests that the Theory of Planned Behavior provides an adequate explanation of cigarette smoking among African-American teenage girls.

SOURCE: Summarized from Hanson, M.J. (1997). The theory of planned behavior applied to cigarette smoking in African-American, Puerto Rican, and non-Hispanic white teenage females. *Nursing Research, 46*(3), 155–162.

a. Axiomatic Derivations

Axiomatic derivations are new statements of relationship logically derived from a given set of assumptions and propositions. An example is provided in Box 2.7 using a set of propositions found in work by Teevan (2000).

Instead of using "low premarital sexual permissiveness" as the example of a "conservative value," one could instead use any number of alternative replacements such as:

- Low likelihood of using drugs
- Deferring marriage
- Choosing traditional careers for one's gender

The new derived propositions should be true if the assumptions, derivations, and original theoretical propositions are accurate. Derivations are made to locate testable hypotheses that then constitute a test of the theory. The reason one makes such derivations is to provide many different tests. The reason one wants to do different tests is that ideally one wishes to identify a theoretically predicted relationship but one that is not obvious.

Why would one want a counterintuitive relationship? Here the answer is psychological rather than scientific. If an unexpected relationship is predicted, and if, indeed, the results of the study confirm it, the evidence is much more convincing. On the other hand, if the predicted relationship is commonsensical, even if it is confirmed, the critic will claim that the results only show what everyone already knew and certainly do not demonstrate any theory. The verification of Albert Ein-

BOX 2.7 *Birth Order and Sexual Permissiveness*

To illustrate axiomatic derivations, Teevan uses the following interrelated set of statements to illustrate the derivation of a testable hypothesis:

1. *First-born children are more closely tied to their parents than are later born (theoretical statement).*
2. *Ties to parents lead to conservative values (theoretical statement).*
3. *Therefore, first-born children have more conservative values than later-born (axiomatic logic)*
4. *Low premarital sexual permissiveness is a conservative value (definition).*
5. *Therefore, first-born children are less sexually permissive (deductive logic).*

SOURCE: Teevan, J.J. (2000). *Introduction to Sociology: A Canadian Focus* (7th ed.). Scarborough: Prentice-Hall Canada. Cited with permission.

stein's simple but counterintuitive prediction that a rapidly moving clock should run slower than a clock that is moving slowly provided powerfully convincing evidence for his theory of relativity.

b. Replacement of Terms

A further way of extending the number of predictions is to use a technique called *replacement of terms*. **Replacement of terms** refers to replacing general theoretical concepts by specific examples of these concepts. For example, if the general concept is health behavior, such a concept could be replaced by a specific instance of health behavior such as seatbelt use, exercise, or meditation. To the extent that one is able to derive new predictions through such replacements, one can provide a virtually unlimited number of testable relationships. One can then select the better ones, choosing those that are counterintuitive and those that

permit one to refine and specify conditions under which the theory does, or does not, hold.

Using a combination of axiomatic derivations and replacement of terms provides powerful, yet simple, methods of deriving interesting testable hypotheses. The student would be well advised, however, to directly test the propositions of a theory and, if that is not possible, to restrict axiomatic steps to a minimum in locating testable hypotheses. Because human relations are so complex and because few relations are extremely powerful, it is problematic to make a large number of axiomatic steps and still have an ironclad connection to the original set of propositions. So, keep it simple!

2. Testing Practice Theory

Routine hospital practices are often the subject of nursing research. Because of the desire to base practice on evidence, graduate students and nurse researchers frequently evaluate current nursing practices. Indeed, many fine master's theses are done evaluating a routine practice. So whether it is assessing the "comfort levels" of patients controlling their pain medication or assessing the impact of the timing of the bathing of newborns on the temperature decreases experienced by newborns, the research can provide evidence for continuing current practice or altering practice. Indeed, one could argue that the key to evidence-based practice is the continuing questioning and evaluation of routines found in nursing practice. Indeed, it is conceivable that future directions in nursing research will include increased efforts at evaluating situation-specific practice theories.

3. Structural Equation Modeling

Structural equation modeling is an advanced statistical method designed to test theories. In a theory, all the concepts are expected to be related. Conceptual maps discussed earlier in the chapter express this web of relationships. Testing the structure of the relationships in a theory as a whole provides more information about the validity of the theory than testing only specific relationships or propositions. This can be achieved using structural equation modeling with path analysis. The researcher anticipates certain outcomes from the structural equations if the model is correct. This consistency does not prove the accuracy of the theory but it does support it. Figure 2.7 illustrates a causal model used by Porter and associates (1996) in their study of influences on the sexual behaviors of elementary and middle school youths. Note the arrangement of the variables and how they are ultimately linked to the dependent variable, self-reported initiation of sexual intercourse. Models such as the Porter et al. one are known as path analysis models. The arrows and lines represent the causal connections between the variables in the model. (Such models are analyzed using techniques in the correla-

tion/regression family of statistical techniques; a preliminary discussion of these techniques is given later in the text.) For a more detailed discussion, interested students are advised to consult an advanced statistics or methods text.

4. Testing Alternative Explanations

The testing of **alternative explanations** is a primitive form of theory testing. This is the case because theory and explanation do the same thing: answer a "why" question. The reason we identify the testing of alternative explanations as a primitive form of theory testing is that such formulations typically fail to fully identify the linkages to the framework that is being used.

The first thing we need in order to test a theory using alternative explanations is a relationship that, we believe, needs to be understood. Then we propose a series of alternative explanations for the relationship. After that, all we have to do is to measure the appropriate variables and do the analysis.

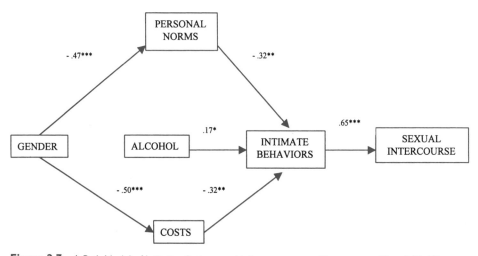

Figure 2.7 A Path Model of Initiation Pathways of influence on sexual intercourse. *$P < 0.05$. **$P < 0.01$. ***$P < 0.001$. Note: the larger the value, the greater the influence of the variable. (From Porter, C., Oakley, D., Ronis, D., and Neal, W. [1996]. Pathways of influence on fifth and eighth graders report about having had sexual intercourse. *Research in Nursing and Health, 19*, 193–204. Cited with permission.)

For example, two possible explanations might be proposed for the connection between the age of initiation of sexual intercourse and socioeconomic background:

- Whether students with higher SESes possess more conservative attitudes and this leads to a deferral of initiation into sexual intercourse; or
- Whether students with higher SESes are more likely to experience less peer pressure to engage in sexual activity.

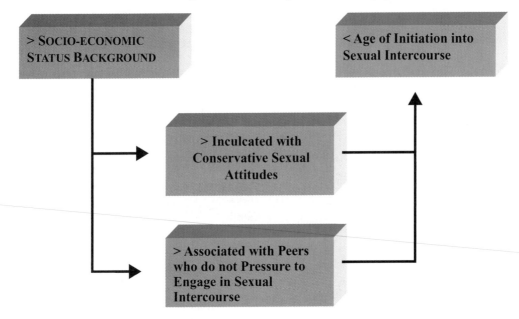

Appropriate research would allow us to evaluate the adequacy of each of the two possible explanations. We would need measures of the student's SES background, age of initiation into sexual activity (if at all), a measure of how conservative their attitudes are, and a measure of the amount of peer pressure they have experienced to engage in sexual activity. The first explanation uses a socialization of conservative values explanation (but connected to what general theory of human behavior?). The second relies on a peer pressure explanation but, again, to what general theory is this connected? Nevertheless, because both explanations are answers to a why question, each may be viewed as constituting a theory of human behavior (albeit an implicit theory).

The advantage of the more formal constructions of nursing theory (middle-range theory) is that we are forced to make explicit our core assumptions of the theory. Without such explicitness, it is difficult to construct truly general, and therefore powerful, theories of human behavior. When we seek to explain particular relationships with highly particularized explanations, we do not advance the general state of knowledge much. Hence, more formal approaches to theory construction are to be encouraged. Nonetheless, especially for beginning researchers, testing alternative explanations for relationships may make important contributions to the discipline.

The basic requirements for the testing of alternative explanations are that:

- One has a relationship between two variables that one suspects will be strong (either positive or negative);
- One has a series of alternative explanations for the relationship;
- That it is possible to get measures for the appropriate variables; and

• That after data are collected, suitable procedures are used for the analysis of the data so that an evaluation can be made of the adequacy of the competing explanations.

5. Theoretical Triangulation

Recently nurse researchers have proposed **theoretical triangulation** as a strategy for theory testing. This involves the testing of two competing or alternative theories within one study. As previously stated, almost all phenomena can be explained using alternative explanations. Hence, a researcher who directly tests alternative explanations using a single sample of subjects is in a position to make powerful comparisons about the utility of competing explanations. Theory triangulation can rule out rival hypotheses, avoid premature acceptance of plausible concepts, prevent ignoring contradictory propositions, and help in refining theoretical systems (Banik, 1993). Bennett (1997) provides a concise example of theory triangulation in her study of nurses' attitudes about AIDS. In this study, Orem's (1995) theory of nursing systems and Travelbee's (1971) theory of interpersonal nursing are used to explore whether patient characteristics and lifestyle are more likely to influence nurses' attitudes than nurses' own caring competencies. Students are encouraged to read this source if they are interested in learning more about this method of theory testing. This example demonstrates how the exploration of related questions not addressed by a single theory may be aided by searching for links among middle-range theories.

F. POINTS OF AGREEMENT ON RESEARCH AND THEORY

Nurse scientists have a variety of perspectives available to them on theory in nursing research. There is a strong tendency for some researchers to be identified with the work of one particular nurse theorist or one methodological approach. And even if people span a variety of approaches, we tend to label them as supporters of one particular theory and paradigm. There are squabbles between the various schools of thought or paradigms over the kinds of evidence that should be used and, indeed, serious arguments over which questions we should be asking as nurse scientists.

On occasion, such debate is carried on with a distinct lack of tolerance for differences. Perhaps it is a measure of the immaturity of our discipline that we are occasionally divided into warring camps. By the end of their university nursing program, most students will witness at least one professor make an unrelenting attack on some theoretical or methodological perspective not shared by that individual. Although debates in universities can be healthy and invigorating, so too can they be destructive and counterproductive if they fail to give the student a balanced view of the various approaches.

But are there also points of agreement? Most nurse scientists would agree that we should:

• **Study the full range of human behavior in health and illness states.** This is to acknowledge that it is equally legitimate to study both social constructions of reality (individual subjective perceptions of reality) and objective, measurable structural patterns found in any society. In short, both qualitative and quantitative methodologies have contributions to make in understanding human responses and behavior.

• **Use the methodology appropriate to the questions asked.** Most people agree that the methodology we apply should be appropriate to the question asked. And although we could never agree that either qualitative or quantitative methodologies are better, we

BOX 3.1 *Nurse Researchers at Work*

NURSE RESEARCHER PROJECTS

These projects were designed by nurse researchers or interdisciplinary research teams with nurse researchers as part of the membership. They were selected from refereed nursing journals and include a variety of research designs. Full references are provided in the reference list at the conclusion of the text.

Research Project Title	Author
Curriculum trends in nurse practitioner programs: Current and ideal	Bellack et al., 1999
Infertility education in baccalaureate schools of nursing	Sherrod, 1998
Competencies of liberal education in post RN baccalaureate students: A longitudinal study	Gillis, MacLellan, & Perry, 1998
Determinants of a healthy lifestyle in new fathers	Walker, Flescher, and Heaman, 1998
Maternal smoking or nonsmoking and feeding choice	Edwards, Sims-Jones, & Briethaupt, 1998
The male experience of caregiving for a family member with Alzheimer's disease	Parsons, 1997
Nerves as status and nerves as stigma: Idioms of distress: And social action in Newfoundland and Norway	Davis & Joakimsen, 1997
Stressors in families with a child with a chronic condition	Ogden-Burke, 1998
Views on assignment of publication credit for scholarly and scientific work	Butler & Ginn, 1998
Courage in middle-aged adults with long-term health concerns	Finfgeld, 1998
Entry into community-based nursing practice: Perceptions of prospective employees	Hahn, 1998
The changing self-concept of pregnant and parenting teens	Alpers, 1998
Care: A value expressed in philosophies of nursing services	Tuck et al., 1998
Hospital nurses and health promotion	Berland, Whyte, & Maxwell, 1995
Women's anger: Relationship of suppression to blood pressure	Thomas, 1997

continued on next page

BOX 3.1 *Nurse Researchers at Work (Continued)*

NURSE RESEARCHER PROJECTS

Research Project Title	Author
Follow-up study of children with growth deficiency	Reifsnider, 1998
Therapeutic touch as a nursing intervention	Meehan, 1998
What a difference a nurse makes—then and now	MacKinnon, 1997
Youngsters caring for adults with cancer	Gates & Lackey, 1998

of research, you simply need to reflect on any practice situation and ponder about discrepancies you see in practice. Simply stated, a **discrepancy** is the difference between the ways things are in practice and the way they ought to be, or between what one knows and what one needs to know to eliminate a problem (Diers, 1979).

Many nursing investigations are born out of a nurse's desire to improve practice situations and eliminate discrepancies so that clients can cope better, feel better, or live life more fully. Discrepancies become relevant sources of nursing problems. For example, you may notice that elderly patients who undergo surgery for a fractured hip experience confusion and delusions after surgery. This is a serious problem because they are often disoriented and attempt to get out of bed on their own. As a nurse, you spend a great deal of time trying to prevent falls, orient them, and reassure them. You mention this to more experienced nurses on the unit, and they may comment that everyone is like that after surgery, that it is an expected effect of the anesthetic. You wonder whether this rationale is based on evidence and, if so, what, if anything, could be done to prevent it. You have the beginning of a highly relevant and clinically significant nursing problem with potential to improve practice. The point here is you need to be open

to seeing discrepancies in practice and not accept "pat" answers to problems that are frequently inappropriately accepted in practice.

b. Exploring a Pattern of Incidents

The previous example provides an important characteristic of research problems—that is, a pattern of incidents in clinical situations that bears a relationship to more general situations. If only one elderly patient was confused and agitated after hip surgery, you would not design a study to address this isolated problem. However, if a problem can be conceptualized at a higher level that will be generalizable to others, it should be investigated. Astute nurses reflect on their practice to identify common patterns of phenomena across client situations that require investigation to be fully understood. Examples of such patterns may include separation anxiety in hospitalized children; effective coping in social support groups; burnout in long-term caregivers of clients with Alzheimer's disease; hopelessness in terminally ill clients; or intuitive decision-making processes in expert nurses. Rather than automatically accepting a pattern as normal, you need to question its existence and ask what can be done to better understand the phenomenon and enhance practice.

c. Testing Folk Wisdom

Interesting projects can often be designed to test systematically the accuracy of some taken-for-granted wisdom. You can have a lot of fun testing knowledge passed on from one generation of nurses to another. If you try it, you might be amazed at some of the results. Consider the following examples:

- Do whirlpool baths consume fewer physiological resources than bedbaths? Traditional wisdom has supported the use of bed baths. Such folk wisdom warrants testing through research.
- Among psychiatric nurses, are female nurses more empathetic to clients' needs than male nurses?
- Is daily vital sign monitoring as effective as monitoring every 4 hours in predicting occurrence of complications in institutionalized elderly recovering from abdominal surgery?
- Does engagement in regular exercise reduce the risk of falls in hospitalized elderly clients?
- Are audio taped end-of-shift nursing reports effective in promoting continuity of care and informed decision making by staff nurses?
- Does it take more energy for cardiac patients to take showers than to brush their teeth?

Spend some time thinking about these and other commonly accepted views of how things work in nursing and then try to think of some way in which these ideas could be tested systematically. Ask yourself how experimental, field, survey, or applied research designs might be used to study the problem. Which design would be ideal and which one would be most practical for each of these topics?

d. Understanding Phenomena from the Insider's Perspective

Many times, a researcher may be interested in exploring a concept or idea from a new perspective, namely from the perspective of those experiencing it. That is, much may be known about a particular experience, procedure, or nursing intervention from the viewpoint of the nurse; however, there may be little or no documentation in the literature about the client's view of the phenomenon. For example, the literature may contain many studies on cardiac stress testing and the best ways to prepare a client for such testing. However, you note that no one has considered this topic from the perspective of the client who is undergoing the stress testing. You may be interested in understanding preparation for stress testing from the client's perspective. Attention to the insider's view on a broad range of phenomena can be a rich and exciting source of topics for nursing investigations. Those interested in exploring qualitative research topics will find this approach particularly useful in generating researchable questions of relevance.

e. Tackling Current Issues

One method of selecting a project is to choose one that is the subject of professional debate. Such topics include nurses as entry point to the health-care delivery system, cost of insured nursing services, expanded roles for nurses, baccalaureate versus diploma or associate degree education for professional practice, and use of alternative therapies by nurses. A word of caution is warranted when selecting such topics for investigation because investigations of these types of topics may be politically motivated. For example, one group may wish to show that nurses can provide services currently delivered by physicians in a more cost-effective and efficient manner than the latter group. Therefore, nurse researchers need to be cautious not to bias the study so that results simply support the desired conclusions (see Chap. 9).

f. Inconsistencies in the Literature

Awareness of the research literature on a particular topic may lead one to note that there are inconsistencies in the reported findings. Such awareness is often a stimulus to design a study to explore the reasons behind such inconsistencies. These projects often are popular because they relate to debates current in the profession and highlight the need for additional research.

g. Testing a Theory

Researchers who have theoretical inclinations may wish to test a current theory of nursing, a theory that appears to be emerging in the nursing research literature but that has not yet been tested, or one of the many theories of human behavior that relate to health or illness situations. Chapter 2 outlines methods for generating testable theoretical hypotheses. The challenge is to examine a relationship between variables that is predicted by a theory but that, at the same time, is not obvious to common sense. For example, building on the previous scenario, you may believe that both the nursing literature and evidence in nursing practice suggest that a relationship exists between confusion in elderly clients and the experience of hip surgery. You decide that this warrants investigation so means may be found to prevent confusion or assist the elderly to cope more effectively. You might be interested in testing a theory that predicts when and which clients experience confusion and agitation and what factors might prevent this in the elderly. Consequently, you might design a study of the variables associated with confusion and agitation in the elderly after hip surgery. Variables might include the patients themselves (e.g., their age, general health state, demographics), the surgical procedure, the anesthetic agents used, post-operative medications, postoperative nursing care, unit routines, skill mix of staff, and so on. The most convincing theory-testing projects are those that make a counter-intuitive (against common sense) prediction that, if it turns out to be true, will be a convincing demonstration of the theory.

h. Testing Practice Theories

A review of the literature may reveal a consistent relationship between two variables, but alternative explanations for this relationship may not have been carefully tested. For example, a relationship is found consistently in the literature between perceived self-efficacy and engagement in health behaviors. In such cases, it is reasonable to propose alternative explanations for the relationship; design a study; and then test which, if any, of the proposed explanations best accounts for the relationship. (See Chapter 2 for other examples.)

i. Exploring Variations in a Dependent Variable

Another approach is to try to understand variations in a dependent variable. Which factors influence engagement in a health-promoting lifestyle by various age groups? What influences engagement in risk-taking behaviors by adolescents? Which variables influence the choice of cancer treatments among female clients with breast tumors? How do children with life-threatening illness nonverbally communicate their desire to terminate a nursing interaction? Here the goal is to understand the factors influencing the dependent variable.

j. Providing an Evaluation

Nurse scientists are frequently called on to provide an evaluation of a nursing intervention or health-care policy. Evaluations are often required for social, community health, health promotion and prevention programs, as well as many hospital-based programs. For example, a nurse researcher may be asked to evaluate the clinical outcomes of premature infants receiving conventional care and those receiving developmental care during their stay in the neonatal intensive care unit. Given the enormous financial and technological resources allotted to neonatal care, this problem is highly relevant to optimize positive developmental outcomes for premature infant survivors. A solid understanding of experimental design and a good deal of imagination and flexibility are qualities well suited to doing evaluations. There is a demand for nurse researchers who know how to do evaluation work.

k. Implementing and Studying a Nursing Action Simultaneously

In today's world of rapidly changing health-care practices, it is important to be able to take action to solve problems and systematically study the effects of the action at the same time. As we discuss in Chapter 8, action research enables researchers to identify whether or not the implemented solution is resolving the problem. Action research leads to the generation of practical knowledge that relates to practice in a particular setting. Action research topics are different from clinical problems in which one expects the results to be generalizable across a range of settings.

l. Replicating a Study

One can choose to replicate, or repeat, some earlier study (following exactly the same procedures as the original study but based on a different sample). Alternatively, one may do an indirect replication by adding a new dimension to the study. In addition to asking the original questions, the indirect replication could take the form of answering a question that was left open by the previous project.

2. How to Identify Problems Not Answerable through Research

Finally, not all problems of interest to nurses are answerable through research. Some problems are philosophical in nature rather than researchable. Problems that involve choosing a moral course of action or that are value questions or policy questions are not answerable through research. For example, should children with terminal illness have extraordinary means used to prolong the dying process? Or, is it ethical to deny a client information about their diagnosis if the family request it? Or, is abortion on demand good practice? These questions cannot be answered through empirical investigation; rather, they are questions for philosophical inquiry and for public policy debates.

It should be understood that although policy questions are not directly answerable through research, research can inform or shape policy development. Numerous professional journals, such as the *Journal of Nursing Scholarship,* regularly publish articles with policy implications.

3. How to Focus the Research Problem and Purpose

Having selected the research topic the next step is to articulate precisely what you wish to investigate. To do this, the researcher must decide on a specific aspect of the research topic that warrants investigation and then proceed to describe the precise problem and develop a statement of purpose. Before we proceed to explain the process of limiting the problem and formulating a statement of purpose, it is helpful to clarify several terms important to the conceptual phase of a research project: research problem, problem statement, research question, and statement of purpose.

a. Terminology

The **research problem** is a situation or circumstance that requires a solution to be described, explained, or predicted. It is an unsatisfactory situation that we want to confront (Norwood, 2000). There is a knowledge gap in an area that needs to be investigated. The research problem identifies the knowledge gap that needs to be filled. Whereas the *research topic* is simply a broad area of interest, the *research problem* identifies what is problematic about the topic.

The **problem statement** is a narrative that elaborates on the research problem and identifies the specific area of concern. It provides direction for the entire study and guides the study toward a quantitative or a qualitative design. Writing the problem statement helps the researcher identify uncertainties that need clarification before the study can proceed (Thomas, 2000). The problem statement includes six elements. These are:

1. Information about the research topic that provoked the study
2. The scope of the problem (e.g., how many people are affected by it)
3. Why it is important to study the problem
4. How nursing science would be influenced by the study
5. General characteristics of the population of interest
6. The overall goal or aim of the study or the question to be answered

The research problem stated in the interrogative form is referred to as the **research question.** It is stated in the present tense. The advantage to stating the problem in the interrogative form is that a question invites an answer. For example, "What is the relationship of maternal and paternal health-promoting lifestyle

to health-promoting lifestyles in adolescent girls?" Or, "What is the meaning of caring for nurses who provide services to disenfranchised patient populations?"

The purpose of a study is the specific aim or goal you hope the study to accomplish. For example, "The purpose of this research is to examine the relationship of maternal and paternal health-promoting lifestyles to health-promoting lifestyle in adolescent girls." Or, "The purpose of this research is to understand the meaning of caring for nurses who provide services to disenfranchised patient populations."

b. Limiting the Problem

The process of limiting the problem involves reflecting on the topic, reviewing the literature to determine the current state of knowledge about the problem, and talking to those in the field who have had experience with the problem. In limiting the problem, the researcher is attempting to pare away all the unrelated information and narrow the problem for investigation to the point where a clear, unambiguous, researchable question will emerge. To illustrate this process, suppose you wished to study the problem of accidental falls in elderly patients. As you start to think about this investigation, determine whether you wish to examine:

- Risk factors for falls in the elderly
- The types of elderly clients who sustain falls versus those who do not
- The relationship between admission assessment (e.g., age, medical diagnosis, level of orientation, functional status) and the incidence of falls
- Whether there are differences in physical environmental factors in hospitals, nursing homes, and private residences that contribute to the incidence of accidental falls in the elderly
- Whether women are less inclined to sustain accidental falls than men, and if so, what accounts for this tendency

The list of issues you might wish to consider could be extended. After a problem has been selected, the work of specifying the precise problem statement or question begins. Suppose that you decided to focus on the first question (identifying risk factors in accidental falls in the elderly); then a thorough review of the literature should be undertaken to find out what other researchers have discovered. The review will also help you determine more precisely what is to be investigated. At this point, it is helpful to specify, as much as possible, the precise question to be studied. This is because the question determines the research design, and one does not want to make unnecessary changes to the design later because of a poorly focused research question.

c. Statements of Purpose

The **statement of purpose** of a study flows from the problem statement and is included in it. One research problem statement may be the basis for several research purposes. The research purpose is usually a single declarative statement that focuses the study and clearly identifies what the researcher intends to do.

Box 3.2 provides examples of research problem statements worded in the declarative and interrogative forms. In nursing research journals, however, you will note that the majority of research problems tend to be expressed as *statements of purpose*. Some authors select to include both a statement of purpose at the beginning of their article and specific research questions at the end of the introductory section of the article. See Box 3.3 for an example of this.

A variety of phrases is used by researchers to indicate the research purpose. Some common ones include:

- The purpose of this study was to describe three classification systems . . .

- The aim of this research was to explicate common life patterns . . .
- This study sought to elicit views of nurses on assignment of publication credit . . .
- The objective of this research was to identify factors associated with maternal–infant bonding . . .
- The purpose of this study was to answer the following questions . . .
- This qualitative study explored the meaning of respect from the perspective of . . .

As research projects are developed, it is normal for the first ideas to be fuzzy and to require an investigation of a rather grand scale. As the researcher reviews the literature, becomes more familiar with it, and becomes sensitive to practical considerations, the project should become more focused and specific and move to something that can be accomplished with the available resources.

B. REVIEWING THE LITERATURE

A **literature review** is a critical step in focusing the research problem and statement of purpose. It is a process of reviewing the current knowledge about the research problem, describing the characteristics of previous studies in the area, noting the similarities and differences in research results, evaluating the strengths and limitations of previous studies, and identifying gaps in knowledge relevant to the research problem. It should culminate in a final product that forms a chapter in a research thesis (usually Chapter 2). In a journal article, it may merit its own heading or be included in the introductory section of a report along with the research problem, purpose statement, and question. (Some qualitative research designs do not include the review of the literature at this stage of the research

---

BOX 3.2 *Nurse Researchers at Work*

RESEARCH PROBLEM STATEMENTS

Example 1. Fall risk factors in an acute-care setting: A retrospective study

Declarative Statement

A major safety issue for patients is the high incidence of falls during hospitalization. Although there is no national database in the United States for falls in the acute-care setting, Morse and Morse (1988) found a fall rate of 2.9 per 1000 bed days in acute care. Falls are the most frequent cause of accidents in the hospital setting (Cathchen, 1983), extend the length of stay (Andrews, 1986), and may be a primary reason for placement in a nursing home (Buchner et al., 1993: Dunn, Furner, & Miles, 1993). The effects of falling range from no physical injury to a major fracture. The proportion of falls resulting in a fracture is low (5%), but the costs of the additional medical treatment can be high (Tinetti, Speechley, & Ginter, 1988). . . . The literature has consistently identified age and medical diagnosis as risk factors for falls. Most research has examined only characteristics associated with fallers and has not compared the characteristics of fallers and nonfallers. The *purpose* of this study was to extend knowledge beyond the known risk factors of age and medical diagnosis by comparing the characteristics of a group of adults who fell while hospitalized with characteristics of a group matched on age and diagnosis who did not fall while hospitalized.

SOURCE: Stevenson, B., Mills, E., Welin, L., and Beal, K. (1998). Falls risk factors in an acute care study: A retrospective study. *Canadian Journal of Nursing Research, 30* (1), 97–113. Cited with permission.

Example 2. Factors affecting acute-care nurses' use of research findings

Interrogative Statement

To date, little research on the influence of organizational factors on research-based practice has been reported. Butler (1995) examined the relationship of organizational support and expectations for research to the use of research findings from the perspective of staff nurses. The following questions were posed:

- What are the nurses' values for, interests in, and experiences with research?
- What are the nurses' expectations of themselves for using research findings?
- What are the perceived organizational expectations to use research findings?
- What is the perceived organizational support for using research findings?
- What is the reported level of research use?
- What are the differences between perceived organizational expectations and staff nurses' expectations of themselves for using research findings in nursing?
- What is the relationship between the nurses' perceptions of organizational support for research utilization and use of research findings?

SOURCE: Butler L. (1995). Valuing research in clinical practice. *The Canadian Journal of Nursing Research, 27*(4), 33–49. Cited with permission.

---

process. These differences in approach are discussed in Chapter 6).

1. Importance of the Literature Review

The literature review should tell us what is known about the research topic and problem and what we need to find out. It places the existing study in the context of prior research studies and current knowledge. The goals of a literature review include:

- Etablishing the significance of the research problem
- Identifying sample characteristics to help identify relevant demographic variables

BOX 3.3 Nurse Researchers at Work

STATEMENT OF PURPOSE AND RESEARCH QUESTIONS

Example 1. Postpartum mothers' return to work: Mothering stress, anxiety, and gratification

More than half of mothers with infants younger than age 1 year are employed (Costello, Miles, & Stone, 1998). Scientific interest in maternal employment has focused predominantly on its impact on child development, especially infant–parent attachment (Bronfenbrenner & Crouter, 1982; Lerner, 1994). Investigators more recently have explored the health experiences of new mothers. However, limited research exists on how employment patterns and maternal health affect mothers' early parenting experiences, such as stress, separation anxiety, and gratification. The *purpose* of this study was to examine parenting stress, separation anxiety, and maternal gratification, in relation to employment patterns and selected health status indicators, of women who return to work during the first postpartum year. Specific questions concerning the first year postpartum included:

- What are the changes in maternal fatigue and depression?
- What are the changes in maternal gratification, parenting stress, and separation anxiety?
- How does the timing of return to employment and hours worked affect maternal gratification, parenting stress, and separation anxiety?
- How do maternal fatigue and depression affect maternal gratification, parenting stress, and separation anxiety?

SOURCE: Killien, M. (1998). Postpartum mothers' return to work: Mothering, stress, anxiety, and gratification. *Canadian Journal of Nursing Research, 30*(3), 53–67. Cited with permission.

Example 2. Evaluation of a home-based traction program for children with congenital dislocated hips and LeggPerthes Disease

Home-based traction (HBT) is an alternative to conventional hospital traction. Health professionals have generally supported the concept of HBT for children. However, widespread implementation of HBT programs has not occurred and research designed to evaluate the safety, effectiveness, and cost of such programs is limited in scope and rigor. The purpose of this study was to evaluate an HBT program for children with orthopedic conditions, including its impact on their parents. Specifically, four questions were posed:

- Is the HBT program acceptable to parents? Why or why not?
- Is the HBT program safe? What are the nature and frequency of untoward effects for the parents and child?
- What are the psychological and social consequences of the HBT program for the child and parents?
- What are the direct and indirect costs of HBT?

SOURCE: Stevens, B., Stockwell, M., Browne, G., et al. (1995). Evaluation of a home-based traction program for children. *Canadian Journal of Nursing Research, 27*(4), 133–151. Cited with permission.

- Identifying gaps in knowledge about the problem
- Identifying limitations of previous studies that may lead to a new study design
- Identifying areas where there seems to be consensus among researchers
- Noting where there are inconsistencies in research findings
- Identifying variables that others have found to be relevant to the problem at hand
- Identifying areas that, if explored, could lead to important new understandings of the phenomenon under examination
- Identifying theoretical frameworks that

others have used to study the phenomenon

- Identifying how other researchers have made connections to theory
- Identifying what other researchers consider to be important to study
- Identifying how other researchers have measured variables and analyzed their data
- Exploring the methods other investigators have used to study the research question

In reviewing the literature, you are trying to get a sense of the state of scientific knowledge about the topic and determine how best to study the research problem.

2. How to Conduct the Literature Review

Many graduate students panic about the idea of creating a "state-of-the-art" literature review on their research topic. This is because they try to do it all in one sitting. We suggest breaking the review into three stages: identifying the literature sources, evaluating the research studies, and writing an integrative review of the findings. Usually the first question posed is, "Where do I start?" Here are some useful steps to get you started.

- If you are part of a university or college, ask professors who work in the area for any ideas they may have on where to get information.
- Check with a reference librarian for sources that may lead you to research done on your topic.
- Check textbooks for leads.
- Check the appropriate discipline's abstracts because they provide brief descriptions of published papers dealing with a variety of topics. Box 3.4 lists some of the relevant abstracts, indexes, and Internet resources available.
- Check journals that are likely to publish work in the area. It is advisable to

begin by checking through the most recent issue. After you have found an article that is close to your topic in either the particular variables treated or the general concepts presented, check it for references to other articles. These references are usually helpful sources to include in the literature review. By starting with the most recent issues, you will identify the latest research. If an older article is referenced frequently, you should read it because it may be considered a classic.

- You may not be able to find published results on the specific relationship or category of individuals you wish to study. If this is the case, focus on variables that researchers have found to be related to the major dependent variable that you propose to examine.
- In many cases, it is appropriate to review research that uses similar methodologies or theories.
- In summarizing the research studies, try to answer the questions "Who?, What?, Where?, and When?" for each study you include in your review.
- Next make a statement about whether the study was sound or not (Chapter 20 provides guidelines for critiquing studies). Use words that reflect an evaluative component in your description of the study. For example, flawed design, robust findings, seminal piece of work, and so on.
- The research question may indicate that it would be appropriate to check various nonprint sources for inclusion in the literature review. These sources include digitized data, photographs, audio tapes, and video tapes.

3. How to Write the Literature Review

Generally, when the literature is analyzed in a report, the authors try to briefly summarize the areas of agreement and dis-

BOX 3.4 *Abstracts, Indexes of Periodicals, and Internet Resources of Relevance to Nursing**

Database/Index	Web Site
Nursing, Health Care, and Related Disciplines	
Cumulative Index to Nursing and Allied Health Literature	*http://www.cinahl.com*
Index Medicus	
MEDLINE CD-ROM (Medicine)	*http://igm.nlm.nih.gov*
HealthSTAR (Health Administration coverage)	*http://igm.nlm.nih.gov*
BIOETHICSLINE (Biomedical Ethics coverage)	*http://www.nlm.nih.gov*
EMBASE (European-based medicine coverage)	*http://erlsevier.com*
CANCERLIT (Cancer coverage)	*http://cancernet.nci.nih.gov*
AIDSLINE (Aids and HIV coverage)	*http://igm.nlm.nih.gov*
Sigma Theta Tau	*http://www.stti.iupui.edu*
National Information Center on Health Services Research and Health Care Technology (NICHSR)	*http://www.nlm.nih.gov/nichsr.html*
Psychology	
Child Development Abstracts and Bibliography	
Psyclit CD-ROM	
Psychological Abstracts	
PsychINFO	*http://www.apa.org/psycinfo*
Education	
ERIC CD-ROM	*http://ericir.syr.edu/eric*
Anthropology	
Abstracts in Anthropology	
	continued on next page

BOX 3.4 *Abstracts, Indexes of Periodicals, and Internet Resources of Relevance to Nursing* (Continued)*

Database/Index	Web Site
Anthropological Literature: Index to Periodical Articles	
International Bibliography of Social and Cultural Anthropology	
Sociology	
Human Resources Abstracts	
International Bibliography of Sociology	
Social Work Research and Abstracts	
SciSearch and Social SciSearch	*http://www.isinet.com*
Sociological Abstracts	
Sociofile CD-ROM	
General Listing (Relevance to Nursing and Other Disciplines)	
Canadian Periodical Index (Canadian content)	
Hospital Literature Index	
Infotrac (Academic Index) CD-ROM	
Social Sciences Citation Index	
Social Sciences Index	
Public Affairs Information Science Bulletin (PAIS)	
Newspaper Indexes	
Canadian News Index	
Canadian Press Newsfiles	
Index de l'actualite	
The National Newspaper Index	
	continued on next page

BOX 3.4 *Abstracts, Indexes of Periodicals, and Internet Resources of Relevance to Nursing* (Continued)*

Database/Index	Web Site
New York Times Index	
The Times Index	
Health-Related Internet Directories and Search Engines	
Health Web	http://www.healthweb.org
Medscape	http://www.medscape.com
National Library of Medicine	http://www.nim.nih.gov
Health Finder	http://www.healthfinder.gov
Evidence-based Nursing	http://www.bmjpg.com/data ebnpp.html
Health Web	http://www.healthweb.org
National Center for Health Statistics	http://www.cdc.gov.nchswww
Yahoo-Health	http://www.yahoo.com/health
AltaVista	http://www.altavista.com
Infoseek	http://www.infoseek.com

*With special acknowledgement to Barbara Phillips of the St. Francis Xavier Library staff who assisted with the preparation of this listing.

agreement in the literature. A critical aspect of reviewing the literature is the authors' interpretations of the various findings and their relationships to the present study. Article summaries may be useful to researchers but are generally not appropriate in a final report. What is required is a description of the current state of knowledge on the topic under investigation. The researchers need to discuss the most significant studies and those that form the theoretical background for the current study. Table 3.1 shows one method of summarizing articles: by using such a grid system, you can make additions to the list, provide a quick summary of areas of agreement and disagreement among researchers, interpret earlier literature in the field, and relate earlier findings to one's own work.

In preparing a discussion of the literature reviewed, it generally seems best to prepare an outline of the major concepts or variables and the relationships of significance to the current study. This allows the researcher to insert material on

Table 3.1 Background Characteristics Associated with Smoking

Variables	DeFronzo & Pawlak (1993)	Willms & Stebbins (1991)	Grossarth-Matieecek et al (1988)	Aloise-Young & Hennigan (1996)	Covey et al. (1992)	Trush et al. (1997)	Pugh et al. (1991)	Kaplan & Weiler (1997)	Glendinning et al. (1997)	Sun & Shun (1995)	Rogers et al. (1995)	Oygard et al. (1995)
Family members smoke	+					+			+		−	
Health problems reported		+	+	+								
Age												−
Education		+		−	−	+			−		−	
Urban community				+	+	+	+			+		
Violence in family	+					+	+		+			
Gender (male)	+										+	
Year of report	1993	1991	1988	1996	1992	1997	1991	1997	1997	1995	1995	1995
Number of subjects	849	NA	5977	1971	8042	2086	NA	NA	627	1320	827	104
Place of study	University of Conn.	McMaster University	London	St. John's	New York	University of Surrey	London	Illinois	Scotland	Florida	Norway	Colorado

+ indicates variable was positively related to incidence of smoking.
− indicates variable was negatively related to incidence of smoking.
Blank spaces indicate the variable was not reported in the study.
Adapted from Gillis, A. (1998). "The trends and variations in smoking." Course paper for Nursing 300, Antigonish, Nova Scotia: St. Francis Xavier University.

each report or study at an appropriate point in the review. It is best to report the findings on one variable at a time.

One suggestion for organizing the review is to divide the variables into clusters as they relate to the major dependent variable in your study. For example, you might have (1) background characteristics of respondents, (2) situational variables, and (3) other factors. Thus, if you were studying factors associated with success on national nursing registration examinations, you might begin by discussing background characteristics (e.g., socioeconomic status, size of home community, gender). These might be followed by situational factors such as family responsibilities or life crises that other researchers have related to success on nursing examinations. Then you might consider general academic factors such as nursing course grades and reading and language skills. In each case, you should summarize the consensus (or lack of it) in the research literature. And if you have provided a summary grid for the literature, readers will be able to review the findings quickly, and the plus and minus symbols will quickly reveal the degree of consensus on the relationship of any particular variable to the dependent variable. Box 3.5 illustrates a literature review statement.

The literature review should have solid informative (who?, what?, when?, and how?), evaluative (e.g., weak, robust, flawed), and integrative components (e.g., findings are consistent, supportive of, contrary to others) that present a balanced perspective of the current state of knowledge on the research topic. It is not necessary to include every article published on the research topic; in many cases, this would make the review too lengthy. However, do make sure that seminal pieces of work and those that focus most closely on the research problem are included.

Be certain to record full bibliographic details of each article or book used. When the final report is being prepared, all the sources should be cited in the reference list. If you have not recorded this information in full, you will waste a lot of time retracing your steps to recover the information.

C. SPECIFYING THE MODEL

Clarity and precision are at the core of successful research. A theoretical or **causal model** is a graphic representation of proposed causal interconnections between variables. In quantitative research, one way to enhance accuracy is to draw a diagram of the causal connections between variables. The advantage of a diagram is that it encourages clear thinking about what you are doing. Thus, drawing a diagram with causal arrows requires you to indicate which variable appears causally before other variables. You are forced to be specific. Such diagrams can also replace stating formal hypotheses; each hypothesis may be reflected in a properly drawn diagram. You may recall from Chapter 1 that *hypotheses* are tentative predictions about the relationships between two or more variables.

1. How to Identify the Variables

As you will recall from Chapter 2, *variables* may be defined as constructs that we intend to measure. Obviously, then, a researcher must identify the specific variables that will be studied in the research project. Variables may be identified by many methods. Most researchers have some idea of the variables that might influence the dependent variable, so it is easiest to begin with these. A review of the research literature also helps you identify the variables that other researchers have used in doing similar research. Studying relevant theoretical frameworks and models and identifying the variables that are implied by the theories are also useful in identifying research variables. Examining

BOX 3.5 *Nurse Researchers at Work*

FACTORS ASSOCIATED WITH NCLEX-RN SUCCESS: A LITERATURE REVIEW

There is a need for more extensive empirical data describing variables that contribute to success on the NCLEX-RN. Until recently, the only reliable factors identified as predictors of success were previous academic achievements, particularly earned grade point average (GPA). However, other factors may be involved.

Academic Nursing Factors

Glick, McClelland, and Yang (1986) found significant simple correlations between grades in clinical nursing courses, cumulative nursing GPA, and NCLEX-RN performance. Froman and Owen (1989) found that GPA in theoretical nursing courses was predictive of performance on NCLEX-RN. Krupa et al. (1988) looked at grades received in the Introductory Nursing course and the Medical-Surgical Nursing course. Their conclusion was that grades from both courses were substantially and directly related to NCLEX-RN performance. Grades in the other practicum courses were not good indicators in their study. Jenks et al. (1989) found that grades in nursing theory courses correlated strongly with NCLEX-RN performance. . . .

General Academic Factors

Some authors have investigated the influence of general academic factors such as reading competency and language skills on NCLEX-RN success. Wolahan (1992) found that reading competency at the 12th grade level and math skills were indicators of NCLEX-RN success among her student population. Johnson (1989) conducted a study with an ethnically and linguistically diverse population and found that language was a major variable predictive of success on the NCLEX-RN. Poorman and Martin (1991) found that test anxiety was inversely related to passing the NCLEX-RN. . . .

Nonacademic Factors

Few studies have considered the influence of nonacademic factors on NCLEX-RN performance. Given the increasing number of minority students, second-career students, adult learners, and students from diverse cultural backgrounds attending nursing programs, it seems appropriate to identify the nonacademic factors that are important in determining students at risk of failing NCLEX-RN. Dell and Valine (1990) examined self-esteem influence on NCLEX-RN scores. Self-esteem and age did contribute to the variance in NCLEX-RN scores. Self-efficacy recently has been found to be an important predictor of NCLEX-RN performance (Owen & Froman, 1990). Tolland (1989) suggested that highly complex interrelationships between intellectual ability and nonacademic variables may determine whether students will succeed. . . .

In summary, it appears that both academic and nonacademic factors are influential in predicting performance on the NCLEX-RN. . . . The current study will try to identify both academic as well as nonacademic variables associated with NCLEX-RN success.

SOURCE: Summarized from Arathuzik, D., and Aber, C. (1998). Factors associated with national council licensure examination: Registered nurse success. *Journal of Professional Nursing, 14*(2), 119–126.

questionnaires for ideas concerning the variables that may be measured if a survey is to be conducted may yield interesting results. Finally, developing your own theoretical models or frameworks and figuring out which sources of spuriousness, intervening, or control variables may be relevant for the study is an exciting means of identifying variables for investigation.

2. How to Develop Theoretical or Causal Models

We will begin with the simplest models and gradually move toward the more complex ones. What all models have in common is that a diagram can represent each of them; each such diagram shows causal direction and the implied hypotheses. The hypothesis or set of hypotheses translates the problem statement into a precise statement that predicts the expected outcomes of the study. In this sense, the research hypothesis is a tentative answer to the research problem or question. The hypothesis is then empirically tested through a process of data collection and analysis. We begin with the two-variable model. Chapter 17 and Appendix A present procedures for analyzing these models.

a. Two-Variable Models

In Chapter 1, the distinction between a dependent and an independent variable was made. The dependent variable is the "effect" in a cause-and-effect relationship or is the result of the influence of an independent variable. Conventionally, we refer to the dependent variable as the Y variable and the independent variable as the X variable. The relationship can be described simply with a diagram:

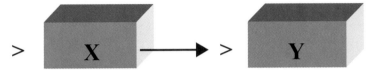

What does the diagram tell us? First, it describes a relationship between two variables known as X and Y. Note that an arrow points from X to Y; this tells us that X is the independent variable and that Y is the dependent variable. The hypothesis reflected by this diagram argues that X influences Y. Next, note the $>$ symbol before the X box. This symbol means "the greater;" the opposite symbol, $<$, means "the less." Putting all these elements together, the hypothesis can be stated as: "The greater X, leads to the greater Y." If we wished to express a negative relationship, the first symbol could be reversed. In this case, the hypothesis would be stated as: "The less X, leads to the greater Y."

If the X and Y were replaced with variable names, we might, for example, be talking about the relationship between participation in health-promoting lifestyles and self-efficacy, suggesting that greater perceived self-efficacy leads to greater participation in health-promoting lifestyles (Gillis, 1994). The wording of the hypothesis indicates that perceived self-efficacy is the independent variable and participation in health-promoting behavior is the dependent variable.

The advantage of drawing a diagram to represent the relationship is that it enables the researcher to:

- Indicate causal direction (the arrow points at the dependent variable); and,
- Indicate if the relationship is positive (note use of $>$ symbol) or negative ($<$ symbol).

Drawing a picture increases precision. There may be times when you cannot formulate a problem in such a way that you are able to say whether the relation is positive or negative. In these cases, one cannot speak in "greater than" or "less than" terms. When you are unable to specify the nature of the relationship, use a "?" to indicate that no prediction is being made.

Occasionally, you will not be in a position to set out a causal order; in these cases, you may be faced with a situation in which variables exist together and influence one another simultaneously. In this event, you can indicate reciprocal causation by placing arrows at each end of the line linking the two variables.

Ideally, hypotheses are deduced from theories, previous research, or logical reasoning. In new areas of investigation, it may be difficult to develop a causal model because there simply is insufficient evidence to support the development of explanatory hypotheses. Many descriptive and qualitative investigations (see Chapters 6 and 7) proceed without a hypothesis statement or a causal model. Such investigations may result in theory building or are precursors to theory generation.

b. Three-Variable Models

Now let us turn our attention to various three-variable models. Some terms need to be reviewed. Besides independent and dependent variables, there are three additional types of variables that will need to be understood: intervening, source of spuriousness, and conditional variables.

(i) An Intervening Variable Model

An **intervening variable** (I) is a variable that links an independent variable (X) to a dependent variable (Y) An intervening variable represents an explanation of how the independent variable influences the dependent variable. The interest here is in understanding the relationship between X and Y—that is, understanding the mechanism by which X is connected to Y. Frequently, a researcher is testing a number of alternative explanations of how X influences Y. In the case of one intervening variable, the relationship could be diagrammed as follows:

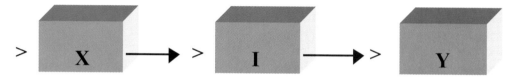

In this diagram, I is the intervening variable, or the linking variable between X and Y. The hypothesis is that variations in X cause variations in I, which, in turn, influences Y. Typically, one would propose a number of possible intervening variables, so the following diagram would be more appropriate:

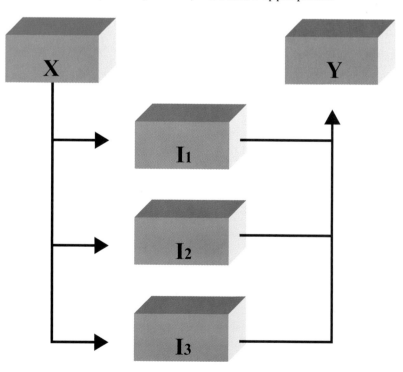

In this diagram, three alternative explanations are suggested for the connection between X and Y. If the X, Y, and I were replaced with variable names, we might, for example, test the relationship between previous health-care experiences (X), utilization of health-care services (Y), and cognitive appraisal (I_1), intrinsic motivation (I_2), and perceived health status (I_3), suggesting that the more positive one's previous health-care experiences, the more positive ones' cognitive assessment of the experiences, leading to greater utilization of health services. Similarly, a second alternative explanation would be that previous positive health-care experiences influenced the intervening variable of internal motivation, leading respondents to seek health-care services. The researcher would collect data that measure each of the variables involved and conduct the appropriate statistical tests to determine, which, if any, of the proposed alternative explanations or intervening variables explains the connection between X and Y. These matters are examined further in Chapter 17.

(ii) A Source of Spuriousness Model

A **source of spuriousness model** is one in which a variable is identified as a possible influence on both the independent variable (X) and the dependent variable (Y) in such a way that it accounts for the relationship between them. In other words, the relationship between X and Y may be "spurious" because it is produced by the influence of S/S on each of them. Here the researcher proposes that, although there is a statistically significant relationship between the variables X and Y, this relationship may be noncausal—that is, only existing because some third variable is influencing both X and Y. Having observed a statistically significant relationship, the researcher will want to ensure that the relationship is not spurious and, therefore, should run a number of spuriousness checks. The source of spuriousness model may be diagrammed as follows:

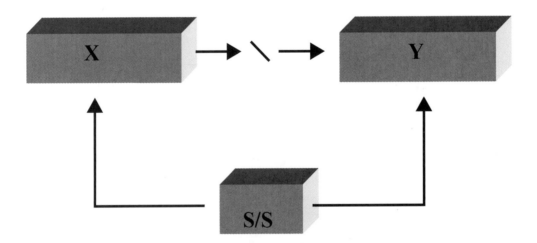

In the source of spuriousness model, the researcher is suggesting that the relationship between X and Y may be spurious. If the variables X and Y were replaced with variable names, we might, for example explore the relationship between socioeconomic status (X) and choice of alternative therapies (Y) in women with breast cancer. We might consider the possibility that rural or urban background is a source of spuriousness (S/S). Possibly the type of community the women come from influences their socioeconomic status as well as influencing their choice of alternative therapies. The techniques for examining such relationships are examined in Chapter 17.

(iii) An Antecedent Variable Model
An **antecedent variable model** is a causal model that proposes a variable that causes variation in an independent variable that, in turn, influences the dependent variable in the model. Thus, the antecedent variable is one that precedes the main independent and dependent variables. This variable may be having an impact on the independent variable that, in turn, may be influencing the dependent variable. An antecedent variable may be diagrammed as follows:

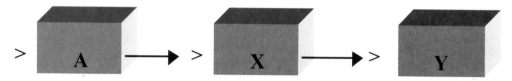

If the *A, X,* and *Y* were replaced with variable names, we might, for example, test the relationships among perceived low job autonomy (*A*), emotional stress (*X*), and smoking behavior (*Y*), suggesting that the greater one's perception of low job autonomy, the greater one's level of emotional stress, leading to an increase in the frequency of smoking behavior.

In a sense, an antecedent variable combines one idea from the source of spuriousness model and one from an intervening variable model:

- It is causally prior to both the independent and the dependent variable (as in a source of spuriousness model).
- It converts the independent variable into one that intervenes between the antecedent variable and the dependent variable.

c. Multivariate Models

Models that use numerous variables are known as **multivariate models.** The first we will consider is the candidate variable model.

(i) Candidate Variable Model
A **candidate variable model** is one that proposes several independent variables as possible causes of variation in a dependent variable. Here the researcher is proposing a number of independent variables that may be influencing the dependent variable. This type of model is illustrated in Figure 3.1.

The variables on the left side of the diagram are the independent variables and are viewed as potential causes of variations in the dependent variable, frequency of smoking behavior (Gillis, 1998). Note that the model uses the symbols > and < to indicate whether the independent variables are positively or negatively associated with the dependent variable. The independent variables are related to the dependent variable either one at a time or simultaneously, through procedures that are outlined in Chapter 18.

(ii) Path Models
A **path model** is a graphic representation of a complex set of proposed interrelationships among variables. A model of this type is shown in Figure 3.2 (Israel and Shurman, 1990).

The following hypotheses represented in Figure 3.2. may be tested empirically:

- Objective conditions conducive to stress have a direct relationship to health outcomes (arrow C).
- Variations in stressors cause variations in perceived stress, which influences health outcomes (arrows A and B).

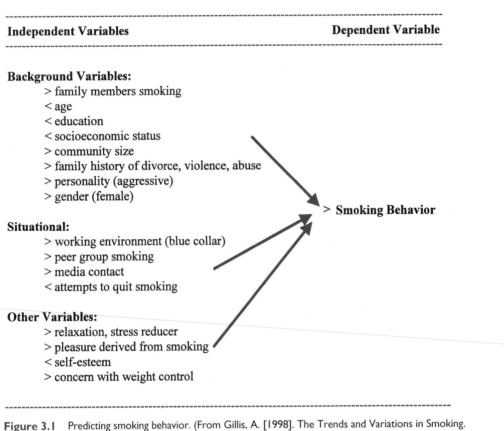

Independent Variables	Dependent Variable

Background Variables:
> > family members smoking
> < age
> < education
> < socioeconomic status
> > community size
> > family history of divorce, violence, abuse
> > personality (aggressive)
> > gender (female)

> Smoking Behavior

Situational:
> > working environment (blue collar)
> > peer group smoking
> > media contact
> < attempts to quit smoking

Other Variables:
> > relaxation, stress reducer
> > pleasure derived from smoking
> < self-esteem
> > concern with weight control

Figure 3.1   Predicting smoking behavior. (From Gillis, A. [1998]. The Trends and Variations in Smoking. Research methods paper. Antigonish, Nova Scotia: St. Francis Xavier University. Cited with permission.)

- Perceived stress directly affects health outcomes (arrow B).
- Supportive relationships and the exercise of control can directly reduce objective stressors (arrow 1) and the perception of stressors as stressful (arrow 2) and directly affect health outcomes (arrow 3).
- Supportive relationships and the exercise of control can influence the effects of stressors (arrow 1a) and perceived stress (arrow 2a) on health outcomes.

All the models discussed reflect the causal thinking of the researcher in such a way that this reasoning can then be tested in later stages of the research project. (See also Box 2.7, which features a path model of influence on the initiation of sexual intercourse.)

D. SPECIFYING HYPOTHESES AND PROCEDURES OF ANALYSIS

We state hypotheses (or diagram them) before data analysis to ensure that the researcher is not tempted to invent ones after the data have been analyzed that will conform to expectations. The specified hypotheses represented in the model in Figure 3.2. are examples of hypotheses that can be tested empirically. After the hypotheses are specified and diagrams of the hypotheses illustrated, it is appropriate to specify the analysis procedures that will be used to test whether or not the data collected support the hypotheses.

Hypothesis testing is central to scientific research. After you have stated the hypotheses and selected your design,

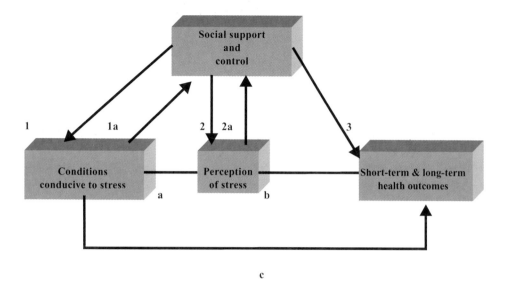

Figure 3.2   Relationships of social support and control. (From Israel, B.A., and Schurman, S. [1990]. *Social Support, Control and the Stress Process.* In Glanz, R., Lewis, F., and Rimer, D. [Eds.], *Health Behavior and Health Education.* San Francisco: Jossey-Bass. Reprinted by permission of Jossey-Bass Inc., a subsidiary of John Wiley & Sons, Inc. Note: See accompanying text for an explanation of the letters and numbers in the figure.

you can proceed to identify your sample, select your data collection instruments, gather your data, and analyze the results. Specifically, your hypotheses are tested during the data analysis stage through statistical procedures.

1. How to Specify Hypotheses

Good diagrams can replace formal hypotheses statements. By using > and < symbols, it is possible to indicate "greater than" and "less than" relationships; arrows may be used to indicate causal direction.

As noted in the hypotheses statements associated with Figure 3.2, a variety of terms are used to express the relationship between the dependent and independent variables in a hypothesis statement. Common expressions include "varies with," "positively influences," "negatively influences," "direct relationship to," "inversely related," and "reciprocal association with." Particularly in candidate variable models, which include a large number of variables, it is easier to diagram the hy-

potheses than to present a written version of each one. Similarly, when many alternative explanations are being tested for a particular relationship, a good diagram clearly shows the causal model and the implied research hypotheses.

In theory-testing projects, it is important not only to state the derived hypotheses but also to indicate the steps that were taken in making the derivation or derivations. You may recall from Chapter 2 that hypotheses in a theory-testing study are derived from the propositional statements in the theory. Only to the extent that such derivations can be traced can one claim to have tested a theory. For example, from the theoretical proposition that social support is related to health outcomes (see Fig. 3.2), the researcher can derive the hypothesis that adolescents with positive peer support will perceive their health status more positively than adolescents with little peer support. Hypotheses are statements specific to an empirical situation. In this example, the hypothesis relating peer support to perceived health status could be tested empirically to establish the validity of the claim. As evidence accumulates to support the proposition that social support is related to health, the worthiness of the theory is established. Remember that one does not *prove* the hypotheses or the theory through hypotheses testing. Conclusions are always considered *tentative;* however, with increasing research evidence to support conclusions, hypotheses come to be accepted or believed.

In stating hypotheses, one should note that although there are two types of hypotheses—the research and the null hypotheses—the researcher is primarily concerned with the research hypothesis, which states the expected outcome of the research. The distinction between the two is discussed in Chapter 12.

2. How to Specify Methods of Analysis

Specifying methods of analysis in advance forces the researcher to be committed to particular procedures. Selecting these procedures also has implications for the way in which variables will be measured. Thus, if cross-tabulation tables are to be used exclusively, it will not be necessary to get ratio level measures on the variables. It is probably unreasonable to require a researcher to specify "cut points" for cross-tabulation tables because of the large number of variables that may be involved (see Chap. 16). However, it is reasonable to indicate the number of categories that will be used and the principle that was used in making the cut points (perhaps by splitting the sample into thirds or at the midpoint).

E. UNDERSTANDING RESEARCH DESIGN

As a creative research student, you have no doubt had some experience following patterns for sewing, recipes for cooking, or blueprints for woodworking. These patterns are directions or guidelines that help you create beautiful masterpieces. This section introduces you to a pattern for designing a research project. A **research design** is like a blueprint for a study. It guides the investigator in planning and implementing the study. It provides a detailed plan for data collection and analysis and is the critical element linking the theoretical framework and questions with the resultant data. The term *research design* is frequently used interchangeably with the term *methodology*. If you think about the research design like a blueprint for a house, it quickly will be apparent how critical the design is to the successful implementation of the study. The blueprint indicates to the contractor, the carpenters, and other tradesmen what parts of the house should be constructed first, and how and what pieces of materials go together to construct the shell and then the walls, and so on. Similarly, research designs indicate the steps and actions the researcher should take and in what order they should be done to carry out the very best investigation of a phenomenon and arrive at an answer to the research question. There are no rigid rules for selecting a research design; rather, the researcher is guided by examining the research question, the purpose of the research, and his or her own philosophical approach to inquiry.

You may recall from Chapter 1 that different types of research (e.g., descriptive, explanatory, predictive) exist. Given different types of research and different research questions, it is necessary to have a variety of research designs. If you decide to explore a phenomenon that is not well understood and has had little empirical investigation, you will most likely use a descriptive research design. For example, the question, "What is the experience of caring for a family member with Alzheimer's disease?" implies a description of the experience that family members go through in the process of giving care to their loved one. A descriptive design such as one of the qualitative approaches discussed in Chapter 6 may be appropriate to answer this query. The question, "What is the relationship between the levels of fatigue in family caregivers of clients with Alzheimer's disease and available social support?" implies a study of the relationships between fatigue in caregivers and social support. A correlational survey design (see Chapter 5) may be appropriate in this example if fatigue and social support have been well described in the literature but the nature of the relationship between the two is not well established.

If the research phenomenon of interest has been well described in the literature and its relationship to other factors is well known, then an experimental design (see Chapter 4) may be appropriate. For example, the question, "What is the effect of a respite care program on the incidence of depression in family caregivers of patients with Alzheimer's disease?" implies an experimental design. Here the researcher would be interested in testing the impact of the respite care program on the incidence of depression in family caregivers who receive respite and comparing them with a group of family caregivers who receive the usual care with no respite program. Chapters 4 through 8 discuss a range of quantitative and qualitative designs useful to addressing a variety of research questions. Each chapter discusses in detail the components of a good research design. As you read each chapter, keep in mind your research question. This will help focus your reading and allow you to evaluate the design's relationship to the research question you wish to answer.

I. How to Describe a Study's Design

Six basic components should be included in describing a study's design. These include:

- **A description of the study participants or the sample.** Most nursing studies include individuals, groups, families, or communities as the elements of the sample (see Chapter 15).
- **A description of the setting.** Some research designs are distinguished by the natural setting in which the research is conducted. The investigator does not alter the conditions of the environment in any way during the data collection procedures (see Chapter 7). Other designs require the investigator to manipulate the environment in such a manner as to control all of the variables except the one major variable whose influence the researcher is interested in measuring (see Chapter 4). This latter type of artificial environment is usually created in a laboratory setting.
- **A description of the variables.** Variables are the main concepts the investigator intends to measure empirically. Research designs may be univariate (one variable) or multivariate (two or more variables). Most nursing investigations are multivariate, reflecting the complexity of nursing practice (see Chapter 2).
- **A description of the data collection methods.** The data collection methods may include the use of self-report data collected by means of researcher developed instruments, questionnaires, standardized instruments, or scales; structured, semi-structured, or nonstructured interview guides; participant or nonparticipant observations; or biophysiologic measures. In some research designs, the data collection plan may also include the use of existing records or data for the purposes of a secondary analysis (see Chapter 13).
- **A description of the time dimension of the design.** The time element is crucial to the design in describing the frequency (how often) and order (when) in which data collection will be conducted. If change over time is an im-

portant component of the study design, it is critical to indicate the timing of data collection procedures to capture the rapid or slow patterns of change. If data are collected at one point in time, it is referred to as **cross-sectional;** if data are collected at different intervals over a period of time, it is referred to as **longitudinal;** if data are collected from the present to some future point in time, it is referred to as **prospective;** and if data collection reflects measures that occurred in the past, it is referred to as **retrospective.**

• **A description of the role of the investigator.** The role of the investigator varies with the research design selected. In some designs, the investigator becomes an active participant in the research project; in other designs, the researcher actively manipulates the variables being studied and assigns participants to different research groups or treatment conditions; and in still other designs, the researcher remains aloof and detached from the variables being studied (see Chapters 4 to 8).

In describing the research design, it is important to provide a detailed description of each component, in much the same way as an architect provides a detailed sketch of the blueprints for a house. This is important in enabling other investigators to replicate your study and determine under what conditions the results of the investigation are applicable in their setting.

2. What Factors Guide Selection of a Study Design?

Many factors influence the choice of a research design. Primarily, it is the nature of the research question asked that determines which design is most appropriate. One should note, however, that there are also pragmatic considerations to keep in mind such as the amount of time and research funds available, access to research participants, availability of research assistants, and constraints imposed by ethical issues, to name a few. Pragmatic considerations should not supercede the primary consideration, which is the research question posed, but they do influence the design decision to a limited extent. In addition to the research question posed, the following factors may be considered in selecting the design:

a. Purpose and Level of Knowledge

The research design needs to be consistent with the research purpose and question. For example, if a health-care facility wants to evaluate the effectiveness of a school-based nurse practitioner clinic, it should try to produce scientific evidence that the clinic produces positive outcomes, such as less substance abuse, fewer missed days because of illness, lower incidence of teen pregnancy, fewer sexually transmitted diseases. The preferred design to get this information is a quasi-experiment using a school district with a nurse-run clinic and a matched control group school district without a clinic. Data could be collected from the two groups and compared on the various outcome measures. On the other hand, if the purpose was to assess student satisfaction with services at the clinic, a descriptive survey design may be more appropriate.

The level of knowledge about the topic is closely related to the purpose and research question. If little is known about a topic, a descriptive or exploratory study is appropriate. On the other hand, if considerable information is known about a phenomenon and the factors that are related to it, an explanatory or predictive study using an experimental design may be appropriate.

b. Nature of Research Phenomenon

Some research phenomena can only be studied in natural settings, requiring the use of field study approaches. For example, the immediate effect on families of mining disasters must be investigated in the settings where they occur. Therefore, a researcher interested in investigating this phenomenon would select a design appropriate to the naturalistic setting, such as one of those outlined in Chapters 6 and 7.

c. Ethical Considerations

Some research questions cannot be addressed in humans because of ethical considerations. For example, to deny clients access to an available treatment for a particular disease would be unethical. In other cases, one may wish to study patterns of illness or disease over time. It would be unethical to induce illness in humans for the purposes of research; therefore, the investigator must find participants in which the disease is occurring naturally.

d. Practical Considerations

Issues such as researcher time, costs, available resources to conduct a study, and available data may strongly influence the selection of the research design. For example, if a study is limited by the researcher's time or is time sensitive because of grant deadlines, it may be more feasible to use ready-made instruments and conduct a survey that can be group administered to the respondents in one sitting rather than select a design that requires in-depth interviews. Similarly, if the only data available to answer a research question are past health records, then the research design necessitates a secondary data analysis approach (see Chapter 5).

e. Feasibility

Sometimes a particular design is the best one to answer the research question but it is not feasible to use it. For example, you may decide that it is best to randomly se-

lect a large sample of women from two rural communities to be interviewed about their birthing experiences at two different health-care facilities. However, you determine that it would not be possible to randomly assign women to a particular institution to receive care because of their health insurance policies. Although it may be desirable to use random assignment, it is not possible in this situation because of the context.

f. Personal Preference

The individual preference of the researcher needs to be considered in selecting a design because every project requires time, energy, and intellectual commitment on the part of the investigator. For this reason, the researchers should consider his or her personal preferences in selecting a design. For example, if a researcher likes to explore concepts or make meaning out of people's experiences, then one of the qualitative designs such as phenomenology may be appropriate. If, on the other hand, a researcher enjoys studying relationships, determine cause-and-effect scenarios, or design and evaluate interventions, then a quantitative approach such as comparative surveys or experimental research may be more appropriate.

3. How to Choose a Research Design

Selection of the most appropriate research design is a critical step in the research process. Now that you know what the components of a design are and which factors to consider in selecting a study design, how do you actually decide what is the best design to answer your research question? The following summarizes some steps to help you decide which research strategy will be followed.

Step 1. What have others done? Do a preliminary review of the literature to get some sense of what has been written about the topic that you wish to explore. As you read the literature, pay attention to the research designs that were used in the studies. Does the author specify a rationale for the design selected? Can you locate any articles that reflect the use of different designs to explore the problem?

Step 2. Review the chapter in this text that introduces the design you have tentatively selected. The following chapters introduce different types of research designs:

- Chapter 4: Experimental and Quasi-Experimental Designs (randomized clinical trials)
- Chapter 5: Survey Designs (surveys, secondary data, comparative studies, meta-analyses)
- Chapter 6: Qualitative Designs (phenomenology, ethnography, grounded theory)
- Chapter 7: Field Study Approaches (participant observation, in-depth interviews, focus groups, field experiments, naturalistic observational studies)
- Chapter 8: New Wave Contemporary Applied Approaches (evaluation research, action research, health promotion research, feminist research)

Recommended readings in each of the chapters may be helpful in gaining additional insights for the design of your study. Students considering a qualitative approach should review Chapters 6 and 7 in detail.

Step 3. Be prepared to reconsider the research design used. As you review the literature in detail, different questions may come to seem more relevant to the purpose and goals of your project. If this happens, be prepared to reconsider the type of research design to be used in the study. Remember that research is never the clean and tidy process that texts on research methods present it to be.

As we have recommended previously, the research design should match the research question and purpose of the study. To reiterate, research is generally conducted for one or more of the following purposes: (1) to identify and describe concepts and phenomena of interest to nursing (descriptive surveys and qualitative designs); (2) to explore differences and associations among variables (exploratory designs such as correlational and comparative studies); and (3) to explain, predict, or control nursing phenomena (experiments, case studies, and evaluation research).

Flexibility and openness are important to good research design. This point is important to remember as the study unfolds. Occasionally, problems arise that are beyond the control of the investigator. Experienced researchers will try to anticipate potential problems and take action to prevent them or solve them after they occur. The following section presents solutions to common problems that may emerge during the process of a research investigation.

F. PREDICTABLE SETBACKS AND CHALLENGES

Few research investigations proceed smoothly. Even after painstakingly evaluating your design options and carefully selecting one, setbacks and problems will emerge. Hence, it is prudent to prepare yourself for some delays and challenges along the way to answering your research question. Seasoned researchers always consider alternatives when faced with difficulties such as those listed below:

- **Time** ("Rats, the project report is due in 3 months!"). Projects always take longer than anticipated, so experienced researchers will plan for delays and unpredictable events in the timeline of the research project. For example, extra time should be allotted for subject recruitment, administration of instruments or an intervention, and follow-up measurement after intervention. It is always wise to allow extra time at the end of a project to deal with any unexpected events that may have caused a delay in the project. If it is not needed, the researcher can relax and enjoy the extra time available to complete the final report.

- **Ethical issues** ("The Ethics Review Board may not approve of efforts to increase recruitment into the study.") If the risk to participants is too high and appropriate steps cannot be taken to protect the participants, maximize benefits, and minimize harm, the study may have to be redesigned (see Chapter 10).
- **Computer resources** ("Our institution does not have the programs that we need to do the analysis.") The feasibility of a project often depends on the availability of facilities and equipment such as computer access, video cameras, recording devices, observation rooms with one-way mirrors, and so on. If resources are not available within your institution, it may be possible to borrow, rent, or have equipment donated from hospital research units or university research centers. This may also be an opportunity to collaborate with researchers in centers that can provide the resources required for your project.
- **Technical competence** ("Regression analysis is beyond me, and to replicate the study, I would need to understand it.") Feasibility of a project depends on appropriate expertise in terms of research skill and knowledge of the substantive area under investigation. When a researcher has deficiencies in either of these areas, experts may

be consulted and invited to join the research team as members or consultants to the project. For example, a statistician and a community health nurse may be welcome additions if you are studying patterns of communicable diseases in low-income families.

- **Availability of research assistants** ("To do this project properly, we would need assistance and there are not enough qualified people available to do the interviewing and observations.") You may need to advertise widely and train your own research assistants if the budget permits.
- **Funding** ("We just don't have enough money to do the project properly.") Research expenses may include printing costs, mailing, telephone or travel costs, space and equipment rental, salaries of research assistants, computer time, and fees to participants. Researchers typically cast a broad net in seeking research funds from government, private, philanthropic, and business sources.

Given difficulties such as these, are there other general alternative strategies that might be used? It may be possible to:

- **Use data that have been generated by other researchers.** You will need to get the material and permission to use it, and you will also have to deal with someone else's operationalizations.
- **Use publicly available data.** For example, (1) university and college research departments often maintain data banks; (2) government agencies sometimes make data of interest available to researchers; and (3) other publicly available data sources exist such as the Human Relations Area Files (see Chapter 6). Typically, data sets are available in the form of computer files.
- **Use information published in hospital databases, medical insurance files, newspapers, or books.** Much seondary data can be gleaned from regularly pub-

lished information. For example, if you were interested in examining the relationship between childhood immunization patterns and childhood disabilities, you could contact the National Center for Health Statistics (NCHS) in the United States; in Canada, contact Statistics Canada to get data appropriate to these variables.

Finally, remember when you think you have exhausted all research possibilities—you haven't! Persistence and determination are invaluable assets for researchers.

G. DETERMINING YOUR READINESS TO START THE PROJECT

Table 3.2 provides a checklist of items that need to be attended to before beginning a project. Not all items will be relevant to your study, but it is worth going through the list to see if all the things that should be done before beginning your project have been completed. As previously discussed, research projects frequently get behind schedule for all sorts of unanticipated reasons. The checklist may help anticipate some of the problems.

The first section of the checklist deals with the development of a research proposal. Researchers preparing theses will have been told by their supervisor that it is possible to develop a draft of the first three chapters of a thesis before any data are collected. These chapters would include:

- A problem statement
- A literature review
- A methodology section

The methods section is usually divided into subsections that deal with the participants, the instruments or measurement, and the procedures. Most nursing research proposals and reports follow the form outlined in the *Publication Manual of the American Psychological Association.* This manual is used by most nursing research journals such as *Nursing Research, Canadian Journal of Nursing Research, Research in Nursing and Health,* and *Image: The Journal of Nursing Scholarship.*

For field studies and other qualitative designs, in which the project usually takes shape in process, proposals can discuss the rationale behind the study and the relevance of the location chosen.

In using Table 3.2, researchers are encouraged to make realistic estimates of the amount of time it will take to complete various elements. Experienced researchers know that unanticipated delays do often occur and will plan for them by adding in some extra time. The more people involved in the project (either subjects, respondents, or informants), the greater the number of delays that may be anticipated. But even projects that involve few others (such as a content analysis of nursing journals) may be delayed because getting some of the material on interlibrary loan may take longer than anticipated. Try to avoid delays, but it is a good idea to assume that they will occur.

How do you know when you are ready to start the data collection phase of your research? A rule to follow is: *You are ready to commence data collection when all the relevant items noted in Table 3.2 have been realistically planned and when all the necessary written materials, permissions, instruments, and equipment are in place.*

There are several products available to assist researchers in managing projects. These range from those that assist in maintaining a file of bibliographic information to those that provide assistance in the overall management of projects. Students may wish to examine the free demonstration program for Reference Manager available from Research Information Systems (*www:http://www.risinc.com*). This program prints indexed bibliographies and imports bibliographic in-

Table 3.2 Project Initiation Checklist

Items to Check	Not Relevant	Initiated Date	Target Date	Completed Date
Preparation of Research Proposal	[ ]			
Statement of problem	[ ]			
Literature review complete	[ ]			
Methodology statement	[ ]			
Written formal hypotheses	[ ]			
Ethics review committee submission	[ ]			
Funding application	[ ]			
Permissions				
From subjects or guardians	[ ]			
For use of copyrighted material	[ ]			
For entry into country or group	[ ]			
For office or laboratory space	[ ]			
Project staff hired	[ ]			
Subjects	[ ]			
Method of contact established	[ ]			
Instruments Completed				
Letters to respondents and others	[ ]			
Questionnaires	[ ]			
Pretesting	[ ]			
Pilot study	[ ]			
Recording forms	[ ]			
Other (list)	[ ]			
Equipment				
Tape recorders	[ ]			
Computers and programs	[ ]			
Other (list)	[ ]			
Sampling procedures determined	[ ]			
Scheduling, Provision for				
Training of staff	[ ]			
Holidays, bad weather days	[ ]			
Data collection period	[ ]			
Time to get last few cases	[ ]			
Data entry time	[ ]			
Data analysis time	[ ]			
Report writing time	[ ]			

formation available from online and from CD-ROM databases, such as CINAHL and MEDLINE. Among its many features, it edits style changes to references. Another product that may prove a good starting point in the search is Microsoft Project, available from Microsoft. This relatively inexpensive program provides basic tools for the overall management of research projects. A product specifically designed for health-related projects is from the National Health Data Systems, Inc., known as *Hii&trade*. Information for this product is available at *www.nhds.com*.

E X E R C I S E S

1. List nine sources of nursing research problems. Which factors would you consider in selecting a research problem for investigation?

2. Choose a dependent variable that is of interest to you and draw a diagram showing the variables that may be influencing variations in the dependent variable.

3. Drawing on propositions of a nursing or health behavior theory, derive a testable hypothesis and draw a diagram of the proposed relationship. You may combine axiomatic and replacement of terms approaches in your derivations. Try for a counterintuitive prediction.

4. Propose and diagram a series of at least three alternative explanations for a proposed relationship.

5. Choose an "applied" nursing problem and diagram relationships that you would explore to solve the applied problem.

6. Diagram the relationship (or relationships) that would be explored if you were to replicate an existing study and indicate and diagram one additional relationship you would explore in the replication.

7. Complete the relevant sections of Table 3.2 for a project that you wish to conduct.

8. Write a problem statement including a statement of purpose and a research question for each of the following research topics:
   * Homelessness in the elderly

   * Osteoporosis in middle-aged women

   * Mother–infant bonding

   * Tobacco use in adolescents

9. Write a research hypothesis statement using the following terms: "greater than," "less than," "positively related," and "negatively affects" to communicate the relationship between two or more variables.

10. Choose a research question of interest and write a brief review of the literature using variables identified in the research question. To complete this assignment, do the following:
    * Identify two indexes used to identify literature sources.

- Identify three publications from each index appropriate to the research question.

- Include articles with conflicting results.

- Write a summary statement at the end of the literature review.

RECOMMENDED READINGS

Brown, S.J. (1999). *Knowledge for Health Care Practice: A Guide to Using Research Evidence.* Toronto: W.B. Saunders. This text covers a broad spectrum of strategies for searching the literature and identifying and relating relevant research evidence to clinical questions.

Edwards, M. (1998). *The Internet for Nurses and Allied Health Professionals.* New York: Springer-Verlag. This is a useful guide for searching nursing databases and information sources that may be useful in completing a literature review.

Martin, D.W. (1991). *Doing Psychology Experiments* (3rd ed). Pacific Grove: Brooks/Cole. Martin includes a useful chapter on knowing when you are ready to commence an experiment.

Sparkes, S., and Rizzoloo, M. (1998). World wide web search tools. *Image: Journal of Nursing Scholarship, 30*(2), 167–171. A good overview of web sources to consider in a review of the current state of knowledge related to a research topic.

Part 2

RESEARCH DESIGNS AND APPROACHES

P art 2 introduces various research designs. Although there is no consensus in the research community on the best way to classify research designs, for purposes of simplicity, this text will classify them into five categories: experimental (including quasi-experimental), survey, qualitative designs, field studies, and new wave contemporary applied approaches.

Part 2 provides beginning researchers with insights into the major research designs used in nursing investigations. As you read this section, you will notice that designs are not always mutually exclusive and each has advantages and limitations that influence the researcher's choice. It is rarely possible to select the perfect design for your study; however, careful selection from a variety of possibilities enables you to choose a design that best fits your study. The experiment is a good starting point because it offers the most straightforward demonstration of causal links among variables. However, because of practical or ethical reasons, many things that nurse scientists want to study cannot be studied experimentally, so other designs have an important place in nursing research. Nonexperimental researchers need to understand the experiment in order to heighten awareness of factors that may be problematic in their own studies.

Chapter 4 introduces students to the basic principles of experimental design and presents examples of experiments and quasi-experiments. Chapter 5 presents survey designs. Chapter 6 introduces popular qualitative research designs, including phenomenology, grounded theory, and ethnography. Chapter 7 discusses qualitative data collection and analysis methods specific to the field study approaches. Chapter 8 presents various new wave contemporary applied approaches, including health promotion, evaluation, action, and feminist research. At the end of each chapter, the Recommended Readings help readers come to a fuller understanding of how to implement these basic designs. Students can select a specific design that can be studied in detail by reading the references provided.

Chapter 4

Experimental and Quasi-Experimental Designs

CHAPTER OUTLINE

A. Basics of Experimental Designs
  1. The Rationale for Experimental Designs
  2. Key Elements in Experimental Designs

B. Pre-experimental Designs
  1. Same Group: Pretest and Posttest Design
  2. Exposed and Comparison Group Design

C. Classic Experimental Designs
  1. Between-Subjects Designs
  2. Within-Subjects Designs

  3. Between- and Within-Subject Designs Compared

D. Quasi-experimental Designs
  1. Nonequivalent Control Group Design
  2. Panel Studies

E. Advantages and Limitations of Experimental Designs
  1. Pre-experimental Designs
  2. Quasi-experimental Designs
  3. Classic Experimental Designs

KEY TERMS

Baseline data	Experiment	Quasi-experimental design
Baseline stability	Experimental group	Randomization
Between-subjects design	External validity	Random variable
Blocking	Instrument decay	Response bias
Classic experimental design	Internal validity	Selection
Confounding variable	Hawthorne effect	Single blind
Control by constancy	History	Statistical regression
Control group	Maturation	Testing
Control variable	Mortality	Treatment levels
Counterbalancing	Panel study	Treatment variable
Crossover design	Precision matching	Within-subject design
Double blind	Pre-experimental design	

A. BASICS OF EXPERIMENTAL DESIGNS

As we saw in Chapter 1, an **experiment** is a scientific investigation that tests cause-and-effect relationships while controlling for the influence of other factors. A key feature of the design is that measures are taken on two or more groups both before and after an experimental intervention. A well-designed experiment should indicate whether or not an intervention (e.g., studying with the radio on) would bring about a measurable change in a dependent variable (e.g., an increase or decrease in grade-point average) with *other things being equal.* This last phrase is critical. It means that an experiment takes into account any number of factors (e.g., hours of sleep, interest in the subject matter, previous performance) to make certain that it is the researcher's intervention and not some other factor that is influencing the change.

1. The Rationale for Experimental Designs

In *A System of Logic,* John Stuart Mill (1806–1873) identified the "Method of Difference" as a key tool in understanding causal relations. Although Mill's rationale for experimental designs was the first to set out the logic of experimentation systematically, experiments, in fact, go back much earlier. Experimentation dates to at least 1648, when Blaise Pascal (1623–1662) had his brother-in-law conduct an experiment testing for the presence of atmospheric pressure (Palys, 1992, pp. 241–244). A special container was taken up a mountain, and it was noted that the level of mercury in the container declined as it was moved higher. As a control, another mercury dish was not taken up the mountain and its level was monitored; its level remained unchanged throughout the observation period.

Nurse researchers use experimental designs to measure if a treatment (intervention) has a particular effect on some outcome. It is important to ensure that other possible reasons for variations in the outcome have been ruled out. In short, we must be confident that it is the treatment and not something else that is effecting the outcome.

If you were studying the effect of listening to instrumental music on a patient's stress level on the day of surgery, one would want to make certain that factors such as the severity of the illness, gender, and age of the patient have been taken into account. These other factors might all be having an impact on reported stress levels. The strength of experimental designs is in their ability to sort out causal relations while taking into account other factors. Indeed, experimental researchers use the term **internal validity** to refer to the extent to which one can demonstrate that one's treatment is having an impact on a given outcome and that other sources of influence have been controlled. **External validity,** on the other hand, refers to the extent to which one can make extrapolations from the particular study to other groups in general.

2. Key Elements in Experimental Designs

Suppose you wish to assess the effectiveness of a CD-ROM in promoting attendance in a university nursing program. Suppose that some students are exposed to a CD-ROM about university attendance and others view a nature CD-ROM. Will seeing the CD-ROM about university nursing education increase the number of high school students wishing to attend a university nursing program? You decide an experiment would be in order. There are a number of elements to such a study, including time, the choice of variables, and the number of levels.

a. Time

A key feature of an experiment is that measures are taken at different points in time (i.e., before and after the treatment is administered). Because the experimental design involves measures of the dependent variables at two points in time (time 1, time 2 measures), the procedure ensures that the measure at time 1 precedes the one at time 2. Second, as we introduce the treatment to the experimental group (the CD-ROM about a university nursing program) but not to the control group (who see a nature CD-ROM instead), and follow this by measuring the dependent variable at time 2, it becomes possible to make an inference about the impact of seeing the university CD-ROM (treatment variable) on the desire to attend a university program (the dependent variable). Thus, because the CD-ROM was shown between the time 1 and time 2 measures, if there is a change in the attitudes toward attending a university nursing program among those seeing the university CD-ROM, we will have made the first step in demonstrating that the CD-ROM caused the change in attitude.

b. Variables in Experiments

Chapter 2 noted that a *dependent variable* is the effect in a cause-and-effect relation; in the CD-ROM study, the dependent variable would be the subject's desire to attend a university nursing program. In an experiment, the dependent variable is the phenomenon measured in order to determine if any change has taken place as a result of some experimental treatment.

The *independent variables* include all the variables taken into account, or manipulated, by the researcher that may influence the dependent variable. Four types of independent variables are relevant to experimental studies:

1. **Treatment variable.** In an experiment, the independent variable whose effect is being studied is known as the **treatment variable.** In our example, the type of CD-ROM shown—either about nature or about a university nursing program—is the treatment variable. An experiment attempts to detect the direct effect of the treatment on the dependent variable. Some experiments include more than one treatment variable. In such cases, the experimenter must determine the effects of each treatment used on the dependent variable. (We might consider the effect of exposure to a multimedia CD-ROM with audio, video, and animated graphics versus a CD-ROM with only video as an additional treatment variable).

2. **Control variables. Control variables** are those specifically taken into account in designing a study. In this case, they would include other major factors which may influence a student's plans to attend a university nursing program such as gender, academic abilities, family role models in health care, and whether the student comes from a family background in which university attendance is expected. These variables need to be controlled, or taken into account, in designing the study to ensure that the study findings accurately reflect reality. By taking control variables into account we are able to eliminate possible alternative explanations for the observed relationships between exposure to a CD-ROM and plans to attend a university nursing program.

3. **Confounding variables.** Experimentalists refer to **confounding variables** as known factors that may unintentionally obscure or enhance a relationship. (Survey researchers use the term *source of spuriousness* to refer to the same idea.) For example, one would not want to measure some students' attitudes toward attending a univer-

sity nursing program on Monday morning, and others on Friday afternoon because it is possible that students' interest in attending a university nursing program varies systematically during the week. If this possibility is not taken into account, it may confound the results of our study.

4. **Random variables. Random variables** are unknown factors that may have an impact on our dependent variable. They are controlled through the random assignment to groups—some students see the university nursing CD-ROM, and others see a nature CD-ROM (see randomization below). It is important to control for these variables; otherwise, we may falsely conclude that it was our treatment that influenced the dependent variable.

c. Treatment Levels

Often, researchers examine two or three different **treatment levels.** These refer to the different treatments to which subjects are exposed. In our example, there are two different possibilities for the type of CD-ROM shown. This two-level study compares the effect of seeing the university nursing CD-ROM with the effect of seeing the nature CD-ROM. A study with three treatment levels might compare the effects of seeing a short, medium, or long CD-ROM. The various control and confounding variables are also exposed to the subject at various levels. The simplest multiple-variable design would be a 2 × 2 one; this refers to a design in which there are two levels of the treatment variable (the first "2") and two levels in a control variable (the second "2"). Thus, when experimentalists talk about designs they might talk of a 2 × 2 × 2 design. This means that the treatment has two categories; similarly, the two control variables each have two levels. A 2 × 3 × 2 experimental design has two levels in the treatment, a three-level

control variable and a two-level control variable. For example, an experiment designed to test the effect of a university nursing CD-ROM versus a nature CD-ROM on the desire to attend a nursing program for high, medium, and low academic achievers of both genders is a 2 (university versus nature CD-ROM) × 3 (high, medium, and low achiever) × 2 (male versus female) design.

B. PRE-EXPERIMENTAL DESIGNS

Pre-experimental designs are considered to be of limited scientific merit because they cannot rule out alternative explanations for observed relationships. However, understanding the problems of making causal inferences from data derived from pre-experimental design studies help us to better understand the rationale and value of experimental designs. For this reason, pre-experimental designs are discussed first in this chapter as a beginning reference point to illustrate weaknesses in these designs that lead to threats to the internal validity of studies and difficulties in interpreting the findings.

A **pre-experimental design** is one that does not permit clear causal inferences about the impact of a treatment on the dependent variable. Although these designs share some of the elements of the experiment, their designs inhibit clear causal interpretations. We will examine two pre-experimental designs, again using the illustration exploring the impact of a CD-ROM on students' desire to attend a university nursing program.

1. Same Group: Pretest and Posttest Design

Suppose you decided that you would need a measure of the students' predispositions toward a university nursing education before seeing the CD-ROM. Having completed this measure, the CD-ROM could then be shown, and the difference between the pre- and posttest scores could be used to measure the change in the desire to attend a university nursing program.

We could diagram the proposed design in the following way:

Same Group: Pretest/Posttest

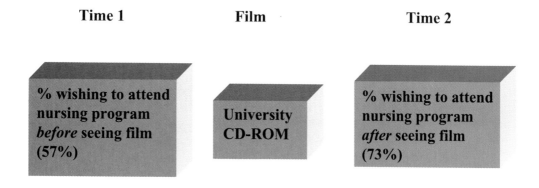

Time 1

% wishing to attend nursing program *before* seeing film (57%)

Film

University CD-ROM

Time 2

% wishing to attend nursing program *after* seeing film (73%)

Suppose that at time 1, 57 percent indicated that they wished to attend a university nursing program and at time 2, after seeing the CD-ROM, the percentage increased to 73. Could we argue that the CD-ROM produced a 16 percent increase in those wishing to attend the university? The answer is no. There are a number of factors that may render such an interpretation incorrect. Campbell and Stanley, in their classic work, *Experimental and Quasi-Experimental Design for Research* (1966), identified threats to internal validity that might confound our interpretations. Readers should note that these threats also apply to nonexperimental designs and should be considered when interpreting study findings.

1. **History.** Any number of events may have happened in addition to the CD-ROM. For example, a local university's nursing school may have established a new community-based health program for high school youth; the university's basketball team may have won a national championship; the university may have announced a new program to prepare nurse practitioners; or a professor may have just won a Nobel Prize. In the context of experimental design, **history** refers to concurrent events that, along with the experimental manipulation, may be influencing variation in the dependent variable.

2. **Maturation.** People change over time. Perhaps the students have become bored with school and, by the time the second measures are taken, systematic changes in attitude may have occurred. Such changes could, in part, be an influence causing the different responses at time 1 and time 2. By 3:00 P.M. on Friday afternoon, grade 11 students may experience a profound drop in their motivation to attend a university. **Maturation** refers to any changes that occur in an individual subject over the course of an experiment, which may, along with experimental manipulation, influence the outcome of the experiment.

3. **Testing.** Even asking identical questions at both tests may influence the responses. Some respondents may want

to appear consistent and, therefore, give the same responses in both tests. Others, suspecting that the study is meant to demonstrate how good the CD-ROM is, might want to help the researcher and exhibit **response bias** by being more positive the second time.

4. **Instrument decay.** Suppose we asked students to indicate their preferences by the strength with which they squeezed a hand dynameter. (A dynameter is a mechanical device with a calibrated dial that permits a researcher to read the indicated intensity.) If, for example, the spring in the device has weakened, the second set of readings will be slightly higher. **Instrument decay** refers to the fact that the dynameter no longer measures reliably.

5. **Statistical regression.** To explain this idea, we will need to alter the example slightly. Suppose, after our pre-test scores had been taken, that we decide to show the CD-ROM just to those with the most negative attitudes toward attending a university nursing program. Could we legitimately say that any gain in the scores of these students is a result of the CD-ROM? The answer is again no. The reason is that when a sample is selected on the basis of extreme scores, retesting will tend to show a **statistical regression** toward less extreme scores. That is, the most negative scores are likely to change in the direction of the mean simply because extreme scores (either positive or negative) are unstable. Even without any CD-ROM, the students' responses

> **BOX 4.1** *Regression Effect: Reading Scores*
>
> Suppose a clinical nurse specialist wants to try out a new program for teaching communication skills to health professionals working in a hospice setting. If the clinical nurse specialist tests the communication skills of all health professionals in the hospice setting and then selects the lowest scoring 10 percent of health professionals for the program, puts them through it, and then retests them, almost certainly the scores will increase. However, the amount attributable to the program versus the amount attributable to regression effects would remain uncertain.

would, on average, be slightly more positive on the second testing. The explanation is that inaccuracies in measurement at the time of the first measurement have tended to distort the data negatively. In short, those subjects with very low scores may have simply given more negative responses on that day because they were in a bad mood. Box 4.1 presents another example of a regression effect.

2. Exposed or Comparison Group Design

After considering the flaws in the previous design, suppose you alter it to provide for a comparison group, as in the following diagram:

Exposed/Comparison Group Design

Time 2

Experimental Group: 75% *After* Seeing University CD-ROM

Comparison Group: 60% *After* Seeing University CD-ROM

In the above design, one group is exposed to the CD-ROM promoting university nursing education, and the other is not. Can we legitimately conclude that the difference in attitude between the exposed group and the unexposed group represents the impact of the CD-ROM? (If 75 percent of the students exposed to the CD-ROM expressed a desire to attend a university nursing program and only 60 percent of those students who did not see the CD-ROM wished to go to a university nursing program, could we conclude that the CD-ROM produced this 15 percentage point difference in measured attitudes?) Again, there are problems. The major difficulty is that we do not know if the groups were the same to start with:

any difference in test results may simply reflect initial differences or differences that emerge during the study but are unrelated to the impact of the CD-ROM. Two additional confounding factors are noted by Campbell and Stanley (1966):

1. **Selection.** It is possible that the students most inclined to go to a university nursing program choose to go to see the CD-ROM; thus, if they score higher in the test, this result may simply reflect their initial predisposition to study nursing at a university. **Selection** thus refers to subjects selecting themselves *into* a study.
2. **Mortality.** Just as people choose to belong to a group, they may choose not to.

Some of those who see the CD-ROM may withdraw from the study before their attitude toward attending a university nursing program has been measured. The effect of subjects' withdrawing from the experiment may be that those who leave are less interested in higher education and hence the proportion for those who stay in the experiment are more likely to indicate a desire to attend a university nursing program. **Mortality** thus refers to subjects selecting themselves *out* of a study. Therefore, mortality may systematically distort the results of the study.

As we have seen, pre-experimental designs have serious problems in making clear causal inferences because of the inherent lack of adequate controls in these designs. Among the problems is whether they have adequately demonstrated: (1) that the test groups were similar before the introduction of the treatment variable; (2) that they have a way of dealing with random, confounding, and control variables. Classic experimental designs deal with these issues.

C. CLASSIC EXPERIMENTAL DESIGNS

To solve the problems in causal inference faced by pre-experimental designs, **classic experimental designs** may be used. We will consider only the most basic of these in this presentation: the between-subjects and the within-subjects designs. When properly executed, these designs are powerful causal inference vehicles.

I. Between-Subjects Design

A **between-subjects design,** also known as the *pretest, posttest control group design,*

contains three crucial elements of the classical experiment: control over extraneous variables, methods of dealing with pretreatment similarity of groups, and manipulation of a treatment. A between-subjects design involves a *control* and an *experimental* group. Measures are taken from members in both groups before treatment and repeated after the treatment has been experienced. Whereas the control group is exposed to a neutral treatment (seeing the nature CD-ROM in the illustration we have been using), the experimental treatment is the focus of the study (the university CD-ROM). Data analysis reveals whether there are differences in the dependent variable as a result of the intervention, while taking into account other factors.

- The **experimental group** is the one that is exposed to the treatment intervention. The researcher attempts to ensure that each subject experiences the intervention in as similar a fashion as possible to deal with extraneous factors that may be influencing the outcome of the study.
- The **control group** is established so that comparisons can be made between the experimental group and the control group. Normally, the control group is exposed to a placebo or some neutral treatment that is similar in the time it takes and the kind of experience it represents. In the case of the CD-ROM example, the control group is exposed to a CD-ROM having a nature theme.

a. Achieving Equivalence of Control and Experimental Groups in a Between-Subjects Design

A key factor in the success of a between-subjects design is that the treatment and the control groups (completely different groups) are made as equivalent as possible before the experimental group is ex-

Between-Subjects Design

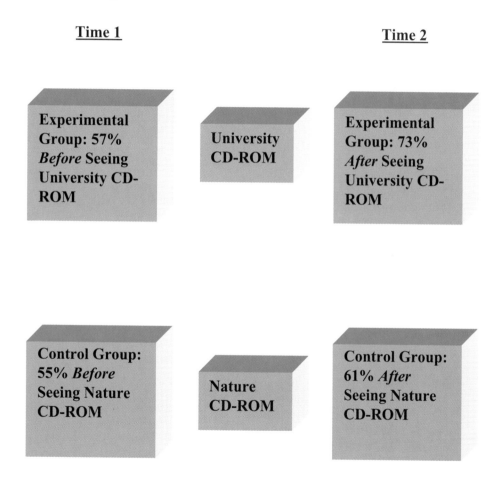

Time 1 — Time 2

Experimental Group: 57% *Before* Seeing University CD-ROM

University CD-ROM

Experimental Group: 73% *After* Seeing University CD-ROM

Control Group: 55% *Before* Seeing Nature CD-ROM

Nature CD-ROM

Control Group: 61% *After* Seeing Nature CD-ROM

posed to the experimental condition. There are three ways of achieving equivalence:

1. Through *randomization* (in which individuals are randomly assigned to either the treatment or to the control group)
2. Through *precision matching* (e.g., matching pairs according to gender, socioeconomic status, and grades, and then assigning one person from each of the matched pairs to the control group and the other person to the experimental group)
3. Through a *combination* of the above two: using precision matching to match pairs and then randomly assign one member of each pair to the experimental group and the other one to the control group

(i) Randomization

Randomization is a process of assigning subjects to a treatment or a control group so that each subject has an equal chance of being assigned to either group. This process of random assignment should not be confused with random selection, which is discussed in Chapter 5. If the numbers are large enough, randomization provides control over both known and unknown factors (the control and random variables). A variety of techniques may be used to accomplish the random assignment. In all cases, we avoid allowing subjects to choose their group assignment. The method selected should assure that each subject has an equal chance of being assigned to the experimental or the control group. Ways of accomplishing random assignment include:

- Random numbers. Computers have random number generators built into them and these may be used to assign individuals to groups. The first number shown by the random number generator is used to assign the first person in the subject pool to the experimental

or control group. Your rule might be to assign odd numbers to the experimental group and even ones to the control group. Using this rule, if the first number generated was a 7, you would assign the first subject to the experimental group. You would continue through the random numbers and subjects until all are assigned. Also, the statistical package SPSS has a procedure for selecting cases at random and may also be used to assign cases to experimental or control groups.

- Tables of random numbers may be used in a similar fashion. Table 4.1 is a table of random numbers. Here the procedure is to close one's eyes and, with pencil in hand, mark the table of random numbers, note the number nearest the mark; establish a rule for proceeding (perhaps, read down column to bottom of page then start at top of next column and read down). Again, using an odd or even rule, you could begin group assignment; if the start number is even, subject 1 is placed in the control group; if the second random number is also even, then subject 2 also goes into the control group. Continue assignment until all subjects are assigned.

  Table 4.2 illustrates the use of a table of random numbers or a computer-generated set of random numbers to assign subjects. In this case, the rule established was that even numbers lead to an assignment to the control groups, odd ones to the experimental group. Thus, if the numbers were odd, odd, odd, even, odd, even, even. The subjects would then be assigned, as shown in Table 4.2.

- A deck of playing cards may also be used to assign subjects to groups. Again, establish a set of rules (e.g., hearts and diamonds mean experimental group, clubs and spades mean control group assignment). Shuffle the cards well. Turn cards up one at a time; if the first card is red (hearts or dia-

Table 4.1 Table of Random Numbers

53	85	34	13	77	36	06	69	48	50	58	83	87	38	59
24	63	73	87	36	74	38	48	93	42	52	62	30	79	92
83	08	01	24	51	38	99	22	28	15	07	75	95	17	77
16	44	42	43	34	36	15	19	90	73	27	49	37	09	39
60	79	01	81	57	57	17	86	57	62	11	16	17	85	76
03	99	11	04	61	93	71	61	68	94	66	08	32	46	53
38	55	59	55	54	32	88	65	97	80	08	35	56	08	60
17	54	67	37	04	92	05	24	62	15	55	12	12	92	81
32	64	35	28	61	95	81	90	68	31	00	91	19	89	36
69	57	26	87	77	39	51	03	59	05	14	06	04	06	19
24	12	26	65	91	27	69	90	64	94	14	84	54	66	72
61	19	63	02	31	92	96	26	17	73	41	83	95	53	82
30	53	22	17	04	10	27	41	22	02	39	68	52	33	09
03	78	89	75	99	75	86	72	07	17	74	41	65	31	66
48	22	86	33	79	85	78	34	76	19	53	15	26	74	33
60	36	59	46	53	35	07	53	39	49	42	61	42	92	97
83	79	94	24	02	56	62	33	44	42	34	99	44	13	74
32	96	00	74	05	36	40	98	32	32	99	38	54	16	00
19	32	25	38	45	57	62	05	26	06	66	49	76	86	46
11	22	09	47	47	07	39	93	74	08	48	50	92	39	29
31	75	15	72	60	68	98	00	53	39	15	47	04	83	55
88	49	29	93	82	14	45	40	45	04	20	09	49	89	77
30	93	44	77	44	07	48	18	38	28	73	78	80	65	33
22	88	84	88	93	27	49	99	87	48	60	53	04	51	28
78	21	21	69	93	35	90	29	13	86	44	37	21	54	86
41	84	98	45	47	46	85	05	23	26	34	67	75	83	00
46	35	23	30	49	69	24	89	34	60	45	30	50	75	21
11	08	79	62	94	14	01	33	17	92	59	74	76	72	77
52	70	10	83	37	56	30	38	73	15	16	52	06	96	76
57	27	53	68	98	81	30	44	85	85	68	65	22	73	76
20	85	77	31	56	70	28	42	43	26	79	37	59	52	20
15	63	38	49	24	90	41	59	36	14	33	52	12	66	65
92	69	44	82	97	39	90	40	21	15	59	58	94	90	67
77	61	31	90	19	88	15	20	00	80	20	55	49	14	09
38	68	83	24	86	45	13	46	35	45	59	40	47	20	59

Table 4.2   Using Table of Random Numbers to Assign Subjects to Experimental and Control Groups

Subject	Odd or Even from Random Number Table	Treatment Condition
Subject 1	Odd	Experimental
Subject 2	Odd	Experimental
Subject 3	Odd	Experimental
Subject 4	Even	Control
Subject 5	Odd	Experimental
Subject 6	Even	Control
Subject 7	Even	Control

monds), the first subject is assigned to the experimental group; if the second card turned over is black, the second subject is assigned to the control group. Continue through the deck assigning each subject.

- An equal number of slips of paper with "Experimental Group" or "Control Group" written on them are placed in a container to be drawn out one at a time. As they are drawn out of the container, the subjects are assigned to either the treatment or control group based on the slip of paper.
- Other techniques could also be used, but with caution. You could not, for example, assign every second person to the control group if your sample was made up of married couples with the man's name first. Even if you start randomly, you would end up with an all-male experimental group and an all-female control group! Be careful that the technique you use provides each individual with an equal chance of ending up in the experimental group and that there are no systematic biases built into the order of your subject pool. If you choose a random number (or a heads or tails coin flip) to determine whether the first subject would be placed in the treatment or in the control group, you could then proceed by placing the next

subject into the opposite group, altering back and forth as subjects arrive. As long as there are no systematic biases in arrivals, this technique should provide each subject with an equal chance of being assigned to the experimental group.

These procedures are some examples of how to increase the likelihood that the treatment and control groups are equivalent before the introduction of the treatment. However, because experiments are often carried out on fairly small samples, researchers often try to enhance the equivalence of the two groups by using a method known as *precision matching*.

(ii) Precision Matching

Precision matching is a method of achieving equivalence between control and experimental groups by ensuring that the groups are matched on certain key variables. The key variables vary depending on the topic being investigated. In the CD-ROM study, one might decide to match on previous computer experience and on gender. A preliminary measure would be taken on the subject's computer experience and the subject's gender would be noted. Subjects could then be arranged from highest to lowest computer experience for the women, and then produce a similar listing for the potential male subjects. The top two women on the computer experience measure would then be randomly assigned—one to the experimental group, the other to the control group. The next pair of women would then be randomly assigned. And so on through each pair, followed by using the same procedure for the male pairs. Following this procedure ensures equivalence in the average computer experience in the treatment and control groups and also matches them by gender composition. Rather than simply trusting that luck (using the randomization process) will balance the two groups, precision matching ensures equivalence on the two key variables. We rely on the random assignment to balance the groups on other control and random variables.

(iii) Blocking

Another technique used in between-subjects designs to reduce within-group variations is **blocking.** A blocked design refers to one in which subjects have been grouped together on some variable that needs to be controlled, and subjects are then randomly assigned to treatment and control groups. For example, if you were testing for the effectiveness of a new health promotion program and you were working in an area with many immigrant children, you might want to use blocking in your experimental design. You would assign immigrant children randomly to either the experimental group (new program) or to the control group (old program); you would then do the same for nonimmigrant children. The blocking does not allow you to measure the influence of immigration status on learning but does increase your chances of detecting a significant effect on your new program. The reason for this is that you have reduced the variation between the treatment and the control groups.

(iv) Baseline Data

Another way in which the pretest equivalence is handled is by taking measures of the dependent variable before the intro-

duction of the treatment. Although the treatment and control groups may be equivalent on many measures as a result of randomization, they nonetheless may be somewhat different in terms of their measures on the dependent variable. Experimenters therefore collect *baseline* data so that we have a stable starting point against which we can make comparisons as we repeat the measures of the dependent variable through the course of the study. **Baseline data** is simply the score a subject has before the introduction of the treatment variable. In some circumstances, several measures are taken and we don't introduce the treatment variable until the measures achieve stability. This is referred to as **baseline stability.** So even if the average baseline scores of the experimental group compared with the control group are somewhat different, we are able to measure how much the scores change from the baseline levels when the measures are repeated after the treatment has been administered.

b. Analyzing the Data

To estimate the impact of the CD-ROM, we could do the following computation on the percent wanting to attend a university nursing program before and after seeing the CD-ROM (Table 4.3):

At time 1, 57 percent of the experimental group planned to attend a university nursing program compared with 55 per-

Table 4.3   Percent Wanting to Attend University Nursing Program by Exposure and Nonexposure to CD-ROM

Group	Patients Wanting to Attend a University Nursing Program, %		
	Time I	Time 2	Difference
Treatment	57	73	16
Control	55	61	6
Estimated impact of CD-ROM:			10

cent of the control group members (baseline measures). The time 2 measures indicate that the experimental group (after seeing the CD-ROM about attending a university nursing program) now had 73 percent planning to attend a university nursing program compared with 61 percent for the control group (viewers of a nature CD-ROM). To estimate the impact of the university CD-ROM on a person's desire to attend a university nursing program, we subtract the time 1 percentage from the time 2 percentage. Here we note a 16 percent difference for those in the experimental group compared with a 6 percent difference among those in the control group. We subtract the control difference (6 percent) from the treatment difference (16 percent) and arrive at an estimate of the impact of the CD-ROM amounting to some 10 percentage points.

The seven factors Campbell and Stanley (1966) identified as confounding interpretations are dealt with in between-subjects designs through:

- Attempting to make certain that the groups are similar to begin with
- Noting that the various factors should influence the treatment and the control groups equally

Thus, between-subjects designs rely on establishing pretreatment similarity of control and experimental groups to minimize the effects of history, maturation, testing, instrument decay, statistical regression, selection, and mortality. Therefore, some form of randomization is a key tool in the experimenter's quest to establish unambiguous causal relationships.

c. Demonstrating a Causal Relationship in a Between-Subjects Design

To show a causal relationship in any research, three conditions must be demonstrated:

1. **Changes in the treatment variable must occur before changes in the dependent variable.** Because the between-group design involves measures of both the treatment and the dependent variables at two points in time (time 1, time 2 measures), the procedure ensures that the measure at time 1 precedes the one at time 2. Second, as we introduce the treatment to the experimental group (the CD-ROM about a university nursing program), but not to the control group (who see a nature CD-ROM instead) and follow this by measuring the dependent variable at time 2, it becomes possible to make an inference about the impact of viewing the university CD-ROM (treatment variable) on the desire to attend a university program (the dependent variable). Thus, because the CD-ROM was shown between the time 1 and time 2 measures, if there is a change in the attitudes toward attending a university nursing program among those seeing the university CD-ROM, we will have made the first step in demonstrating that the CD-ROM caused the change in attitude.

2. **The variables must be associated; as values on the treatment variable are increased, the dependent measures vary correspondingly.** A variety of techniques may be used to illustrate that the variables are associated. For example, we might show that those who saw the CD-ROM are more likely to indicate that they are planning to attend a university nursing program than those who did not see the CD-ROM. To say that the dependent variable varies systematically indicates that either:
   - The proportion of respondents saying that they plan to attend a university nursing program is higher among those exposed to the university CD-ROM; or
   - The proportion of respondents saying that they plan to attend a uni-

versity nursing program is lower among those exposed to the university CD-ROM; or

• The proportion of students saying that they plan to attend a university nursing program increases as the length of the CD-ROM increases. However, there may appear, for example, to be a leveling off in the proportion of students planning on attendance when the CD-ROM is longer than 23 minutes.

3. **Nothing but the treatment variable can have influenced the dependent variable.** To ensure that it is only the treatment variable that is causing variation in the dependent variable, steps must be taken to rule out, or control, various sources of contamination:

Step 1: Ensure that the context in which the experiment is carried out is the same for all subjects. To guarantee the similarity of the experimental situation, researchers take great pains to ensure that physical conditions (e.g., temperature, humidity, lighting conditions) all remain the same; similarly, instructions to the subjects are standardized, even recorded, to be certain that each respondent gets the same information in the same manner. As much as possible, all subjects should have a similar experience in participating in the experiment.

Step 2: Balance the background characteristics of the subjects. Typically this control is accomplished through some combination of precision matching (matching a woman with a woman; high computer experience person with another who is also experienced with computers) and randomly assigning each person to the control or to the experimental groups. The goal is to try to populate both groups with similar kinds of people.

Step 3: Neutralize any confounding variables. The researcher must be careful that the experience of the experiment is

not having an impact on the results. For example, if you were testing the impact that the intensity of color (treatment variable) has on the speed of recovery from a major depressive episode, you should not simply move systematically from low color intensity (soft white, beige) through to intense color (bright yellows, bright pinks, lime greens). Subjects will probably recover from their depressive reaction as they go through their regular treatment regimen, and you should therefore vary the presentation of different color conditions for each subject randomly. In this way, the order of presentation would not in itself systematically influence the speed of recovery. If you do not deal with this potential confounding factor, you would not be able to tell how much of the increase of speed in recovery was caused by increasing the intensity of color in the clients' environment and how much was caused by a response effect to the regular protocol of care for depressive clients. Confounding variables of this sort are dealt with by:

• Varying the way the treatment is administered to the subjects; one strategy for doing this is known as **counterbalancing.** Here a treatment level is introduced, changed, maintained, and then returned to the first level to control for effects of learning on the subject's performance.

• Statistical controls in which subgroups are analyzed separately to take into account potential confounding variables (perhaps analyzing the male subjects separate from the female subjects).

Step 4: Deal with random variables. Random variables include all other unknown factors that might influence the dependent variable, none of which you can control. Subjects are assumed to be different on all dimensions. Knowing this, experimenters do not let subjects choose which group they will go into (they might think it more fun to be in a experimental group than in a boring control group; or they might choose to be in the same group as their friends). The randomization process used in the assignment of subjects to groups increases the likelihood that the two groups are similar on both known and unknown variables before the introduction of the treatment variable. When sample sizes exceed 30 in each group, random assignment is likely to result in reasonable balancing of the groups on random factors.

Box 4.2 presents a classic between-subjects experiment in nursing, Ciliska's investigation of two nondieting interventions for obese women. This study is of interest for its design, its anticipated findings, and its clarity of presentation. It uses a randomized trial to determine the efficacy of new weight paradigm interventions as alternatives for dieting in obese women.

2. Within-Subjects Designs

An alternative to the between-subjects design is a *within-subject design* (also known as *repeated measures* designs). Sometimes these designs use a single subject, sometimes just a few subjects, and sometimes large samples. What is the idea behind this kind of design?

We have stressed the importance of controlling possible sources of contamination. Matching groups and randomly assigning subjects to treatments were noted as ways of ensuring pretreatment similarity. Without such controls, it would be impossible to distinguish treatment effects from the effects of other factors.

Sometimes, however, one can use an alternative strategy, which provides for the ultimate in control of extraneous factors. Suppose that instead of assigning people to different treatments, we instead

expose *each subject to the different treatments*. Because the subject is the same person, the background characteristics, attitudes, and intelligence are all perfectly controlled. In a control group design, on the other hand, the researcher counts on randomized assignment to groups (or precision matching) to adjust for known and unknown variations between the two groups. With large samples, the assumption that sources of contamination have been satisfactorily addressed is reasonable; with smaller samples, one has less faith in the ability of randomization to deal with such contamination.

The key advantage of a **within-subject design** is that it provides convincing evidence for the impact of the treatment variable on the dependent variable. The evidence is all the more convincing because, by using the same subject under different levels of the treatment variable, one can be confident that most of the possible extraneous influences, such as gender, age, socioeconomic status, type of background, and values, have been controlled. Sometimes the control achieved in within-subject designs is called **control by constancy.** The term stems from the idea that because the same subject experiences different levels of the treatment, the subject acts as his or her own control. In contrast, the between-subjects design has to try to control these differences by random assignment or precision matching. Especially in studies using relatively small samples, such controls are somewhat suspect because there are always going to be some random fluctuations, which may mask true effects.

a. Crossover Designs

Suppose we were interested in the effect of two smoking cessation treatments (i.e., the nicotine patch and Zyban) on number of cigarettes smoked by cardiac clients. A within-subject design could be chosen to study this effect. In this design,

BOX 4.2 *Nurse Researchers at Work*

EVALUATION OF TWO NONDIETING INTERVENTIONS FOR OBESE WOMEN

Many women have a long history of failure at attempted weight loss and experience an accompanying self-appraisal of being fat and a failure. Recently, feminist critiques of the biomedical paradigm have contributed to a new paradigm that encourages no further attempts at weight loss but instead focuses on self-acceptance, improved body image, better nutrition, and more physical activity. Because little research exists on the effectiveness of such nondieting approaches, the primary purpose of this project was to evaluate them.

A *randomized trial* design was used in which consenting women were *randomized,* using a table of random numbers, into three groups: education alone, psychoeducation, or a no treatment (wait-list) *control group.* Measures were taken at pretest, posttest, and 6 months and 1 year posttests, although this article reports only the pre- and posttest results.

Three hypotheses were tested:

1. Participation of obese women in a group education intervention program increases self-esteem, decreases body dissatisfaction, and decreases restrained eating patterns.
2. Participation of obese women in a group psychoeducation intervention program increases self-esteem, decreases body dissatisfaction, and decreases restrained eating patterns.
3. Participation in a psychoeducation intervention will result in increased self-esteem, decreased body dissatisfaction, and decreased restrained eating patterns, which are of greater magnitude than results of participation in the education intervention.

A variety of scales were used to measure self-esteem; feelings of social inadequacy; body dissatisfaction; restrained eating patterns; and factors in eating behaviors, including cognitive restraint, disinhibition, and susceptibility to hunger. After signed, informed consent was obtained, the pretest questionnaires were completed. The same questionnaires were used after testing, immediately after the 12-week intervention session.

Inclusion criteria included: women, age 20 years or older, 120 to 200 percent average weight. Women who were pregnant or had a medical or psychiatric disorder self-disclosed were excluded. A total of 78 subjects had data collected on the primary outcome variables at pre- and posttest time. There were no statistical differences in the intervention and control groups in mean ages, mean weights, mean height, mean body mass indexes, or means of percent average weight, indicating that *randomization* was successful.

The *treatment interventions* consisted of meeting once a week for 12 weeks. The education group consisted of a lecture format with 16 to 21 people that met for 1 hour per week and included only the educational content such as the cultural imperative for women to be thin, strategies to achieve a nondieting style of eating, and the importance of regular physical activity. The psychoeducation group was a more intensive, small group (6 to 8 women) that met for 2 hours every week and included the educational content plus cognitive therapy strategies, assertiveness, body image exercises, and a group support component. The *control group* received no intervention.

In relation to the three hypotheses tested, results suggest:

1. Participation of obese women in a group education intervention did not increase self-esteem or reduce body dissatisfaction, nor did it decrease restrained patterns of eating compared with a control group.
2. Participation of obese women in a group psychoeducation intervention increased self-esteem, decreased body dissatisfaction, and decreased restrained patterns of eating in comparison to a control group.
3. Participation in the psychoeducation intervention resulted in increased self-esteem and decreased restrained patterns of eating, which are of greater magnitude than results of participation in the education intervention. The changes in body dissatisfaction did not reach the level of statistical significance.

In conclusion, this study established that a 12-week group intervention can be effective in improving self-esteem, encouraging a nonrestrained pattern of eating, and, in the short term, improving body dissatisfaction. For a complete description of this study, consult the original source.

SOURCE: Summarized from Ciliska, D. (1998). Evaluation of two nursing interventions for obese women. *Western Journal of Nursing Research, 20*(1), 119–135.

both treatments are given to the *same individuals* rather than separately to two different samples. An obvious advantage in this type of design is the saving in the number of subjects required because the same group is used twice (or more often if necessary). Because the subjects serve as their own controls, the sample size required to detect a significant effect is considerably less.

A drawback does exist in within-subject designs: Because two treatments are being tested, there may be an effect from the first treatment that the subjects underwent. One may argue that the subjects who receive the second treatment are not exactly the same as the group of subjects who received the first treatment. To cancel out the effects of any carry-over from treatment A to treatment B, a within-subject **crossover design** (also called a *counterbalanced design*) is used. Crossover designs assign subjects randomly to a specific sequencing of treatment conditions. In this case, half of the subjects (group 1) receive treatment A (the nicotine patch) followed by treatment B (Zy-

ban), and the other half (group 2) receive treatment B, (Zyban) followed by treatment A (the nicotine patch). This distributes the carry-over effects equally across all conditions of the study, thus canceling them out. It can be argued that any difference found between groups 1 and 2 cannot be attributed to the fact that treatment A always followed treatment B or vice versa. To prevent an effect related to time, the same amount of time needs to be allocated to each treatment. The design must also allow for a *washout period*. This is an adequate interval of time between the two treatments to eliminate the effect of the first treatment. Figure 4.1 illustrates a within-subject, crossover design.

In this design, a group of heavy smokers are selected from a cardiac clinic. They are randomly assigned to two groups, 1 and 2. Before the experiment begins, an initial *baseline* assessment of the number of cigarettes smoked by each subject is made over a 1-week period. The baseline measure is an essential element in any experimental design because it represents the situation existing before any experi-

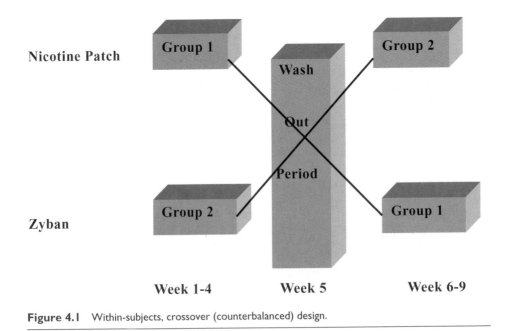

Figure 4.1   Within-subjects, crossover (counterbalanced) design.

mental treatment is introduced. Group 1 then receives the nicotine patch for 4 weeks followed by Zyban for 4 weeks. Group 2 receives Zyban for the first 4 weeks followed by the Nicotine patch for 4 weeks. The design specified that each subject would crossover to the alternate smoking cessation treatment after a 1-week washout period. Throughout the 9 weeks of the study, the subjects recorded the number of cigarettes smoked per day.

If all the smokers had received Zyban followed by the nicotine patch and if Zyban had proved to be superior in reducing the number of cigarettes smoked, the conclusion would be open to criticism that it was simply the fact that Zyban was tried first that explained the results. Giving half the sample Zyban first and the other half of the sample the nicotine patch first overcomes this criticism. This solution to the problem of order and carry-over effects is known as counterbalancing. A disadvantage to this design is the fact that subject dropouts may increase because the data collection period is longer.

b. Hawthorne Effect

A limitation of the experimental design that may influence the study design in Figure 4.1 is a phenomenon known as a **Hawthorne effect.** This phenomenon refers to any differences in the dependent variable that are not the direct result of changes in the treatment variable. This phenomenon is named after one of the experiments done in the Hawthorne Western Electric plants in Chicago by Roethlisberger and Dickson (1939). In their study, workers' output was monitored under varying intensities of lighting. (The hypothesis was that worker productivity would increase with increasing levels of illumination.) The experimenters noted that as lighting intensity *decreased,* worker output *increased.* It looked as if simply dim-

ming the lights in the workplace would be the way to increase productivity. However, when the experimenters then increased lighting intensities to the baseline levels, they noted that worker productivity continued to increase. Woops! Something other than the intensity of illumination was having an impact on the speed of work. A possible interpretation of this result is that the workers knew that they were being observed, so they tried hard to please the observers by increasing their productivity (Roethlisberger and Dickson, 1939). Whenever an outcome cannot be reversed, you have to suspect that some factor (or factors) other than the treatment is influencing the dependent variable (in this case, the speed of work).

In nursing research, an investigator may have to contend with a double Hawthorne effect. For example, if an orthopedic unit is interested in testing the impact of a new ambulation protocol on client recovery rates after hip replacement surgery, nurses, patients, and other hospital staff may be aware of their participation in the study. This may lead to both groups' altering their behavior accordingly. This is why **double-blind** experiments, in which neither the subjects nor those who administer the treatment are aware of who is in the experimental or the control group, are so powerful. Unfortunately, it is often difficult to disguise nursing interventions in the same way that medication or medical treatments can be disguised. Hence, for some nursing investigations, a double-blind approach is not feasible.

3. Between- and Within-Subjects Designs Compared

Let's compare a between-subjects approach with a within-subject approach to the same research question: *What is the efficacy of therapeutic touch (a specialized type of healing touch often used in nursing practice) on situationally induced stress in healthy adult women?* We will approach the question by looking at two different between-subjects studies and one within-subject study. Table 4.4 compares fictitious data on these studies.

- **Student nurses comparison: a between-subjects design.** Suppose nursing students in a research methods course are asked to volunteer for an experiment. They are asked to report to the nursing school laboratory on Saturday afternoon. Students are given basic instruction on the procedure of therapeutic touch, a demonstration of it, and an opportunity to practice it on each other for 20 minutes. The students are then randomly assigned to either laboratory A or B. In laboratory A are healthy adult women who will receive *therapeutic touch* from student nurses while being subjected to artificially induced stress. In laboratory B are healthy adult women who will receive *casual touch* from student nurses while being subjected to artificially induced stress. The women receiving the touch therapy are not aware of the type of touch they will be administered. This is called a **single-blind** study and is used to minimize the possible effects on the subject of knowing which intervention is being used. Each student first records a blood pressure reading (a physiological indicator of stress) for the subject. Students then administer the touch intervention to the women who have been subjected to artificially induced stress and then record the blood pressure of the subject a second time. The results of the difference in diastolic pressure readings are shown in section I of Table 4.4. Note that there is considerable variation in the scores. Even though the average reduction in diastolic blood pressure readings for subjects in the therapeutic touch group is higher, we are not comfortable in concluding that therapeutic touch is effec-

tive in reducing stress that is situationally induced—there is simply too much variability in the pressure values. Had one or two persons ended up in the opposite group, the results might change substantially. (A test of significance confirms our suspicion because the difference between the diastolic readings achieved with therapeutic touch and the diastolic readings of subjects receiving casual touch is not statistically significant. See Chapter 12 for a discussion of what these tests tell us.)

- **Experienced nurse practitioners: a between-subjects design.** The second experiment is identical to the previous one, except we will use expert nurse practitioners who have been specially prepared to administer therapeutic touch and have varying years of experience in doing so. Using each nurse's history of administering therapeutic touch permits us to rank-order all the nurses by skill level in therapeutic touch. Assignment to laboratory A and B is done in pairs: using a coin flip, the ranked nurses are randomly assigned to either laboratory A (therapeutic touch) or laboratory B (casual touch) until 20 nurses have been assigned. Once again, each expert nurse records the blood pressure reading for the subject and then administers the touch intervention to the participant who has been subjected to artificially induced stress, and then records the blood pressure of the subject a second time. Section II of Table 4.4 shows much less variation than was apparent among the student nurses. Nonetheless, some of the variation between the expert nurses may still be caused by differences in nursing skill, the female subjects, or the touch interventions. The results indicate that the reduction in diastolic blood pressure readings of subjects who received therapeutic touch are somewhat greater than those of subjects who received casual touch. The nagging problem, how-

Table 4.4   Results from Three Studies to Test Therapeutic Touch versus Casual Touch on Blood Pressure

Experiment	Therapeutic Touch		Casual Touch	
	Name	Change in BP	Name	Change in BP
I. Student nurses:	Kathleen	10	Paula	12
Between-subjects	Li	9	Marlies	7
design; random	Danielle	11	Vanny	6
assignment to	Kim	8	Paula	6
groups	Kevin	12	Sandra	11
	Mary	4	Marius	1
	Yvonne	5	Chris	2
	Tara	7	Andrea	4
	Ursula	8	Tony	7
	Holly	10	Carol	8
Mean		8.40		6.40
Standard deviation		2.547		3.502
Mean difference		2.00		

Experiment	Therapeutic Touch		Casual Touch	
	Name	Change in BP	Name	Change in BP
II. Expert nurses:	Eve	12	Mary	11
between-subjects	Joan	12	Ted	11
design; pairs	Freda	11	Gladys	10
matched on	Carlie	10	Ronelda	9
known skill level;	Jill	12	Molly	10
random assignment	Neil	11	Emily	10
to groups	Hazel	10	Sara	9
	Iris	11	Edwina	9
	Frank	10	Zoe	9
	Betty	11	Brenda	9
Mean		11.00		9.70
Standard deviation		0.816		0.823
Mean difference		1.30		

Experiment	Therapeutic Touch		Casual Touch	
	Name	Change in BP	Name	Change in BP
III. Expert nurses:	Jamie	12	Jamie	10
within-subject design	Petra	11	Petra	10
	Margo	11	Margo	11
	Jill	13	Jill	12
	Sandra	13	Sandra	12
	Dale	12	Dale	11
	Paula	11	Paula	10
	Teresa	11	Teresa	10
	Linda	11	Linda	10
	Melanie	12	Melanie	11
Mean		11.70		10.70
Standard deviation		0.823		0.823
Mean difference		1.00		

ever, is whether differences in the subjects themselves and their reaction to stress may have been responsible for some of the differences in the diastolic readings. However, because of the small sample of only 10 expert nurses in each group, we lack confidence with the results. (The test of significance, however, does indicate a statistically significant difference in diastolic blood pressure for the two touch interventions.)

- **Expert nurse practitioners: a within-subject design.** Given some uncertainty about the results, could we get even greater confidence in our results by changing our design? Suppose we simply have *each nurse run two trials with the same subject,* once administering therapeutic touch and once administering casual touch? We now have control over the subject who will be subjected to artificially induced stress, as well as the skill of the nurse. We have control by constancy—the nurse and the subject are the same for the test with therapeutic touch and casual touch. As before, the subjects are not aware of which type of touch they will receive first (single blind). They are randomly assigned to the different orderings of the touch treatment. The results, reported in section III of Table 4.4, show about the same variability as the results of the previous experiment, but now we have greater confidence that we have controlled both nurse and subject variability. (The differences by touch intervention are statistically significant.) As a nurse practicing in the specialized and controversial field of therapeutic touch, which of these tests would you trust more?

The goal in experimental research is to isolate and measure treatment effects. To demonstrate an effect convincingly, one wants clear differences in the dependent variable (diastolic blood pressure values) by treatment categories (therapeutic touch versus casual touch). To make a study as convincing as possible, we should have lots of variations between the categories (average diastolic pressure should vary consistently by type of touch) but little variation within the category (diastolic pressure readings for those subjects receiving the same type of touch). In the three designs presented here, note how the first design had a lot of within-group variation (the nursing students varied considerably in their therapeutic touch skills); the second and third designs had less within-group variation (all expert nurses).

Although it is not always possible to use a within-subject design, the advantage of such a design over a between-subjects design is that you need fewer subjects, require less time to train and run your experiment, and exercise almost perfect control over extraneous influences on your dependent variable.

D. QUASI-EXPERIMENTAL DESIGNS

Often we want the power of an experimental design in making causal inferences but find that it is not possible to conduct an experiment. Sometimes this happens because we cannot manipulate the required variables for ethical or for practical reasons; sometimes we cannot randomly assign people to different treatments. When these situations arise, researchers modify the experimental approach and design a quasi-experiment. A **quasi-experimental design** is one in which it has not been possible to meet all of the following requirements:

- Randomly assign subjects to a treatment or control group
- Control the timing or nature of the treatment

An important feature of the quasi-experimental design is its attempt to compensate for the absence of either the random assignment or the control group component by introducing other controls. The quasi-experimental design comes as close as possible to the experimental design in order to measure the impact of a treatment.

There are a number of quasi-experimental designs available to nurse researchers. These include the nonequivalent control group, the one-group pretest-posttest (also called pre-experimental), the time series design, and the one-time case study design, to name a few. This section discusses the most basic quasi-experimental design: the *nonequivalent control group*. To illustrate this approach, we will examine a study using this design.

1. Nonequivalent Control Group Design

To illustrate the nonequivalent control group design, we will examine an imaginative study done by Smeenk and associates (1998) that makes an important contribution to nursing knowledge in the area of palliative care and quality of life. The objective of this study was to investigate the effects of a home care intervention program for terminal cancer patients on the quality of life of direct caregivers, compared with standard care programs. It is an important investigation because it is the first documented controlled study that has investigated the effects of such an intervention program on the quality of life of direct caregivers of terminally ill cancer patients.

In a nonequivalent control group design, the control and experimental groups are not drawn from the same population. It is used in situations in which subjects cannot be randomly assigned to the experimental and control group. Consequently, the researcher cannot assume equivalency of the two groups. Usually in a nonequivalent control group design, the groups are naturally occurring; for example, nursing students at two different universities or clients from two fitness clubs are used. The Smeenk study is a good illustration of how the limitations of a quasi-experimental design can be addressed in a study. As you read the summary of the study in Box 4.3, pay particular attention to the means used by the investigators to deal with the issue of the nonequivalence of the two groups and possible confounding variables.

This study is convincing because it is a quasi-experimental study that compensates for the fact that it is not a classic experimental design. The investigators could not assume the equivalence of the two groups because they were drawn from two different natural collectives and not randomly assigned. To address this, the researchers made a point of showing the similarities between the two geographical areas from which the sample was drawn. The areas were similar in terms of population and accessibility to hospitals and home care services. Hence, it is unlikely that the different residential areas could explain the findings. Furthermore, a broad spectrum of patient and direct caregiver characteristics were collected at time 1. The groups proved to be fairly comparable on these characteristics. The data were examined for confounding variables. Potential confounders were entered into the regression analyses with the preintervention OQOLI (at time 1). As a result of these precautions, one can have confidence that the final results of the study are convincing.

2. Panel Studies

Panel studies monitor specific organizations or individuals over time. Because the participants in panel studies are monitored over time, these designs are included in this section on quasi-experimental designs. Panel studies frequently use survey data collection techniques (questionnaires or interviews) to investi-

BOX 4.3 *Nurse Researchers at Work*

TRANSMURAL CARE OF TERMINAL CANCER PATIENTS: EFFECTS ON CAREGIVERS

Few studies in the nursing literature have investigated the effect of a home care program on the quality of life of direct caregivers of cancer patients. This article describes an intervention program called transmural care, which was developed specifically to meet the individual needs of patients with cancer, and was offered by professional caregivers from hospitals and primary care teams in the Netherlands. Its purpose was to provide supportive care at home for patients and their direct caregivers.

It was hypothesized that transmural care may lead to a better quality of life for direct caregivers of terminal cancer patients. Because of practical and ethical reasons, the study used a *quasi-experimental design.*

The sample consisted of 116 direct caregivers of terminal cancer patients whose estimated prognosis was less than 6 months. Patients and their caregivers were included from January 1994 until February 1995. All caregivers living in Eindhoven, the Netherlands, were assigned to the intervention group ($n = 79$), and those living in the urban surroundings of Eindhoven were assigned to the control group ($n = 37$). (The experimental and the *nonequivalent control group* were natural collectives.) Considering the study design, one should note that the two areas are very similar. The population of both Eindhoven and the suburban area is 200,000 each. The maximum travel time to a hospital in both sites is approximately 30 km (20 miles), and the availability of home care service in each area is comparable. Furthermore, a pilot study using the database of the Comprehensive Cancer Center showed no significant difference in the incidence of the various cancer types, mean age, and genders of cancer patients in these two populations.

After discharge from the hospital to the home, subjects in both groups received the standard care available in the Netherlands. In addition, patients and caregivers in the experimental group received the intervention program. This consisted of four main elements: (1) access to a specialist nurse coordinator, (2) a 24-hour telephone service in the hospital with access to a transmural home team, (3) a collaborative home care dossier (case file), and (4) protocols designed by a multidisciplinary team to standardize and support caregivers when using specific skills and actions such as intravenous therapy or epidural and spinal pain relief.

The outcome variable was the direct caregivers' quality of life. It was measured in a multidimensional way using four instruments that measured four dimensions, namely, daily functioning, fear, loneliness, and general well-being. Data were collected 1 week before (T1), 1 week after (T2), and 4 weeks (T3) after the patient's discharge from the hospital, as well as 3 months after the patient had died (T4). Discharge from the hospital marked the starting point of the intervention. Two trained interviewers using structured questionnaires collected the data. They were *blinded* to the study design. To yield an aggregate score for the quality of life measurements, a factor analysis was conducted at each assessment stage. This yielded one factor and was considered the primary outcome variable called the overall quality of life index (OQOLI).

Before assessing whether the intervention contributed positively to the direct caregivers' OQOLI, a search for possible confounding variables in the relationship between the experimental condition and the outcome measure was performed. Correlations between the direct caregiver and patient characteristics and the outcome measure yielded only two potential confounders: the patient's being treated with chemotherapy and the direct caregiver's also being the patient's partner. To control for the confounding variables they were added to the experimental condition as independent variables in the regression analyses.

To assess whether the intervention contributed positively to the direct caregivers' OQOLI, hierarchical backward multiple regression analyses were performed on the outcome measure. A total of 71 direct caregivers withdrew from the study at various times because they found it too burdensome. No significant differences could be found when comparing dropouts

continued on next page

BOX 4.3 *Nurse Researchers at Work*

TRANSMURAL CARE OF TERMINAL CANCER PATIENTS: EFFECTS ON CAREGIVERS (*CONTINUED*)

with the direct caregivers, who could be evaluated on their initial characteristics. The results suggest that the intervention contributed positively to the direct caregivers OQOLI at T2 (1 week after hospital discharge) and T4 (3 months after patient's death). At T3, no significant difference was found between the two groups. The lower number of direct caregivers that could be analyzed for this time period may explain this.

In conclusion, this study supports the value of transmural care of terminal cancer patients and their caregivers. Such programs can be effective in lessening the burden of care for terminal cancer patients and in reducing the negative effect on the direct caregivers' quality of life. For a complete description of the study, consult the original source.

SOURCE: Summarized from Smeenk, F., de Witte, L., van Haastregt, J., et al (1998). Transmural care of terminal cancer patients: Effects on the quality of life of direct caregivers. *Nursing Research, 47*(3), 129–213.

---

gate a particular group but collect data about the respondents a minimum of two times. Panel studies are also referred to as *longitudinal studies*. Panel studies allow the researcher to assess not only change over time but also the differences and similarities in two or more cohorts or groups over time.

a. Rationale for Panel Studies and Examples

Why would one choose to do a panel study rather than an experiment or a survey? The answer is that experimentation is frequently not possible, or judged not to be relevant, for the examination of some relationships. Surveys, on the other hand, might not provide a sufficient basis for making causal inferences. Clairmont and Jackson (1980) were interested in studying the impact of working for large companies rather than small companies. In this case, the researchers needed to establish what the individuals were like at time 1; next, the researchers needed to monitor changes in these individuals over time. These are complex issues that require the individuals' being compared to be roughly similar at the beginning of the

study and that the two groups compared over time be exposed to different types of employers. A carefully designed panel study provided a naturalistic experiment and led to a better understanding of the impact of the workplace on workers (Clairmont and Jackson, 1980).

Harton and Latané (1997) used a panel study to examine the impact of social influence (defined as popularity) on development of mature lifestyle attitudes in five cohorts of school children, age 9 to 15 years. The main purpose of the study was to examine the development of mature adolescent attitudes in older children and to look at how these attitudes relate to popularity with the same and other gender. (See Box 4.4.)

b. Tips for Keeping Track of Respondents in a Panel Study

On occasion, respondents are contacted at different points in time. When the time between contacts is a year or two and the population being studied is fairly mobile, special problems are posed for the researcher. With an initial sample of 538, Clairmont and Jackson (1980) were able to locate and interview 96 percent of respon-

BOX 4.4 *Nurse Researchers at Work*

SOCIAL INFLUENCE AND ADOLESCENT LIFESTYLE ATTITUDES

In this panel study, mature attitudes were defined as favorable attitudes toward activities that adolescents become increasingly interested in as they age. Both "deviant" behaviors such as smoking cigarettes and consuming beer and wine (illegal for children in the study age group) were considered, as well as normal developmental activities such as wearing make-up and kissing. The study examined longitudinally, fourth- through eighth-grade students' lifestyle attitudes and sociometric status (popularity), once each semester. Group-administered questionnaires were used to collect data on lifestyle attitudes and sociometric status. The current study reports on data collected over 2 years.

The study examined grades and gender effects on lifestyle attitudes and popularity. Specifically, it examined whether popularity is related to lifestyle attitudes and whether increased popularity leads to greater adoption of lifestyle attitudes. Complete data for both semesters of year 1 were obtained for 201 students, and a total of 193 students completed both semesters of year 2. Complete data from all four waves were obtained from 128 students (30 fourth graders, 31 fifth graders, 35 sixth

graders, and 32 seventh graders, subtracting out the graduating eighth graders from year 1), representing 62 percent of the total eligible population, and 76 percent of those for whom permission had been given in year 1.

Results indicated that approval of both healthy and deviant mature lifestyle attitudes increased linearly with grade for both boys and girls. By eighth grade, gender differences in attitudes had almost vanished. Students with more mature attitudes were more popular with the opposite gender, but there was no relationship between same-sex popularity and attitudes. In this situation, the panel study design enabled use of the repeated measures over 2 years to study attitude measures, to trace the development of mature lifestyle attitudes over time and simultaneously to test measures of same-sex and cross-sex popularity and its relationship to development of mature lifestyle attitudes in five cohorts of students. On the basis of this investigation, the researcher can generate several hypotheses about adolescent attitude development and the role of social influence. The same panel design could be used for purposes of testing these hypotheses in future studies.

SOURCE: Summarized from Harton , H.C. & Latané, B. (1997). Social influence and adolescent lifestyle attitudes. *Journal of Research on Adolescence, 7*(2), 197–220.

dents in the second wave of interviews, some two years after the initial interview. The following techniques were used in that study to locate the respondents:

1. At the time of the first interview, request that the respondent provide the name of a relative or friend who will always know how to get in touch with him or her. These names prove invaluable later in efforts to contact individuals.

2. Try the original phone number; even though the respondent has moved, the same phone number may have been maintained. If the phone has been dis-

connected, the operator may be able to provide the new number.

3. Phone directories for the original year and for the current one are helpful; check how the person was listed in the original directory. If the person is still in the area, the chances are that the name will be listed identically.

4. Contact the employer of the respondent. Also contact coworkers in an effort to locate the individual.

5. Contact neighbors. Especially in smaller cities and towns, neighbors can be helpful in tracing respondents.

6. Now you are desperate! Call people in

the directory with the same last name and hope you will get lucky by finding a relative of the person involved who might be able to give you an address or phone number.

E. ADVANTAGES AND LIMITATIONS OF EXPERIMENTAL DESIGNS

The forte of the experiment is in demonstrating that a treatment variable has an impact on an outcome measure. To do this well, an experimentalist has to rule out possible sources of contamination, deal with control variables, and deal with the effect of random variables. These challenges are met in greater or lesser degrees by experimental designs.

1. Pre-Experimental Designs

a. Limitations

The pre-experimental design involving a *same group: pretest and posttest* discussed earlier in this chapter had problems in that in this design all kinds of other random factors may have influenced the change in outcome measures. On the other hand, the *exposed comparison group design* was seen to be flawed because it could not demonstrate that the experimental and control group were similar before the introduction of the treatment. In short, the groups may have been different from one another, and the treatment effect cannot be convincingly documented.

2. Quasi-Experimental Designs

a. Advantages

Quasi-experimental designs are typically done when the topic dictates that an experiment is not possible. Thus, they are often the best that can be done given certain ethical or practical constraints.

Sometimes quasi-experimental designs involve representative samples. In such studies, a group of individuals (usually called a panel) is monitored over time. The panel may have been selected as a representative one and thus the results may enable the researcher to make sound causal arguments than can, at the same time, lead to extrapolations to the larger population. Quasi-experimental designs thus can sometimes fuse strong causal inferences and also be strong on external validity.

b. Limitations

Given limited control over the context in which the study is conducted, quasi-experimental studies lack the causal inference power of the classic experiment. It is sometimes not possible to control the treatment variable or to place individuals in experimental and control groups. Thus, these studies often represent a compromise between what the ideal study would look like and what is feasible.

3. Classic Experimental Designs

The classic experimental designs seek to remedy the problems of causal inferences by establishing randomly matched comparison groups (experimental and control groups) along with before-treatment and after-treatment measures on the dependent variable. These designs are referred to as *between-subjects designs*. A second approach discussed dealt with problems of causal inference by exposing the same subjects to different treatments. Control over random variables is achieved in the latter design through *control by constancy*—the use of the same subject in the comparisons.

a. Advantages

The advantage in both these designs is that they can provide powerful, convincing evidence for the effect of a treatment variable. Through statistical analysis and through the use of randomization and precision matching, control over random and confounding variables is enhanced. A nurse researcher who wishes to assess whether a given nursing intervention is better than some current practice may well turn to an experimental design to shed light on the question. Thus, classic experimental designs produce the clearest view of causation. This is accomplished through the application of a treatment to subjects under conditions in which extraneous variables are controlled. Furthermore, through the use of *double-blind* designs, in which neither subjects nor researchers know which subjects are under what condition, there is considerable control over bias on the part of subjects and researchers. However, there are some limitations of experimental designs.

b. Limitations

(i) External Validity

Few experiments are conducted using samples that can be viewed as representative of a larger population; therefore, one cannot make extrapolations to the general population. This is the issue of *external validity*. In short, can a study on a single ward in Kansas City be extrapolated to wards across the country? Clearly one would need to repeat the study in many different locales to determine the extent to which valid generalizations may be drawn from a single study. In our therapeutic touch experiment, significant differences were found in the stress levels of subjects who received therapeutic touch. These differences, however, may well hold true only for older nurses experienced in therapeutic touch protocols but not for younger ones (all of the nurses in the test were older than age 40 years). Thus, we

should not conclude that therapeutic touch performed by nurses of all ages is effective in reducing stress.

(ii) Limits to Predictability in Experimental Studies

The fact that experimental studies do a better job than surveys in predicting outcomes should not be misinterpreted. For example, suppose that a treatment variable X (therapeutic touch) controls 10 percent of the variability in the dependent variable Y (stress level). Ideally, an experiment is designed to control all external factors that influence the dependent variable. Surveys can only exercise such control through statistical adjustments. Thus, the ability of experimental and nonexperimental designs to predict outcomes is not comparable. In principle, experiments should produce higher predictability than that achieved by nonexperimental designs using the same variables. A robust variable in an experiment, however, may be relatively impotent outside the laboratory setting.

(iii) Artificiality Issue

The third major concern is that there is an element of artificiality in laboratory experiments that is difficult to detect, interpret, or control. In the nursing world, the natural environment in which the client is situated bears heavily on health outcomes. Controlling all factors, as you do in a classic experiment, may not yield results that are applicable in the real world, where you are unable to control the same set of factors.

In addition, a "good subject" may try to respond by giving the researcher what he or she thinks the researcher wants. The subject may also be intimidated and act atypically. To what extent do people modify their behavior when they know that they are being studied? Although more is said about this topic in Chapter 9, researchers need to take into account the effects of expectations on the responses

Table 4.5   Advantages and Limitations of Alternate Designs

Research Design Category: Experimental Designs	General	Validity	Causal Inference	Multivariate	Probing
Pre-experimental	–	–	–	–	–
Experimental	–	–	+	–	–
Quasi-experimental	±	–	+	–	–
Panel studies	±	–	+	±	±

In each category, a plus sign means that this is an advantage of the technique; a minus sign means this is a possible limitation; a plus or minus sign (±) means that in some conditions it is a limitation, but in others, it is an advantage.
- **General** refers to the extent to which extrapolations to larger populations may be made using each of the design or data collection procedures.
- **Validity** is the extent to which indicators clearly measure what they are intended to measure.
- **Causal Inference** refers to the ease with which inferences about causal relations among variables may be made.
- **Multivariate** refers to the ease with which information on many variables is collected, leading to the possibility of multivariate analysis.
- **Probing** refers to the extent to which responses may be probed in depth.

of subjects. Because subjects can manage their presentation of themselves to the experimenter, questions can be raised about the validity of some experimental results (e.g., are you measuring what you claim to measure?).

(iv) Limitations on Number of Variables

For practical reasons, experimental designs can only deal with a few variables simultaneously. (Multiple-variable designs are possible, but with several treatment and control levels, one would soon need far too many subjects to run the experiment. For example, a $3 \times 3 \times 3 \times 3$ design produces 81 treatment conditions and, if there were 10 subjects per condition, would require 810 subjects.) When a large number of variables require simultaneous analysis, it is advisable either to use a different experimental design or to simplify the experiment by using fewer variables or fewer levels in each variable.

(v) Experiments Cannot Study All Topics

It is neither practical nor ethical to experiment on all aspects of human behavior; therefore, other designs remain important tools for nurse researchers. For example, in a study exploring the effectiveness of a new birth control method, it would be impractical and entirely unethical to randomly assign half the clients at a well women's clinic to use no birth control while the other half would be assigned to use the new method. Beginning researchers should have some understanding of experimental designs because their great strength is their ability to control many of the confounding factors that influence outcomes. When experimentation is not possible, it is more difficult to produce convincing inferences about causal relationships. Table 4.5 summarizes the advantages and disadvantages of experimental and quasi-experimental designs.

E X E R C I S E S

1. Suppose you wished to investigate the impact of a school nutrition program on the grade performance of students. What research design or designs would be appropriate to deal with such a question? Outline the rationale for your choice.

2. Outline a within-subjects experimental project. Be sure to identify all variables and the number of levels that will be used and indicate how the dependent variable will be measured. Comment on the method by which controls will be achieved on possible contaminants.

3. Outline a between-subjects experimental project. Be sure to identify all variables and the number of levels that will be used and indicate how the dependent variable will be measured. How will control over possible sources of contamination be achieved?

4. Outline a quasi-experimental project. Be sure to identify all variables and indicate how the dependent variable will be measured. How will control over possible sources of contamination be achieved?

5. Review a current nursing research journal and select a pre-experimental, experimental, or quasi-experimental study of interest to you. Identify the type of design and the major steps in the design. Also, compare the advantages and disadvantages of the design. Formulate design remedies to deal with potential disadvantages or weaknesses in the design.

RECOMMENDED READINGS

Brink, P.J., and Wood, M.J. (1998). *Advanced Design in Nursing Research* (2nd ed). London: Sage. This advanced text explores three levels of research based on knowledge of the topic: experimental, survey, and exploratory-descriptive. The text begins with the experimental design and subsequent designs are contrasted with the classic experiment.

Campbell, D.T., and Stanley, J.C. (1966). *Experimental and Quasi-Experimental Designs for Research*. Chicago: Rand McNally. This is considered by many to be the classic statement on confounding variables in different types of research designs.

Ciliska, D. (1998). Evaluation of two nursing interventions for obese women. *Western Journal of Nursing Research, 20*(1), 119–135. Ciliska's experimental design compares two non-dieting interventions to the problem of obesity in women.

Mitchell. M., and Jolley, J. (1997). *Research Design Explained* (3rd ed). Orlando: Harcourt Brace Jovanovitch College Publishers. This is an excellent text that explains experimental design and the analysis of results.

Smeenk, F., de Witte, L., van Haastregt, J., et al. (1998) Transmural care of terminal cancer patients: Effects on the quality of life of direct caregivers. *Nursing Research, 47*(3), 129–136. An example of a quasi-experimental design testing the hypothesis that transmural care may lead to a better quality of life for the direct caregivers of cancer patients.

Survey Designs

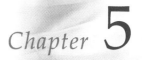

A **survey design** is one in which a researcher collects information from respondents on some topic at *one point in time.* It is similar to a snapshot of the phenomenon under investigation. Unlike an experiment, which involves some *treatment* and includes measures both before and after the treatment, survey designs do not include an experimental manipulation. Instead, surveys measure many variables, and statistical techniques are used to make inferences about causal relations among variables. A survey design is similar to the pre-experimental *exposed or comparison group* design reviewed in the Chapter 4. Much nursing research falls into this category.

The most common forms of the survey design include censuses, polls, and a whole range of situations in which respondents are asked to provide answers to a set of fixed questions. A survey design is generally used to collect data from large, representative samples on the prevalence, distribution, and interrelationships of variables within the sample. The variables of interest can be classified as knowledge, attitudes, attributes, opinions, or behaviors. Survey data are typically collected by means of questionnaires or interviews. Examples of survey topics include lifestyle practices of middle-aged adults, health-care services accessed by disadvantaged women, nutrition practices of female adolescents, factors influencing public opinion on euthanasia, health-care needs of clients with AIDS, attitudes of high school students toward abortion, and family planning practices in low-income communities, to name a few.

Survey designs are sometimes used to do comparative studies between countries or other groupings, and these generally rely on *secondary data* (these are data collected by other researchers). But because the techniques used to analyze such data are modeled after survey research, they are discussed in this chapter. In addition, *meta-analysis* researchers, who review the findings of many researchers on some topic, frequently use survey analytical techniques; therefore, this category of research is also included in this chapter.

A. A SHORT HISTORY OF THE SURVEY

Surveys have been around for a long time—there are biblical references to the counts of the children of Israel, and censuses were taken of the population of ancient Egypt. However, Charles Booth, who conducted three major surveys, laid the foundation for the modern survey in 19th century England. Booth was concerned with providing an accurate count and description of poor people living in London. He was the first to work out operational definitions (the indicators he used to measure poverty); the first to draw color maps to reflect the social characteristics of an area; and the first to attempt to show how variables were related to one another, thus beginning efforts to understand the association between social variables.

More recently, survey research developed in this century partly through the efforts of pioneer pollsters George Gallup and Elmo Roper to provide an accurate profile of Americans, partly from efforts of market researchers to understand consumer behavior better, and partly from the interests of journalists, government agencies, and political organizations, all of whom understood the advantages that could be gained if one could accurately gauge public opinion. Survey research was just too powerful a tool to be left to scholars alone.

During the post–World War II era, Samuel A. Stouffer and Paul F. Lazarsfeld did much to make survey research a legitimate academic and practical pursuit. *The People's Choice* (Lazarsfeld, Berelson, and Gaudet, 1948) was a sophisticated analysis of voting intentions and behavior. It was the first study to interview members of a panel several times leading up to an election. *The People's Choice* marks the beginning of voting studies in political science and was the first study to take control variables into account systematically.

From the 1950s onward, survey research became a key approach in nursing and several social science disciplines. Many universities support survey research centers. These centers typically offer consulting services and coordinate surveys being conducted by university scholars. They are excellent resources for professionals, community groups, and beginning researchers who need assistance with aspects of survey design.

In the new millennium, survey designs will remain particularly important to social, health, and nursing research investigations because they can economically provide a wealth of surprisingly accurate data on a wide range of phenomena important to professionals working in these areas. Currently, academic researchers in many disciplines, including psychology, political science, sociology, education, and business, also commonly use surveys. Public opinion pollsters, community groups, and professionals doing evaluations of applied programs all make frequent use of survey methods.

This chapter discusses the major types of surveys and provides practical guidelines for using them. Let us first examine the rationale for surveys to see how it contrasts with that of experiments.

B. THE RATIONALE FOR SURVEYS

Survey designs often involve collecting information to describe, compare, or explain knowledge, attitudes, attributes, or behaviors. To do so, researchers frequently have respondents complete a questionnaire. A **questionnaire** is made up of a series of set questions and either provides a space for an answer or offers a number of fixed alternatives from which the respondent makes a choice. Questionnaires can be completed in group settings, mailed to respondents, or read to respondents by interviewers, either over the phone or in person.

As indicated in Chapter 1, surveys are typically associated with the positivist approach to knowledge. But it is to be noted that both Marx and Weber used surveys. Marx developed a questionnaire to measure French worker experiences (using the conflict approach; cited in Bottomore, 1988), and Weber surveyed attitudes toward work (using the interpretive approach).

Surveys can be a relatively inexpensive method of collecting much information from a large number of people. Survey researchers frequently draw a sample to make estimations about some population. As used by researchers, the term **population** refers to a collection of individuals, communities, or nations about which one wishes to make a general statement. To save time and money, the researcher draws a **sample** from the population, which is interpreted to represent the population. Although including the whole population could prove to be more accurate (as in a census), the costs may be prohibitive. If a researcher wishes to make extrapolations from a sample to a larger population, then a fairly large sample is required; therefore, it is likely that a survey design will be used. Because human behavior is often highly complex and subject to the simultaneous impact of many variables, a research strategy that measures many variables simultaneously is often appropriate.

1. Appropriateness of Surveys

Surveys are appropriate for descriptive and correlational studies. Unlike experiments, in which researchers are interested in demonstrating a link between a treatment and an outcome of that treatment, the survey presents a picture of events, people, and phenomena as respondents report them. Thus, in a survey, a researcher explores the prevalence and interrelationships among variables in a population without introducing a treatment variable. This is again in contrast to experiments, in which researchers introduce a treatment variable (e.g., a low-fat diet versus a high-fat diet) that is manipulated and then measure its effect on another variable (serum cholesterol level). Notice that the same research question, on the relationship between a low-fat diet and serum cholesterol levels, can be studied using a survey. Such a survey may include a large number of participants who already consume a low-fat diet and a similar number from a population known to consume foods high in fat content. Results of data analysis may indicate that those who consume foods high in fat content have a higher serum cholesterol level than those who consume low-fat diets. In this situation, the researcher did not introduce participants to a low-fat diet or manipulate the amount of daily fat intake; the researcher simply investigated the relationship that occurred after fat was consumed. This type of survey is known as a **retrospective** or **ex post facto study,** meaning that "after the fact," the researcher attempts to link present events (serum cholesterol) to past events (amount of fat in diet).

2. Validity of Surveys

With both experimental and survey designs, there can be difficulty in establishing the validity of the measures used. In the case of surveys, respondents are asked to report their own attitudes, behavior, and backgrounds. Some of the data requested require respondents to recall episodes from their pasts (e.g., "How anxious were you when you were first diagnosed?") And because questionnaires probe into sensitive areas, they permit respondents to manage their responses so they can appear in a favorable light. Suppose one was attempting to measure attitudes toward minorities. In such cases, one has to understand that some people may try to appear tolerant—perhaps more tolerant than they actually are. There is not a one-to-one relationship between what people say they believe and how they actually behave when confronted with real situations. For example, adolescents who are concerned about public perceptions or negative consequences of behavior may underestimate their engagement in unhealthy lifestyle practices such as consumption of alcohol or drug products, or conversely, overestimate their engagement in healthy practices on surveys to make a favorable impression.

An initial field study conducted by Richard T. LaPiere (1934) highlights the discrepancy between what people say and what they do. In his classic work, he showed that only one overnight lodging establishment out of 251 directly refused accommodations to a Chinese couple. Yet when LaPiere asked the same businesses some 6 months later in a mailed questionnaire whether or not they would accept as guests members who were Chinese, only one business indicated that it would. Deutscher (1966) also reminds us that the relationship between attitudes expressed on a questionnaire and subsequent behavior can be problematical (Box 5.1). Sometimes there may be little relation between the two. This is an important point for nurses and other health professionals to consider if they are depending on the results of survey data to guide program planning, design, and evaluation.

Nonetheless, questionnaires can produce reliable and valid responses on many issues. And if one wishes to measure attitudes, there is no good alterna-

BOX 5.1 *Irwin Deutscher: Words and Deeds*

Deutscher argues that much of our work as scientists has to do with predicting behavior. However, the predictions we make are derived from responses interviewed people have made or from answers prompted by questionnaire items. The key issue is the extent to which we can rely on such responses to accurately reflect behavior.

In his review of the relationship between attitudes and behavior, Deutscher identifies considerable evidence that frequently shows an inverse relationship between the two. Deutscher notes that:

. . . this discrepancy between what people say and what they do is not limited to the area of racial or ethnic relations: it has been observed that trade union members talk one game and play another, that there is no relationship between college students' attitudes toward cheating and their actual cheating behavior, that urban teachers' descriptions of classroom behavior are sometimes unrelated to the way teachers behave in the classroom, that what rural Missourians say about their health behavior has little connection with their actual health practices, and that the moral and ethical beliefs of students do not conform to their behavior (Deutscher, 1966:246).

SOURCE: Deutscher, I. (1966). Words and deeds: social science and social policy. *Social Problems,* 13,235-254. Cited with permission.

tive to asking people about them. One simply has to live with the problems of measurement if the variables are to be measured at all. According to conventional wisdom, survey designs are considered **cross-sectional** studies in that they provide *point-in-time data* and are therefore poor at measuring changes over time. Although it is no doubt risky to assume that people will recall their past reliably, most questionnaires include items about a variety of points in time, such as the year of the respondent's birth, the type of community the respondent grew up in, or how old the respondent was when getting his or her first full-time job. Once again, although problems do exist with recall data, sometimes there is no practical alternative for measuring some variables.

Questionnaires are restrictive because they can only be used with a literate population. The wording of questions must be straightforward so that all—or at least most—of the respondents are able to handle the language. Also, the requirement that all respondents be able to understand the questions prevents certain areas from being probed in depth. Everyone is given the same set of questions, and although it is advantageous to have all respondents reply to the same question, it does mean that interesting responses cannot be pursued. For in-depth probes, a personal interview is necessary.

Students frequently conduct surveys. Box 5.2 lists some recent studies completed by nursing and sociology students under the supervision of the authors of this text. As can be seen by the titles of the projects, many topics can be addressed. The questionnaires were designed and the data collected in consultation with the instructor. Many of these questionnaires may be seen by checking the Web site *http://www.stfx.ca/people/wjackson.* By clicking on *Questionnaires,* some 160 project questionnaires may be viewed. Appendix B includes a questionnaire designed by nursing students.

This chapter provides a general orientation to survey research. Anyone who wishes to know how to carry out a survey needs to consult two additional chapters in the book: Chapter 14 provides guidelines for developing a questionnaire, and Chapter 15 discusses how one goes about selecting a sample and determining how large it should be.

BOX 5.2 *Student Surveys*

The following is a list of recently completed surveys conducted by sociology or nursing students. Each project was designed by a research team in consultation with the instructor in a research methods course. The student who submitted the best paper in the research team is identified as the author. Copies of the questionnaires may be viewed at the Web site *http//www.stfx.ca/people/wjackson*. Click on *Questionnaires.*

Project	Author
Premarital Sex Among University Students	Michelle Chisholm (1999)
Contraceptive Usage Among Males	Andrea Brophy (1999)
The Effect of Program of Study on Health Seeking Behaviors	Christina Vanhorn (1999)
Attitudes Toward Voluntary Active Euthanasia and Physician-Assisted Suicide: Are Nursing Students Supportive of These Practices?	Donna Beiswanger and Cathy Richard (1999)
Experiences of Sexual Harassment Among Females Living on Campus	Jan Murray (1999)
The Self-Acceptance of Homosexuality	Michelle Murray (1999)
Occupational Ranking: Prestige and Cultural Diffusion	Ray MacIssac (1999)
The Consequences of Shiftwork: Physical, Psychological, Social, and Economic	Michelle Chisholm (1998)
Health Promoting Behaviors at St. Francis Xavier University	Sarah LeBlanc (1998)
Alcohol Consumption of University Students	Alison Fisher (1998)
Attitudes Toward Women in Competitive Sports	Alanna MacNeil (1998)
The Punitiveness of Students at St. Francis Xavier University	Kristine Cameron (1998)
The Trends and Variations in Smoking	Amy Gillis (1998)
Illegal Drug Use Among Young Adults within a University Setting	Wendy Chisholm (1998)
Eating Disorders	Linda Jane Liutkus (1998)

continued on next page

BOX 5.2 Student Surveys (Continued)

Project	Author
Nurses' Attitudes Toward Student Nurses	Shauna M. Grant (1997)
Students' Attitudes Toward Campus Health Care Facilities	Tanya M. LeBlanc (1997)
Homesickness Among First-Year University Students	Elsa Arbuthnot and Laura Rogal-Black (1997)
Illegal Drug Use at University	Tracey Pye (1996)
Perception of Risk of Sexual Assault Among Freshman Women at St. F. X. University	Alicia Van De Sande (1996)
Suicidal Ideation on Campus	Laurie Fraser (1996)
Attitudes Toward Euthanasia	Tracey MacMillan (1996)
The Effects of Gender on Self-Esteem	Kathleen Lumsden (1996)

C. STEPS IN SURVEY RESEARCH

There are various types of survey research. The main differences are determined by how the data are collected. The range may include face-to-face interviews; phone interviews; individually delivered, group, or **mailed questionnaires**; and secondary data studies. Regardless of the data collection method used, the steps in survey research are the same. Wilson (1993) outlines a simple series of steps to follow in survey design.

1. Formulate the research question.
2. Determine that the survey is the appropriate design to address the research question.
3. Select the type of survey to be used (e.g., interview, questionnaire, phone survey).
4. Translate the objectives of the survey into categories of questions or items (see Chapter 14).
5. Identify the population of participants or settings (see Chapter 15).
6. Develop sampling procedures to select a representative and appropriately sized sample (see Chapter 15).
7. Design data collection procedures.
8. Plan for data analysis (see Chapter 16).
9. Pilot test the approaches to data collection and data analysis procedures.
10. Modify the procedures as necessary.
11. Collect and analyze the data (see Chapters 16, 17, and 18).
12. Write descriptive, comparative, or evaluative findings and draw conclusions (see Chapter 19).

D. GUIDELINES FOR THE ADMINISTRATION OF SURVEY QUESTIONNAIRES

In this section, general rules are provided for administering questionnaires in a variety of ways. In all cases, the suggestions should be used with common sense because there are times when they should be violated. A summary account of a nursing survey study is provided in Box 5.3 and comments on the application of administration guidelines as they relate to this study are noted.

Permissions from parents, school administrators, and ethics review committees are typically required in order to distribute questionnaires; researchers need to take this fact into account in planning surveys. Pursuing permissions takes time and usually requires a statement of the problem under investigation and a copy of the proposed questionnaire. Researchers must plan for extra time.

1. General Rules for the Administration of Questionnaires

The following rules are intended to increase response rates for all types of surveys. Later sections suggest approaches for particular types of surveys.

Rule 1. Establish legitimacy. Establish the legitimacy of the research by noting who is sponsoring it, describing why it is being done, and presenting it in such a way as to make it seem credible and competent. The cover letter and the questionnaire must look professional.

Rule 2. Keep it simple. Keep questionnaires, interview guides, and phone interviews as simple and as nonthreatening as possible. Questionnaires should be easy to respond to and should avoid asking questions that pry unnecessarily into the respondent's personal affairs. (Chapter 14 provides additional ideas for making questionnaires easy to complete.)

Rule 3. Provide a report to the respondent. When individuals are to be interviewed more than once during the course of a study (as in a *panel study*), report findings to respondents. In all cases in which a report has been promised to the respondents, it must be provided; otherwise, the researcher makes it less likely that the respondents will cooperate in the future.

Rule 4. Pay respondents. When reasonable and financially possible, pay respondents for their time and cooperation. The fee helps establish the legitimacy of the study as well as a reciprocal relationship with the respondent. Such payments appear to have a modest impact on the willingness of respondents to participate (Heberlein and Baumgartner, 1978). Payments help establish reciprocity between researchers and respondents and help to avoid the respondents' perception that they have been "ripped off" for their data.

Rule 5. Do not pressure respondents to participate. Although researchers have powerful interests in getting everyone selected to complete the survey, it must be indicated that although cooperation in completing the questionnaire or interview is appreciated, it is, nonetheless, optional. Particularly in face-to-face encounters, unintended pressure may be placed on individuals to participate in the study. In the case of questionnaires administered to a gathering of individuals, there may be considerable informal pressure from peers in the room to complete the survey. Researchers must exercise self-discipline and avoid putting undue pressure on individuals in an attempt to coax participation. (See the discussion on research ethics in Chapter 10.)

Rule 6. Do not reveal research hypotheses to those involved in a study. Generally, it is not advisable to inform respondents, interviewers, or data collection assistants about the hypotheses of the study. Interviewer expectancy bias (see Chapter 9) may be reduced if the hypotheses are not known. Respondents who are made aware of the research hypothesis may also try to help the researcher by

BOX 5.3 *Nurse Researchers at Work*

WILL EVIDENCE-BASED NURSING PRACTICE MAKE PRACTICE PERFECT?

Little is known about the kinds of evidence that nurses use in their practice. This study explores the sources and types of knowledge on which nurses base clinical decisions. Important discoveries are revealed about both the nature and structure of nursing knowledge as it is applied in practice. This information is important to the profession as it strives to adopt evidence-based nursing (EBN), and base decisions on empirical evidence.

The Alberta Association of Registered Nurses (AARN) membership list was used to draw a random sample of 1500 nurses for a cross-sectional mail survey. All participants were required to be actively engaged in the delivery of nursing care. Following initial receipt of the survey instrument reminders were mailed at approximately 3, 6, and 9 weeks. With the six-week reminder a replacement questionnaire was included. The final sample consisted of 600 (40%) questionnaires. The sample of nurses was representative of the population from which it was drawn based on a comparison of it with demographic data about nurses in Alberta.

The 16-item survey questionnaire developed for this investigation was adapted from the 12-item Research Utilization Questionnaire (Baessler et al., 1994). The 16 questions began with the transition statement: "The following questions relate to the kind of knowledge you use in your nursing practice." A pilot study was conducted on a convenience sample of 23 postbaccalaureate and master's level nursing students.

Mean scores were reported for each item and scores were ordered from most to least frequent. Results indicated that the two most frequently used knowledge sources were experiential followed by nursing school, workplace sources, physician sources, intuitions, and what has worked in the past. Literature, either in textbook form or journal articles, was found in the bottom five for frequency.

This survey study has important implications for nursing. First, it suggests that nurses use a broad range of practice knowledge, much of which is experientially based rather than research based. Secondly, we can infer that traditional scientific journals are not very effective as dissemination vehicles. A third issue is that basic nursing education continues to play an important ongoing role as a source of practice knowledge for nurses.

Comments on Mailed Questionnaire

1. This survey provided a relatively cheap way of contacting a large number of nurses.
2. A cover letter was included to explain the survey to the respondents.
3. The survey topic was likely to be salient and of interest to the participants.
4. The questionnaire was brief, easy to respond to, and professionally presented.
5. Additional contacts were made by the researcher with the participants at 3, 6, and 9 weeks after the original mailing to increase the response rate.
6. A replacement questionnaire was included at week 6 to nonrespondents.
7. A 40% response rate was achieved and the researcher noted that a comparison of the sample with the total population of 15,000 nurses on major demographic and related variables suggests that the sample was representative of the population from which it was drawn.

SOURCE: Summarized from Estabrooks, C.A. (1998). Will Evidence-Based Nursing Practice Make Practice Perfect? *Canadian Journal of Nursing Research, 30*(1), 15–36.

skewing their responses in a direction to favor the hypothesis. Respondents have the right to know why the study is being done and who is sponsoring it.

Rule 7. Do quality control spot checks. It is critical to do spot checks to ensure that administrative procedures are being followed. Research directors are sometimes negligent on this point. Conducting interviews and handing out questionnaires is not many people's idea of fun. Research assistants occasionally cut corners; these range from ignoring the random sampling procedures that should be used to select which person in a household is to complete the questionnaire to inventing respondents and their answers. Checks can be run on the representativeness of the sample (to see how well the respondents and their answers match known characteristics of the target population) or to see if the person who was supposed to have been interviewed actually was. However, by the time checks are run, field research funds may be expended and you may not be able to redo the work. And if any data have been falsified, it will take a lot of time to distinguish the genuine data from the bad. Be cautious of interviewers who are doing much more than other interviewers. Watch out for systematic differences in response rates to sensitive questions. Sometimes, for example, interviewers are too embarrassed to ask about someone's income, so they preface their question by saying, "You don't have to answer this one if you don't want to, but could you tell us your family income last year?" By giving this cue to the respondent, it is easier for the respondent to say, "I'd rather not answer that." So, if an individual interviewer is missing data more often than other interviewers, try to go through the part of the questionnaire affected to see if

the presentation can be improved. The quality of one's research can be no better than the quality of the data collected. Monitor the process carefully.

As previously discussed, there are many variants of the survey, but only the major approaches are explored here. Each method has a distinctive set of advantages and disadvantages, as well as rules that apply to its administration. Let us begin with the questionnaire that is personally handed to a respondent.

2. Individually Delivered Questionnaires

Individually delivered questionnaires are delivered to a respondent by a researcher. A brief explanation is offered, questions are answered, and arrangements are made for the return of the completed questionnaire. This method of handing out questionnaires is typically used in community surveys in which the form is dropped off at selected houses, in college dormitories, where questionnaires are handed to selected respondents (usually the researcher tries to obtain a systematic sample of campus dormitory rooms), and in studies of organizations (e.g., surveys of hospital staff, university faculty, or employees of a private firm) in which the target respondents are approached individually.

In cases in which a survey of a systematic sample of patients in a hospital is being conducted, care should be taken to provide everyone with an equal chance of participating in the survey if there is a mixture of single and double rooms. This means that, in the case of double rooms, both patients should be asked to complete the questionnaire. In this way, all patients have an equal chance of being selected to participate in the survey. (In this case, rooms are the units being selected. See more details on the systematic sampling procedure in Chapter 15.)

a. Rules for Individually Delivered Questionnaires

In addition to the general rules for conducting surveys (see previous section), there are some rules that should be considered in situations where respondents are approached on a one-to-one basis.

Rule 1. Make personal contact with the respondent. When feasible, contact respondents in person to explain the survey and let them know when you will pick up the completed form. In a door-to-door survey, it should be possible to get more than 80 percent to agree to complete the form. Avoid having third parties handing out your questionnaires; a member of the research team can better explain the survey and answer questions that might be raised. In particular, avoid having teachers, workers' supervisors, or coworkers hand out questionnaires. The extra effort needed to have a member of the research team hand out the questionnaires avoids many problems associated with a third-party delivery. In short, *the greater the personal contact, the greater the response rate.*

Rule 2. Avoid mailed and drop-box return methods. When possible, avoid mailed returns or having respondents drop their completed questionnaires into a box in a dormitory, staff office, or other convenient spot. If at all possible, the researcher should pick up completed forms at a time agreed to with the respondent. Such arrangements encourage respondents to complete the forms by the prearranged time. Do not be tempted to violate this rule; if you do, you will pay a heavy price in lost and missing questionnaires.

Rule 3. Record place and time information. It is critical to record where questionnaires have been dropped off and when they are to be picked up. Pick up the questionnaire on time; respondents will be annoyed if it is not picked up. A form for recording this information should be developed and then used faithfully (Table 5.1). Besides information regarding place and time, the form should also have space to list dates when an attempt was made to contact the individual and to record times when it would be convenient to return to meet the person. After the data have been collected, these sheets will prove invaluable in calculating the response rate to the survey and in identifying the problems that were encountered.

Rule 4. Provide envelopes to help maintain privacy. Generally it is a good idea to provide respondents with an envelope into which they can seal their completed questionnaires. Sometimes questionnaires are left around waiting to be picked up, and unwanted eyes may peruse the responses. A sealed envelope foils most snoopers. In introducing the survey to the respondent, the researcher can indicate that the envelope is a means of protecting the anonymity of the respondent. This makes respondents feel safe.

Rule 5. Use a slotted return box. To help convey the sense of anonymity, it is a good idea to use a box with a slot cut in one end (a box measuring 9" × 12" is a good size), and respondents' questionnaires can be slipped into the box as they are returned. In especially sensitive studies, this return procedure can be pointed out when the questionnaire is delivered to the respondent.

3. Group-administered Questionnaires

Group-administered questionnaires almost always have good response rates.

Table 5.1   Sample Drop-Off Form

#	Address	Try 1 Date	Try 2 Date	Try 3 Date	Pick Date	Pick Time	Done	Notes
1								
2								
3								
4								
5								
6								
7								
8								
9								
10								
11								
12								
13								
14								
15								
16								
17								
18								
19								
20								

This form of administration involves handing out questionnaires to an assemblage of persons—be it a class, at a public meeting, or any other setting where people can be asked simultaneously to complete a questionnaire. There is considerable informal pressure (from peers in the room) to cooperate with the researcher and, normally, between 90 and 100 percent of potential respondents will complete questionnaires in group settings.

One caution when using group-administered questionnaires is that typically probability sampling procedures (see Chapter 15) are not used and, therefore, the data collected cannot be used to extrapolate to some larger population. What this means is that the groups selected are usually done on the basis of convenience; they cannot be taken as representative of some larger population.

a. Rules for Group-administered Questionnaires

In addition to the general rules for the administration of surveys, there are some rules that apply to situations in which a researcher distributes questionnaires to an assembled group.

Rule 1. Indicate the voluntary nature of survey. Researchers should acknowledge this informal pressure and be sure to inform the potential respondents of their complete freedom to refuse to answer any or all questions; participation is voluntary. The person administering the questionnaire can briefly explain what it is about and be available to answer any questions that may be raised.

Rule 2. Arrange well in advance. It is frequently necessary to gain permission from the person in charge of the group meeting to have a questionnaire administered, so it is a good idea to make arrangements well in advance. And just before the questionnaire is to be administered, it is also a good idea to remind the person concerned that you will be coming.

Rule 3. Explain the survey to those present. The researchers should explain who is doing the research and why it is being done, and respondents should be encouraged to ask any questions about the survey in general or about particular questions.

Rule 4. Administer the questionnaire at the end of the session. For practical reasons, it is usually best to administer questionnaires at the end of a meeting, group session, or class, rather than at the beginning. If, for example, one goes into a classroom with a questionnaire at the beginning of a class, problems will arise because not all the students will finish at the same time. Hence, from the teacher's point of view, valuable class time will be wasted as the researcher waits for the last forms to be completed. Similarly, at a meeting, avoid handing out a questionnaire before the meeting begins; administer it at the end, or before a break during the meeting. This allows people who work at different speeds to complete the questionnaire without feeling rushed. However, administering a questionnaire at the end of a meeting or class probably loses a little in terms of the quality of replies. At the end of sessions, respondents may be tired or bored and wish to leave as soon as possible. But, given the researcher's desire to maintain cordial relations with those giving permission to administer the questionnaires, it is generally less disruptive to administer them at the end of the session.

Rule 5. Take steps to identify bad questionnaires. One hazard to watch out for is that a few within the room may decide to make a joke of the questionnaire and start making silly responses. This happens rarely, but watch out for such responses. Normally any questionnaires that appear not to have been taken seriously are reviewed by the research team and withdrawn if judged to be frivolous.

4. Mailed Questionnaires

Although researchers try to avoid doing so, often there is no choice but to use the mail system. Long-distance phone interviews may be too expensive and travel costs would quickly eat up a research budget if the researcher attempted to deliver the questionnaires by hand.

Mail surveys are popular because they provide a relatively cheap way of contacting a large number of respondents. And despite the reputation mail surveys have for producing low *response rates,* it is possible to have the majority of questionnaires returned. The **response rate** measures the percentage of delivered questionnaires that are returned. In mail surveys, we normally deduct from the total number of questionnaires sent out the number that are returned because of an incorrect address. In other words, the number of delivered questionnaires is equal to the number sent out minus the number returned as undeliverable.

Because our major concern with the mail survey is the response rate, we will consider the factors that influence whether a questionnaire will be returned. John Goyder has done extensive work in examining survey research response rates. Using a regression-based method of analysis (see Chapter 18), he developed a nine-variable model for predicting final response rate

(Goyder, 1982, 1985a, 1985b; Goyder and Leiper, 1985c; Box 5.4). Two factors are involved: those largely beyond the control of the researcher and those the researcher can control.

a. Factors Beyond the Control of the Researcher

These factors are of interest in trying to predict the likely response rate to a mailed questionnaire. The type of respondent receiving the questionnaire is important; as Heberlein and Baumgartner have noted (1978), students, employees, and military personnel are more inclined to return a mailed questionnaire than are members of the general public. The type of sponsoring agency also has an impact that favors government-sponsored research over market research. (Perhaps the response rates in government-sponsored projects are higher because some citizens may believe that they are legally required to participate in the same way that they are required to participate in the census.) Finally, we need to consider the **salience of the topic** to the respondent; subjects that are important to the respondent are more likely to produce a positive response than those of less importance to the respondent.

b. Factors Under the Control of the Researcher

Although the quality of the questionnaire is not identified as a factor in the Goyder model, it should be noted that his research group was examining published studies that had passed various reviews before publication, so it would be reasonable to assume that all were highly professional. Common sense dictates that every effort be made to make the questionnaire look as professional as possible. For the convenience of the respondent, include a stamped return envelope. A cover letter should be included that explains the survey to the respondents. The legitimacy of the survey is enhanced if the questionnaire is well presented, the sponsoring agency identified, and the worthiness of the research established.

Among the variables examined, the evidence indicates that monetary incentives do increase response rates. Follow-up contacts in the form of letters, postcard reminders, registered mail, and long-distance phone calls all enhance the likelihood of a positive response. However, with each contact, one can expect slightly reduced effectiveness. Registered mail and long-distance phone calls seem to impress on respondents the importance of the study and their role in it; using these approaches pays off well in increased participation. One of the follow-up contacts should contain a replacement copy of the questionnaire in case the first one has been misplaced. Although follow-up contacts are worthwhile, one must always be careful not to harass potential respondents.

Given the many factors involved, it is difficult to estimate a response rate with precision before the survey is undertaken. However, a first-round response rate of about 50 percent should be considered good; three follow-up contacts can be expected to increase the response rate to about 75 percent. Any response rate above 75 percent should be considered excellent. In Canada, one can expect somewhat lower response rates (Eichner and Habermehl, 1981; Goyder, 1982). Goyder has suggested that there may well be cultural factors working to lower response rates to mail questionnaires in Canada. His research indicates that in Canadian studies, researchers should anticipate a response rate about 7 percent lower than is likely in the United States (Goyder, 1982, 1985a).

It is useful for the researcher to estimate response rates by using Goyder's formula presented in Box 5.4. To illustrate

BOX 5.4 Eight-Variable Model for Estimating Response Rate to a Mailed Questionnaire or Interviews

John Goyder and his associates identified factors that influence response rates to mailed questionnaires or interviews. His work is useful to anyone planning to do interviews or a mailed survey to calculate an estimated response rate (ERR). This box will provide you with the steps necessary to do the estimation for the example in the textbook. A worksheet is provided in Box 5.5 to do the calculation for the study you propose.

Response Rate Factors	(A) Coefficient	(B) Scoring	(A) × (B) = (C) Total
Constant	1.146	1	1.146
Post-1970 field work (constant)	−0.059	1.000	−0.059
a. Data collection mode (0,1)	−0.349	0	0.000
b. Number of contacts (logged)	0.856	0.477	0.408
c. Salience of topic (0,1,2)	0.272	1.000	0.272
d. Special third contact (0,1,2,3)	0.130	1.000	0.130
e. Incentive (0,1,2,3,4)	0.148	0.000	0.000
f. Type of sponsor (0,1)	0.260	0.000	0.000
g. Population type (0,1)	−0.099	0.000	0.000
Total			1.897

Steps in Completing the worksheet.

Step 1. For the proposed study, assign a scoring value for points a through g; using the following guide, enter the score in column B.

a. Data collection mode: **0** = mailed questionnaire; 1 = interview
b. Log value of number of contacts, where 1 = 0.000; 2 = 0.301; 3 = **0.477**; 4= 0.602 (be sure to include your initial contact as part of the total number)
c. Salience, where 0 = not salient; **1** = possibly salient; 2 = salient
d. Special third contacts, where 0 = none; **1** = regular mail; 2 = special mail; 3 = telephone or personal contact
e. Incentive, where **0** = none; 1 = less than 25¢; 2 = 25¢; 3 = 50¢; 4 = $1.00 or more

f. Type of sponsor, where **0** = nongovernmental; 1 = government
g. Population type, where **0** = special subgroup 1 = general population

Step 2. For each row, multiply Coefficient (A) by Score Value (B), enter result in Total Column (C). Note that the first two rows are already entered; treat these as constants but include them in your calculations.

Step 3. Add the values in column (C).

Step 4. To calculate the Estimated Response Rate (ERR), use the following equation (Goyder, 1985c: 58): TOTAL = 2 arcsine ($\sqrt{\text{ERR}}$), where TOTAL is the total value calculated by summing the values in the table above. (In the case of our example, the value is 1.897.)

continued on next page

BOX 5.4 *Eight-Variable Model for Estimating Response Rate to a Mailed Questionnaire or Interviews (Continued)*

Step 5. Using a *scientific calculator* do the following calculations:

Notes:*	
1. TOTAL = 2 arcsine $(\sqrt{\text{ERR}})$	Goyder formula
2. $1.897 = 2$ arcsine $(\sqrt{\text{ERR}})$	Use value calculated above (1.897)
3. $\dfrac{1.897}{2} =$ arcsine $(\sqrt{\text{ERR}})$	Divide by 2
4. $0.9485 =$ arcsine $(\sqrt{\text{ERR}})$	To get rid of arcsine, take sin of value (use calculator radian mode)
5. $\sin(0.9485) = \sqrt{\text{ERR}}$	
6. $0.8125 = \sqrt{\text{ERR}}$	Square both sides
7. $0.66 = \text{ERR}$	66% expected to respond

Step 6. After the ERR is calculated, decide if you need to alter procedures to increase the expected response rate. To do so, examine the Goyder coefficients to decide which procedures would be most feasible in your case.

---

*The use of the arcsine in computing the response rate prevents the predicted response rate from exceeding 100 percent. This can be problematic if steps are not taken to take into account the diminishing returns of additional contacts with respondents. Heberlein and Baumgartner (1978) regression estimate of response rate, for example, can lead to estimates of returns of over 100 percent.
SOURCE: Adapted from John C. Goyder (1985b). Face-to-face interviews and mailed questionnaires: The net difference in response rate. *Public Opinion Quarterly, 49,* 234–252.

the use of Goyder's formula, suppose a study is designed to survey graduates of a university nursing program to determine their job experiences since graduation. The survey is sponsored by the university school of nursing, the subject is regarded as "possibly salient" to the respondents, and two follow-up contacts are planned. In this case, we estimate the response rate by simply plugging in the values presented. The predicted response rate is shown in Box 5.4.

Meeting the predicted response rate should be considered an excellent result. To be within 20 percent of the predicted response rate should be considered acceptable. If the researcher thinks that the estimated response rate will be insufficient, then additional steps should be taken to increase the likelihood of a response. An examination of the last column of Box 5.4 suggests that the most important factors in determining response rate include:

- The number of contacts the researcher has with the respondents
- The importance of the subject matter to the respondent
- Special third contacts such as phone calls or special delivery letters
- The use of a monetary incentive

One might wish to consider trying to make the questionnaire more salient for the respondents, using phone call follow-ups, or include a 25-cent coin as a token of appreciation. Although many researchers would feel uneasy (the authors included) about sending money to try to encourage a positive response because some potential respondents would be insulted by the gesture, it would, nonetheless, probably be effective in increasing the response rate. It has been shown, for example, that the use of incentives as small as ten cents increase the response rate. For example, in one classic study of top corporate executives, 40 percent of those receiving no incentive responded and 54 percent of those receiving 10 cents responded. However, among those who received a 25-cent piece, 63 percent returned their questionnaires (Erdos, 1983). Would you have guessed this result if you knew that the value of the token sent was all that differentiated the various surveys and that the respondents were among the highest-paid executives in North America?

c. Tips for Increasing Response Rate

Assuming that the questionnaire looks professional and that the appropriate cover letter is included, the following tips are suggested as methods for increasing the likelihood of response to a mailed questionnaire:

1. The envelope should identify the sponsoring organization's name. By identifying the sponsor, an effort is made to increase the perceived legitimacy of the project.
2. The name should be typed or even handwritten using the full name, rather than initials.
3. The mailing should be sent by first class mail and should use stamps rather than metered postage. The idea is to make the package seem as personal as possi-

ble. Avoid the mass produced look; do not use mailing labels.
4. A stamped envelope for the return of the completed questionnaire should be enclosed with the original material.
5. If the questionnaires are to have identification codes placed on them, place them on the top right-hand corner of the first page and indicate in the accompanying letter that the number is there to assist in following up on respondents who have not returned the questionnaire. Do not use secret codes.
6. If an incentive is being used, use new currency enclosed in plastic envelopes.
7. You can follow up by sending a postcard, thanking respondents if they have returned the questionnaire, and reminding them that returning the form would be much appreciated if this has not already been done.
8. A second follow-up, including a copy of the questionnaire, may be sent 3 weeks after the original has been mailed.
9. A third follow-up after 6 or 7 weeks, using either registered mail or a phone call, is worthwhile and increases the response rate. Most researchers do not go beyond the third follow-up.

Generally, returns will be quick at first and then slow down. After 1 week, expect to receive about 30 percent of all the questionnaires that will be returned, and expect to receive about 85 percent within 2 weeks. By the end of 4 weeks, about 96 percent of the questionnaires that will be returned will have arrived (Erdos, 1983; Jackson, 1999).

Box 5.3 reports on a study by Estabrooks (1998) that used a mailed survey to collect information from nurses in Alberta, Canada, on the use of evidence-based decision making. The survey achieved a 40 percent response rate (600 out of 1500 returned the questionnaire), and the results indicated that in this random sample, nursing practice was informed more by experience than by research-based knowledge.

BOX 5.5 *Worksheet for Estimating Response Rates for Mailed Questionnaires and Interviews.*

The following worksheet may be used to do the calculations to estimate the response rate for mailed questionnaires or interviews. To deter- mine the scoring for each of your proposed approaches, see Box 5.4.

Response Rate Factors	(A) Cofficient	(B) Scoring	(A) × (B) = (C) Total
Constant	1.146	1.000	1.146
Post-1970 field work (constant)	−0.059	1.000	−0.059
a. Data collection mode (0,1)	−0.349		
b. Number of contacts (logged)	0.856		
c. Salience of topic (0,1,2)	0.272		
d. Special third contact (0,1,2,3)	0.130		
e. Incentive (0,1,2,3,4)	0.148		
f. Type of sponsor (0,1)	0.260		
g. Population type (0,1)	−0.099		
TOTAL			

The values for the constant and post-1970 field work should be left as is and included in your calculations. See Box 5.4 for details on calculating the estimated response rate (ERR).

Furthermore, the study indicated that there are problems in how scientific evidence is communicated to practitioners.

5. Phone Surveys

Like all surveys, **phone surveys** rely on information reported by respondents and are therefore vulnerable to image management. Questions and response categories must be kept simple because they are presented verbally. In-depth probes are difficult and, as with other surveys, it is always difficult to make causal inferences. The interviewer's expectations may inadvertently influence the responses that are recorded into the computer. Today most phone interviews use computers to present the questions to the interviewer on the screen as well as the possible response categories into which respondents' answers are to be fitted. Care must be taken, however, to monitor the reliability of interviewers in placing respondent's answers in the categories provided.

a. Advantages and Disadvantages of Phone Surveys

Phone surveys are gaining in popularity. They are widely used by polling organizations and academic and applied researchers, and they represent a technique of data collection that will almost certainly increase in years to come. Phone surveys are a relatively cheap and quick way to collect data. Because no travel time is included, phone interviewers can do many more interviews in a day than would be possible if the interviewer had to travel to each respondent's home. Moreover, phone interviewing can provide cost-effective access to people with whom it is very difficult to arrange interviews (such as physicians) or with those that are not concentrated in one area (such as the blind).

In national studies, it is estimated that phone surveys cost about 45 percent as much as personal interviews (Jackson, 1999). Recently, there has been some troubling news regarding the willingness of people to participate in telephone interviews. In 1993, some 7 out of 10 respondents in the Toronto area refused to cooperate in pre-election polls. If these levels of nonparticipation become widespread, it will be more difficult to justify using the phone for collecting such information (Sheppard, 1993; Fisher, 1993).

But there are disadvantages to phone surveys. First, they are not the best means of gathering data if probing is required or if complex response categories are to be presented. Second, the distribution of phones is uneven. The less well off and the mobile are less likely to have a phone or a phone number listed. However, as phones become more universally available, there is less need to avoid phone surveys on principle as long as researchers recognize the possibility of sample distortions. Indeed, it is possible to weight samples to adjust for underrepresented categories in a survey. Respondents interviewed over the phone are slightly less at ease than respondents being interviewed in person. As a result, phone interviews generally produce slightly higher refusal rates on sensitive issues, such as income or political preference (Jackson, 1999).

Phone interviews also have some special problems related to assessing response rates. It is not always easy to determine how many numbers called are connected to "live" phones; there are a fair number (generally about 20 percent) of phones attached to businesses. Furthermore, phone interviews have lower completion rates than questionnaires; typically, the completion rate does not exceed 70 percent (Jackson, 1999). Studies based on rural populations generally have greater success in phone surveys because lower levels of mobility mean that fewer phones are disconnected.

b. Creating a Sample

In conducting a phone survey, one may work with a list of potential respondents (e.g., a list or from the names listed in the phone book). In such cases, one usually proceeds by using a systematic sampling procedure (see Chapter 15 for this sampling method).

It is also possible to create a sample by identifying the various residential phone exchanges in the area and then using a table of random numbers to determine the numbers to be called. Typically phone numbers are assigned in five-digit blocks, the first three determining the exchange. The numbers might start 863–21xx. A table of random numbers may be used to determine the last two digits to be used. If it is possible to get the information from the phone company, one attempts to find out the percentage of phones in each block and then a sample is drawn to represent each block proportionally (Abrahamson, 1983; Jackson, 1999).

Computer-assisted telephone interviewing is an important tool for polling organizations and market researchers. A computer dials a sample of respondents and then guides the interviewer through the data collection by presenting the questions on the screen and, depending on the response, it proceeds to show the

b. Interview Schedule

Interview schedules outline the major questions that are to be raised. The interviewer has greater autonomy in exploring questions in detail. Interviews require much skill on the part of the interviewer and care must be taken not to "lead" the respondent. Furthermore, the responses are filtered through the interviewer; therefore, if there are a number of interviewers, one must realize that some of the variations in response will be caused by differences between interviewers and not solely by differences between the respondents. Interview schedules are used for in-depth interviews in field studies (see Chapter 7).

c. Advantages and Disadvantages of Interviews

Because interviews are expensive, they are normally done when not too many are required and when in-depth information is needed. One major advantage is that good rapport is often built up between interviewers and respondents so that if repeated interviews are required, as in a panel study, it will be possible to maintain high response rates. A second major advantage of interviews is that they permit the respondents to clarify any questions that they have about the interview. One of the disadvantages is that interview studies are expensive (more than double the cost of phone interviews) and time consuming (Jackson, 1999).

d. Selection and Training of Interviewers

Although it is beyond the scope of this book to discuss the selection and training of interviewers, we will make some brief comments on this subject. Research done by NORC (National Opinion Research Center) indicates that the quality of work done by interviewers is related to the length of time spent working for NORC, high grade point averages in high school, liking two or more science subjects, intelligence, and the completion of college. In addition, those who scored high on "need achievement" and manipulativeness (Machiavellianism scale) are more likely to do well when interviewing. Of note is that happiness, financial need, religious behavior, perfectionism, and size of home community were not found to be related to the quality of interviewing that a person does (Sudman, 1967; Jackson, 1999).

Interviewers need to be trained. They need to gain knowledge about ethical issues, the survey being conducted, appropriate dress, how to introduce themselves to the respondent, gaining rapport, organizing the interview setting, how to present questions, how to react to responses, which issues to probe and how to probe them, how to keep the respondent on topic, and how to gracefully end the interview. In addition to some of these issues, research directors need to provide potential interviewers with experience in a few simulated interviews.

Interviewers are frequently paid on a "per interview" basis. This method is often preferred because it allows researchers to control costs. Also, it seems that many interviewers "burn out" after 6 or 8 weeks. Interviewing is an especially challenging task, requiring great concentration, and it is not easy to remain alert after having walked many respondents through the interview process. Expect high turnover among interviewing staff.

E. COMPARATIVE STUDIES

Whether we are doing an experiment comparing time 1 measures on some variable with time 2 measures, or whether we are trying to figure out why inner city crime rates are higher than those of suburban rates, we make comparisons. Thus, comparison is integral to the research process itself. *Comparative surveys* involve comparing two or more samples on one or more variables, at a single point in time, and they use standard survey techniques of analysis; therefore, they are included in this chapter. But there is an important distinction between experiments, surveys, and other designs that allow us to draw comparisons and **comparative research studies** whose very *purpose* is to compare. It is this latter group of studies that we examine here.

Comparative research may be quantitative, qualitative, or a combination of both. Comparative researchers use the full range of standard techniques, including surveys, interviews, field studies, and experiments, but, in particular, they use published information. Cross-cultural studies and historical studies are two of the most common examples of comparative studies; these look at the similarities and differences between cultures or within the same culture over time.

When the modern social sciences were emerging in the 19th century, comparative studies were a central concern of social research. During the early years of the 20th century, after arguments against a **unilineal model** (that proposes that the same patterns of development are followed by all societies), comparative studies shifted to intensive studies of exotic cultures by anthropologists such as Bronislaw Malinowski (1925) and Margaret Mead (1935). In the closing decades of the 20th century, many comparative studies have been undertaken. Later in this chapter you will read about a study comparing the experience of girls coming of age in Jerusalem with those in Toronto (Box 5.6).

There is, then, a long comparative tradition in social science research. Because many early nurse scientists received their research training in schools of social science, it is not surprising that a number conducted studies using cross-cultural comparative analyses. As nursing has become increasingly concerned with providing culturally competent care in all sectors, such studies have taken on greater importance. And although these studies do not have a distinct methodology associated with them—they use historical material, surveys, secondary data, experiments, and field studies—what they have in common is that they attempt to make comparisons between cultures or within cultures over time.

Because nurses are frequently curious about the efficacy of different approaches and treatments to client problems and conditions, comparative studies enable them to test these differences as well as compare and contrast the impact of various interventions on different client groups. For example, a comparative study may be used to answer the following types of research questions:

- What caring behaviors are identified by oncology nurses compared with oncology patients on an active treatment unit?
- Do clients who receive care for hypertension in a nurse-run clinic do better in reducing their blood pressure levels than clients who receive care through their doctor's office?
- What is the experience of school-aged children admitted to a hospital day care unit compared with those admitted to a general pediatric unit for treatment of asthma?
- Do psychosocial differences exist in adaptation to pregnancy for Latin-American, African-American, and Anglo-American ethnic groups?
- What differences exist in the career interests of nurses educated in a baccalaureate program, an associate degree, and a diploma program?
- What is the pattern of folk healing beliefs and practices among Korean and Chinese refugees who move to the United States?
- What differences exist in the health

BOX 5.6 *Nurse Researchers at Work*

COMING OF AGE IN THE METROPOLIS

Findings

The results indicate similarities and differences between girls from the two cities. The most striking similarities included:

- Requests from girls in both cities for continuing, systematic opportunities for guided discussion on their personal development and well-being
- A shared perspective on the social function of schools
- The need to be trusted, to have greater freedom of action, and not to be overprotected or controlled
- The perspective, whether realistic or not, of professional aspirations
- The need and desire to be free of teasing and harassment by boys
- The embarrassment about and rejection of the role of grandparents in their lives

The differences were equally striking:

- *Primary concerns.* Despite their existence in an unstable part of the world, girls in Jerusalem expressed concerns mainly about their positive biopsychosocial development. More than anything else, the girls from inner city Toronto articulated their insecurities and risks concerning rape, AIDS, pregnancy, and sexual pressures.
- *Tasks and chores.* The girls in Jerusalem could not discuss this even when prompted. This suggests that they were negligible. The girls in Toronto, without exception, reported de-

manding, relenting domestic chores and care-giving tasks, differentiating themselves clearly from their brothers, who were free of regular responsibilities.

- *Ideals and aspirations.* The girls in Toronto were preoccupied with wealth and Barbie dolls. This may suggest some deprivation in their lives, compensated by fantasizing about the lives of TV soap and drama characters. The girls in Jerusalem cited a fashion model as their ideal and also stressed intelligence and inner strength.
- *Fathers.* The girls from Jerusalem described some egalitarian tasks and roles of fathers; the girls from Toronto mentioned fathers mainly as authoritarian figures.
- *Discussion style.* Responses from the girls in Toronto were short, sometimes almost monosyllabic; group dialogue and interaction were minimal. The group from Jerusalem freely engaged in debate and discussion. It is difficult to know if this difference is cultural or situational.

Conclusions

A better understanding of this critical period of life is needed to support these young girls through this developmental phase toward their future goals as women. Policy development that is relevant to age and gender is needed to strengthen and enhance health and lifestyle decisions for the girls themselves but also because women everywhere are the major health-care providers and users. This would ultimately contribute to the health status of countries.

SOURCE: Summarized from Paltiel, F., Ross, E., and Neill, M. (1998). Coming of age in the metropolis: The Toronto experience. *The Canadian Nurse, 94*(10), 22–30.

---

promotion role for nurses working in urban versus rural hospital settings?

When conducting a comparative study, researchers must pay special attention to the sampling procedure used. Usually the sample for a comparative study is drawn from *two or more* populations that are be-

ing contrasted. For example, if a nurse researcher is interested in conducting a comparative survey of health promotion practices of nurses working in large urban hospitals and nurses working in small rural hospitals, two samples would be obtained, one from a population of nurses working in urban hospitals and one from a population of nurses working in small, rural hospitals. This is in contrast to other surveys in which the researcher is interested in studying how variables are related (correlational surveys) rather than how populations differ on a variable. For example, if the researcher were simply interested in examining the factors or variables related to health promotion practices by nurses, the study sample could be drawn from a *single* population of nurses. In a comparative survey, the emphasis is on how two or more populations *differ* with respect to the variables of interest. It usually involves measurement of one or more variables in two or more groups at one or more points in time (Woods and Cantazaro, 1988).

Let us consider some examples of comparative studies in nursing.

1. Examples of Comparative Nursing Studies

Two nursing studies are presented to illustrate the comparative approach. The study by Paltiel and associates (1998) compares perimenarchal girls from two different cultures. This qualitative study was reactive in nature, using focus groups to elicit data for comparison purposes. We also include an exploratory study using open-ended interviews to collect data on prenatal adaptation to pregnancy of women from three different cultural groups.

a. Coming of Age in the Metropolis: An International Study on the Needs and Concerns of Girls 10 to 14

Palteil and associates (1998) investigated the differences and similarities among two urban groups of early adolescent girls residing in different parts of the world in terms of their identified needs and major concerns. A collaborative, qualitative, action-oriented study was

conducted to identify cross-cultural universal and culturally unique needs of young adolescent girls. Data were collected by means of nurse-facilitated focus groups that lasted for 2.5 hours. The first focus group was conducted in Jerusalem with 19 girls from the ages of 10 to 14 years. These girls shared aspects of the biological, social, and psychological aspects of their lives. The second focus group was conducted in Toronto with 24 girls ages 12 to 14 years (see Box 5.6).

A discussion guide was developed for use in the focus groups by the principal investigator. The guide covered a wide range of topics, including education, health, friendship, sexuality, ideal women, spirituality, recreation, and family. The focus groups were intended to provide a forum in which the experiences, feelings, perceptions, values, and judgments of the adolescent girls could be expressed. In each focus group, the nurse facilitator could adapt the guide for ease of use with the local group. The opening question in each group was a general one, *What are the major concerns of girls your age?* A round robin technique was used to promote discussion. Girls could pass if they did not wish to speak. In Toronto, the focus group took place in a large inner city school. In Jerusalem, the focus groups were held in a health center. In addition to the adolescent girls, the principal investigator, the facilitator, and two observer-recorders were present in the focus groups.

The Toronto sample was selected from one school and reflected the multiculturalism of Toronto and, especially, the neighborhood in which the school was located. The group was multiethnic with origins from Burma, the Philippines, the Caribbean, Vietnam, China, Iran, India, and African countries. Two of the 24 girls were of European descent. The Jerusalem sample came from four different schools in four different neighborhoods. The socioeconomic range of the Jerusalem sample was wider because of the range of neighborhoods used for selection.

b. Adaptation to Pregnancy in Three Different Ethnic Groups: Latin-American, African-American, and Anglo-American

This comparative study used a qualitative approach to investigate adaptation to pregnancy in three ethnic groups—Latin-American, African-American, and Anglo-American women (Lederman and Miller, 1998). The research question addressed was: *Do psychosocial differences exist in adaptation to pregnancy for Latin-American, African-American, and Anglo-American ethnic groups?* The purpose of this study was to produce knowledge that would improve the prenatal health care and the counseling of women from different cultural groups. The goal was to create a survey that would target differences in cultural groups so that the success of future interventions could be enhanced (Box 5.7).

Thirty Latin-American, 34 African-American, and 30 Anglo-American women were recruited from a low-risk prenatal clinic at a university medical center in the southwestern United States. Participants were interviewed face-to-face in the latter half of pregnancy by trained interviewers using open-ended questions. The interviews ranged from 45 to 90 minutes in duration. The interview schedule focused on five dimensions: acceptance of pregnancy, identification with motherhood role, relationship with mother, relationship with partner or husband, and preparation for labor. The interview schedules were translated into Spanish using a forward-and-backward method of translation (from English to Spanish and back to English). The interviewers of the Latin-American participants were fluent in Spanish; most interviews, however, were conducted in English.

A goal of this study was the development of a psychosocial adaptation questionnaire for different cultural populations; therefore, response categories were prepared for all questions after the interviews were completed by creating mutually exclusive categories based on subject responses. Results and conclusions of this study are provided in Box 5.7. The results have implications for providing culturally sensitive and relevant health care to pregnant women in the three ethnic groups studied. By identifying the reproductive concerns of minority ethnic groups and providing culturally competent care to respond to these needs, the anxiety and stress experienced by pregnant women can be reduced. This study suggests that culturally informed data be used for research development, policy decisions, and program implementation.

2. Challenges in Comparative Research

Comparative research, particularly studies that focus on cultural differences, has potential to contribute significantly to nursing's body of knowledge. Culture has an important impact on one's interpretation of health and illness and one's response to health care. Nurses and all health-care professionals must make a commitment to expand their knowledge base and competence in cultural concepts and care. A critical area for comparative research in nursing is the impact of cultural diversity on health outcomes in various populations. Nursing actions must be based on systematic investigations of cultural groups and not on cultural myths. Cherry and Jacob (1999) call for research that examines normal life processes of growth and development, birth, death, pregnancy, as well as well-designed studies that examine the biological, psychological, sociological, and spiritual differences within, between, and among cultural groups. Comparative designs can yield such information.

BOX 5.7 *Nurse Researchers at Work*

ADAPTATION TO PREGNANCY IN THREE DIFFERENT ETHNIC GROUPS

Results

Women in all three ethnic groups were pleased with their pregnancies, despite the unplanned nature of the event and the associated changes in life plans that resulted. Less than 30 percent of the pregnancies were anticipated. Many women commented that their feelings toward the pregnancy changed as they progressed through the various stages moving from disappointment to anticipated pleasure. It appears the women had come to accept their pregnancy by the time the interviews were conducted in the third trimester.

Childcare was an issue for all three groups. Family, friends, and day-care centers were sources used to provide assistance. Contrary to reports in the literature about support for childcare in Latin-American families, the women in this study were not able to depend upon family care to the same extent. A possible explanation for this finding may be that the women were first generation Americans and hence did not have easy access to their families who resided elsewhere.

Differences were noted among the groups in terms of aspects of pregnancy that brought pleasure. The Latin-American women were happier than women in the other two groups with their pregnancies and stated more frequently that their families were happy. Whereas, Anglo-American women made comments that reflected a valuing of their children; African-American women did not reflect this sentiment in their comments.

The ability to stay at home and provide child care was explored, as well as anticipated life changes that would result from the birth of a child. Plans to stay at home were expressed strongly by Anglo-Americans and less so by African Americans. Anglo- and Latin-American women anticipated more life changes than African-American women as a result of giving birth. African-American women more often ex-

pected to receive help from their extended family and other family members, whereas Anglo- and Latin-American women depended more upon their partner. Latin-American women reported that they wanted to be like their own mother although they thought less about the kind of mother they wanted to be.than the other groups.

In reflecting upon childhood patterns of seeking help it was noted that the Latin-American women sought assistance most often from their mothers, Anglo-Americans from their fathers, and African-Americans turned to a range of family members.

Patterns of sexual activity underwent changes for all three groups. An increase occurred for a small number of African- and Anglo-American women but for the majority in all groups there was a decrease reported. Anglo-Americans reported the greatest satisfaction with the frequency of intercourse, while the other two groups of women would have preferred a further decrease. Different forms of pleasure were explored most frequently by Anglo-Americans.

Conclusions

This study is important because it addresses an area understudied in nursing research. It highlights the unique concerns and needs of three ethnic groups of pregnant women. This information can be used to provide culturally sensitive and responsive counselling and health teaching in the area of family nursing and prenatal care. It points out that future research should address "ethnic and cultural differences relevant to prenatal care should address representative samples of populations at risk and prominent psychosocial and health problems, and should use related assessment and intervention approaches to produce culturally informed data for research development, policy decisions, and program implementation."

SOURCE: Summarized from Lederman, R. and Miller, D. (1998). Adaptation to Preganancy in Three Different Ethnic Groups: Latin-American, African-American, and Anglo-American. *Canadian Journal of Nursing Research, 30*(3), 37–51.

Although it has much to offer nursing, comparative research also presents some interesting challenges because it deals with different cultures and often a different language. A number of authors identify issues concerning equivalence in concepts, indicators, and language (Warwick and Osherson, 1973; Jackson, 1999).

a. Equivalence of Concepts

Although ideas such as incest and health are cultural universals, there is no precise agreement about what is meant by these concepts. What is incest in one culture may be defined as a preferred marriage partner in another; what is considered normal, healthy behavior in one culture may be labeled as bizarre in another. So although we may have similar concepts, their content and meaning may vary considerably from culture to culture. Moreover, even within a culture there may be subtle variations in how concepts are defined.

In all research, but particularly in comparative research, it is important to define concepts carefully, noting any variations between the cultures being studied. The search for appropriate indicators is facilitated by attention to the definition of the concepts. Only if a researcher is satisfied that there is an equivalence of concepts can direct comparisons between cultures be drawn.

b. Equivalence of Indicators

The evidence collected in different countries is rarely based on identical definitions and collection procedures. For example, if one country defines a school drop out as anyone under age 14 years not attending school but another defines a drop out as anyone under age 16 years not attending school, do we dare use the information to compare the two societies? Similar problems arise if we wish to compare health status: given different definitions, recording methods, and, indeed, the different interests of the parties involved in the data collection (would they benefit by showing an increase in morbidity?), can we legitimately make comparisons across jurisdictions? For most measures, there are problems with a lack of equivalence indicators as we move from one jurisdiction to another.

How might we go about limiting the effects of such disparities? One suggestion is that we use data trends rather than absolute measures (e.g., the rate of crime, the school drop-out rate). For example, if you are comparing the United States and Canada in school drop-out statistics, you could minimize the effects of alternate measures by simply using the change in school drop-out rate over periods of time. Then, even if definitions vary between the countries, at least they are comparable across time spans within the country (unless, of course, definitions or procedures have changed within the country). Just as we standardize data within a country by calculating rates and ratios to deal with units of unequal size, when between-country data are required, consider computing trend data. And although such trend data would not provide the absolute measures desired, at least one should be able to detect whether the rates are converging or diverging.

c. Equivalence of Language

In the study Adaptation to Pregnancy in Three Different Ethnic Groups, the investigators attempted to provide for equivalence of language by having the interview guides translated into Spanish using a forward-and-backward method of translation. In addition, the interviewers of the Latin-American participants were fluent in Spanish. This greatly facilitated the participants' ability to communicate appropriately with the interviewer. Such precautions, however, are no guarantee of successful equivalency of language, as the following anecdote suggests.

Box 5.8 describes a problem that can arise when trying to provide for language equivalence. Several years ago, Clairmont and Jackson were doing a study in Moncton, New Brunswick, Canada. They were comparing people who worked for large companies and government agencies with a matched sample of workers in smaller companies. Because Moncton has a bilingual community, the researchers hired a translator to develop a French version of the interview. A number of bilingual interviewers were employed to conduct the interviews with some 600 residents in Moncton. Box 5.8 reports on the experience.

BOX 5.8 *Don Clairmont and Winston Jackson: Attempting Equivalence of Language in the Field*

Moncton, New Brunswick, is a bilingual community. Thus, when Clairmont and Jackson were planning a research study comparing Moncton's workers, they decided to make their interview questions available in both English and French. However, during the interviewing process, some of the French-speaking respondents seemed to be having difficulty understanding the interviewer's questions. On checking, the researchers discovered that their translator had done a fine job of converting their simple English version into Parisian French, not the Moncton dialect. Additionally, when they found a respondent was having difficulty understanding a question, the resourceful interviewers translated the question into English. The respondent would reply (usually in English) and the interviewers would then dutifully translate the answer back into French. Ah, the pleasures and problems of data collection!

SOURCE: Winston Jackson, personal memories of the Moncton Project (Jackson, W. [1999]. Methods: Doing Social Research. Scarborough: Prentice-Hall Canada. Cited with permission.)

---

d. The Problem of Selecting Evidence

Although the problem of researchers' choosing among alternate indicators is relevant to all types of research projects, this is especially the case in comparative studies. Given the vast amount of information available, what is the best way, for example, to measure health status in a country? (Some may use morbidity statistics as number of hospital admissions, days spent in the hospital, or rates of chronic illness as indicators; others may select community health outcomes such as infant or child mortality rates or immunization rates; others may use health-related quality of life indicators such as quality-adjusted life years [QALYs]; and still others may use social outcomes that relate to health such as school absence rates and status indicators such as employment, income, and living arrangements). The problem is that it is possible to demonstrate almost anything if you are free to search around for possible indicators. The general point here is that the selection of evidence is an especially problematic issue in comparative research. Not only can we question whether the indicators reflect what they are intended to, but we can also question whether the same variable will have the same meaning in different cultural contexts. This was demonstrated in the cross-cultural study of adolescent girls in Toronto and Jerusalem concerning family chores. Despite the best prompting efforts by the group facilitator, the girls in Jerusalem would not discuss this, leading one to conclude that they were either negligible or the participants did not understand the meaning of the question. The opposite situation existed for the girls in Toronto, who spoke without exception about the demanding family chores and domestic responsibilities they were expected to assume.

It would be difficult for most nurse researchers to avoid selecting indicators that produce results conforming to the researcher's preferred outcomes, ruling out the indicators not selected as insufficient in some way. There is no easy solution to this problem. One check is simply that researchers be forthright about which indicators were used and perhaps even public about which indicators were rejected and why they were rejected. It would not be practical to ask researchers to explain all of their decisions or to list all the alternatives considered. To do so would be akin to asking a chess player to explain all the alternatives considered before making a move. The chess player's information processing is highly complex and the player, in fact, probably could not provide much useful information about how the choice was made. The same would be true of the researcher. But if we are up front about the choices that have been made, then critics can reexamine the issue using the same or alternate indicators.

Researchers have not always paid sufficient attention to identifying precise indicators before beginning data analysis. Such precision is required because otherwise the researcher may inadvertently bias the outcome of the study. Moreover, the exact cut-points that are to be used in collapsing categories should also be identified before beginning analysis (e.g., where will the line be drawn between large and small communities when looking at the relationship between prevalence of sexually transmitted diseases and community size?). Again, if commitments are not made, the researcher may inadvertently select cut-points that result in an analysis showing what the researcher anticipated or wanted.

Realistically, these two suggestions are unlikely to be applied routinely by scientists. It is sometimes a challenge to get researchers to state hypotheses formally, let alone provide details of exact operational procedures. At present, there is little awareness that there is a problem in this area. Issues raised in Chapter 12 and in Chapter 9 are also related to the issue of committing oneself to operational procedures and operational hypotheses.

F. SECONDARY DATA ANALYSIS

A range of researchers, including nurses, economists, political scientists, historians, and, to a lesser degree, sociologists, anthropologists, and psychologists, frequently conduct research based on available material. These sources may include virtually any data, including published statistical data, national census track surveys, medical records, health data from personal health records, business data, and unpublished diaries of important historical figures. With the exception of those who record oral histories, historians rely on secondary data sources and the resulting studies are based entirely on secondary data analysis. **Secondary data analysis** is the analysis of an existing data set, or documents, for some research purpose other than the one originally intended. It involves re-analysis of data collected by another investigator to answer the same research question or a different question or to apply a different method of analysis. Secondary data analysis is included in this chapter because it most resembles survey designs in terms of the analytical procedures used.

Meta-analysis is the statistical analysis of a large collection of results from individual studies for the purpose of integrating findings (Onyskiw, 1996). The subject and the unit of analysis in a meta-analytic study is the individual research report. Meta-analysis is often referred to as *analysis of analysis* because it depends on the findings of primary research for its data. This approach provides a mechanism for nurses to make sense out of the growing body of nursing research so it can be used to guide practice. For example, Gillis (1993) conducted an integrated review and meta-analysis of the research literature on determinants of a health-promoting life-style. The meta-analysis allowed her to summarize mathematically the results of the studies to determine the effect of a range of independent variables on the dependent variable of health-promoting behavior. The ranges and pooled correlation values were determined for the independent variables to provide an index of effect magnitude. For a discussion of meta-analysis using the correlation statistic (r), interested readers are referred to Rosenthal (1984). The review summarized the findings of 23 separate research studies on determinants of health-promoting behavior and showed interesting patterns across the studies.

Box 5.9 lists some recent projects in secondary data analysis completed by our students in a one-term course.

1. Purpose

There are several purposes for conducting secondary data analysis (Jackson, 1999; Woods and Catanzaro, 1989; Hinds et al., 1997). These include:

- The identification and focus on a sub-sample or subset of cases not considered in the original study. For example, in a study of health-promoting lifestyles in childbearing families, you may wish to do a secondary analysis of the lifestyle profiles of only the adolescent girls in those families sampled in the original study.
- The analysis of variables or concepts not analyzed in the original study. For example, if the original study focused on the impact of social support as a critical determinant of success in smoking cessation for single mothers, you may wish to analyze the impact of a related variable, the peer network that appeared to be discussed in the original study but was not analyzed.
- The investigation of relationships or hypotheses not considered in the orig-

inal study. For example, Humenick and associates (1998) used secondary data analysis to partially replicate and extend Morton's (1994) research to examine additional risk factors with mediating potential on the relationship of elevated breast milk sodium (BM [Na+]) to breastfeeding outcomes. The primary research question was, "Do elevated levels of BM [Na+] at postpartum day 6 by themselves serve as a marker to predict low frequency of breastfeeding at week 4?" In addition, Humenick et al. asked a new question: "Do the psychosocial risk factors of (1) perceived insufficient milk supply (IMS); (2) the number of best friends who breast fed their babies in the past 3 years; and (3) the mother's own perception of her breastfeeding skills mediate the relationship between elevated BM [Na+] and the breastfeeding outcome?"

- To use a unit of analysis that is different from that used in the original data analysis. For example, in the study on health-promoting lifestyles in childbearing families, a researcher may elect to focus on the mothers' lifestyles and subsequently see the mother rather than the family as the unit of analysis.
- To use different analytical strategies from those used in the original study. For example, in a study titled *Examining Emotional, Physical, Social, and Spiritual Health as Determinants of Self-rated Health Status,* the researchers Ratner and associates (1998) used different statistical procedures to conduct a secondary analysis of data from the Yukon Health Promotion Survey. The purpose of the secondary analysis was to determine if individuals' perceptions of their emotional, physical, social, and spiritual health constitute elements of their self-rated health status operationalized with a commonly used single indicator (the EGFP, or ex-

BOX 5.9 *Student Researchers at Work*

SECONDARY DATA ANALYSIS PROJECTS

Project	Student or Students	Brief Summary
Conformity to Thinness in Women	Kelly Yorke (1995)	This project was a content analysis of television ads in terms of the degree of thinness by type of commercial.
Portrayal of Women in *Seventeen* magazine	Robyn MacConnell (1995)	This project examined the female models used in the 1960s, 1970s, 1980s, and 1990s in terms of body type.
Pay, Performance, and Productivity	Sean Barret (1995)	Using published information, the project related team pay levels to win and loss records.
Change in the Portrayal of Women, 1950–1995	Kathleen Lumsden (1995)	Using Maclean's ads published over 4 decades, the study examined changes in the portrayal of women.
Personal Ads	Shelley Conners (1996)	Using the *Halifax Chronicle Herald's* personal ads, the study did a content analysis (what people were looking for) in heterosexual ads, 1994–1995.
NHL Penalty Minutes	Scott Gardner (1996)	Using published hockey results material, the project examined the relationship between penalty minutes and the success of teams.
Romance in Alcohol, Car, and Cologne Ads	Deborah E. Farr (1996)	Continue analysis of the use of romance to promote cars and cologne.
Content Analysis of Advertisements in *Vogue Magazine,* 1982 to 1991	Logann McNamara (1997)	This project examined changes in the extent to which women in advertisements were portrayed in sexually permissive or dominant positions.
Faceism and Gender Roles	Wendy Chisholm, Rita Gillis, Michelle Waye, and Flora Murphy (1997)	This project examined changes in the extent to which women in advertisements are portrayed with "full body" shots but men are more likely to use "face" shots: *Time* magazine in the 1950s, 1970s, and 1990s.

cellent, good, fair, poor indicator). The sample was made up of 742 women and 713 men. The key finding of the analysis was that the EGFP indicator, as a measure of self-rated health status, measures only physical health status and does not appear to tap the emotional, social, and spiritual dimensions of health.

2. Sources of Data

Secondary analysis involves using data in a variety of forms and from a variety of sources. Both quantitative and qualitative data can be subjected to secondary analysis. It may be raw data in the form of tapes, interview transcripts, videos, completed questionnaires or interview schedules, a database, or archival material. Computerized databases are becoming popular sources for secondary analysis of data in health-care settings. They are excellent data sources for nurses wishing to explore clinical questions, particularly those that require information over time, without gathering new data (Querker, 1997).

A vast range of health information and data sources is available to nurse researchers for secondary data analysis. Examples include the databases of national, provincial, and state nursing associations; clinical databases from health maintenance organizations (HMOs); Canadian Medical Services Insurance databases; records of Medicaid and Medicare (USA); reportable disease registers of the Centers for Disease Control and Prevention and the World Health Organization, as well as those of provincial and state health departments; local and regional hospital databanks; the Vital Statistics Registers, which record events such as births, deaths, divorces, and marriages; and an array of national databases. In Canada, several national population surveys have yielded interesting data. These include the Canada Health Promotion Survey; Statistics Canada Violence Against Women Sur-

vey; Statistics Canada National Census Data; the National Population Health Survey; and The National Institute of Nutrition's Tracking Nutrition Trends Survey. In the United States, comparable surveys exist such as the National Health Survey; the Annual Survey of Hospitals conducted by the American Hospital Association; the National Survey of Personal Health Practices and Consequences; and the Health Records Survey, which contains information from medical and residential institutions providing health care, to name a few.

3. Challenges in Conducting Secondary Data Analysis

a. Using Clinical Databases

Most large health-care institutions have some type of computerized data collection system. These databases are rich resources for answering nursing questions, but some issues need to be dealt with before using them for research purposes. With careful planning, many of the limitations of databases can be overcome, making them viable and economical sources of data as research funding continues to shrink. Querker (1997) identifies the following issues:

- The research question must be framed in a manner that enables the researcher to answer it using the available data. The researcher must be familiar with the nature of the data collected, as well as who collected it and how. This helps the researcher determine if the data set is appropriate to answer the research question. To fully understand the limitations of the database, the researcher should be familiar with the clinical setting from which the data emerged.
- Terminology of the database may be idiosyncratic. For example, the term "unit of care," which has many meanings ranging from a physical space or a caring episode to a period of time, may be

used in the database. Therefore, the researcher must become familiar with the vocabulary, data entry procedures, and any associated documentation about the system.

- The group of interest must be adequately represented in the database. If the researcher wishes to examine a subpopulation of the data set, he or she must determine that sufficient information on the subset exists. The nature of the sampling and measurement in the database may seriously constrain a secondary analysis.

- Adequacy of method is a major concern with an established database. The researcher must accept the method used to collect the original data and has no recourse to redesigning the initial study.

- Permission must be obtained to use the database for research purposes if it is not in the public domain. Subjects who gave permission when the data were collected originally usually do not have to be asked again for permission unless the risk to participants' confidentiality is significant. Human subjects committees will determine this.

- Many databases are not originally designed for research purposes, so the researcher must structure the data in a usable format. This involves compiling a workable data set from the database; checking the quality, accuracy, and reliability of information; eliminating redundant and duplicate entries; completing missing data that may be available from earlier records in the database; and learning the meaning of any special vocabulary or codes in the data. The best way to correct redundant entries, missing data, and other errors is to visually inspect a printout of the data.

b. Using Qualitative Data Sets

Although secondary analysis of quantitative data such as a national census survey has gained wide acceptance in the research community as a cost-effective approach to fully using previously collected data, secondary analysis of qualitative data sets has not been as enthusiastically endorsed. In attempting a secondary analysis of qualitative data, several major challenges come to mind. These concerns are identified and addressed by Hinds and associates (1997, pp. 409–423) and summarized as follows.

- The first issue to resolve is the appropriateness of qualitatively generated data for re-analysis. Because the large volumes of qualitative data generated in a single investigation must be reduced as part of data management, the researcher selectively samples the data. The result is that potentially important data may not be considered in the final analysis if it does not contribute to the emerging patterns or themes in the primary analysis. Hinds and associates (1997) suggest the fit may best be determined by the extent of missing data. Missing data are those that did not find their way into the analysis process. For example, if an issue is explored in one interview but not in previous or subsequent interviews, it may be that the topic emerged spontaneously or that the researcher decided to narrow the study's scope and refine the interview questions; therefore, the topic is not addressed again. A secondary analysis of a qualitative data set does not enable the researcher to answer his or her research question if the phenomenon of interest is not uniformly addressed in the primary study. The researcher must determine this before proceeding further.

- Assessing the quality and appropriateness of the qualitative data from the primary study for secondary analysis involves having direct access to it and to members of the research team. Access can be negotiated to include taped interviews; hard copies; disk copies;

and copies of field notes, memos, and interpretive notes. Negotiated access is crucial to determining if the data can be validly used for a secondary analysis. Figure 5.1 illustrates a tool for assessing the appropriateness of a data set for secondary analysis.

- The similarity between the question in the primary research study and the question for the secondary analysis must be significant. If the difference between the two questions is considerable, it is unlikely that the primary data set will yield an answer because it will lack appropriate depth and detail related to the secondary analysis question.

- A pilot study using data from the primary study will help determine if the data are capable of meeting the research objectives of the secondary analysis. Usually three randomly selected interviews are sufficient to determine if the study purpose can be achieved or if it needs to be revised.

- Permission from participants in the primary study to have their data reanalyzed by other researchers must be sought either at the time of the initial study consent or subsequently. Figure 5.2 provides an example of a consent form to use data for secondary analysis. It is ideal if this can be sought with the initial study, but often researchers do not anticipate doing a secondary analysis until after the primary study is complete and additional phenomena not represented in the study findings are noted in the data.

- Researchers must be sensitized to the context of the primary study. The process of qualitative data collection and analysis is affected by the context in which it occurs; therefore, secondary analysis needs to consider the context and try as much as possible to get as close to the experience of having been there.

- Researchers must determine whether primary data sets are still current and if the timing (either concurrent with the primary analysis or after it) is appropriate for secondary analysis. Factors to consider in doing so include whether the context in which the data were collected has changed. If the phenomenon of interest has changed significantly since the primary study, a secondary analysis may yield very little new and relevant information. If done concurrently, the researcher has easier access to participants if conceptual clarification of secondary analysis is required but if premature sharing of findings between the two studies is done, one set may unduly influence the other.

4. Examples of Research Using Secondary Data Analysis

This section illustrates two examples of secondary analysis, one using qualitatively generated data and the other using quantitatively generated data to investigate a nursing issue.

a. Emancipatory Potential of Storytelling in a Group

In this qualitative investigation, Banks-Wallace (1998) examined the health-promoting function of storytelling in a group of women through the use of secondary analysis. All of the information was made available through analyzing a subset of 115 stories derived from the transcripts of 28 women of African descent who participated in the original study titled *Sisters in Session (SIS): Focus Groups as a Research Tool and Intervention for Working with Women of African Descent*. The purposes of the original study were to increase awareness of barriers to women's participation in or conducting of research, to identify research priorities for people of African descent, and to explore the therapeutic potential of focus groups. The secondary data analysis enabled the re-

CRITERIA FOR DETERMINING GENERAL QUALITY OF PRIMARY STUDY DATA SET

Ready access to stury documents/team	Yes	No
Tapes of interviews	——	——
Hard copies/disk of interviews	——	——
Field notes	——	——
Memos to interpretive notes	——	——
Principal investigator/team member	——	——

Training of primary team	Satisfactory	Unable to determine	Unsatisfactory
Credentials of team members to conduct primary study	——	——	——
Training of members for role in primary study	——	——	——

Completeness of data set	Yes	No
Available documents are complete (i.e., no missing papers/tapes)	——	——
Accuracy of transcription	——	——
Minimal typographic errors	——	——
Appropriate use of software	——	——

Able to assess quality of interviewing	Satisfactory	Unable to Determine	Unsatisfactory
Interviewing quality	——	——	——
Interviewing format allowed			
Responses of descriptive depth	——	——	——
focus/meaning/subject of responses can be determined	——	——	——

Able to assess sampling plan Type of sampling plan (e.g., convenience, purposive, theoretical, etc.) is clear	Yes ——	No ——

CRITERIA FOR DETERMINING FIT OF SECONDARY RESEARCH QUESTION

	Present in sufficient depth	Unable to determine	Not present in sufficient depth
Able to determine extent to which concept of interest is reflected in data set	——	——	——
Able to estimate validity of new question	Likely	Not sure	Not likely
Study sample could be expected to experience this concept/situation	——	——	——
	Similar	Somewhat similar	Not similar
Proposed research question is similar to that in primary study	——	——	——

AGGREGATE IMPRESSION Data set of sufficient quality, completeness, and fit with secondary research question	Yes ——	No ——

Figure 5.1   Example of an assessment tool: criteria for use in a secondary analysis of qualitative data. (From Hinds, V, Vogel, R, and Clarke-Steffen, L [1997]: The possibilities and pitfalls of doing a secondary analysis of a qualitative data set. *Qualitative Health Research* 7[3] 408–424. Cited with permission.)

In coding the interviews, our research team has coded only those sections of the interviews that are directly about the caring experiences of pediatric oncology nurses. But what we have noticed is that other valuable information about what is meaningful to pediatric nurses was present throughout the interviews even though not directly in response to our interview questions about caring experiences. Because we do not want to lose any of that information, we have decided to conduct a secondary analysis of the same interviews. A pediatric nurse researcher who is not a member of our research team will do this secondary analysis. Would you consider giving your permission for this nurse researcher to do a secondary analysis of your interview?

Yes, my interview may be included in the secondary analysis. ___ Signature ————————

No, my interview may not be included in the secondary analysis. ___ Signature ————————

Date:_____

Time:_____

ID code:_____

Figure 5.2   Example of a consent form for permission to use data for secondary analysis. (From Hinds, V., Vogel, R., and Clarke-Steffen, L. [1997]: The possibilities and pitfalls of doing a secondary analysis of a qualitative data set. *Qualitative Health Research* 7[3] 408–424. Cited with permission of Sage Publications, Inc.)

searcher to answer a research question that was closely related to one of the purposes of the initial study, namely, "What is the role of storytelling in promoting health among SIS participants?" (Box 5.10).

b. Breast Milk Sodium as a Predictor of Breastfeeding Patterns

The quantitative study by Humenick and associates (1998) was designed to replicate and extend the work of Morton (1994) which reported that elevated BM [Na+] during early lactogenesis was predictive of poor breastfeeding outcomes. Humenick and associates were able to meet their research objectives by conducting secondary analysis of 6-day postpartum breast milk and maternal data collected from a subset of 41 mothers that were part of the original study. The original study consisted of 340 subjects selected for inclusion in a longitudinal, prospective study of insufficient milk syndrome (IMS). Original study consent forms allowed for additional unspecified analysis of the milk samples. Humenick et al. were interested in studying variables that mediate the relationship between elevated BM [Na+] levels and breastfeeding outcomes. Although the number of variables they could study were limited to those present in the original data, the secondary analysis enabled them to explore the influence of important psychosocial risk factors on breastfeeding outcomes. Box 5.11 provides a discussion of the findings of this secondary data analysis study.

G. ADVANTAGES AND LIMITATIONS OF SURVEY DESIGNS

Sample surveys are the major tools in studies attempting to represent large popula-

BOX 5.10 *Nurse Researchers at Work*

EMANCIPATORY POTENTIAL OF STORYTELLING IN A GROUP

Therapeutic benefits of storytelling were noted in the nursing literature more than 60 years ago. Recently there has been a renewed interest in the scientific value of storytelling. The current project used a descriptive, secondary analysis design to examine the health-promoting functions of storytelling in a convenience sample of 28 African-American women.

Data were audiotaped in four focus groups convened during a 6-week period. The six-part narrative analysis included (1) providing information about the historical setting for the study, (2) demarcating transcripts into individual stories, (3) analyzing the context in which the stories occurred and the content of specific stories, (4) grouping stories according to themes and functions, (5) comparing story themes and functions across sessions, and (6) reviewing stories for conspicuous absences.

Six major functions of storytelling in the group were identified: (1) to provide contextual grounding, (2) to provide a means of bonding with other participants, (3) to provide a means of validating and affirming women's experiences, (4) to provide a means of catharsis, (5) to provide a means for resisting oppression, and (6) to provide a vehicle for educating other participants. (For a detailed description of each of these functions with illustrative stories, interested readers should check the original source).

Storytelling was used as both a means of learning more about factors affecting the well-being of women of African descent and as a tool for improving the lives of study participants. The stories shared by women provided insight into factors that constrained their choices or enabled them to move further along their journey. Listening to the women and designing a study that centered their experiences resulted in a project that not only provided answers to the researchers' questions but also allowed participants opportunities to learn and grow. Through storytelling, participants were better able to make decisions related to living as a woman of African descent. Group storytelling is a tradition that continues to sustain communities of African descent and other cultures throughout the world.

SOURCE: Summarized from Banks-Wallace, J. (1998). Emancipatory potential of storytelling in a group. *Image: Journal of Nursing Scholarship, 30*(1), 17–21.

---

tions. They often attempt to deal simultaneously with many variables and attempt to describe the complexity of human behavior. Surveys also permit researchers to construct new variables by combining a number of characteristics; status integration or status crystallization are examples of such constructed variables.

Despite the many advantages of survey research, it is difficult to make clear causal inferences from such data. Most of these difficulties derive from the nature of the data. Survey data are normally based on self-reports and frequently involve data based on recollection. Although it is probably not difficult to recall factual information (e.g., reporting the community you were born in or the salary of your first full-time job), it may be very difficult to recall how well you got along with your mother when you were 6 years old. Another fundamental issue has to do with the connection between words (what people say they will do) and deeds (what they actually do). There are therefore doubts about the extent to which surveys reflect ideal behavior as opposed to real behavior. To what extent, then, can we claim to reflect reality with survey data?

Table 5.3 summarizes the advantages and limitations of the first two approaches to research design that we have considered so far, experiments and surveys. Causal inferences are clearest when exper-

BOX 5.11 *Nurse Researchers at Work*

BREAST MILK SODIUM AS A PREDICTOR OF BREASTFEEDING PATTERNS

Findings

Consistent with the findings of the original study, 80 percent of those with a BM [Na+] of 16 mmol/L or lower at day 6 sustained a high level of breastfeeding at week 4, compared with only 50 percent of those with an elevated BM [Na+] ($\chi^2 = 4.05$, df = 1, $P = .04$). This difference was even greater in a subgroup of mothers predicted to be at risk for insufficient milk supply on the basis of support density and self-perception variables. Of the latter group, 75 percent with low BM [Na+] sustained a high level of breastfeeding at 4 weeks postpartum, compared with only 22 percent with an elevated BM [Na+] ($\chi^2 = .65$, df = 1, $P = .01$).

In contrast, among the low-risk mothers, BM [Na+] levels were not associated with any difference in breast milk sustainment (89 percent and 82 percent sustainment for low- and high-sodium groups, respectively). Thus, a normal decrease in BM [Na+] is predictive of higher sustainment of breastfeeding. However, the predictive validity of this marker appears to be enhanced by combining it with the psychosocial variables of support density and self-perception of breastfeeding by the mother.

Summary

In summary, this secondary analysis provided the following answers to the research questions:

- Elevated levels of BM [Na+] at postpartum day 6 do predict a significant decrease in breastfeeding sustainment at week 4.
- When Insufficient Milk Syndrome (IMS) risk group was used as a mediating variable, high-risk mothers showed a striking decrease in sustained breastfeeding at week 4 (75 percent compared with 22 percent) for low and elevated BM [Na+] groups, respectively.
- For mothers who had been judged to be at low risk for IMS, level of BM [Na+] showed no prediction of future breastfeeding patterns.
- Thus, BM [Na+] appears to be a marker predicting poor breastfeeding outcomes only for mothers at high risk for perceived IMS.

SOURCE: Summarized from Humenick, S., Hill, P., Thompson, J., and Hart, A. (1998). Breast-milk sodium as a predictor of breastfeeding patterns. *Canadian Journal of Nursing Research*, 30(3), 67–81.

imental and, to a lesser degree, panel data are used. Generalizing about larger populations is the forté of survey designs.

Although neither surveys nor experiments rate high on validity, this does not mean that they are, by nature, invalid. The negative sign simply means that this is a problem area in these designs. It is difficult to demonstrate that respondents have not altered their behavior or their answers on a questionnaire in response to the fact that they know they are being studied. Both experimentalists and survey researchers take the problem of validity seriously and try to minimize distortions. The negative sign for group-administered questionnaires in the generalization column is there because such groups are typically selected in the most convenient way. Probability procedures have therefore not been followed in the way that would be necessary if one wished to make extrapolations to the general population. (See Chapter 15 for details on sampling.)

The major limitation of research based on secondary data is that the necessary information is often unavailable, incomplete, or inappropriate for the purposes of the secondary analysis. But with imagination, excellent work can be done. Health researchers are impressively adept, for example, at locating "indirect indicators" in available data (e.g., using the number of hits on the dietary or cholesterol educa-

Table 5.3 Advantages and Limitations of Alternate Designs

Research Design Category	General	Validity	Causal Inference	Multivariate	Probing
Experimental Designs	–	–	–	–	–
Pre-experimental	–	–	+	–	–
Experimental	±	–	+	–	–
Quasi-experimental					
Survey Designs					
Individual questionnaire	+	–	–	+	–
Group administered	–	–	–	+	–
Phone survey	+	–	–	+	–
Interview	+	–	–	+	+
Comparative analysis	+	–	–	+	–
Secondary data	+	–	–	+	–
Meta analysis	+	–	–	–	–

In each category, a + means that this is an advantage of the technique; – means this is a possible limitation; ± means that in some conditions it is a limitation, but in others it is an advantage.

- **General** refers to the extent to which extrapolations to larger populations may be made using each of the design or data collection procedures.
- **Validity** is the extent to which indicators clearly measure what they are intended to measure.
- **Causal inference** refers to the ease with which inferences about causal relations among variables may be made.
- **Multivariate** refers to the ease with which information on many variables is collected, leading to the possibility of multivariate analysis.
- **Probing** refers to the extent to which responses may be probed in depth.

tional page of the American Heart Foundation's Web site as an indirect measure of the usefulness of that page as an educational tool). And if the data are reported at different points in time, a researcher who is interested in tracking and explaining health trends may be able to build and test elaborate causal models. So, whether they are attempting to understand the link between diet and health status or between cardiac disease and utilization of health care resources, many researchers make efforts to understand the world by using secondary data.

Secondary data analysis is cost effective and, providing the data are relatively complete, can lead to sound general statements about the world. Many major research costs (e.g., personnel salaries and data collection costs) have already been assumed by the initial study. Larger and more geographically dispersed samples can be studied through the use of existing databases rather than limiting the sample to what a researcher's funds can support for an original study. Finally, the collecting and tracking of longitudinal data and trends over time are made reasonably affordable with the use of secondary analysis of databases and archival materials.

Whatever research design is selected, it is important to understand the strengths and limitations of each of the approaches. Such knowledge helps researchers select appropriate designs and try to deal with the weak points of each design. When a decision has been made to use a survey design, Chapters 13, 14, and 15 contain information of particular relevance to the survey researcher; measurement, questionnaire construction, and sampling methods are all covered there.

E X E R C I S E S

1. Suppose you wished to understand the factors that influence the grade performance of university nursing students. What kind of design would you recommend for such a study? Outline the rationale for your choice.

2. Suppose you wished to investigate four alternative explanations for the relationship between social support and adolescents' perceptions of stress. What kind of design would you recommend? Outline the rationale for your choice.

3. Suppose you are interested in exploring gender differences in attitudes concerning the acceptability of permissive parenting practices. What design would you recommend to explore such a question? Outline the rationale for your choice.

4. Suppose you wished to explore the frequency and the intensity with which female undergraduates have experienced sexual harassment in their lives. What variables would you wish to measure in such a study?

RECOMMENDED READINGS

Brentro, M., and Hegge, M. (2000). Nursing faculty: One generation away from extinction? *Journal of Professional Nursing, 16*(2) 97–103. A state-wide survey of nurses with graduate degrees was undertaken to understand the career paths and intentions of nurses in one midwestern state.

Clark, D., Clark, P., Day, D., and Shea, D. (2000). The relationship between health-care reform and nurses' interest in union representation: The role of workplace climate. *Journal of Professional Nursing, 16*(2) 92–96. This is an example of an exploratory survey design using a mailed instrument to 1500 registered nurses.

Fain, J.A. (1999). *Reading, Understanding, and Applying Nursing Research.* Philadelphia: F.A. Davis. This text and workbook provide a brief but useful discussion of the survey as a data collection method.

Fowler, F.J. (1993). *Survey Research Methods* (2nd ed.). Newbury Park, CA: Sage. This text provides a comprehensive overview of survey design, the process, advantages, disadvantages, and practical examples.

Humphris, D. (1999). Types of evidence. In Hamer, S., and Collinson., G (Eds.). *Achieving Evidence-Based Practice: A Handbook for Practitioners.* Edinburgh: Harcourt Publishers. This chapter explores the survey as a method of providing evidence-based information for use in practice. In addition, it explores how to make judgments about the quality and usefulness of such evidence.

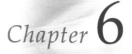

Chapter 6

Qualitative Research Designs

CHAPTER OUTLINE

A. **Entering the World of Qualitative Research**

   1. Defining Qualitative Research
   2. Core Activities in Qualitative Research

B. **Qualitative Research Designs**

   1. Characteristics of Qualitative Research Designs
   2. Phenomenological Research Perspective

   3. Grounded Theory Perspective
   4. Ethnographic Perspective

C. **Scientific Adequacy of Qualitative Research**

   1. Traditional Standards of Quality
   2. Contemporary Standards of Quality

D. **Advantages and Limitations of Qualitative Approaches**

KEY TERMS

Audit trail

Bracketing

Componential analysis

Confirmability

Constant comparative method

Core variable

Credibility

Culture

Cultural scene

Cultural themes

Dependability

Domain analysis

Emic

Ethnography

Ethnonursing

Etic

Gatekeeper

Grounded theory

Holistic ethnography

Informant

Intersubjectivity

Key informant

Lived experience

Maxi ethnography

Mini ethnography

Participant

Phenomenological perspective

Qualitative research

Saturation

Simultaneity paradigm

Symbolic interactionism

Taxonomy

Themes

Theoretical memos

Trustworthiness

Totality paradigm

Transferability

The previous two chapters presented introductions to experimental and survey approaches to nursing research. Both are predominantly quantitative (using numbers to summarize the findings of the research) and are associated with the positivist, scientific approach that emphasizes careful measurement, sampling, rationality, objectivity, prediction, control, and the logic of hypothesis testing. A vast number of research questions can be posed and answered using these approaches. So whether it is attempting to describe and explain the patterns surrounding the relationship between gender and suicide or trying to determine the effectiveness of a prenatal education program in improving maternal and infant outcomes, a quantitative approach is likely to be used. When well done, these studies have high levels of credibility because they are using scientific techniques that are fairly well understood and respected in our culture.

The problem with limiting oneself to positivistic approaches is that there is a whole range of human activity that is not easily understood using positivistic approaches. For example, if you wanted to know what it is like to be a terminally ill client on a hospice unit, one would be quite limited in getting a real understanding of the hospice experience by conducting a survey on client perceptions and attitudes toward hospice care. A great deal of information could be gleaned from such a study, but could you really understand the experiences of the terminally ill? Could you understand the complex relations between the clients, nurses, family members, physicians, and other care attendants? A reality is ignored if one limits oneself to survey or experimental approaches. In this example, can you make much sense out of how the hospice unit works within the health-care institution or the complexity of how a client experiences the transition from active treatment into hospice care? These kinds of questions beg for a holistic perspective, one that attempts to tap into clients' perceptions of themselves and of how they see others and for a description on the process of how they learn to act, live, and die in a hospice setting.

Fortunately, some qualitative perspectives in nursing science pay attention to such matters. Qualitative approaches are defined as those that use words rather than numbers to describe findings, assume a dynamic reality, and emphasize seeing the world from the eyes of the participants being studied. The goal of qualitative approaches is understanding rather than prediction and they emphasize the subjective dimensions of human experience. They are holistic (i.e., studying the whole institution, group, or culture) rather than reductionistic. Generally, they are associated with the interpretive approach, which is discovery oriented, explanatory, descriptive, and inductive in nature (see Chapter 1).

This chapter introduces the most frequently used qualitative approaches in nursing research, including phenomenology, grounded theory, and ethnography. Most qualitative researchers do not subscribe to the broad classification of research designs proposed in this text. Although some may refer to their designs as *case studies* (i.e., exploration of a single entity bounded by time and activity using a variety of data collection procedures) or *field studies* (i.e., observations of behavior in natural settings, in which participants are acting as they usually do), many simply describe their perspective as grounded theory, phenomenology, biography, and so on and go on to explain what they do

Data collection and analysis methods specific to the approaches discussed in this chapter are described in Chapter 7. These include participant observation studies, in-depth interviewing, focus group interviews, observational studies, and field experiments. Let us begin by defining qualitative research and comparing the core research activities required for doing a qualitative investigation with those required for a quantitative study. Common characteristics of qualitative designs are discussed as a means of establishing a foundation for describing the three approaches discussed in this chapter. Examples of qualitative designs are provided from the research literature. The examples are useful models for research students who are interested in designing a qualitative study.

A. ENTERING THE WORLD OF QUALITATIVE RESEARCH

Several leading authors have written personal perspectives on qualitative research (Creswell, 1994, 1998; Denzin and Lincoln, 1994; Marshall and Rossman, 1995; Munhall and Oiler, 1986; Parse et al., 1985; Silverman, 1997). Their work has been instrumental in advancing our understanding of this research tradition. It is a field of inquiry that cuts across disciplines, fields, and subject matter and has much to offer nurses and others who are interested in gaining a holistic understanding of human experiences.

I. Defining Qualitative Research

To understand the place of **qualitative research** requires discussion of the two major paradigms that are reflected in nursing science today. Parse (1987) has named these belief systems the *totality paradigm* and the *simultaneity paradigm*. In the **totality paradigm,** reality exists independent of the knower, humans are viewed as the sum of their parts, persons adapt to an external environment through cause-and-effect relationships, and health is viewed along a continuum from illness to wellness. The totality paradigm is best suited for the quantitative research approach and is associated with the positivist tradition.

In the **simultaneity paradigm,** reality is characterized by a mutual process of human and environment, and persons exist in open participation with the universe and are more than and different from the summed parts studied in the totality paradigm. The wholeness or unitary nature of the human being is primary in this paradigm. Thus, nurse scientists study the universal lived experiences of health or patterns of the whole. A study in this paradigm is conducted not to control the human being and the world but to gain insights into human living. The researcher believes in the personal meaning individuals give to their lived experience. The simultaneity paradigm is best suited for the qualitative research approach and is associated with the interpretive tradition (see Chapter 1).

Parse and associates (1985) offer a definition of qualitative research that is rooted in nursing's simultaneity paradigm. They state:

Qualitative research identifies the characteristics and the significance of human experiences as described by subjects and interpreted by the researcher at various levels of abstraction. In qualitative research the researcher's interpretations are intersubjective, that is, given the researcher's frame of reference, another person can come to a similar interpretation. Qualitative data are processed through the creative abstractions of the researcher as the subjects' descriptions are studied to uncover the meaning of human experiences (p. 3).

From this definition, we see that the aim of qualitative research in nursing is an understanding of what it means to be human. Nursing science needs to be open to the variety of ways of knowing and learning that are evolving from the two paradigms. Each presents challenges to researchers who are working to ground nursing practice in nursing science.

A generic definition of qualitative research is proposed by Denzin and Lincoln (1994, p. 2). They note:

It is multimethod in focus, involving an interpretive, naturalistic approach to its subject matter. This means that qualitative researchers study things in their natural settings, attempting to make sense of, or interpret phenomena in terms of the meanings people bring to them . . . It involves the use of a variety of empirical materials-case study, personal experience, introspective, life story, interview, observational, historical, interactional, and visual texts—that describe routine and problematic moments and meanings in individuals' lives. Accordingly, qualitative researchers deploy a wide range of interconnected methods, hoping always to get a better fix on the subject matter at hand (p.2).

They go on to discuss the qualitative researcher as a *bricoleur,* which is a "Jack of all trades" or do-it-yourself person. The multiple methodologies of qualitative research are defined as a *bricolage* or a pieced-together, close-knit set of practices that provide solutions to a problem in a concrete situation. This metaphor is helpful in concretely illustrating the complex and multifaceted nature of qualitative research. Box 6.1 summarizes their description of *bricoleurs.*

The field of qualitative research is far from a unified set of principles that are promoted by scholars with shared visions. Rather, Denzin and Lincoln discovered that the field is defined primarily by a series of essential tensions, contradictions, and hesitations. These tensions work back and forth among competing definitions. Although there are differing

---

BOX 6.1 *The Qualitative Researcher as* **Bricoleur**

The multiple methodologies of qualitative research may be viewed as a *bricolage* and the researcher as the *bricoleur.* The *bricoleur* is adept at performing a large number of diverse tasks, ranging from interviewing to observing, to interpreting personal and historical documents, to intensive self-reflection and introspection. The *bricoleur* reads widely and is knowledgeable about the many interpretive paradigms (e.g., feminism, Marxism, cultural studies, constructivism) that can be brought to any particular problem. He or she may not, however, believe that paradigms can be mingled or synthesized— that is, paradigms are overarching philosophical systems denoting particular ontologies, epistemologies, and methodologies and cannot be easily moved between. The researcher as *bricoleur* theorist works between and within competing and overlapping perspectives and paradigms

The *bricoleur* understands that research is an interactive process shaped by his or her personal history, biography, gender, social class, race, and ethnicity, and those of the people in the setting. The *bricoleur* knows that science is power because all research findings have political implications. There is no value-free science. The *bricoleur* also knows that researchers all tell stories about the worlds they have studied. Thus, the narratives or stories scientists tell are accounts couched and framed within specific storytelling traditions, often defined as paradigms (e.g., positivism, postpositivism, and constructivism).

The product of the *bricoleur's* labor is a *bricolage,* which is a complex, dense, reflexive, collage-like creation that represents the researcher's images, understandings, and interpretations of the world or the phenomenon under analysis. The *bricolage* connects the parts to the whole, stressing the meaningful relationships that operate in the situations and the social worlds studied (Weinstein and Weinstein, 1991, p. 164).

SOURCE: Adapted from Denzin, N.K., and Lincoln, Y. (1994). *Handbook of Qualitative Research.* London: Sage.

views on how one may define qualitative research and its many perspectives, most would agree that its essence includes a commitment to the naturalistic, interpretive approach to its subject matter. Denzin and Lincoln's definition espouses this *a priori* perspective, which is grounded in the philosophical assumptions of the interpretive worldview, and highlights the importance of multiple sources of information available to researchers.

The work of Denzin and Lincoln (1994) has been expanded by Creswell (1998, p. 15). His definition emphasizes the complex, holistic picture created by qualitative research. He writes:

> *Qualitative research is an inquiry process of understanding based on distinct methodological traditions of inquiry that explore a social or human problem. The researcher builds a complex, holistic picture, analyzes words, reports detailed views of informants, and conducts the study in a natural setting.*

This definition incorporates the idea that the researcher is an instrument of data collection who focuses on the meaning of participants' experiences in social contexts. The use of descriptive language that emerges from the complex narrative of participants is critical to Creswell's perspective. His definition adds the dimension of "distinct methodologies within the traditions of inquiry." For Creswell, these traditions include the historian's biography, the psychologist's phenomenology, the sociologist's grounded theory, the anthropologist's ethnography, and the political scientist's case study. Although some of these traditions are explored in this chapter, a full discussion is beyond the scope of this text. For a complete description of each tradition, interested readers are directed to Creswell's text in the Recommended Readings at the end of this chapter.

A significant number of researchers define qualitative research by comparing it with quantitative research (Brink and Wood, 1998; Burns and Grove, 1997; Fain, 1999; LoBionda-Wood and Haber, 1998). These distinctions are helpful in contrasting assumptions and values that are profoundly different in each perspective. Table 6.1 summarizes the distinctions reported by these authors. The table is not intended to be exhaustive; rather, it highlights the key differences for each research tradition.

Having defined qualitative research, it is important to note that it is complementary to quantitative research. Both processes produce different kinds of nursing knowledge that are valued by the profession and both are needed to promote excellence in practice. Qualitative and quantitative methods enable nurses to engage in the systematic collection and analysis of data on the organization, delivery, and outcomes of nursing care for the purpose of enhancing the client's health and understanding the meaning of health and the health-care experience from the perspective of the client (Parahoo, 1997). Both qualitative and quantitative research contribute significantly to the knowledge base required for the provision of quality care and excellence in practice.

2. Core Activities in Qualitative Research

In many ways, the format for a qualitative investigation follows the traditional research approach of asking a question or presenting a problem, collecting data, analyzing the data, and presenting findings. There are, however, important distinctions in the manner in which a qualitative investigation is designed and conducted as compared with a quantitative study. Figure 6.1 illustrates the formats for designing a qualitative and a quantitative study. Streubert and Carpenter (1999) identify several core activities that are

Table 6.1   Qualitative and Quantitative Research Contrasted

Qualitative	Quantitative
Multiple realities	Single reality
Reality is socially constructed	Reality is objective
Reality is context interrelated	Reality is context free
Holistic	Reductionistic
Strong philosophical perspective	Strong theoretical base
Reasoning is inductive	Reasoning is deductive and inductive
Discovery of meaning is the basis of knowledge	Cause-and-effect relationships are the bases of knowledge
Develops theory	Tests theory
Theory developed during study	Theory developed a priori
Meaning of concepts	Measurement of variables
Process oriented	Outcome oriented
Control unimportant	Control important
Rich descriptions	Precise measurement of variables
Basic element of analysis is words	Basic element of analysis is numbers
Uniqueness	Generalization
Trustworthiness of findings	Control of error

different in the two approaches. These are summarized next.

a. Literature Review

A quantitative investigation involves an extensive review of the literature early on in the research process to establish the need for the investigation. The researcher must be familiar with what others in the field have reported about the research topic. This information is important so the researcher can have confidence that this investigation is the next appropriate one to advance the particular field of knowledge. The literature review helps the quantitative investigator refine the research question and situate the question within a larger theoretical framework.

In qualitative investigations, the literature review is usually conducted *after* the research has been conducted and the data analyzed. Although some qualitative investigators accept that a cursory review may be conducted initially to help focus the study, purists argue that the review should not occur until completion of the study. The rationale for this is to prevent the researcher from leading participants in the direction of what has already been discovered about the phenomena of interest. The purpose of the literature review in qualitative studies is to show how the current findings fit into what is already known about the research topic.

b. Explicating Researcher's Beliefs

Before beginning most qualitative investigations, the researcher engages in a process known as *bracketing*. This does not occur in quantitative studies or in qualitative research done using Hermeneutics (a type of phenomenology attrib-

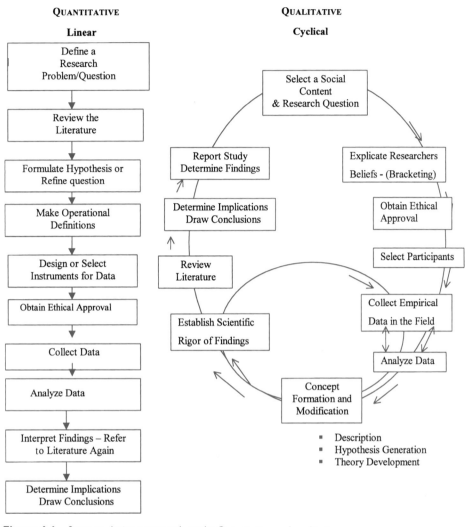

Figure 6.1   Steps to design a research study: Quantitative and qualitative.

uted to Heidegger). **Bracketing** is a cognitive process used by researchers to set aside one's biases and personal perspectives about the research topic. Its purpose is to make known what the researcher believes about the research topic so that the researcher can then approach the topic honestly.

Bracketing is a critical step in most qualitative investigations because of the subjective nature of the investigation and the close relationship of the investigator

to the phenomena studied. To bracket one's ideas about the research phenomenon, the investigator may keep a diary in which he or she writes personal thoughts and feelings about the topic. After these ideas are disclosed, they can be set aside. Through bracketing, the researcher is made aware of when data collection and analyses reflect personal beliefs rather than those of the participants. For example, you may be interested in exploring the phenomenon of meaning in life in el-

B. QUALITATIVE RESEARCH DESIGNS

The use of qualitative methods to study human phenomena has taken on important significance in nursing. Indeed, some would say that a quiet revolution has taken place in nursing research over the past decade. This has been marked by an increase in the number of qualitative studies reported in nursing journals and research textbooks, as well as an increase in the number of qualitative research conferences at both national and international levels, and an increase in the number of nurse researchers who are presenting reports of qualitative investigations in such forums. Many nurses are now focusing on qualitative perspectives to enhance understanding of the human experience of health and illness and subsequently to improve practice. This chapter examines three perspectives to qualitative research: phenomenology, grounded theory, and ethnographic methods. Although these perspectives are quite different, they do share a common essence—that of understanding and examining meaning in human experiences.

1. Characteristics of Qualitative Research Designs

Streubert and Carpenter (1999) identify six characteristics of qualitative investigations. Each warrant comment before examining the three qualitative designs selected for discussion in this chapter.

1. **Multiple realities exist.** There is not just one reality, one truth. Rather, all qualitative researchers believe there are many realities—those of the researcher, the participants being studied, and the readers of the research report. Through social interaction, participants come to know and understand phenomena in different ways and construct their realities. Different people come to know things differently in various social contexts. Researchers must come to know these different realities and report them through use of extensive quotations and identification of **themes** that reflect the descriptions of the participants.

2. **The researcher is committed to identifying a perspective to understanding that will support the phenomena studied.** Qualitative researchers address questions about the phenomena of interest by using multiple methods or perspectives to answer the question. Therefore, the discovery leads the choice of method rather than the method leading the discovery. In many qualitative investigations, a combination of methods, such as focus groups, unstructured interviews, and observations, are required to fully understand the phenomena of interest. Method and data collection strategies may change as the study unfolds because the researcher is committed to using whatever perspective best enables an understanding of the phenomena of interest.

3. **The researcher is committed to the participants' points of view.** Qualitative researchers are co-participants in the inquiry process. They seek to understand the participants' life experiences as constructed in their social worlds. Qualitative researchers become deeply involved with participants immersing themselves in the field to understand the phenomena of interest from the participant's perspective. Extensive interviews and observations are conducted to provide a view of reality that is important to those studied rather than what is important to the researcher. The researcher gains an insider perspective. For example, Lee (1997) conducted a phenomenological study of the meaning of menopause as experienced by modern Korean women. To understand this human health experience, in-depth interviews were conducted with 65 women ages 40 to 60 years to reveal

the covert meaning of menopause. Participants were asked to reveal their thoughts, feelings, perceptions, and expectations related to menopause and how they were coping with them. Four patterns emerged from the lived experience of the 65 women: (1) from suffering to comfort, (2) from oppression to freedom, (3) from being a good wife and mother to becoming a woman, and (4) from a productive life to a transformed life.

4. **Inquiry is conducted in a way that does not disturb the natural context of the phenomena studied.** Researchers collect data in natural settings where people are acting as they usually do. There is considerable onus on investigators to be as nonintrusive as possible. Researchers try to limit the distance between themselves and those being studied. Prolonged time is spent in the field to reduce the objective separateness that exists in quantitative studies. For example, Anderson (1996) spent extensive time in the field to discover how adolescents make decisions about substance abuse while in juvenile detention. An ethnographic design was used to learn, interpret, and describe perspectives of adolescents as they go about the business of living their lives and making sense out of their world in detention. The researcher became the data collection tool, learning how things worked in the closed institutional setting of a detention facility by living and working in the setting. Participant observation, focus group interviews, and individual interviews were used to explore the dynamics among young women in juvenile detention as they discussed their resolutions for the future. The presence of the investigator in the natural setting over time (in this case, the detention center) usually enables the investigator to establish an inclusive understanding of the particular phenomena of interest.

5. **The researcher, as a participant—observer, is considered to be an insider.** As the previous example illustrated, the researcher is considered to be the research instrument. This requires an acceptance of the investigator as part of the research study. The researcher plays a role as observer, interviewer, and interpreter of data; therefore, qualitative investigators accept the subjective bias inherent in qualitative investigations. The acknowledgment of the subjective nature of qualitative research is fundamental to the conduct of qualitative inquiry.

6. **The research report is written in a literary style rich with participants' comments.** The findings of qualitative research focus on the experience of the participants. The use of first person (i.e., "I"), metaphors, and a focus on personal stories add to the richness of the report and to the understanding of the meaning of the social interaction of those studied. The language is very personal and emerges as the participants tell their stories.

Qualitative research is well suited to many nursing investigations in which the goal is to develop a deep understanding of human experiences and the meanings participants attribute to these experiences. Life processes such as maturing, parenting, grieving, adapting to change, coping with stress, and dying are all phenomena of central concern to nurses as they work with individuals and family members experiencing these processes. Qualitative exploration of these processes provides nurses with critical insights and a deep understanding of participants' experiences. Such insights could not be gleaned from a reliance on strictly quantitative approaches.

Developing an understanding of the full range of human experiences that one encounters in the nursing world requires a multitude of methods. Following is a discussion of three frequently used qualitative approaches in nursing science. Each is discussed in terms of its definition, philosophical tenets, and application of the method. Unique features of each perspective are highlighted and research examples are provided. Table 6.2 presents a comparison of the three qualitative methods.

2. Phenomenological Research Perspective

The **phenomenological perspective** is a qualitative research method that describes the meaning of a lived experience from the perspective of the participant. **Lived experiences** are the everyday human experiences that are real to the individuals who experience them. Phenomenology seeks to achieve a deep understanding of the phenomenon being studied through a rigorous, systematic examination of it. Its purpose is to describe the essences of lived experiences. *Essences* are

elements related to the true meaning of something that gives common understanding to the phenomenon under study (Spiegelberg, 1975; Fain, 1999). For example, in a phenomenological investigation of how nurses experience caring for dying patients, the researchers reported that four themes formed the essence of the experience of caring from the nurses' perspectives: knowing the patient, preserving hope, easing the struggle, and providing for privacy (Rittman et al., 1997). It is phenomenologists' role to uncover and convey the true meaning or essence of the experience through the use of descriptive language.

a. Philosophical Tenets

Central tenets of phenomenology evolve around the idea of social action. Phenomenology is predicated on the belief that each person has a unique view of the world and each person's social reality is as valid and true as any other view (Munhall and Boyd, 1993). It focuses on the every-

Table 6.2 Comparison of Qualitative Methods

Method	Focus	Foundations	Question
Phenomenology	The meaning of the lived experience	Philosophy	What is essential for social dancing in caring for persons with dementia in a nursing home? (Palo-Bengtsson & Ekman, 1997)
Grounded theory	To generate or discover a theory about a basic social process	Sociology symbolic interaction	What is the process used by families to manage the unpredictability of heart transplantation? (Mishel & Murdaugh, 1987)
Ethnography	Description and interpretation of a cultural group or system	Cultural anthropology	What are the meanings of health to adolescents within their subculture? (Rosenbaum & Carty, 1996)

day way in which people make sense of their being in the world. The philosophical basis for phenomenology lies in existentialism. Existentialism refers to the way one views the world and stresses the personal "here and now" experience and the demands they place on the person as a free agent in a deterministic universe (Smith, 1997). Phenomenology is concerned with the nature of being, the here and now as it is—the lived experience.

Phenomenology has been impacted by philosophers such as Kant, Hegel, Lambert, Husserl, and Heidegger (Schmitt, 1972). Husserl (1859–1938), known as the father of phenomenology, held unique beliefs about what it means to be human. He introduced two ideas that are central to phenomenology: lifeworld and intersubjectivity. *Lifeworld* is the world of lived experience, and **intersubjectivity** describes how subjective awareness and understanding can be reached in a common world (Fain, 1999). Phenomenologists believe that whatever is known must appear to consciousness; whatever does not appear to consciousness cannot be known. Consciousness then provides access to the world. To be conscious is to be aware of the lived experience of some phenomenon. Husserl believed consciousness and the lived experience were in relationship, that is, consciousness was the means that constituted the objects of experience. Everything that appears to one's consciousness constitutes an object. This is referred to as *intentionality*. Heidegger (1889–1976) advanced the concept of being in the world from the conception of consciousness as intentionality. He believed the nature of being human was concern or awareness of one's own being in the world.

All phenomenologists believe in multiple realities that are constructed by individuals within the social context of their lives. Reality is constructed from human experiences that emerge from the relationship between human consciousness and

phenomenon. The phenomenological view enlarges the experience and tries to understand it in the complexity of its context. Phenomenologists believe any experience is a valuable and valid source of knowledge. They also believe that intuition (i.e., developing one's consciousness through looking and listening) is important in knowledge development (Smith, 1997).

b. Application of Method

For each perspective discussed, this section addresses the following topics: developing the research question, the role of researcher, selecting participants, data collection, data analysis, review of the literature, and reporting the findings.

(i) Developing the Research Question

The focus of a phenomenological investigation is to describe the meaning of the lived experience from the perspective of the participants. Any experience that presents itself to consciousness can be a focus of phenomenological investigation. The nursing world, which confronts the experiences of human health and illness, offers a rich source for phenomenological questions. Examples include being a patient, surviving breast cancer, receiving a terminal diagnosis, giving birth, and even experiencing laughter.

The research question is usually quite broad. This is to allow the participants to provide the answer. It usually takes the form of "What is the meaning of one's lived experience?" From this, the researcher may develop a central overarching question and several subquestions that follow from the central question. Phenomenological researchers avoid using hypothesis statements so as not to sway the participants toward a desired answer.

Suggested steps for formulating the question have been developed by a number of nurse researchers (Munhall and Oiler, 1986; Omery, 1983; Parse et al.,

1985). The steps may vary depending on the phenomenological perspective followed. Moustaka (1994, p. 99) suggests four subquestions that may be useful in explicating the meaning of the lived experience. They focus on what is important about the experience to the participant and how the experience impacts on what it means to be human:

1. What are the possible structural meanings of the experience?
2. What are the underlying themes and context that account for the experience?
3. What are the universal structures that precipitate feelings and thoughts about the experience?
4. What are the structural themes that facilitate a description of the experience?

Holldorrsdottir and Hamrin (1997) conducted a phenomenological study to explore caring and uncaring encounters with nurses and other health-care professionals from the perspective of cancer patients. The research question was, "What is the essential structure of caring and uncaring encounters with nurses and other health professionals from the cancer patients' perspectives?" Participants were asked three questions that followed from the research question:

1. Can you tell me of your personal experience of a caring nurse or health-care professional whom you have encountered during your illness experience?
2. Describe what the nurse or health-care professional did and try to analyze why you felt that he or she was caring.
3. Could you describe how you felt during the encounter?

The same questions were posed for the uncaring experiences.

(ii) Role of the Researcher

The phenomenological researcher enters into the experience of the research participant. The researcher is the instrument for data collection and therefore must be an effective communicator and an empathetic listener. It is critical that the researcher establishes a good rapport with the participants and listens attentively with of all her or his senses to the participants' stories. The meaning of the lived experience can only be revealed when the investigator understands and interprets correctly the participants' stories.

Researchers usually explicate their beliefs about the research topic through the process of bracketing, which was previously discussed. This process is important in phenomenology in which the researcher develops a close relationship with the participants and engages in prolonged dialogue. Through bracketing, the researcher identifies personal biases, making it easier to attend to issues introduced by the participants instead of leading the participant in the direction of issues deemed relevant to the researcher.

An example of a researcher's bracketing her perspective on the research phenomenon is provided by Parse (1993) in her phenomenological investigation of laughter. Parse, who was interested in uncovering the structural definition of the experience of laughing, bracketed her personal biases and perspective on laughing by articulating her views in writing. She explicitly describes her perspective on the lived experience of laughing. By doing so, she provides the reader with an opportunity to assess how her perspective may influence the research findings.

It is to be noted, however, that some researchers believe that it is impossible to "set aside" one's beliefs and personal biases. This is particularly true of Hermeneutic phenomenology, in which the researcher's self-understandings must be identified, but they claim it is unrealistic— if not impossible—to set them aside.

(iii) Sample

A phenomenological investigation requires a purposive sample composed of individuals who have experienced the phenomenon of interest. It is essential that participants are able and willing to talk about their experience of the phenomenon and describe their inner feelings associated with it. The sample size may vary, but usually a small number of participants are selected because of the extensive documentation that results from the participants' narratives. One cannot easily predict the required sample size. It must be large enough to produce a rich and comprehensive description of the phenomenon under investigation. This occurs when the data are saturated; that is, when the inclusion of new participants does not lead to new information but rather confirms the previously collected data. Sample sizes typically range from 5 to 15 participants, but this may vary considerably depending on how quickly saturation is reached.

(iv) Data Collection

A variety of methods are used for data collection, including in-depth interviews, written descriptions of specific experiences in diaries or journals, and observation. Interviews are usually tape recorded and transcribed verbatim and last varying lengths of time ranging from 1 hour to several hours. It is often necessary to conduct several interviews with the same participants to ensure that the phenomenon is fully described and reflects the meaning of the lived experience for the participants. Saturation of data helps determine the number of interviews required.

(v) Data Analysis

A number of techniques are available for analyzing data in phenomenological studies. These include the methods of Colaizzi (1978), Georgi (1985), Patterson and Zderad (1976), Streubert (1991), Van Manen (1990), and Van Kaam (1959). For detailed information on a specific method, research students are advised to consult the original source. Although each method presents unique aspects, commonalities exist in the process of analyzing phenomenological data. Regardless of perspective, data collection and analysis occur simultaneously and the researcher immerses her- or himself in the data. This requires the researcher to "dwell with the data" by reading and rereading the transcripts in their entirety to get a sense of the lived experience as a whole. Depending on the technique chosen, the data analysis process may require returning to participants to get further clarification or more descriptions of the phenomenon. The researcher synthesizes the descriptions of participants and reduces the data into a smaller and smaller number of categories to arrive at a consistent description of the meaning of the lived experience for all participants. The steps usually involve:

1. Reading and rereading the transcripts in their entirety.
2. Identifying key statements of participants that have a bearing on the phenomenon.
3. Identifying and naming the themes in the identified statements; it may be helpful to write these in the margins of each transcript.
4. Identifying the essential structure of the phenomenon in the transcribed data. This involves taking all of the themes and trying to identify the commonness or essential structure of the phenomenon in each of the dialogues.
5. Identifying the essential structure of the phenomenon. This involves comparing the different dialogues to find similarities and differences in the dialogues to construct the overriding theme as well as the essential structure of the phenomenon.
6. Comparing the essential structure with the data. After the essential structure of the phenomenon has been identified, it is compared with the transcripts to make sure it fits the data. The researcher looks for themes in the transcripts that are not accounted for in

the description. A decision must be made as to whether they should be included or excluded and why.

7. Sharing the analytic description of the phenomenon with the participants for verification. Participants should be able to recognize their own experiences in the description.

This way of doing phenomenology has been referred to as the Vancouver School of Phenomenology. It is adapted from Colaizzi's method (Fig. 6.2). Box 6.2 demonstrates Halldorsdottir and Hamrin's (1997) adaptation of Colazzi's framework to identify themes from cancer patients' perspectives of caring and uncaring encounters with nurses and health-care professionals.

(vi) Review of the Literature

In phenomenology, the literature review is conducted after the data collection and analysis are complete. The purpose of the literature review is to place the study findings within the context of what is known about the phenomenon. Parse (1993) used the review of the literature to relate her findings on the lived experience of laughing to other investigators' views of laughing. A cursory review may be conducted to verify the need for the study; however, the concern with examining the literature too early in the process is that it may bias the researcher in the investigation of the phenomenon.

(vii) Reporting the Findings

Phenomenological findings report the essential structure or essence of the experience. The researcher describes the unifying meaning of the experience that is recognized by participants as their experience. For example, Parse (1993) described the experience of laughter as "a buoyant immersion in the presence of unanticipated glimpsings prompting harmonious integrity which surfaces anew through contemplative visioning." The reader of a phenomenological report should come away from the report with a better understanding of what it is like to experience the phenomenon that was investigated.

c. Example of Phenomenological Research

An account of the findings from a phenomenological study is provided in Box 6.3. The following comments are offered about the study in Box 6.3:

A phenomenological perspective is particularly appropriate for this study that sought to gain an understanding of the process of developing a mother–child relationship in the preadoptive period from the perspective of women who became mothers through international adoption. Because this process is not well understood and there is little investigation of it in the nursing literature, the phenomenological perspective is particularly appropriate for exploring people's preadoptive experiences from their own perspective. The women in this study recently lived the experience and are a rich source of data.

An open-ended interview was used that included a semistructured guide to focus discussion on the mother–child relationship rather than the adoption process. A questionnaire or structured interview would have imposed the researcher's perspectives on the women and would have been inappropriate. The early interviews were used to inform questions for the later interviews. The respondents talked freely and asked impromptu questions reflecting what they thought was important rather than what the researcher thought was important.

Data were analyzed inductively using a method developed by Strauss and Corbin (1990). Themes that reflected the experience of the participants in the preadoptive stage were identified. The literature was reviewed to compare the study findings with what was already known about

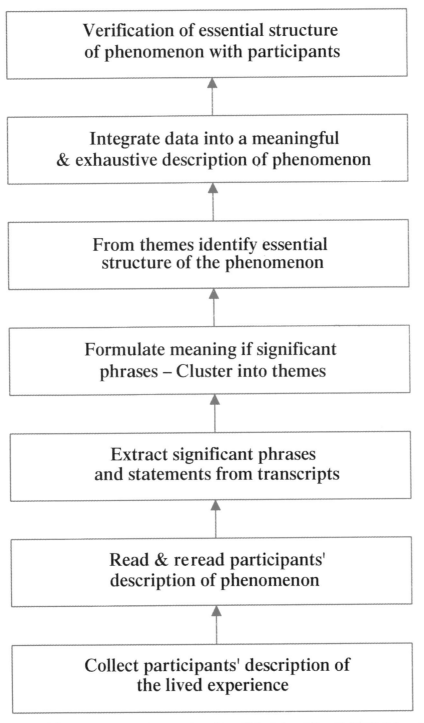

Figure 6.2   Phenomenological data analysis. (From Valle, R.S., and King, M. [1978]. Existential-Phenomenological Alternatives for Psychology. Oxford University Press, England. Cited with permission.)

BOX 6.2 *Theme Clusters That Constitute the Essential Structure of Caring and Uncaring Experiences*

Essential Structure of a Caring Encounter Embodied in Three Themes

1. The nurse or health-care professional is perceived as caring and as an indispensable companion on the cancer trajectory.
2. The result is mutual trust and caring connection.
3. The perceived effect of the caring encounter is a sense of solidarity, empowerment, well being, and healing.

Essential Structure of an Uncaring Encounter Embodied in Three Themes

1. The nurse or health-care professional is perceived as uncaring and as an unfortunate hindrance to the perception of well being and healing.
2. The result is a sense of mistrust and disconnection.
3. The perceived effect of the uncaring encounter is a sense of uneasiness, discouragement, and a sense of being broken down.

SOURCE: Adapted from Halldorsdottir, S., and Hamrin, E. (1997). Caring and uncaring encounters within nursing and health care from the cancer patient's perspective. *Cancer Nursing, 20*(2), 120–121.

the process of mother–child relationships. Women's narratives demonstrated the strength, commitment, and resilience inherent in the journey to create a family. Qualitative investigations such as this one contribute to the field of nursing's knowledge base on the experience of waiting for the adoptive child and can increase nurses' sensitivity to and understanding of the needs of preadoptive mothers. The study can also educate and inform other women who are waiting to adopt.

3. Grounded Theory Perspective

Grounded theory is an inductive, qualitative research method that seeks to understand and explain human behavior. The goal of this method is the development of theory that explains underlying social and psychological processes. It is different from phenomenology in that the researcher is not seeking to describe the phenomenon under investigation but rather to develop a theory about the dominant processes in the social scene under investigation (Stern, 1980). In the social situation studied, the researcher is interested in understanding how people interact, take action, or engage in the process in response to the phenomenon. For example, in their grounded theory investigation of family adjustment to heart transplantation, Mishel and Murdaugh (1987) studied the processes used by family members of heart transplant recipients to manage the unpredictability evoked by the need for and receipt of a heart transplantation.

Grounded theory is useful in areas in which little research has been conducted or in gaining a new perspective in areas that have an extensive research background. It is particularly appropriate in exploratory and descriptive studies (Glaser and Strauss, 1967) and is now among the most influential and widely used modes of qualitative research when the researcher's goal is generating theory (Strauss and Corbin, 1997). It is making an important contribution to knowledge development in nursing because of its ability to produce middle-range theory. Middle-range theory is the most useful to nursing because it can be empirically tested (see Chapter 2). It is the level of theory that fits between the broad, grand theories and the narrow practice or partial theories. Glaser and Strauss (1967) made the bold claim that after a grounded theory study has been conducted in an area, little additional research is done because of the density of the the-

BOX 6.3 *Nurse Researchers at Work*

ANTICIPATING THE ADOPTIVE CHILD: A PHENOMENOLOGICAL STUDY

This phenomenological pilot study explored the experiences of three women who became mothers through international adoptions. The study sought to gain an understanding of the women's experiences of developing a mother–child relationship in the preadoptive period.

Findings provided a description of seven themes that describe the process of developing a mother–child relationship in the preadoptive period. The themes include taking control, creating a family, celebrating the pictures, honoring the child's origins, investing personally, and bonding.

Taking control encompasses the mother's process of beginning to develop a mother–child relationship. Mothers took control of their lives and their environments in order to make a place in the world for a family purposely created through adoption. All made conscious decisions not to pursue pregnancy, seeing adoption as a natural, proactive choice that put them in control of their reproductive health and desire to be parents.

Creating a family was the second theme that emerged. All mothers stated clearly that their goal was to create a family, be a parent, and have a child. One mother summed it up nicely:

It's a feeling, like you have been on this road all your life and everything that came before was bringing you to this point. These were the kids meant to be in this house, in this home, to be our children. I have no doubt about it. This is the way and the time they had to come to us.

Anticipating, the third theme, was charged with emotion, preparation, and expectancy. They prepared for their children by sharing their anticipation and the adoption process with family, friends, acquaintances, and even strangers who were willing to listen.

Celebrating the pictures was a significant component of developing the relationship. All mothers described the pictures of their child as something to hold onto, share with others, and help them prepare for the arrival of their child. The photographs became tangible connections to their babies a world away, similar to a pregnant belly to rub and smooth.

Honoring the child's origins and learning about their child's land and culture were ways of paying tribute to the country that was giving them their child. They saw the child's time in their country of origin and with their caretakers as worthy beginnings.

Investing personally went beyond money, time, and resources of the mothers. They invested themselves and pursued adoption with blind determination. After they began, stopping the pursuit to adopt seemed no longer an option.

Bonding was the term used by mothers to describe what they did during the preadoption period. It was a significant theme running throughout their experience of developing a relationship with their adopted child. One mother summarized:

The bonding starts with all the preparation you make in your home, just psychologically, all the anticipation, having the pictures. What is that like? Maybe it is like parents who first feel their child kicking. The things that we did to bond, many of them are the same as the couple who are pregnant. I mean you paint a room, you get a crib, you have a baby shower. Many of those things are the same, and then some of the other things are different.

The narratives of the women describe themes in the process of preparing to welcome a child. These were different from those that emerge during pregnancy, yet there are parallels between the preadoptive process and pregnancy.

The stories of these women demonstrate the strength, commitment, and resilience inherent in their journeys to create families. Future research may focus on providing adoptive mothers with validation of both their journey and the processes inherent in it, credibility for this alternative but natural path to motherhood, and recognition of the beauty of the adoptive mother's development of a deep, loving, lifelong mother–child relationship.

SOURCE: Summarized from Solchany, J.E. (1998). Anticipating the adopted child: Women's preadoptive experiences. *Canadian Journal of Nursing Research, 30*(3), 123–129.

ory that emerges. Because the generated theory emerges from the data, it is said to be grounded in the data and useful to practice.

a. Philosophical Tenets

Grounded theory emerged from the discipline of sociology and has its theoretical foundations in **symbolic interactionism,** a theory about human behavior and human group life. Symbolic interaction focuses on the meaning of events to people in everyday settings. It is this meaning created by the people in the situation that guides behavior, action, and the consequences of that action (Chenitz and Swanson, 1986). At the core of symbolic interaction is an examination of how people define events or reality and how those beliefs shape their actions. George Herbert Mead (1934) and Herbert Blumer (1969) advanced the symbolic interaction tradition. Mead described the process whereby a person develops a sense of self through social interaction with others. Blumer believed symbolic interaction rested on three premises: (1) humans react to things on the basis of the meanings that the things have for them; (2) meanings are derived from the social situations that one has with others; and (3) meanings are altered and shaped through an interpretive approach used by individuals in dealing with things they encounter (Blumer, cited in Chenitz and Swanson, 1986).

For social life to emerge, group meanings must be shared among the group. Communication provides the mechanism for such sharing. Meaning of the event emerges through both verbal and nonverbal behavior; therefore, the interaction becomes the focus of the investigation to discover the true meaning. Through interaction, human beings are changed and influence each other. Through interaction with others, humans create meaning about life and themselves. Social interac-

tionism focuses on the nature of the dynamic social interaction occurring among persons and seeks to understand it.

b. Application of Method

(i) Developing the Research Question

A grounded theory investigation is conducted to identify concepts and propositions about the relationships between them, as they relate to a basic social psychological phenomenon. Unlike most methods, the researcher approaches the study without a specific well-defined question in mind. Instead, the question initially is broad and general in nature. It serves to focus the study. It identifies the phenomenon to be investigated in a particular social context. The question emerges, is refined, and may change several times as the data are collected and analyzed. The basic social process is usually a *gerund* (a noun ending in "ing") indicating change across time as a social reality is realized (Lo-Bionda-Wood, 1998). For example, Greenberg (1998) in a grounded theory study of humor within the nurse–client relationship posed the question, "What is the experience of humor in the nurse–client relationship from the perspectives of the professional nurse and the client involved in the nurse–client relationship? *Therapeutic playing* was the basic social process or core category that emerged. It was used by study participants to integrate humor within the relationship. The question may not be explicitly stated in the research study but can be implied from the study's purpose or goal statements. Other examples of questions appropriate for grounded theory studies include (1) how do family members who have survived an adolescent suicide experience healing? (Kalischuk, 1998); (2) what is the process used by nurses to deal with the problem of "being stymied" in their person-related interactions in the presence of technology?

(Alliex, 1998); or (3) What is the process of living with fibromyalgia syndrome for women? (Hughes, 1998).

(ii) Role of the Researcher

In grounded theory research, the investigator is intimately involved with the investigation. The researcher aims to describe social behavior as it takes place in natural settings. This means the researcher must not only study the behavior but the social setting that influences the interaction. The researcher plays an integral role in the investigation as a participant in the world and an observer of that world. Chenitz and Swanson (1986, p. 7) described the role of the researcher as follows:

> The researcher needs to be able to understand behavior as the participants understand it, learn about their world, learn their interpretation of self in the interaction and share their definitions. In order to accomplish this the researcher must take "the role of other" and understand the world from the participant's perspective. The researcher, therefore, must be both a participant in the world and an observer of participants in the world. Finally, in order for the knowledge to be understood and accepted by the researcher's discipline, the researcher, as observer, must translate the meaning derived from the researcher as participant into the language of the research discipline.

The researcher needs to be able to collect and analyze data, recognize and avoid bias, and think abstractly. The investigator must set aside his or her own perspectives and theoretical notions so that the theory can emerge from the data. This is critical to the method; the theory must be grounded in the data. In addition, the researcher needs to possess keen interpersonal and observation skills, powerful analytical abilities, and the art of accurately crafting a good narrative to de-

scribe the theory that has emerged from the process.

(iii) Sample

The researcher selects participants who are experiencing the social process under investigation. For example, in their study of caregiving to persons with cancer and AIDS, Stetz and Brown (1997) recruited 26 family caregivers of persons with cancer or AIDS from newspaper advertisements and announcements at home care agencies and public health departments. The sample size is not predetermined as in statistical sampling used in quantitative research; rather, it is determined by theoretical sampling. This is a process whereby the researcher collects, codes, and analyzes the data simultaneously and then decides what additional data are needed to enhance the theory. Similar to phenomenology, data collection continues until *saturation* is reached. In this situation, saturation refers to the inability of new data to add new codes or expand existing codes. At this point, the researcher concludes that the data are saturated and the theory has emerged. As a rough estimate, saturation typically requires about 20 to 30 interviews and several visits "to the field," although it varies depending on the quality of the data that emerges and the phenomenon and social process being investigated.

(iv) Data Collection

Astute observation of participants in the social group and skilled interviewing are the primary sources of data collection available to the grounded theorist. Interviews are usually audiotaped and transcribed verbatim and field notes of observations are transcribed as soon as possible on return from the field. Documents such as journals and diaries may also be used, but they are not typical of grounded theory. The researcher participates in the social group and observes and records information relevant to the study purpose. Interviewing may be informal or formal using a semistructured interview guide or topical outline. Such guides are not rigidly adhered to rather the questioning emerges from the data and becomes more focused as the study progresses. Questions are broad, open-ended, and general in nature. For example, Stetz and Brown (1997) used the Caregiver Outreach Interview Guide to collect qualitative data on the caregiving experience. The guide contained open-ended questions about the overall experience, as well as specific questions on the caregivers' perceptions of their role, and the demands of that role on their lives. Sample questions included:

1. Tell me about your family member's illness.
2. How was the decision made that you would be a caregiver?
3. Sometimes persons caring for their family member encounter situations that are a concern for them. What things about this experience are of concern for you?
4. How has caring for a family member changed your life?

Researchers need to be careful that the questions they pose do not limit them from hearing what the participants have to say or restrict the participants from having their own perspectives. One useful technique is to ask participants to share stories of their experiences in life. This can provide rich detail and add depth and texture to the data (Carla Mueller, personal communication, 2000).

(v) Data Analysis

A unique feature of grounded theory research is that data collection, coding, and analysis occur simultaneously from the beginning of the study. The process is systematic but fluid, allowing the researcher to respond to new information that emerges from the data. The **constant comparative method** is used when each piece of information is coded and compared with other pieces for similarities and differences in the lives of those interviewed. Figure 6.3 illustrates the fluid and cyclical nature of data analysis in grounded theory research. It requires detailed record keeping of interviews, field notes, and memos. It follows a standard format that has been described by a number of experts in the field (Beck, 1993; Creswell, 1998; Glaser, 1978; Stern, 1980; Strauss and Corbin, 1990; Streubert and Carpenter, 1995; Chinitz and Swanson, 1986). The steps are briefly summarized below using the process outlined by Stern (1980) and Streubert and Carpenter (1995, pp. 155–161).

1. **Concept formation: coding.** The researcher reads the transcripts and looks for an underlying pattern in the data. *Coding* occurs at three levels. Level I coding involves studying the data line by line and identifying key processes in the data. Level I codes are called *substantive codes* because they codify the substance of the data and use the words of participants (Stern, 1980).

   Level II codes assign data to categories according to obvious fit. A *category* is a unit of information composed of events, happenings, and instances (Strauss and Corbin, 1990). They emerge from condensing level I codes by comparing each level 1 code with all other level I codes. Each category is then compared with every other category to ensure that they are mutually exclusive.

   Level III codes identify the **core variable** or the *basic social psychological process* (BSP). A core variable is one that focuses the theory and accounts for most of the variation in a pattern of behavior that is both relevant and problematic for the participants involved. It is central to the other categories (Beck, 1993). BSPs usually represent the title given to the themes that emerge from the data. They are processes that occur

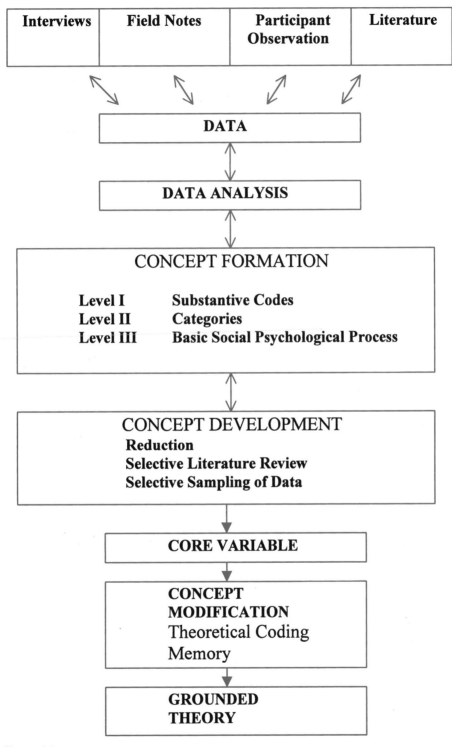

Interviews	Field Notes	Participant Observation	Literature

DATA

DATA ANALYSIS

CONCEPT FORMATION

Level I   **Substantive Codes**
Level II   **Categories**
Level III   **Basic Social Psychological Process**

CONCEPT DEVELOPMENT
Reduction
Selective Literature Review
Selective Sampling of Data

CORE VARIABLE

CONCEPT MODIFICATION
Theoretical Coding
Memory

GROUNDED THEORY

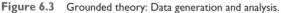

Figure 6.3   Grounded theory: Data generation and analysis.

over time and involve changes over time. For example, "Redesigning the Dream" was the BSP that emerged from Mishel and Murdaugh's (1987) study of family adjustment to heart transplantation. Table 6.3 illustrates examples of BSPs discovered through grounded theory research.

2. **Concept development.** Three steps are involved in the development of the core variable: reduction, selective sampling of the literature, and selective sampling of data. *Reduction* is a vital step in identifying the core variable or BSP. In reduction, each category is compared to see if there is a higher order or umbrella category under which a number of the existing categories can be merged. It is similar to clustering items in factor analysis (see Chapter 18). The researcher identifies theoretical links among the categories and collapses them to form more general categories. For example, in their study of family adjustment to heart transplantation, Mishel and Murdaugh perceived the three categories of freeing self, symbiosis, and trading places all mean to promote the welfare and comfort of the patient while they waited for a heart.

Table 6.3   Nurse Researchers at Work Selected Examples of Grounded Theory Studies

Title	Basic Social Psychological Process	Stages
"The Invisible Burden: Women's Lives with Fibromyalgia"	Bearing the invisible burden	1. Dealing with traumatic life 2. Yearning for affirmation 3. Searching for relief 4. Adjusting to limitations
"HIV-Positive Women: Double Binds and Defensive Mothering"	Defensive mothering	1. Preventing 2. Predicting 3. Protecting
"Transforming: The Process of Recovery from Schizophrenia"	Transforming	1. Battling 2. Connecting 3. Determining 4. Committing
"Handling the Hurt: Women Who Use Cocaine and Heroin and Lose Child Custody"	Handling the hurt	1. Numbing out 2. Giving up 3. Running away 4. Cleaning up 5. Dealing with feelings
"Inner Strength in Women: A Grounded Theory"	Learning to live a new life	1. Dwelling in a different place 2. Healing in the present 3. Giving and allowing nurturance 4. Connecting with the future 5. Being spiritual
"Integration: The Experience of Living with Insulin Dependent (Type 1) Diabetes Mellitus"	Integration	1. Having diabetes 2. The turning point 3. The science of one
"Loss and Bereavement: HIV/AIDS Family Caregiving Experiences"	Personal work	1. Reconciling 2. Making life-and-death decisions 3. Letting go

Thus, it was possible to reduce these three categories to form the broader category of immersion (a process whereby family members pledge themselves to the welfare of the patient).

Selective sampling of the literature occurs simultaneously with, or follows, data analysis. The literature review is conducted to determine what is known about the concepts that are emerging from the data. The literature is considered data and used to fill in the gaps in the emerging theory and add completeness and clarity to the theoretical description.

Selective sampling of the data occurs after the main concepts have emerged. At this point, additional data are collected in a selective manner to develop the hypothesis statements further, identify the properties of the main variables, and ensure saturation of the categories. The researcher generates hypotheses about categories and their relationships and interrelationships and then tests these hypotheses with selective data that either support or fail to support the hypotheses. Researchers stop collecting new data when they are satisfied that they are not hearing anything new about the category or the emerging hypothesis. At this point, one *core category variable* emerges that can explain the relationship between all of the others. This core variable best explains how a problem is processed (Chenitz and Swanson, 1986).

3. **Concept modification and integration.** This phase of data analysis involves two processes: theoretical coding and memoing. **Theoretical coding** forms theoretical linkages or connections between the data categories. Whereas the substantive coding that occurred at level I fractured the data into pieces, theoretical coding helps weave the fractured pieces back together again, by introducing level II code (Beck, 1993). Glaser (1978) has identified 18 *families of theo-*

retical codes to sensitize researchers to the subtleties of their data and the possibilities for integration of data. Three examples of Glaser's coding families (and their constituent members) include (1) the consequences family (i.e., the six C's: causes, contexts, contingencies, consequences, covariances, and conditions); (2) the interactive family (i.e., mutual effects, reciprocity, mutual trajectory, mutual interdependence, interaction of effects, and covariance); and (3) the strategy family (i.e., strategies, tactics, mechanisms, manipulations, maneuvering, dealing with handling techniques, ploys, means, and goals).

Stetz and Brown (1997) used the above three coding families to connect the categories and subcategories of "taking care" that emerged from the data. Box 6.4 illustrates the strategies, consequences, and interactions that constitute the process of "taking care."

Theoretical memos are the ideas the researcher holds about codes and the relationships as they strike the researcher during analysis. Memos vary in length from one line to several pages. Their purpose is to help the researcher put the fractured data back together. Glaser (1978) identifies three roles for memos: (1) to raise data to a conceptual level, (2) to develop the properties of each category, and (3) to generate hypotheses about relationships between the categories. Memos are sorted into a theoretical outline to assist the researcher in writing up the grounded theory that was discovered. Glaser's rule of sorting memos is to begin sorting categories and their properties *only* as they relate to the core category or BSP. Memos that do not fit are saved until such time as a new focus of the study is considered. Sorted memos become the basis of the research report.

(v) Review of the Literature

Grounded theory research contrasts with quantitative investigations in that there is

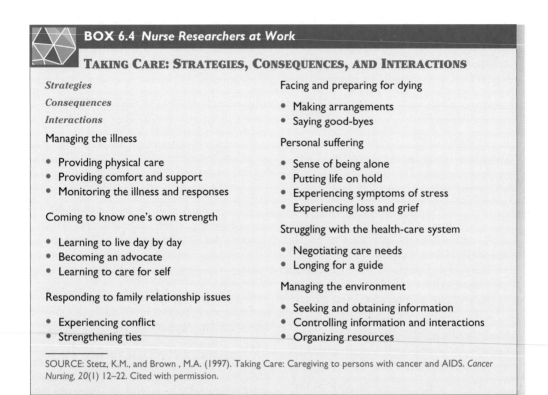

no review of the literature in the substantive area of the study before data collection. Indeed, the dictum in grounded theory research as stated by Glaser, cited in Beck (1993, p. 7) is: "There is a need not to review the literature in the substantive area under study." The rationale for this dictum is to avoid biasing the researchers' efforts to create concepts and hypotheses from the data that truly fit the data. The review of the literature is reserved until the theory begins to emerge from the study data. At this point, the researcher integrates the literature with the emergent theory during saturation, sorting memos, and the writing of the final report.

(vi) Reporting the Findings

The findings of grounded theory research include a substantive theory that describes the phenomenon under investigation supported by study data. Rich narratives of the study process and findings are provided to show how the theory is embedded in the data. A review of the literature and numerical results are not included in a grounded theory report.

c. Example of Grounded Theory Research

An account of a grounded theory study is provided in Box 6.5. The following comments are offered about the study in Box 6.5:

A grounded theory perspective is particularly appropriate for this study, which sought to develop a theory of the process engaged in by families to manage the unpredictability of cardiac transplantation.

"Redesigning the Dream" is the core variable or basic social psychological process that accounts for the pattern of behavior among participants as they adjust to the reality of the treatment envi-

---

BOX 6.5 *Nurse Researchers at Work*

A GROUNDED THEORY STUDY: FAMILY ADJUSTMENT TO HEART TRANSPLANTATION

The processes family members of heart transplant recipients use to mange the unpredictability evoked by the need for and receipt of a heart transplant were explored in a grounded theory study. The sample consisted of 20 family members of patients who received heart transplants. The subjects were labeled as partners to designate the significant other relationship to the patient. The partners were participants in three separate support groups, each of 12 weeks' duration. The groups consisted of 14 wives, five mothers, and one sister.

Data were collected from the three support groups over a period of 2.5 years. The investigators collected and audio taped all data from the 12 weekly group sessions that lasted approximately 1.5 hours each week. The investigators recorded content discussed as well as the participants' reactions, group dynamics, and the investigators' thoughts about the processes that occurred during the group meetings. A total of 36 transcripts were analyzed using the constant comparative method. Data collection and analysis continued until theoretical saturation was achieved.

"Redesigning the Dream" was the main theme emerging from the data that explained family adjustment to heart transplantation. Through this process, family members learned to readjust their cognitive thinking and behaviors in a manner that enabled them to cope with the situation of heart transplantation in their loved one. Their initial dream that life would return to normal after the patient received the transplant had to be revised to reflect the reality of the medical–technological treatment environment. The theory that emerged contained three major concepts: immersion, passage, and negotiation. These concepts parallel the stages of waiting for a doctor, hospitalization, and recovery. This study makes an important contribution to nursing in the area of middle-range theory related to the psychosocial needs of patients and families awaiting cardiac transplantation.

SOURCE: Summarized from Mishel, M.H., and Murdaugh, C.L. (1986). Family adjustment to heart transplantation: Redesigning the dream. *Nursing Research, 36*(6), 332–338.

---

ronment. This core variable focuses the development of the theory in the study. The theory contains three main concepts: immersion, passage, and negotiation and a number of subcategories.

Data were collected over a 2.5-year period and analyzed using the constant comparative method previously described. This study shows the promise that grounded theory yields for accurately depicting the participants' real world and the processes that participants use to deal with problems in that world. Theories such as "Redesigning the Dream," which are grounded in data, hold promise for a deeper understanding of nursing knowledge.

4. Ethnographic Perspective

Ethnography is a qualitative research method that attempts to understand human behavior in the cultural context in which it is embedded. It provides a description and interpretation of a cultural group that is gleaned from the researcher's prolonged examination of the observable and learned patterns of behavior, language, customs, interactions, and ways of life of the culture-sharing group (Creswell, 1998). Its aim is to understand the way in which people live from the **emic** (insider or native's) point of view, and how they derive meaning from their experiences (Spradley, 1980). The emic view is in contrast to the **etic** view, which is the view of a researcher or an outsider.

Ethnography is the work of describing a *culture* (Spradley, 1980). Leininger (1970), a nurse anthropologist, defines **culture** as a way of life belonging to a designated group of people. It includes all the ways a group of people solve problems, as reflected in their language, dress, food, traditions, and customs. It is a pattern of living that guides the group's thoughts, actions, and sentiments. The purpose of ethnographic research is to make *explicit* what is *implicit* within a culture by studying various cultural characteristics. The ethnographer's role is to paint a portrait of the culture-sharing group.

Within anthropology, a number of ethnographic interpretations have emerged over the years, including holistic, semiotic, behavioristic, cognitive, and ethnonursing perspectives. The proliferation of schools of ethnography has led to a lack of orthodoxy in method; therefore, it is important for investigators to identify which school they espouse when discussing their methods. **Holistic ethnography,** which defines culture as a way of life and studies it as an integrated whole (Fain, 1999), and *ethnonursing* are the two perspectives most frequently found in nursing investigations. A discussion of all the subtypes of ethnography is beyond the scope of this chapter; however, ethnonursing requires some comment because of its important contribution to nursing knowledge and its popularity among nurse researchers.

The **ethnonursing** tradition developed by Leininger (1978, 1985, p. 38) is defined as "the study and analysis of the local or indigenous people's viewpoints, beliefs, and practices about nursing care phenomena and processes of designated cultures." The goal of ethnonursing is "to discover new nursing knowledge as perceived or experienced by nurses and consumers of nursing and health services" (Leininger, 1985, p. 35). The focus in ethnonursing is the systematic documentation, description, explanation, and interpretation of the comprehensive meanings of both obscure and obvious nursing phenomena related to care, health, prevention of illness, and recovery from illness or injury. Ethnography is a viable research method for nurses because it provides a means to study cultural variations in health and illness and nurses and their clients as subcultures of society.

Two types of ethnography are useful for answering nursing questions: *mini* and *maxi* ethnographies. A **mini ethnography** is defined as a small-scale ethnography focused on a narrow area of inquiry. An example is the study by Holroyd and associates (1997) that explored the cultural practices of women in Hong Kong during the postpartum period (see Box 6.7). In this study, the researchers interviewed seven women about their self-care practices within the family home during the month after the birth of their first child. The number of participants in the study is small and the focus is limited to postpartum practices in the first month after delivery. The small sample size and the limited focus on one aspect of cultural practices over a 1-month period qualify this study as a mini ethnography. This is in contrast to a **maxi ethnography,** which is defined as "a large and comprehensive study of general and particular features of a designated culture" (Leininger, 1985, p. 35). Most maxi ethnographies have a broad focus of inquiry, extend over a long time period (e.g., several years), and are published in book form. Mini ethnographies are well suited to investigations by nursing students who wish to study cultural aspects of health situations but do not have the time to engage in extensive field work required in maxi ethnographic studies. Mini ethnography enables the student to experience the challenges and richness of doing work in the field within a reasonable time frame.

a. Philosophical Tenets

Ethnography has its roots in cultural anthropology—the study of the origin of people, their past ways of living, and their strategies for surviving through time. The philosophical underpinnings of anthropology are still evolving, but there is consensus that culture is the central concept of interest and ethnography remains central to the study of culture within anthropology. Anthropologists seek to discover the interrelationships between all the parts that make up a culture so that a picture of the wholeness of the culture emerges. These parts include the material culture consisting of manmade objects associated with a given group; the ideas, beliefs, and knowledge expressed in language; social networks; social and political institutions; and the ideals that the group holds as desirable goals (Burns and Grove, 1997).

Ethnography involves learning from people rather than studying people. This important distinction means that the researcher must become a student and the participants of the culture become the teachers. By observing and studying what people do (cultural behavior), what people say and know (cultural knowledge), and the things people use and make (cultural artifacts), the ethnographer comes to learn about the culture by making cultural inferences (Spradley, 1980). The ethnographer attempts to discover the insider's view (emic) of the world. To do this, the ethnographer must set aside the idea of naïve realism—the belief that all people define the real world in a similar way. Ethnography requires the researcher to adopt an attitude of conscious ignorance about the culture under investigation (Spradley, 1980).

In seeking to describe a culture at a particular moment in time, ethnographers strive to learn the meanings of life experiences and events to the people studied. This is best expressed by Spradley (1980, p. 5), who states:

> The essential core of ethnography is this concern with the meaning of actions and events to the people we seek to understand. Some of these meanings are directly expressed in language; many are taken for granted and communicated only indirectly through word and action. But in every society people make constant use of these complex meaning systems to organize their behavior, to understand themselves and others, and to make sense out of the world in which they live. These systems of meaning constitute their culture; ethnography always implies a theory of culture.

b. Application of Method

Implementation of the ethnographic method involves three phases of research activity: prefield work, fieldwork, and postfield work (Fain, 1999). Within each stage, specific steps must be followed. These have been described by authors such as Atkinson and Hammmersley (1994), Leininger (1985), and Spradley (1980) and are listed in Box 6.6.

(i) Developing the Research Question

Formulating the research question requires that decisions have already been made about the phenomenon to be investigated, the scope of the study, and the site and cultural group. The phenomenon of concern usually focuses on some pattern of behavior, lifestyle, custom, or belief of the culture-sharing group. The researcher selects a group of people to study and a site where an intact group has developed shared values, beliefs, and assumptions. Table 6.4 highlights phenomena nurse researchers have chosen to study using ethnographic methods. In addition to reading Table 6.4, research students who are

BOX 6.6 *Nurse Researchers at Work*

POSTPARTUM PRACTICES IN CHINESE WOMEN

An ethnographic study was conducted to determine the cultural practices of Chinese women in Hong Kong during the postpartum period. Seven multiparous women were interviewed and asked to reflect on their self-care practices within the family home during the month after the birth of their first child. The interviews were translated from Chinese to English and then transcribed. Nonverbal behaviors observed during the interviews were described in field notes immediately after the interviews. The data were coded and then analyzed using content analysis, constant comparative techniques, and a code-mapping category described by Morse (1991). Categories and themes were identified that described the daily enactment of the postpartum practices of the Chinese women and to what extent other people influenced these.

Results indicated that this group of Chinese women demonstrated customary beliefs and behaviors. Most women perceived that following traditional Chinese practice would speed their recovery after childbirth. They believed that if the cultural rules were violated, ill effects would result in their older age as a result of an imbalance of the Ying and Yang in their body. In addition, significant others acted as potent reinforcers of cultural mores, often stirring salient associations with past memories.

According to the Chinese belief system, the postpartum period lasts for 30 days after delivery, during which time the mother must perform a variety of avoidance rituals and remain at home. This is called "doing the month." These specific practices are regarded as not only curative but also preventative. To a new mother, the degree of importance attached to these customs serves to indicate her importance in her husband's household, with increased significance if the woman has produced a son.

Analysis of categories and themes revealed five major postpartum practice areas that Chinese women adhere to:

1. Good food and bad blood. Food was used as a tonic to restore the balance of the good blood in the body and was also seen as aiding in the expulsion of bad blood.

2. Dirt and prohibitions. Bathing and hair washing were not permitted because they would open the pores and allow the wind in, leading to harmful effects in later life. Preventative rituals were thought to restore youth and insulate against the crushing effects of old age.

3. Rest and appeasing the placenta god. Bed rest was essential after delivery to appease the placenta god.

4. Housework: variations and variety. Women made modifications in doing housework. In many situations, family members (e.g., mother and father-in-law) did this work. These acts demonstrated care and respect by family members.

5. Poisonous sexual intercourse. Sexual intercourse was delayed for at least 1 month after childbirth. It was implied that intercourse was unclean and had the potential to pollute the mother. In general, women resumed sexual activity 3 months after delivery, more aptly described by the Chinese lunar calendar as 100 days.

6. Competing loyalties. Some women expressed not really wanting to follow traditional cultural practices but did so because of family pressure. Mothers-in-law were seen as potent reinforcers of tradition and the act of checking on their daughter-in-law was present in nearly every dialogue describing a customary practice. The older people still reinforce beliefs that they once practiced themselves, yet the reality of modern-day Hong Kong and women's changing perception of their place in society pose conflicting demands on the young women.

This study highlights the importance of culturally sensitive and congruent nursing practice. It suggests that nurses have unique opportunities to support and provide culturally sensitive interventions such as hot–cold dietary guidelines, hygiene suggestions, and activity and leisure recommendations that can help women and their families restore their optimal health without violating cultural norms, standards, or beliefs.

SOURCE: Summarized from Holroyd, E., Katie, F., Chun, L., and Ha, S. (1997). "Doing the month": An exploration of postpartum practices in Chinese women. *Health Care for Women International, 18,* 301–313.

Table 6.4   Phenomena Investigated in Ethnographic Studies

Culture-Sharing Group	Site	Phenomenon	Researchers
Women in western Kenya and Somali refugees in the United States	Western Africa and a Somali section of San Diego	Practice, beliefs, and attitudes toward female circumcision	Morris (1996)
Health professionals with the National Health Service of Scotland	Telemedicine sites in Scotland	Diffusion of telemedicine across Scotland	Ibbotson (1999)
Adolescents	Juvenile detention facility	Decision making about substance abuse	Anderson (1996)
Adolescent peer subculture	Local community youth center	Meanings and experiences of care and health within peer subculture	Rosenbaum and Carty (1996)
Hutterites	Dariusleut and Lehrerleut groups in Alberta, Canada	Concepts of health and empowerment in health promotion	Brundt, et al. (1997)

composing ethnographic questions may find it helpful to consider the five areas identified by Fain (1999) as appropriate for ethnographic investigation:

1. Description of a cultural group that has not yet been described. (e.g., a first-generation group of immigrants to a new country). This would entail a maxi ethnographic study that would be long term and involve complex observations and interviews with multiple informants.
2. An aspect of culture that has not yet been described among a given group of people (e.g., Native American children's beliefs about death and dying).
3. A theoretical problem that requires investigation (e.g., health beliefs in conflict with cultural practices).
4. A practical problem needs some solutions identified (e.g., high rates of cardiovascular disease among Hutterite community members).
5. A society previously studied needs to be reexamined to see the changes that have occurred (e.g., Hong Kong's change of sovereignty).

Spradley (1980, p. 31) suggests that an ethnography is usually conducted with a single general problem in mind: "to discover the cultural knowledge people are using to organize their behavior and interpret their experience." However, many ethnographers design their studies to address more limited problems. Nursing investigators tend to focus on one or more aspects of life in a community that impact the health experience of its members. Nurses are interested in asking questions about how one's cultural knowledge, values, norms, and standards influence one's health experience (LoBionda-Wood, 1998). Questions may be asked about health and illness beliefs, self-care practices, lifestyle decisions, life events, health values, and attitudes as one's cultural group impacts them. Often the question in an ethnographic report is implied in the purpose statement of the study rather than explicitly stated. For example, Holyrod and associates (1997) crafted their study to answer the question: "What are the self-care practices of Hong Kong Chinese women within the family home during the first month after the birth of their first child?" This question is implied from the purpose statement of the study.

(ii) Role of the Researcher

The role of ethnographic researchers is to be interpreters of the experience of others. Researchers enter that world for an extended period of time, asking questions, observing, participating in the respondents' experiences, and collecting whatever data are available about the study question. Ethnographers observe behavior but go beyond it to inquire about the *meaning* of that behavior. Similarly, ethnographers see artifacts and record emotional states but go beyond these to discover the *meanings* people attribute to these objects and feelings. It is the researcher's role to make inferences from their observations and then to test these inferences over and over again with their population of interest until they are confident that they have an adequate description of the culture (Spradley, 1980). Ethnographers attempt to learn, interpret, and transcribe perspectives of individuals and groups of people as they go about the business of living their lives and making sense out of their world (Aamodt, 1991). As the primary data collection tool, the researchers are integral to the study.

To understand the study phenomenon from the participants' perspective (emic view), the ethnographer must explicate his or her own beliefs and set aside or bracket personal biases. For example, in their study of the health-care beliefs in the subculture of adolescence, Rosenbaum and Carty identified Leininger's (1991) theory of culture care diversity and universality as the framework that guided their study. This perspective defines care in relation to assisting, supporting, or enabling experiences that lead to an improved human condition or lifestyle.

(iii) Sample

The investigator selects a cultural group that has experience with the phenome-

non of interest. **Informant** rather than *subject* is the term used to refer to participants in an ethnographic investigation. The term "informant" implies that the person has special attributes such as knowledge or experience that are important to the investigation. Creswell (1998) suggests it is best to select a group of informants that the researcher can gain access to and one to which the researcher is a *stranger.* Unless a compelling case can be made to study people in one's "*own backyard,*" it should be avoided because of the difficulties that can arise. Studying those well known to the ethnographer can create expectations for data collection that may compromise the value of the data and cause individuals to withhold information or slant it in a way to please the investigator (Glesne and Peshkin, cited in Creswell, 1998). Students are often attracted to do ethnographic investigations of this type because of the easy access to participants. It is a procedure, however, that should be discouraged because of the difficulties inherent in making known to others what is only implicitly understood by the investigator.

Access to the cultural group is usually gained through a **gatekeeper,** an individual with special group status who can lead the researcher to other *key informants.* **Key informants** are the group members who are most knowledgeable about the study phenomenon. They are representative of the culture and have potential to yield substantive data about the study phenomenon. Key informants are willing to teach the ethnographer about the study phenomenon and refer him or her to general informants who also have knowledge of the phenomenon under study. Leininger (1985) suggests that depending on the study scope and purpose and the phenomenon under investigation, about 10 to 15 key informants and 30 to 60 general informants constitute a desirable number of informants for ethnonursing or ethnographic studies. In Rosenbaum and Carty's study of the subculture of adolescence, 27 key informants were interviewed. They were effective key informants because they were knowledgeable about their own subculture and they could teach the investigators about their meanings and experiences with health and care. In addition, 44 general informants were interviewed to reflect on the meanings expressed by the key informants.

(iv) Data Collection
Participant observation, formal and informal interviews, and collection of artifacts and documents are all means of gathering data in ethnographic research. Of these methods, participant observation and interviews are the most popular forms. Through the process of fieldwork, the researcher spends prolonged periods of time in the natural settings of the participants and observes members of the culture in their everyday lives. Field notes are written and provide descriptions of the researcher's observations and experiences in the field. They become valuable sources of data as the study unfolds. The steps for conducting a participant observation study, writing field notes, and doing in-depth interviews are described in detail in Chapter 7.

During the fieldwork phase, investigators may decide that additional information is required about what they are observing in the field. For example, collection of basic demographic data may be accomplished through census taking; mapping may be used to identify the location of people and understand how they interact with their physical environment; genealogies may be collected to study the kin relationships of informants; and life histories may be collected to show how general cultural patterns are integrated into a person's life (Fain, 1999).

Anderson (1996) provides a useful example of ethnographic data collection. She used participant observation, in-depth interviews, and small focus groups to collect data on the content of teenagers' decisions; the meaning of substance abuse in their lives; and the interactional dynamics among young women in juvenile detention as they discussed their resolution for the future related to substance abuse.

In this example, the critical first step was to establish a working relationship with the teens and staff. This required the investigator to learn how things worked in the closed setting of a juvenile detention facility (JDF). Daily routines, such as meal and bed times, attendance at classes, and events such as Sunday morning church services and Thursday evening co-ed dances, all provided opportunities to learn the folkways at JDF. As Anderson commented, "Participant observation during these activities helped me to learn what it means to live and work behind locked gates."

Data collection began with focus groups designed to obtain perceptions on a defined area of interest in a permissive, nonthreatening environment in which the teens had an opportunity to present their own perspective about substance abuse decisions. Each focus group session lasted 1 to 1.5 hours. One-hour participant observation sessions were carried out on the dormitory units where the informants lived both before and after the focus groups. Observations were recorded in field notes along with notations regarding nonverbal behaviors during the focus group discussions. During the focus groups, talk about decisions regarding past and future substance use became a dynamic process. The girls made resolutions and plans, offering them to each other, and in their interactions they shaped and reshaped their decisions. General questions were used such as, "How do teenagers usually solve their problems?" and "How do teenagers decide to use drugs or alcohol?" Questions that repeated some of the discussion during the focus groups were asked in individual interviews to discover the individual participants' perspectives. Focus groups and interviews were audiotaped and transcribed verbatim by a linguistic anthropologist who specialized in the slang of inner city teenagers. Three months were required to collect the data.

(v) Data Analysis

Analysis of data in ethnographic inquiry follows a cyclical pattern whereby the researcher goes back and forth collecting ethnographic data, recording the data, analyzing the data, and returning to the field to collect more data. It is a process of question–discovery (Spradley, 1980). Unlike quantitative researchers, who go into the field with specific questions in mind, ethnographers analyze the field data compiled from participant observation and interview to discover more questions that bring the researcher back to the field for more data collection, more field notes, and more analysis, and the cycle continues.

After each session in the field, the researcher analyzes the data in order to know what to look for in the next period of participant observation. The analysis proceeds through four levels as the researcher learns, describes, and interprets the meaning of cultural symbols on the informants' language. The experienced researcher conducts the four levels of analysis simultaneously throughout the research project; however, it is recommended that the research student learn to do each in sequence before moving on to higher levels. The suggested sequence includes domain analysis, taxonomic analysis, componential analysis, and theme analysis (Spradley, 1980). Throughout the analysis, the researcher is looking for patterns in the data. The goal is to discover the cultural patterns people are using to organize their behavior, to make and use objects, to arrange space, and to make sense out of their experience. These patterns make up the culture (Spradley, 1980).

1. **Domain analysis.** In the **domain analysis,** the researcher is moving from observing a *social situation* (a set of behaviors carried out by people in a social situation) to discovering a *cultural scene.* A **cultural scene** is an ethnographic term used to refer to the culture under study (Spradley, 1980). Cultural domains are categories of meaning that include other smaller categories. The first step in a domain analysis is to select a situation to observe. For example, the researcher may observe a pediatric unit. The category, people on the unit, is the first domain to be analyzed. The researcher asks the question, "Who are the people on the unit?" She refers to her field notes and easily identifies the various categories of people (e.g., children, parents, family members, doctors, nurses, ward clerks, cleaning staff). Spradley suggests that it is important to identify the *semantic relationships* in the observations made in your particular cultural scene. He identifies a list of universal semantic relationships. For example, x is a kind of y; x is the result of y; x is a part of y. Children are a kind of patient on the unit. Furthermore, another analysis can be done to explore the types of children admitted to the pediatric unit. By creating the domain analysis, the researcher identifies additional questions and makes more focused observations that lead to exploring the roles and relationships of other members in the cultural scene.

2. **Taxonomic analysis.** A *taxonomic analysis* is a more in-depth analysis of the domains. The researcher is searching for larger categories to which the domain may belong. A **taxonomy** is a set of categories organized on the basis of a single semantic relationship. The major difference between the two is that the taxonomy shows more of the relationships among the things inside the cultural domain (Spradley, 1980). You are moving from the general to the particu-

lar. For example, children are a type of patient on the pediatric unit. One way the children can be categorized further is based on their treatment requirements: medical patients, surgical patients, mental health patients, and so on. These can be further broken down based on the specific diagnosis (e.g., surgical patients may be those undergoing tonsillectomies, appendectomies, hernia repairs, and so on) assigned to them in the particular culture under study. After this analysis is complete, the ethnographer looks for relationships among the parts or relationships to the whole (Streubert and Carpenter, 1999). Based on these new categories, additional questions and observations are made. For example, are surgically classified children treated differently than children with mental health problems? Are there different types of nurses who care for children with different diagnoses?

3. **Componential analysis.** Cultural meaning comes not only from patterns based on similarities but also from patterns based on contrasts. **Componential analysis** looks for all the contrasts among the cultural categories in the domains. Spradley defines it as "the systematic search for the *attributes* (components of meaning) associated with cultural categories" (p. 131). He uses the domain of mail to exemplify componential analysis. Think about all the different kinds of mail you receive. You get junk mail (i.e., flyers, notices, and advertisements), bills, magazines, personal letters, and so on. A person from a culture without mail would find it more difficult to classify the mail than you would because he or she would not see the differences. This person would see all the paper as mail. Although it is true that they are all kinds of mail, they each have a unique cluster of *attributes* that convey the cultural meaning of the mail to you. For example, whereas bills are usually impersonal printed forms, personal letters are often hand addressed and often use your first name. All these different bits of mail have components of meaning (attributes) attached to them that make them meaningful. You act on the implicit cultural meanings without even thinking about them. You know to discard the junk mail, pay your bills, and save your personal letters to respond to them.

The attributes for all the cultural domains are represented in charts known in ethnography as *paradigms*. A sample paradigm for the domain of mail is provided in Table 6.5. It highlights the differences (attributes) for the three cultural categories of e-mail directed toward (1) everybody in the company, (2) members of your department, (3) you personally.

To complete a componential analysis, ethnographers should carry out the eight steps outlined by Spradley (1980, pp. 133–139). These include:
• Select a domain for analysis (e.g., people on a pediatric unit).

Table 6.5 Ethnographic Paradigm for the Domain of E-Mail

Domain	Attributes and Responses		
	Target	Action	Feeling
General e-mail	All employees	Scan & delete	Boring! Anger
E-mail to group	Dept members	Read & print	Okay: I need this
Personal e-mail	Personal	Read & save	Nice to get thanked!

Spradley, J.P. (1980). *Participant Observation.* New York: Harcourt Brace College Publishers. Cited with permission.

- Take an inventory of all contrasts previously listed (e.g., some people are patients, some people are professional staff, some are support staff).
- Prepare a paradigm worksheet.
- Identify dimensions of contrast that have binary values (e.g., pediatric patient, yes or no).
- Combine closely related dimensions of contrast into ones that have multiple values (e.g., nurses and doctors are professional staff who provide care to patients).
- Prepare contrast questions for missing attributes.
- Conduct selective observations to discover missing information.
- Prepare a complete paradigm.

The final paradigm may be used as a chart in your ethnography. It enables you to present a great deal of information in a concise manner.

4. **Theme analysis. Cultural themes** are recurrent patterns in the data that are used to connect domains. Spradley defines them as "any principle recurrent in a number of domains, explicit or tacit, and serving as a relationship among subsystems of cultural meaning. . . . They usually take the form of an assertion such as men are superior to women" (p. 141). Themes are assertions that apply to numerous situations and have a high degree of generality. To identify themes, an ethnographer must immerse him- or herself in the data. Spradley suggests that if you are not able to live in another society for a year or two (as many nurses are not able to do), you can still immerse yourself in the data by blocking several days to immerse yourself in the cultural setting and look for themes and then take several days to review your field notes in an intensive manner. This type of immersion often reveals patterns and themes that relate to the domains previously identified.

One way to search for themes is to look for similarities and differences across domains. This focuses your attention on the cultural scene as a whole. Another strategy to identify themes is to compare different cultural scenes. A third strategy is to make a schematic diagram of the cultural scene, identifying relationships among the domains. Spradley suggests a list of *universal themes* that may be used as a basis for scrutinizing your data. The list is not intended to be exhaustive; rather, it simply suggests possible themes that you may find in studying your cultural scene. The universal themes include:

- **Social conflict.** In every social situation, conflicts emerge; identifying these conflicts helps researchers interpret the culture. For example, conflict may arise in a pediatric unit between nurses and physicians concerning treatment plans.
- **Cultural contradictions.** Every society has contradictory messages. What inherent contradictions have people learned to live with and how?
- **Informal techniques of social control.** What formal and informal means are used in the group you are observing to get people to conform to the values and norms that make social life possible? For example, nurses may get physicians who continually forget to reorder their clients' drugs to conform to the hospital policy of reordering clients' medications every 5 days by phoning those who refuse to do so late at night to request the reorder.
- **Managing impersonal social relations.** How do people in the cultural scene you are observing deal with people they know well and those they do not know well?
- **Acquiring and maintaining status.** What cultural symbols and icons convey status and prestige, and how are they acquired and maintained?

- **Solving problems.** A person's cultural knowledge is often designed to solve problems. Ethnographers seek to discover the cultural problems that exist and find out about the knowledge that is used to solve them. For example, within the nursing culture, much professional knowledge is focused on helping clients solve problems related to their health or illness states. Much of what nurses know deals with promoting the health of an individual or family or community.

The final step of thematic analysis is to write a summary overview of the cultural scene. The goal is to condense everything you know down to essentials and deal primarily with the relationships among the parts of the culture. Although ethnographers examine small details of a cultural scene, at the same time they seek to understand the broader cultural landscape. Through the analysis process and writing of the ethnographic report, the researcher is hoping to provide an in-depth analysis of selected domains, an overview of the cultural scene, and a description that conveys a sense of the whole.

(vi) Reporting on the Findings

Ethnographic studies yield a great deal of data. They include voluminous field notes; transcripts of interviews; artifacts; and miscellaneous information such as photographs, charts, and maps. The researcher must compile all of these items in a way that meaningfully describes the observed culture. Spradley suggests that this be done in two steps: first, writing a cultural inventory and then proceeding to write the descriptive report. The cultural inventory organizes the data for the researcher. After it is completed, the researcher is ready to write the final report. It includes nine steps:

1. Make a list of cultural domains.
2. Make a list of analyzed domains.
3. Collect all the sketch maps you have drawn such as maps of places, activities, and interactions.
4. List all the major and minor themes.
5. Take an inventory of all the examples of descriptions of events or experiences (many examples will be included in the final report because they bring the analysis to life and make it meaningful to the reader).
6. Identify organizing domains (there may be one or more domains that tie together many facets of a cultural scene).
7. Complete a table of contents.
8. Complete an inventory of miscellaneous data (e.g., memos, newspaper clippings, photographs, and other artifacts related to the cultural scene).
9. Suggest areas for future study (Spradley, 1980).

These steps organize all of your data, influence your thinking about the cultural scene, and prepare you to write the final report.

If you are conducting a maxi-ethnographic study, the final report may take the form of a book or monograph that describes a particular culture. If you are writing a mini-ethnographic study (as many nurses who use the ethnographic method do), you will probably present your findings in a scholarly journal. It is important to know who your audience will be. One of the best ways to know how to present an ethnographic report is to look at good examples of what others have done.

c. Example of Ethnograhic Research

An account of an ethnographic study is provided in Box 6.7. The following comments are offered about the study in Box 6.7.

Emphasis in this ethnographic study is placed on obtaining the emic perspective of Chinese women regarding the self-care practices in which they engaged in the family home during the month after the

BOX 6.7 *Phases of Ethnographic Research*

Prefield

- Identify the phenomenon to be studied and establish the scope of the study.
- Select the culture and site to be studied.
- Identify significant variables within the culture to be studied.
- Review the literature and gather information on the culture and the specific phenomenon to be studied.
- Prepare interview guides, instruments, data collection equipment, and so on.
- Obtain ethical approval.

Fieldwork

- Gain entrance to the cultural group.
- Identify key informants.
- Gain cultural immersion in group.
- Gather data (i.e., participant observation, interviews, artifacts, and documents).
- Identify major themes.
- Collect additional data that is more focused and selective.
- Continue with participant observation and interviewing, raising more sensitive issues.
- Double check data and probe for meanings.
- Refine themes.
- Determine how representative findings are of the culture as a whole.

Postfield

- Finalize analysis and findings.
- Develop a cultural inventory.
- Write an ethnography.

to observe, describe, document, and analyze the lifestyles or patterns of a culture or subculture (Leininger, 1991).

The main method of data collection in ethnography is participant observation. The act of participating gives opportunities for the researcher to have conversations with or interview people as he or she interacts with them. These are referred to as informal interviews. As in this case, formal interviews can also be arranged. In this study, the researchers carried out formal interviews and observations during the interviews that were recorded in field notes. The interviews used open-ended questions and then semistructured questions to explore both anticipated and unanticipated information and were tape recorded. In addition, a demographic profile was used to collect data.

The sample size of seven was appropriate for this mini-ethnography. The study was short term and limited in scope. It addressed the phenomenon of "doing the month" in a subunit of the Hong Kong Chinese culture (postpartum women).

This ethnographic study sheds light on an important area in nursing—the need for culturally congruent nursing care to Chinese people in Hong Kong. It is likely that the advent of Hong Kong's recent change of sovereignty will exacerbate this concern and nurses will need to deliver care to a large proportion of clients who hold more traditional Chinese beliefs with minimal Western influence.

birth of their first child. This was achieved by getting personal accounts from the women themselves of the complex issues that contemporary Chinese women in Hong Kong face in trying to follow traditional Chinese practices in a changing world.

An ethnographic design is appropriate for this study that explored postpartum practices in Chinese women. This perspective is considered a systematic way

C. SCIENTIFIC ADEQUACY OF QUALITATIVE RESEARCH

In quantitative research, the canons of validity and reliability are critical to the confidence we put in research findings. Similarly, in qualitative research, it is just as important to assess the rigor of qualitative studies to know how much faith one can have in the findings. Multiple approaches exist for defining and assessing the trustworthiness of qualitative studies and there is a "gulf of distance" among those engaged in this discourse (Creswell, 1998). **Trustworthiness** relates to the process of establishing the validity and reliability of qualitative research. Many researchers argue that the use of positivist language is no longer appropriate or adequate to a discussion of rigor in qualitative research (Creswell, 1998; Lather, 1993; Webb, 1993; Denzin and Lincoln, 1994; Sandelowski, 1993). They reject the notion of objectivity, reliability, validity, and generalizability as applied to qualitative methods. They believe it is as inappropriate as using the rules of one religion to judge the behavior of people from another religion: certain behaviors can be seen as sinful when judged through the eyes of one religion but not another (Parahoo, 1997). Lincoln (1995) has proposed a new approach to quality; her views are presented after the traditional approach discussed next.

I. Traditional Standards of Quality

In their classic statement, Lincoln and Guba (1985) shed some light on the issue of assessing truth in qualitative research. They outlined four questions that any investigation (quantitative or qualitative) into the human condition should consider if the trustworthiness (quality) of the project is to be properly assessed:

1. How truthful are the particular findings of the study? By what criteria can we judge them?

2. How applicable are these findings to another setting or group of people?
3. How can we be reasonably sure that the findings would be replicated if the study were conducted with the same participants in the same context?
4. How can we be sure that the findings are reflective of the subjects and the inquiry itself rather than the product of the researcher's biases or prejudices?

When appropriately addressed, these questions establish the trustworthiness of a study, its applicability, its consistency, and its neutrality. These terms are associated with terms from the positivist paradigm of internal validity, external validity, reliability, and objectivity. Lincoln and Guba are among the many researchers who believe it is inappropriate to rely on positivist's concepts of validity and reliability to evaluate qualitative research that operates within a different paradigm from the positivist perspective. They identify four alternative concepts that more accurately reflect the assumptions of the qualitative paradigm: credibility, dependability, transferability, and confirmability (Lincoln and Guba, 1985, p. 300). Taken together, these criteria establish the trustworthiness of qualitative findings. Table 6.6 illustrates the concepts of validity and reliability in qualitative research. A discussion of threats to validity and reliability in quantitative and qualitative studies is found in Chapter 13.

Credibility refers to the accuracy of the description of the phenomenon under investigation. The portrayal of the reality must be faithfully represented and

Table 6.6　Concepts of Rigor in Quantitative and Qualitative Research

Quantitative Research	Qualitative Research
Validity	Credibility (authenticity)
Generalizability (external validity)	Transferability (fittingness)
Reliability	Dependability (auditability)
Objectivity	Confirmability

plausible to those who have experienced that reality. Credibility can be enhanced by prolonged time in the field collecting data and repeatedly observing and interacting with participants. *Triangulation* of data sources (e.g., different persons, times, and places) methods (e.g., observations, interviews, documents), data type (e.g., qualitative, quantitative, recordings) investigators (e.g., researcher A, B), and theories is a popular means of establishing credibility. Triangulation was defined in Chapter 1 as the use of multiple referents to draw conclusions about what constitutes the truth. Triangulation leads to trustworthiness of the data by enabling the researcher to look for patterns of convergence as well as counter patterns or negative cases in the data. Essentially, triangulation is supposed to support a finding by showing that independent measures of it agree with or, at least, do not contradict it (Miles and Huberman, 1994). Other techniques suggested to gain accurate and true impressions of the phenomenon being studied include conducting member checks. This involves having participants involved in the data analysis—that is, the participants or "subjects" who were observed actually read the analysis and then refine it to be congruent with their experience. Collaborative research also improves the credibility and believability of results. This is accomplished by having other investigators verify the effectiveness of data collection procedures, the comprehensibility of descriptions, the inclusivity of samples, and the logic of arguments. Credibility is enhanced by an accurate description of the setting, participants, and events observed.

Dependability refers to both the stability and the trackability of changes in the data over time and conditions. The issue of dependability in qualitative investigations reflects the reality that situations constantly change and people's realities differ. In assessing dependability, the researcher is interested in determining the extent to which another investigator with similar methodological training, rapport with participants, and knowledge of the field would make the same observations. This is determined by an **audit trail,** in which a researcher does an audit of the research process, documenting all the raw data generated as well as methods and sources of data generation and analysis decisions. By reading the audit trail, another researcher should arrive at comparable conclusions given the same setting.

Transferability is concerned with the generalizability or fittingness of study findings to other settings, populations, and contexts. In assessing transferability of findings, the research consumer hopes to show that the results are not context bound. To enable the research consumer to do this, the researcher must provide sufficient detail in the study report so that readers can assess the appropriateness of the findings to other settings. The lack of transferability of findings to other settings is often viewed as a weakness of qualitative methods.

Confirmability refers to the objectivity of the data. Meanings emerging from the data have to be tested for their plausibility, their sturdiness, and their "confirmability" so that two independent researchers would agree about the meanings emerging from the data. Otherwise we are left with interesting stories about what happened, but they are of unknown truth and usefulness (Miles and Huberman, 1994). The basic issue here is one of neutrality. In other words, do the conclusions depend on the subjects and conditions of the inquiry rather than on the researcher (Lincoln and Guba, 1981; 1985)? To assess confirmability, the audit trail is used. The researcher must be explicit about how personal biases, assumptions, and values may have come into play in the study. The researcher considers the plausibility of alternative conclusions and rival hypotheses. To a certain extent, the researcher is trying to limit the influence of the Hawthorne effect (see Chapter 4), which is an inevitable part of doing research. Box 6.8 contains some useful questions that can help qualitative researchers assess the trustworthiness of their findings. These are not rules to be applied stiffly but simply test questions that may help researchers focus on the central question: Do the results of the inquiry fit and make sense and are they true to the understanding of ordinary people in the everyday world?

Drawing conclusions from qualitative research data requires careful assessment and involves the processes of forming patterns in the data, looking for contrasts, clarifying relationships, posing rigorous test questions (such as those posed in Box 6.8), and collecting respondent and peer

---

BOX 6.8 *Questions to Be Asked of Qualitative Research to Assess Rigor*

Test for Credibility (Validity)

- Do the findings make sense to the people studied and do they consider them accurate?
- How context rich and meaningful are the descriptions?
- Does the account "ring true" and enable a vicarious presence for the reader?
- Did triangulation among complimentary methods and data sources produce converging conclusions? If not, is there an adequate explanation for this?
- Was negative evidence sought? Found? What happened then?
- Are the data well linked to the categories of the emerging theory?

Test for Transferability (Generalizability and Fittingness)

- Are the characteristics of the original sample of persons, settings, processes, and so on fully described to permit adequate comparisons with other samples?
- Is the sampling theoretically diverse enough to encourage broader applicability?
- Does the researcher describe the scope and the boundaries of reasonable generalization from the study?
- Do many readers report the findings to be consistent with their own experiences?
- Are the findings congruent with, connected to, or confirmatory of prior theory?
- Have the findings been replicated in other studies to assess their robustness? If not, could replication be done easily?

Test for Dependability (Reliability and Auditability

- Are the research questions clear and are the features of the study design congruent with them?
- Did data collected across the full range of appropriate settings, times, and respondents suggest the research questions?
- Do multiple field workers have comparable data collection protocols and do their accounts converge in areas where they might be expected to?
- Were data quality checks made (e.g., for bias, deceit, and informant knowledgability)?
- Were any forms of peer or colleague review in place?
- Were coding checks made, and did they show adequate agreement?

Test for Confirmability (Objectivity)

- Are the study's methods and procedures described in sufficient detail so that an audit trail can be followed?
- Can the actual sequence of how data were collected, analyzed, condensed, transformed, and displayed be followed for the drawing of conclusions?
- Has the researcher been explicit about personal biases, assumptions, and values and how these may have come into play in the study?
- Were competing hypotheses considered?
- Are study data retained and made available for reanalysis by others?

SOURCE: Adapted from Miles, M., and Huberman, A. (1994). *Qualitative Data Analysis*. London: Sage.

feedback. In their investigation of family adjustment to heart transplantation, Mishel and Murdaugh (1987) demonstrated how the trustworthiness of their data was assessed using the traditional criteria outlined by Lincoln and Guba (1985) for determining rigor in qualitative investigations. Box 6.9 illustrates the procedures followed by the researchers to test the scientific rigor of their study findings.

2. Contemporary Standards of Quality

More recently, Lincoln and Guba (1994) have noted that although the traditional criteria (referred to previously) have been well received, their parallelism to positivist criteria make them suspect. Lincoln and Guba continue to call for additional critique of the issue of quality in

---

BOX 6.9 *Nurse Researchers at Work*

TESTING SCIENTIFIC RIGOR OF QUALITATIVE RESEARCH: FAMILY ADJUSTMENT TO HEART TRANSPLANTATION

"Redesigning the Dream" was identified as the integrative theme in the substantive theory that emerged from interviews with 20 family members of heart transplant recipients. The trustworthiness of the study findings was assessed using the criteria for determining rigor in qualitative investigations.

Six methods were used to assess credibility. These included:

1. Prolonged engagements at the site
2. Persistent observations during lengthy data collection periods
3. Peer debriefing and exposure of the investigator's thinking to a jury of peers by scheduling discussions with the transplant team members who worked closely with the patients and their families
4. Triangulation was accomplished by comparing the emerging perspective with lay articles on transplant recipients, professional articles on life after transplantation, literature on spouses' experiences living with a chronically ill partner, and television documentaries.
5. Investigators' findings were compared with recorded information from consultants who worked with family members and patients.
6. Member checks to verify or modify concepts that emerged were conducted during the group meetings.

In relation to transferability of findings, the sample covered all adult age groups, education levels, and adult role activities. Therefore, the subjects, content, and range of data were adequate to provide the basis for assessing the relevancy to related contexts and care providers. Because the partners provided the data on patients, the generalizability of the findings is limited to the perspectives of the partners.

Dependability of the findings was determined by an audit trail. To do this, a research assistant reexamined a portion of the transcribed data from the group sessions. The research assistant was able to draw comparable conclusions given the same data, perspective, and context.

Confirmability was established by gathering data from the heart transplant team members in addition to the subjects. In addition, alternative explanations for the data were explored with the team members. The researchers also reflected on detailed notes depicting the initial directions in the organizing and processing of the data, enabling changes in the early formulations. Through the means identified by Lincoln and Guba (1985), the researchers of this investigation can have confidence in the trustworthiness of their findings and conclude that their description of "Redesigning the Dream" reflects the true state of human experience for family members of heart transplant recipients.

SOURCE: Adapted from Mishel, M.H., and Murdaugh, C.L. (1987). Family adjustment to heart transplantation: Redesigning the dream. *Nursing Research, 36*(6), 332–338.

qualitative research. Although many researchers continue to observe the four traditional criteria (Miles and Huberman, 1994; Streubert and Carpenter, 1999), some argue there is no longer a need to defend the value and rigor of qualitative research with criteria that parallel those in quantitative research. This has led to an effort to determine more appropriate methods of determining quality in qualitative research (Creswell, 1998; Sandelowski, 1993). Lincoln (1995) traces her own thinking on the issue of quality and the scientific adequacy of qualitative research. She has moved beyond the traditional parallel criteria of the classic work by Lincoln and Guba (1985) to her current perspective. It includes a commitment to emergent relations with respondents, a commitment to a set of stances, and a commitment to a vision of research that promotes justice (Lincoln, 1995). Flowing from these commitments are eight standards found in Box 6.10 for assessing the quality of qualitative research. Adherence to these standards helps the researcher answer the all important question— "Did we get it right?" And, as Sandelowski noted (1993):

> . . . we can preserve or kill the spirit of qualitative research; we can soften our notion of rigor to include the playfulness, imagination, and technique we associate with more artistic endeavours, or we can further harden it by the uncritical application of rules. The choice is ours: rigor or rigor mortis.

D. ADVANTAGES AND LIMITATIONS OF QUALITATIVE APPROACHES

Qualitative research approaches have made important contributions to knowledge development in nursing during the past decade. Phenomenology, grounded theory, and ethnographic methods are

BOX 6.10 *Lincoln's Standards of Quality*

1. Diverse inquiry communities exist with unique traditions of research with their own standards of rigor. These serve to either exclude or legitimize researchers.
2. Positionality: A balanced and honest reflection of the participant's and the author's stance.
3. Community: All research takes place in a community and serves that community's purposes.
4. Voice: Qualitative research gives multiple or alternative voices to participants that must be "heard" in the text.
5. Critical subjectivity: The researcher should have a heightened self-awareness before, during, and after the research encounter, leading to personal transformations.
6. Reciprocity: The relationship between the researcher and participant should be one of mutual respect, trust, and intense sharing.
7. Sacredness of the relationship between researcher and participant: There is an inviolate relationship between the researcher and the participant that is both egalitarian and collaborative.
8. Sharing privileges: Qualitative researchers share the benefits of their research with the participants. This may take the form of authorship, rights to publication, and royalties.

SOURCE: Adapted from Lincoln, Y. (1995). Emerging criteria for quality in qualitative and interpretive research. *Qualitative Inquiry, 1*, 275–289.

examples of qualitative research perspectives used to describe and explore phenomena of concern to nursing. These methods share similar characteristics that include:

1. Attention to the social context in which events occur and have meaning.
2. Emphasis on understanding the social world from the participant's point of view.

3. The perspective is primarily inductive.
4. Data collection techniques include participant observation, interviewing, and printed documents.
5. Data collection tools and procedures are subject to change in the field. Concern is primarily with discovery and description of phenomena.
6. Hypotheses are developed during the research rather than a priori.
7. Analysis is presented in narrative form.

Qualitative methods are congruent with the field of nursing's philosophy of holistic, humanistic caring. Such methods enable a holistic understanding of the patterns, characteristics, and meanings of the phenomenon under study. They attempt to focus on the experiences of people and seek to describe the uniqueness of participants' human health experiences. Similarly, nurses hope to focus on the client as an individual requiring holistic care that encompasses biological, psychological, social, cultural, and spiritual dimensions. Because qualitative methods focus on the whole of the human experience and the meanings ascribed to them by clients, they provide nurses with deep insights into the experiences of clients that would not be possible using quantitative methods exclusively.

The major strength of qualitative research is the validity of the data it produces. Because researchers collect data primarily by means of in-depth interviews and participant observation in natural settings, the participant's true reality is more likely to be reflected in the rich descriptions that result than would be reflected in data collected in contrived settings using quantitative instruments. The *major limitation* of qualitative research is its perceived lack of objectivity and generalizability. It is argued that because qualitative researchers become the research tools, they become so intimately involved with the data collection process that they cannot be objective.

Researchers are likely to be subjective in deciding which participants to select and which data to accept or reject. The small and unrepresentative samples and the analytic procedures that rely on subjective judgments make qualitative methods appear to be weak in terms of reliability and generalizability.

Qualitative researchers have devised their own terminology such as truth value and have established their own procedures to assess the scientific rigor of their work. Rigor in qualitative research is less about adherence to rules than about fidelity to the spirit and standards of qualitative work (Sandelowski, 1993).

Some researchers believe it is appropriate to integrate quantitative and qualitative data within a single study or a cluster of studies on a particular phenomenon. Not everyone agrees, however, that methods can be mixed in the same study. Creswell (1994) suggests that there are three positions on the subject of integration: the purists, who believe methods and paradigms should not be mixed; the situationalists, who believe certain methods are appropriate for certain situations; and the pragmatists, who support integrating methods in a single study.

Table 6.7 summarizes the advantages and limitations of the qualitative designs discussed in this chapter. There are obvious strengths in the areas of validity and in the ability to probe in depth the human experience.

The authors of this text believe there are advantages to mixing methods as we work toward the common goal for research of understanding of the world in which we live. Both quantitative and qualitative methods are complementary processes. The Oxford Dictionary defines complementary as "to make complete"— that is, one perspective completes or makes up for the lack or deficiency in the other perspective. Hence, by mixing perspectives to address an area of inquiry, the weakness of a single perspective may

Table 6.7   Advantages and Limitations of Alternate Designs

Research Design Category	General	Validity	Causal Inference	Multivariate	Probing
Experimental Designs					
Pre-experimental	−	−	−	−	−
Experimental	−	−	+	−	−
Quasi-experimental	±	−	+	−	−
Survey Designs					
Individual questionnaire	+	−	−	+	−
Group administered	−	−	−	+	−
Phone survey	+	−	−	+	−
Interview	+	−	−	+	+
Comparative analysis	+	−	−	+	−
Secondary data	+	−	−	+	−
Meta analysis	+	−	−	−	−
Qualitative Designs*					
Phenomenology	−	+	−	−	+
Grounded Theory	−	+	−	−	+
Ethnographic	−	+	−	−	+

In each category, a + means that this is an advantage of the technique; a− means this is a possible limitation; ± means that in some conditions a limitation, others an advantage.
- **General** refers to the extent to which extrapolations to larger populations may be made using each of the design or data collection procedures.
- **Validity** is the extent to which indicators clearly measure what they are intended to measure.
- **Causal inference** refers to the ease with which inferences about causal relations among variables may be made.
- **Multivariate** refers to the ease with which information on many variables is collected, leading to the possibility of multivariate analysis.
- **Probing** refers to the extent to which responses may be probed in depth.

*Note: this table is intended for comparisons with previously considered designs and uses criteria quantitative researchers typically use. See body of text for alternative criteria used by qualitative researchers.

be overcome or reduced. Neither perspective on its own can establish the truth about phenomena of interest to nurses. Rather, each serves a unique purpose; taken together, they can provide a rich repertoire for building nursing knowledge. The successful blending of methods in a single investigation requires resolution of epistemological biases, budgeting for higher costs, and researcher training in both quantitative and qualitative methods. Many believe the benefits to knowledge development that result from integrating methods outweigh the hassles of blending methods and encourage nurse researchers to make the effort to consider integration if it is appropriate to the study question.

E X E R C I S E S

1. Suppose you are interested in exploring the meaning of healthy lifestyle choices for adolescent girls. What type of qualitative design would you chose to study this phenomenon? How would you go about selecting your sample? What setting would you select to conduct the study? Explain your choices. search question? Does the researcher address issues related to scientific rigor? Comment on how the credibility, transferability, dependability, and confirmability of findings are handled by the investigator. What suggestions would you make for enhancing the rigor of the study?

2. You are working with cancer patients who are waiting to receive bone marrow transplants. You are interested in understanding the processes that their family and they use to cope with the ordeal of receiving the bone marrow transplant. Which research design would you select to investigate this phenomenon? Explain your choice and describe the steps you would follow in conducting the study.

5. Read an article that uses only quantitative data to respond to the research question. Discuss how the addition of qualitative data may enhance the validity of the findings. What suggestions, if any, would you recommend to the study's designer to strengthen the study?

3. Formulate a research question from the practice setting that is appropriate for a mini-ethnographic investigation. Suggest the type and size of sample that might be appropriate for this investigation. Discuss how you came to your decision on sampling. Describe the setting for data collection and how you would go about the process of collecting data to answer your research question.

6. Identify a lived experience from a phenomenological study. List your assumptions and beliefs about the experience. What means would you use as a researcher to deal with your preconceived notions and ideas about the phenomenon under study? Elaborate on the process.

4. Review a recent issue of a qualitative nursing research journal such as *Qualitative Health Research* or the *Western Journal of Nursing Research*. Select an article of interest to you and assess the scientific adequacy of the design. Is the design appropriate to answer the re-

7. Review a qualitative nursing research article that uses a grounded theory perspective. Pay particular attention to the process of data analysis. Comment on how the researcher identified themes or common patterns in the data. Describe the core variable. What steps were involved in identifying the basic social psychological process?

RECOMMENDED READINGS

Creswell, J.H. (1998). *Qualitative Inquiry and Research Design.* London: Sage. Provides an excellent overview of five different traditions of qualitative inquiry—biography, grounded theory, ethnography, phenomenology, and case studies.

Denzin, N.K., and Lincoln, Y.S. (1994). *Handbook of Qualitative Research.* London: Sage. This comprehensive handbook synthesizes the existing literature on qualitative methods and helps to shape the future direction of qualitative research. Written from the perspective of sociology and education, it is a springboard for new thoughts on this research tradition. It is a key addition for the library of serious qualitative researchers.

Leenerts, M., and Magilvy, J. (2000). Investing in self-care: A midrange theory of self-care grounded in the lived experience of low income HIV-positive white women. *Advances in Nursing Science, 22*(3), 58–75. This is a good example of how midrange theory emerges in a grounded theory project.

Miles, M.B., and Huberman, A.M. (1994). *Qualitative Data Analysis.* London: Sage. This is a practical sourcebook that describes a rich variety of approaches for analyzing qualitative data. It contains numerous examples and is appropriate for beginning researchers as well as practicing researchers who are dealing with qualitative data analysis issues.

Nelms, T. (2000). The practices of mothering in caregiving an adult son with AIDS. *Advances in Nursing Science, 22*(3), 46–57. A phenomenological investigation of mothering and how it informs our understanding of what it means to be women, mothers, nurses, and human beings.

Spradley, J.P. (1980). *Participant Observation.* New York: Harcourt Brace College Publishers. An excellent guide to conducting participant observation studies.

Streubert, H.J., and Carpenter, D.R. (1999). *Qualitative Research in Nursing* (2nd ed). Philadelphia: J.B. Lippincott. This clearly written text presents the essentials of qualitative research as it relates to nursing.

Zerwekh, J. (2000). Caring on the ragged edge: Nursing persons who are disenfranchised. *Advances in Nursing Science, 22*(4), 47–61. The voices of seven nurses in their fearless caring for the disenfranchised are heard in this phenomenological study. The words of the nurses reveal the meaning of their work and the life experiences of their clients.

Chapter 7

Field Study Approaches

CHAPTER OUTLINE

KEY TERMS

Analytic files

Coefficient of reliability

Content analysis

Field experiment

Field notes

Field studies

Focus group

Grounded theory

In-depth interviews

Index system

Master field file

Master table

Naturalistic observational study

Nodes

NUD*IST

Participant observation study

Proxemics

Tally sheet

Chapter 6 presented a general introduction to three popular qualitative approaches to nursing research: phenomenology, grounded theory, and ethnography. This chapter discusses field studies, which are the data collection and analysis methods most commonly associated with these qualitative approaches. However, quantitative field research, in the form of field experiments and naturalistic observational studies, can also be conducted in unaltered social environments and is also discussed in this chapter.

Field studies are among some of the most admired work in nursing; they include investigations in which the researcher observes and records the behavior of individuals or groups in their natural settings. Part of the appeal of such studies is that humans are being directly observed in everyday situations; as a consequence, these studies are more convincing because they ring true to the reader. Field studies tend to pay more attention to the qualitative dimensions of the phenomenon being studied. So whether researchers are observing who is more likely to exhibit supportive behavior in crisis situations; monitoring trends in the portrayal of nurses in popular literature; or comparing baccalaureate, associate degree, and diploma-prepared nurses on caring behaviors, their studies are likely to focus on the context in which the phenomena occur and to quote from cases to illustrate the generalizations emerging from the studies.

The three main types of qualitative field studies explored in this chapter are participant observation studies, in-depth interviews, and focus group interviews. Two types of quantitative field studies, including field experiments and naturalistic observational studies, are also considered in this chapter. Finally, this chapter closes with a closer look at the analysis of qualitative data. Here, readers are introduced to the use of computers in analysis of qualitative data. The chapter then briefly explores the technique of content analysis, which can enrich findings from any of the types of field studies covered or even function as a study method on its own.

The information in Chapters 6 and 7 together is adequate to provide an understanding of the process and the steps involved in doing a qualitative investigation, as well as give you a feel for the experience. If you elect to design a study using one of the methods discussed, you should seek additional sources of guidance for analyzing data. Sources by Coffey and Atkinson (1996), Hanna (1997), Kidd and Parshall (2000), Maynard-Tucker (2000), Miles and Huberman (1994), and Silverman (1993), referenced at the end of this chapter in the Recommending Readings, are useful resources for beginning researchers. It is also suggested that you find a mentor, someone experienced in the appropriate method of data analysis to assist you to develop the necessary skills and judgment required.

A. PARTICIPANT OBSERVATION STUDIES

A participant observation study ordinarily involves an intensive examination of a particular culture, community, organization, or group. It is the method used in *ethnographic* and *ethnonursing* studies, which are discussed in Chapter 6. Normally, such a study is based on a careful and complete exploration of one case and involves having the researcher join the group for an extended period. For example, in studying a preliterate society by living with the group, the anthropologist adopts an emic perspective (see Chapter 6). Because the researcher is living with the group and is involved in the daily lives of its members, such studies are called **participant observation studies.** The researcher is a participant in the lives of the group's members, sharing their joys and pains. Such studies frequently take much time to complete, which is not surprising given the need to learn a new language and to absorb the intricacies of the culture.

Classical anthropology led the way in developing participant observation techniques; the names of Bronislaw Malinowski, Margaret Mead, and Oscar Lewis come immediately to mind. Nurses associated with this tradition include Mary Breckinridge, Madeleine Leininger, Toni Tripp-Reimer, and Jan Morse. Working in this qualitative tradition, researchers have studied everything from health-care systems and exotic cultures to prisons (Gresham M. Sykes, 1968), hobos (Nels Anderson, 1929), and the world of punk rockers (Baron, 1989). Erving Goffman's study on mental institutions, *Asylums* (1962), William F. Whyte's analysis of a street gang, *Street Corner Society* (1955), and Becker and associates's *Boys in White* (1961) are classic participant observation studies.

I. Rationale for Participant Observation Studies

The method of participant observation can best be understood by comparing it with different research approaches. We have seen in Chapter 4 that the experiment examines causal relations among a limited range of variables and that it typically identifies treatment effects of one or two variables on a dependent variable. Surveys (see Chapter 5) focus on measuring a large number of variables and exploring the statistical relationships among them. In contrast, participation observation studies try to understand institutions, groups, communities, and even whole cultures or subgroups within a culture. These studies are holistic because they attempt to understand the whole group. Typically, researchers using this approach do not begin with a limited number of variables like survey researchers or experimentalists; instead, they immerse themselves in the everyday

lives of the people they are studying, attempting to provide accurate descriptions and explanations of their activities. The important characteristics of these activities emerge during the course of field observations. Surveys and experiments begin with specific variables and proceed to analyze them; participant observers begin with the more ambitious goal of understanding how a whole group functions.

The rationale of such studies is that only through sharing in the daily lives of a group can a researcher fully understand the behavior that is manifested. Researchers doing participant observation attempt to minimize the effect of preconceived ideas by trying to see the world from the points of view of the members of the group they are studying. By spending a good deal of time within the community, the researcher gains first-hand knowledge of social behavior as it unfolds over time. The fundamental point is that the conclusions of a participant observation study are grounded in the data—that is, based on direct and careful observations of everyday life within the group.

To the extent that we wish to study commonsense understandings—the social construction of reality—then it is clear that we have to try to understand the world from the point of view of the humans involved in these constructions. A researcher doing experiments on the people involved or conducting a survey of them may fail to document adequately the social construction created by them. Participant observation studies try to capture both the subjective and the objective complexity of human behavior, trying to penetrate the inner lives of the people being analyzed. Nurse scientists challenge themselves when they attempt to understand the subjective dimensions of human activity. Doing participant observation studies is one of the ways in which nurse scientists attempt to meet this challenge.

2. Steps in Conducting a Participant Observation Study

Each participant observation study is different, depending on the research question, design selected, study sample, context, and setting (see Chapter 6). However, the following steps are necessary in most studies: gaining entry to the group, establishing a working rapport, creating field notes, analyzing observations, and writing the report.

Step 1: Gaining Entry into the Group

Gaining entry is sometimes a simple matter but is more difficult at other times. For starters, the type of group has to be taken into account: if the researcher wishes to enter a formal organization (e.g., hospital, religious group, prison, bureaucracy, business organization, or school) the entry methods will differ from those used when attempting to study an informal organization (e.g., community response to a crisis, street clinic for gays and lesbians, homeless people, street gangs, or the business lunches of young executives). But no matter what the researcher studies, entry should be viewed as an ongoing and reciprocal relationship between the researcher and the population being studied. The researcher has to negotiate a relationship with each person in the study population.

In entering a formal organization, it is probably best to begin by finding out as much as possible about the organization. Who are the key actors? Are there any critical issues (e.g., strike threatened, new methods introduced for care delivery, required technology and equipment becoming increasingly expensive) currently facing the organization? What are the best times of the week or month to approach the leadership of the organization?

Having determined that the intended study would be appropriate, informal contact should be established with the persons whose permission will be required to gain entry. A brief written statement that outlines the goals and methods of the proposed study should then follow this initial contact. The preparation of this document assists the researcher in defining the problem more clearly (in participant observation, the precise problems studied emerge through the research process and are not necessarily present from the beginning of the project). The letter outlining the project should:

- Establish the legitimacy of the project. This may be achieved by using the stationery of the sponsoring organization, and mentioning the sponsors of the project.
- Indicate that the project has been approved by the institutional ethics review board.
- Indicate the goals and methods of the study. This provides the leadership of the target organization with a simple statement that can be used to communicate the project to others in the organization.
- Indicate how the goals of the organization may be enhanced through participation in the project.
- Specify the length of time that researchers will be on site. This provides the organization's leaders with important information as to how long the researchers will be present.
- Indicate the amount of time that will be spent interviewing various members of the organization.
- Indicate the extent to which anonymity and confidentiality will be possible for various participants.
- Indicate the form in which feedback on the project will be provided to the organization. This may take the form of informal verbal reports, seminars, or formal reports.

Research reports typically mask the location of the site and the names of participants. However, the researcher should assume that published reports circulate among those studied. When studying a group, it may be difficult to disguise the identity of some of the individuals behind the pseudonyms—especially those whose role is occupied by only one person. One must be careful, therefore, in promising anonymity before starting a study because it may not be possible to mask everyone's identity adequately in the final report even though steps are taken to disguise identities. These steps may include using pseudonyms or fictitious names of organizations; modifying descriptive data to mask the identity of the organization; and when using direct quotes, stating the reference as "one subject stated . . ."

In studying informal organizations, it is usually not necessary to get an official's permission to enter the group; one simply has to establish cordial relations with the people being studied. For example, to do observations among homeless people, one would simply need to establish a solid working relation with them. To keep things simple, one would probably just say that a book (or an article) is being written about the lives of the homeless, that the researcher would be talking to the homeless in the area, and that the identities of individuals will not be revealed in the publication.

Gaining entry to the group is a critical step in participant observation studies. There are no hard and fast rules to follow because much depends on the personality and skill of the investigator in gaining access and minimizing the effects of intrusion on the group observed. Three general guidelines are proposed for those planning a participant observation study:

- First, it is probably wise to keep one's explanations simple. For example, a nurse studying health-care utilization patterns in a Native American tribal community may simply state that she is writing about how Native Americans use the health-care system (this will most likely be accepted because the nurse will be seen by most residents many times during the day as they visit the health center).

- Second, it is usual for a social gap to exist between the researcher and the subjects being studied. Complete acceptance by a community is not a requirement for successful fieldwork. Indeed, there are advantages to remaining somewhat of an outsider in that the researcher can adopt the role of a naive learner.

- Third, it is helpful to enlist the aid of local "sponsors" to legitimize the researcher's presence in the community. For example, if a member of the tribal council approves of the presence of the researcher, it is likely that the tribe will cooperate in the study even though the members may consider the researcher an exotic addition to their community. The development of a trusting relationship between the researcher and the community is key to a successful project.

Although most participant observers are open about their studies, sometimes *covert entry* is used to become part of a group. Although arguments have been advanced (see the discussion of ethics in Chapter 10) that all research should be done openly, with the knowledge and consent of those being studied, there have been times when this was not feasible. Festinger and associates (1956), for example, wished to study a group predicting the end of the world. However, because the group initially avoided publicity, observers joined the group covertly to conduct the study. It should be noted that it is highly unlikely that a similar project would ever receive the approval of an ethics review board today.

The following are some of the *advantages* of covert entry:

- Entry is gained in circumstances in which it might have been denied.
- Those being observed are less likely to alter their behavior to please a researcher (as in overt entry studies), hence increasing the validity of the observations.
- If the people studied think they are dealing with a regular member of the group, they may be more open in sharing their thoughts and feelings than they would with someone known to be a researcher.

The following are among the *disadvantages* of covert entry:

- There may be ethical reservations about doing research on individuals without having their consent. Indeed, as research continues and the observer develops a rapport with the group, considerable guilt may arise on the part of the researcher because of the deception involved; today it would be rare to be able to get an ethics review board to approve a project involving covert entry.
- The researcher must play the role of a regular member and therefore may not have the freedom or time to roam about, ask questions, and collect data.
- By becoming more intimately involved, it may be more difficult for the researcher to remain objective.
- The researcher may have a difficult time finding a way of leaving the group gracefully.

When entry has been made without deception, the observer has the advantage of being able to ask questions, move about, and explore issues to a greater degree than might be appropriate in everyday social relations. Moreover, the observer need not expend effort to disguise the fact that research is being carried out.

The role of the observer is a marginal one: the researcher is in the group but not really part of it. There is always dis-

tance; whereas the researcher is in the group temporarily, the regular participants are there longer, often for life. The commitment of the researcher in the eyes of the group is therefore suspect.

There are times when gaining entry is extremely difficult, taking weeks or even months to accomplish (Morse, 1992; Morse and Field, 1995; Streubert and Carpenter, 1999). In the case of nurse researcher Evaneshko (cited in Leininger, 1985), who was studying diabetes in an American Indian tribe, she found that it took months to achieve success in overcoming the fear locals who spoke no English had of outsiders. She explains the process of seeking approval from innumerable subcommittees, the tribal council, the Department of Indian Affairs, and the local health authorities, as well as the Navaho people themselves.

Step 2: Establishing Rapport

One challenge that participant observation researchers face is to develop good relationships with the people being studied. Maintaining these relationships is sometimes strained because the subjects may wish to "capture" the researcher to their points of view. The researcher must be careful to not become overly attached to one faction because this would make it more difficult to get information from members of other factions. The researcher may also be blamed for difficulties that the group encounters. Furthermore, the researcher's objectivity may be strained if an unequal amount of time is spent with each side.

Step 3: Creating Field Notes

Another challenge of participant observation is the creation and recording of detailed and comprehensive field notes. **Field notes** attempt to capture, with as much accuracy as possible, descriptions and interpretations of individuals, inter-actions, and events. The exact time and location of observations should be recorded, along with other descriptions to help the researcher recall the events (e.g., weather conditions, other signifi-cant events going on in the community or in the world that day). Emphasis should be placed on reflecting exactly what peo-ple say and how they say it and describ-ing the reactions of others to what is said. As a practical suggestion, Strauss and as-sociates (1964), in their seminal presen-tation, distinguished types of quotations:

- Words recalled verbatim enclosed within " . . . "
- When there is less certainty about the exact wording ' . . . '
- When meaning is clear but wording not exact: no quotation marks

Field notes should also distinguish clearly between *descriptions* of events and people and *interpretations* of them. A suggestion for doing this is to organize field notes so that there is a wide column for descriptions and a narrow column for interpretations. Note, too, that there are two kinds of interpretations: (1) the sub-jects' own interpretations of their behav-ior and the behavior of others and (2) the interpretation that the observer places on these same activities.

The emphasis, particularly in the ini-tial stages of research, should be on de-scriptive accuracy. Field research is a dy-namic process in which ideas develop, are refined, and are then tested and mod-ified throughout the observational pe-riod. The writing of theoretical memos is encouraged to help the observer system-atically develop explanations (see Chap-ter 6). These tentative interpretations emerge and are tested during the obser-vational period. Indeed, participant ob-servers do well to concurrently carry out both observations and theoretical reflec-tion about these observations (Strauss and Corbin, 1997).

In order to make sense of field experi-ences, the researcher interprets the data continuously. For example, if the observer sees a person explaining something to an-other person, this may be thought to indi-cate the dominance of the person doing the explaining. Such dominance may be re-flected in a variety of ways, and all of these may be thought to reflect dominance and submission behaviors. Grounded theories, Corbin and Strauss argue, are built out of conceptualizations of behavior, not out of the actual incidents themselves; obser-vations are generalized, and behaviors are interpreted as reflections of concepts (Strauss and Corbin, 1997).

In deciding which situations, or per-sons, are to be observed, Corbin and Strauss suggest that researchers should *sample* according to concepts and their properties and not try to locate represen-tative individuals. They argue that in **grounded theory** "representativeness of concepts, not of persons, is crucial" (1990, p. 9). Thus, if you want to study peer sup-port in urban adolescent girls, you would go to where adolescent girls hang out and watch how they interact and support each other. You may visit schools, shopping malls, video arcades, youth centers, and local spots frequented by youths. While at these locales, the observer would note events that occur and begin classifying them according to some general princi-ples. What techniques do girls use to initi-ate contact with peers? What is the nature of the interaction? How are friendships negotiated? How is support offered and re-ceived? Perhaps the researcher would then try to observe some of the most and least popular girls to note differences in how they interact in offering and accept-ing support.

Field notes should be made as soon af-ter field observations as possible, prefer-ably on the same day. At the very latest, notes should be made the morning after an evening's observations. Expect to spend as much time writing up field notes as you spent in the field. Three hours of observation is usually followed by 3 hours of writing up the observations. The use of a laptop computer is most helpful in compiling field notes. It is also possible to tape field interviews and then have these interviews transcribed. Some researchers even prefer to dictate their observations and then have them transcribed. Field notes tend to be lengthy. The field notes for *When Prophecy Fails,* combined with transcriptions of recorded information, came to well over 1000 typewritten pages (Festinger, 1956). *Boys in White* produced about 5000 single-spaced typewritten pages of field notes and interview material (Becker, 1961). When writing the report, the challenge will be to condense the field notes into a coherent document of reasonable length.

Step 4: Analyzing the Observations

It is recommended that field notes be entered into a word processor. Then a printout of the complete journal of these notes, called the **master field file,** should be placed in a binder and retained.

Before you can begin analyzing the data, you should make several additional copies of the master field file to use as raw material for building up *analytic files.* **Analytic files** are files relating to a specific topic or relationship explored in the study. For example, you may wish to build up a subfile on interactions between status unequals. You would cut out all the field notes pertaining to such interactions. These will frequently be ordered along some dimension (in this case, perhaps along the degree of status difference between the two persons interacting). Each piece cut from the copy of the master file should have its original (master copy) page number on it. You may also want files related to the methodology of the study, the history of the institution or area being studied, or

particular people you interviewed. On the other hand, it may well be the case that not every part of the master file will make it into any of the subfiles you create. In summary, your files will typically include:

- **Master field file.** This is the original complete file of the field notes. Pages are numbered and each entry is dated. This represents the raw data to be analyzed.
- **Analytic files.** These files each deal with a particular type of observation or relationship (e.g., descriptions of interactions between status unequals, interactions across gender lines, interactions of strangers).
- **Background or history file.** This subfile contains information drawn from the master field file as well as from other sources.
- **Key character files.** Individual files may be established on key players in the organization or group being observed. These files attempt to reflect the personality, mannerisms, and typical behaviors of central characters.

In addition to qualitative analysis of field data, there will be occasions when some quantitative analysis is appropriate. Where the analysis involves few variables and not too many cases, a quantitative analysis can be done by hand. Chapter 16 provides suggestions for how to proceed without the use of a computer and gives tips for how the data set should be prepared if computer processing is anticipated. At the end of this chapter, we discuss the use of computers in analyzing qualitative data. *Content analysis* is a method for analyzing qualitative data but because it involves counting and the use of numbers, some qualitative researchers do not consider it a qualitative analysis technique. It is discussed at the end of this chapter as a means of quantitatively analyzing qualitative field data.

BOX 7.1 *Nurse Researchers at Work (Continued)*

ROSE WEITZ: LIVING WITH THE STIGMA OF AIDS

deserved AIDS as punishment for his sins, reported that initially his family 'wouldn't come in the room unless they had gloves and a mask and they wouldn't touch me . . . [And] for a time I couldn't go over to somebody's house for dinner. And they still use paper plates [when I eat there].' Even PWAs who feel such precautions are necessary still miss the experience of physical warmth and intimacy. They report feeling stigmatized, isolated, and contaminated.

Although PWAs fear that their families will reject them once their illness becomes known, they also hope that news of their illness will bring their families closer together. A 38-year-old store manager who had never had a particularly close relationship with his family described his fantasy 'that something like this—an experience where you come this close to death or the reality of death—is when you realize what's really important and not who's right and who's wrong.'

For the lucky ones, this fantasy materializes. The oldest man I interviewed, a 57-year-old lawyer, had always considered his father a cold and selfish man, and had never been on good terms with him. This situation changed, at least partially, when he became ill. As he described it:

We've gotten closer . . . There's the verbal "I love you," there's the letters. One of the nicest things that's ever happened to me . . . is my father sent me a personal card. In the inside he wrote "God bless you. I love you son". . . It meant the world to me.

Another man described how, despite their disapproval of his lifestyle, his fundamentalist Christian family had provided him with housing, money, and emotional support once they learned of his illness. As he described it, in his family, when 'little brother needed help . . . that took priority over . . . They were right there.'

Diagnosis can also bring families together by ending previous sources of conflict. Whether to preserve their own health, protect others from infection, or because they simply lose interest in sex once diagnosed with a deadly, sexually transmitted disease, PWAs may cease all sexual activity. For health reasons, PWAs may also stop smoking and drinking. As a result, families that previously had disapproved of PWAs' lifestyles may stop considering them 'sick' or 'sinful,' even if the PWAs continue to consider themselves gay. Consequently, some PWAs achieve a new acceptance from relatives who attach less stigma to AIDS than to their former behaviors."

SOURCE: Rose Weitz (1990). Living with the Stigma of AIDS. *Qualitative Sociology*, 13(1), pp. 26–29. Adapted with permission.

marize the experiences of the 23 men in her study population.

High-quality journalism and studies based on in-depth interviews are quite similar. Although nurse researchers typically are more concerned with how representative their respondents are of some social category, they share with journalists a concern for accurate description. A report written by a journalist and one by a nurse researcher on the plight of the homeless, for example, might not be that different. However, one would expect that the researcher would display greater care in arriving at conclusions and would spend much more time in exploring the theoretical and methodological issues in such a study.

C. FOCUS GROUP INTERVIEWS

Compared with in-depth interviews, an approach that is becoming popular again in academic research is the use of focus groups. A **focus group** typically consists of 6 to 12 individuals who are asked to discuss topics suggested by a facilitator.

The idea is for the researcher to observe the interactions among focus group members and detect their attitudes, opinions, and solutions to problems posed by the facilitator. On some occasions, even the topic to be discussed is left up to the focus group, but, the facilitator typically provides some structure.

1. Evolution

The use of focus groups in academic research dates back to the 1940s, when, according to Bruce L. Berg (2001), they were used to assess the effectiveness of radio programs designed to boost morale among military personnel. During these sessions, members of the focus group were asked to press either a red button to indicate something they did not like or a green one if they were responding positively to the program. Later the participants were asked to indicate the reasons for their responses. But the technique was not used much after the war years.

Since the 1970s, market researchers have found it useful to use focus groups in assessing the effectiveness of product marketing strategies. But because the technique was largely seen as a tool of the corporate world, academic researchers shied away from using focus group techniques for another decade. It was only in the 1980s that the technique grew in popularity among academic researchers. Today it represents an important approach that one encounters frequently in the literature.

2. Rationale for Focus Groups

There are many appealing aspects of focus group interviews. Respondents may be asked, for example, to discuss their experiences taking a distance education nursing program that is presented using multimedia CD-ROM technology to present course materials to the students. Although questionnaires may be used as part of the evaluation, there is the danger that key issues may not be anticipated by the researcher and may therefore not come to light. With a focus group approach, respondents are likely to mention fears they had about doing a course that requires a certain level of computer literacy. Or it may be that students found they spend a lot of time exploring the materials rather superficially and they were overwhelmed by the volume and found it hard to decide what was critical to know for examinations versus what was supplementary material. In short, the focus group interviews are likely to bring to the surface a number of issues that would prove helpful in improving the method of delivering a distance course using multimedia technology.

Although important information may be revealed in one-on-one interviews, the rationale of focus groups is that they provide a dynamic in which participants learn from one another and develop ideas together. The researcher is able to detect whether there seems to be wide agreement on a point or whether a view being expressed is limited to one or two individuals. Similar to open-ended questions in a questionnaire, the responses may well lead into important issues initially unanticipated by the researcher.

3. How a Focus Group Works

Focus groups appear to work best with from 6 to 12 participants. The information collected represents the work of the group and may be somewhat different from what would be obtained in separate interviews with participants. Some issues that would be raised in individual interviews may never be expressed in a group setting; on the other hand, as group members talk about issues, they may come up with suggestions and solutions that may not emerge from separate interviews.

4. Selecting Focus Group Members

Standard sampling techniques (see Chapter 15) may be used along with a variety of research designs. In the example used previously on testing the effectiveness of a multimedia CD-ROM presentation of course materials, the researcher would probably wish to compare the CD-ROM participants (experimental condition) with students enrolled in the same course that is being delivered using traditional methods (control condition). One way in which the differences between the two groups could be measured is through the use of focus groups, questionnaires, test scores, and individual in-depth interviews. By using multiple approaches (known as triangulation), one should be in a good position to assess the effectiveness of the new course delivery method.

5. Recording Data

Focus group discussions are typically recorded either manually by having someone take notes on what is said or by tape recording the proceedings. If taped, the discussion may then be transcribed. It is useful to record the names of the speakers so that the discussion may be tracked precisely during the analysis stage. Simply writing down the name of the speakers in the order in which they speak is helpful. It is also helpful for the facilitator to note any comments that will help in the evaluation of the discussion. Qualitative notes on attitudes and interactions are useful additions that may prove helpful in interpreting the results.

6. Analyzing the Data

The transcript of the discussion becomes the data in a focus group interview. Because the data constitute the transcript of the discussion, plus the accompanying notes, the researcher may use the techniques associated with content analysis. Normally the results are presented in terms of quotations from the transcript of the discussions. Care should be taken to reflect the qualitative dimensions of the participants' interactions.

7. Example of a Focus Group Study

Box 7.2 presents an example of a study using the focus group technique. Stewart and associates (1996) reported on the causes and cessation of smoking among disadvantaged women. The study involved women from 10 Canadian provinces and used a variety of techniques to gather data. Besides phone interviews and in-depth personal interviews, the research team also used focus groups. Note that the reporting style for the focus group information is similar to that used in in-depth interviews. The generalizations that emerge from the study are illustrated by using many direct quotations from the participants. One gets a good sense of the frustrations and difficulties disadvantaged women have in quitting smoking. What emerges from the study is the crucial role that social support plays in smoking cessation (Stewart et al., 1996).

8. Advantages and Disadvantages of Focus Groups

Focus groups present researchers with opportunities to observe how a small group responds to an issue posed by the facilitator. In a sense, focus groups are similar to an open-ended question on an in-depth interview. The difference, however, is that researchers do not probe for meaning; rather, the group is left to pursue the topic. The researchers allow the group to spontaneously deal with the issues rather than having the facilitator di-

BOX 7.2 *Nurse Researchers at Work*

SMOKING AMONG DISADVANTAGED WOMEN: CAUSES AND CESSATION

Miriam J. Stewart, Angela Gillis, Gerry Brosky, Grace Johnston, Susan Kirkland, Gillian Leigh, Vena Persaud, Irving Rootman, Susan Jackson, and Betty Anne Pawliw-Fry

Research teams at two Canadian health-promotion research centers engaged in several sequential data collection activities during the six phases of the project. These included:

- Phase 1: A comprehensive literature review
- Phase 2: A secondary data analysis of the Ontario Health Survey and the Atlantic provinces' Hears Health Surveys
- Phase 3: Telephone interviews with representatives of 13 women-centered cessation programs in Manitoba, Ontario, Quebec, Nova Scotia, and Prince Edward Island
- Phase 4: Focus group interviews with 254 disadvantaged women and individual interviews with 134 disadvantaged women in 10 provinces
- Phase 5: Telephone interviews with representatives of 29 nontraditional support agencies in 10 provinces
- Phase 6: Telephone interviews with 22 disadvantaged women using these nontraditional support services

This paper focuses on the Atlantic component of the fourth and sixth phases, which involved interviews with disadvantaged women.

The three specific objectives of the consultations with disadvantaged women were to (1) record their recollections and reflections about their experiences with smoking; (2) elicit their opinions and beliefs about smoking cessation; and (3) explore the psychosocial factors associated with smoking and smoking cessation. A total of 126 women participated in the Atlantic region interviews: 84 in the nine focus groups and 42 in individual interviews. Disadvantaged women smokers over age 20 years who were poor, unemployed, or single parents; had low levels of formal education; and lived in rural and isolated communities were included as participants. Consistent with qualitative methodologies, the sampling was purposive.

At each focus group, the facilitator was assisted by an observer/recorder. During the introductory portion of both the group interviews and the individual interviews, the facilitator/interviewer clarified the objectives of the study, provided a brief overview of the procedure, and assured participants that all comments were confidential and that their names would not be used in the report.

The focus group guide included eight questions focusing on the reasons why these women began to smoke and continued to smoke; two questions about the perceived impact of non-smoking messages in the media, in public places, and so on; eight questions on their opinions and experiences with smoking cessation or curtailment; and six questions regarding strategies, services, and support that would help them stop or reduce smoking. The questions were exploratory, open ended, and accompanied by probes.

The research team conducted content analysis of themes and subthemes in the qualitative data. The researchers identified themes and categories and attempted to achieve consensus.

Findings: Factors Influencing Smoking

A summary of findings is presented with exemplar quotations to illustrate some themes and subthemes. . . . Disadvantaged women began smoking to project an image. The participants' stories about their first smoking experiences as adolescents focused on their attempts to establish an identity consistent with those of their peers and usually at variance with the expectations of parents or other members of society. The picture changed when the participants talked about being adult smokers. In the reasons they gave for smoking and the feelings they expressed about being smokers, the women revealed a deep ambivalence about a behavior

continued on next page

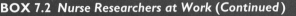

BOX 7.2 *Nurse Researchers at Work (Continued)*

SMOKING AMONG DISADVANTAGED WOMEN: CAUSES AND CESSATION

they knew was dangerous in the long term but that was compelling for the immediate sense of relief it brought to their daily lives. They spoke of the "hold" that smoking had on their lives. Addiction was a pervasive theme. Disadvantaged women experienced the psychological aspects of addiction and the physical manifestations of addiction and perceived that they smoked more after a cessation attempt.

Nonsmokers who have never smoked, or even ex-smokers who are faithful at it—I don't think they fully understand how hard it is and how much cigarettes play on your mind when you are not smoking. I've never been a drug addict, but it has to be along the same line.

I'm sorry I ever picked up that first cigarette again . . . I said just this one won't hurt; I'll never go back to smoking what I used to. But you're lying to yourself. You go back, and you're smoking twice as much.

Because of the pressing nature of the participants' life circumstances, many were caught in a daily struggle for survival. Consequently, the long-term benefits of quitting had little relevance for them. Disadvantaged women continued to smoke to cope with the moment. Many stressors and few resources with which to respond to stressful situations characterized their lives. Coping mechanisms predominated in all the explanations women gave for their smoking behavior. They smoked to cope with the stress, chaos, and crises in their lives.

Let people in government try to live on $800 a month with two kids. See how far they get with it. Rent, heat, lights and all that. If my kid gets sick, I can't afford to go out and get medicine for him. But because I smoke [they say], "Don't smoke any more. That's four dollars you're spending . . . " It's [smoking's] about the only thing that I can afford that does relax me . . . But I have quit in the past . . . and I didn't find I had a lot more money to do anything constructive with. I still couldn't go out and buy my own home.

Most women had multiple role demands that offered little space and time for themselves, and they smoked as a break from the monotonous, burdensome routine of their days. They smoked as an antidote to boredom or inactivity and to relieve their sense of isolation, loneliness, and limited social opportunities. These women also smoked for social and recreational reasons because others were smoking, and they used cigarettes as a reward and for pleasure.

Findings: Factors Influencing Cessation

Participants were unanimous in their dislike of smoking. All participants stated that they would like to be ex-smokers, and almost all had attempted to stop at least once. However, participants had different motivations for changing their smoking behavior. The level of impact of antismoking messages in the media was related to the woman's Stage of Change (Prochaska, Velicer, Guadagnoli, Rossi, and DiClemente, 1991).

. . . Participants frequently mentioned lack of social support as a key barrier to smoking cessation. Lack of support from partners and immediate family posed the biggest problem. Lack of support from friends and acquaintances was also cited as a barrier:

I used to have temper fits and everything . . . I was a contrary person. My husband said, "You're going to have to take up smoking again. I can't live with you."

Friends? They all begged me not to quit. My girlfriend said to me, "You're some friend, telling me not to smoke." I said, "Go ahead, it doesn't bother me if you smoke." They said, "No, we don't want you with us if you don't smoke" . . . I had a hard time.

Participants unanimously acknowledged the positive role played by social support during cessation attempts.

My father, he's a reformed smoker, he's my hero. Every time I quit smoking, his praise was good. He never put me down for smoking, but whenever I would go and tell him I hadn't had a cigarette in a few days his praise made me feel better.

Summarized from Stewart H.J., Gillis A., Brosky G., et al. (1996). Smoking among disadvantaged women: Causes and cessation. *Canadian Journal of Nursing Research, 28*(1), 41–60.

rect the discussion. In this way, it is the group that determines the direction of the discussion. However, a good facilitator is always prepared with questions in the event that the group gets too far off the topic or has difficulty getting started.

A further advantage is that of cost. If the researcher organizes the focus groups and runs them, costs should be relatively modest, both in terms of time spent and money expended. However, if numerous sessions are done or if recording equipment and transcriptions of dialogue are done, the costs increase accordingly. But generally the cost per inference made should be relatively low compared with that of other research methods.

Focus groups have some distinct disadvantages. Although sampling techniques may be used in establishing focus groups, the number of groups exposed to the research questions will generally be small; therefore, the extent to which generalizations may be made is limited. One should expect fewer original ideas from the focus group members than from individual interviews (Jackson, 1999), and the ideas expressed in the focus group may be somewhat more extreme than those reported from surveys of the same respondents (Sussman et al., 1991; Jackson, 1999).

Compared with participant observation studies, focus groups are, in fact, contrived creations of a researcher; therefore, they lack the advantage of the natural setting observations. Participants know that they are being studied, so they may alter their presentations of themselves to fit the situation. In this way, focus groups are more similar to experiments or surveys—they lack spontaneity.

One persistent difficulty in focus group work is to limit the influence of strong-willed individuals to dominate and control the directions that group discussion take. One must be aware that although focus group data represent group data, it almost certainly is skewed toward the opinions and attitudes of the more ver-

bally aggressive individuals in the group (Berg, 2001).

In summary, focus group interviews are important qualitative tools for advancing our understanding of human behavior. It is a cost effective method particularly for evaluating the responses of people to new products, assessing the effectiveness of programs and for sounding out people for ideas on improving products or programs.

D. FIELD EXPERIMENTS

Recall that, in a laboratory experiment, the researcher introduces a treatment variable and measures the response. The same occurs in a **field experiment;** however, the researcher's intervention occurs in a natural setting rather than a laboratory, and the study is usually simple, limited, and quickly completed. Suppose, for example, that a nurse researcher greets a stranger while walking along a street and then records the type of response (if any) that results. In this case, the researcher is intervening in a natural environment and is interested in recording the response to a mild form of nonconformity (greeting a stranger). The kinds of observations that the researcher can make here are quite limited; however, as in most observational studies, fairly accurate measures may be recorded concerning the subject's age, gender, dress, and type of response.

In Chapter 4, we pointed out that laboratory experiments attempt to maintain as much control as possible over the treatment variable (or variables) and over the conditions under which the experiment takes place. Because observations are being made in a natural environment in field experiments, the researcher cannot exercise as much control. But what is given up in control may be compensated for by the fact that the subjects are probably not aware that they are part of an experiment and hence react normally. Both field and laboratory experiments attempt to understand the relationship between a treatment variable and a measurable outcome, exercising as much control over conditions as possible. A researcher conducting a field experiment simply takes conditions and events as they occur naturally, intervenes in some way, and observes the response to the intervention.

The following example illustrates a field experiment. Notice that an environment is set up under controlled conditions and systematic observations are made of the people who pass through the space. This experiment investigates **proxemics,** the norms surrounding personal space and the conditions under which such space will or will not be violated. It is a particularly important concept in the area of mental health and illness and counseling. The researcher positions two partners (i.e., people working with the researcher) facing one another, apparently discussing some issue, in a narrow corridor. A space about 18 inches wide is left between the wall and the back of one of the partners; the other partner stands against the opposite wall. As people pass through the corridor, an observer records information about the subjects: perhaps their age, whether they are alone or with others, and whether they cut between the investigators or squeeze through the 18-inch space along the wall. If the subjects cut through, do they acknowledge this by saying, "Excuse me" or bowing their heads slightly as a nonverbal apology? After a number of observations of this sort, the distance between the researchers could be increased or decreased. As a control, the research partners could be replaced by large trashcans with 18 inches between them (Jackson, 1999).

Over the past few years, a number of the authors' students in a first-level, one-semester methods course have completed field experiments as part of the course requirements. In one, a research partner sat right next to a student of the opposite gender who was working in a library where many other seats were available. This process was repeated a number of times. The responses of the target students varied, but many erected a barrier with books to mark off territory; only rarely did the subjects flee.

In a related study, a female research student invaded a group of male students who were standing in a public area chatting between classes. The researcher was not known by the male students. Once again, this intrusion was repeated with a number of all-male groups. Typically these violations produced a moment of silence: the men looked at one another in bewilderment, and then they turned and fled! So far, no group of male students has volunteered to see if the same phenomenon occurs with female target groups.

Box 7.3 lists more student studies that were completed within the time constraints of a one-term course. In each of the studies, students were encouraged to pay particular attention to the nonverbal dimensions of their observations. They were encouraged to carefully describe how various target subjects responded to the situation created by the researchers. The project reports used qualitative descriptions to add depth to the report. Typically the reports also tested a number of hypotheses related to differences in response to the situation, such as if elderly adults are more likely to be "helpful" than young adults.

The major advantage of these types of studies is that behavior is observed in natural settings and is therefore not contaminated by the artificiality inevitable in laboratory experiments. Such studies can be relatively inexpensive to do and, because conditions can be altered systematically by the researcher, some control can be maintained over the experimental conditions. One of the disadvantages of these studies is that only a limited number of variables can be measured. The

BOX 7.3 *Student Researchers at Work*

STUDENT FIELD EXPERIMENTS*

Project	Student or Students	Brief
Racial Discrimination in the Service Industry	Alicia Van De Sande (1995)	This project compared speed of response in various local stores with a young female African American student to that of a young white female student.
Nonverbal Communication at Public Telephones: The Effects of Personal Space Invasion	Mary E. Gillis (1996)	Observed the impact of researchers encroaching upon the personal space of target subjects using a public telephone; nonverbal responses noted.
Proxemic Violations in the Library	Corine MacDonald (1996)	This study compared nonverbal responses to different levels of personal space violations in a library reading room.
Greeting Behavior	Maureen Keough (1996)	This study compared the nonverbal responses of target subjects with a greeting from a university-aged woamn stranger to that of a 38-year-old female stranger.
Cutting Through Behavior: Who Cuts Between Interacting Pairs?	Kelly Hannay (1997); Chris Parsons (1997)	Students set up different gender combinations of interacting pairs and observed who would or would not cut between them.

*These projects did not include recording information that would allow for the identification of individual subjects, involved minimal risk to the subjects, and could not be carried out practically without the waiver of informed consent.

samples used are usually not representative and one cannot, therefore, generalize the findings.

E. NATURALISTIC OBSERVATIONAL STUDIES

A **naturalistic observational study** is one in which the people being studied are unaware that they are being observed. Typically these studies simply involve recording everyday behavior that occurs in public places. Because the behavior occurs in public and the subjects are usually not known by the observer, the issue of anonymity does not arise. Given the absence of free and informed consent by the subjects, one might question whether such observations are within legitimate ethical boundaries. Our view is that such studies are ethically acceptable if the observation process poses no danger to the observer or to the observed, no attempt is made to encumber those observed by reporting their behavior to authorities, the observation is not staged, and the anonymity of the individuals or group observed is protected. So whether you are observing the age and gender of those who wear or do not wear their seat belts when driving a car or observe nonverbal behaviors in a public meeting, the research appears to be within legitimate ethical boundaries.

In discussing the role of research ethics boards in approving naturalistic observational studies, the Tri-Council Policy Statement *Ethical Conduct for Research Involving Humans* (1998) notes that "naturalistic observation that does not allow for the identification of the subjects, and that is not staged, should normally be regarded as of minimal risk." The document presents the case that some or all of the elements of informed consent could be waived when:

- The research involves no more than minimal risks to the subjects.
- The waiver is unlikely to adversely effect the rights and welfare of the subjects.
- The research could not practicably be carried out without the waiver alteration.
- Whenever possible and appropriate, the subjects will be provided with additional pertinent information after participation.
- The waivered or altered consent does not involve a therapeutic intervention.

An additional discussion of research ethics is presented in Chapter 10.

1. Rationale for Naturalistic Observational Studies

The goal of naturalistic observational studies is to observe and to record behavior that occurs in natural settings. Unlike field experiments, naturalistic observational studies do not attempt to alter the social environment in any way. The researcher observes and records behavior that occurs in natural settings. Similar to field experiments, naturalistic observational studies have high levels of validity (measuring what they claim to measure). However, with both field experiments and naturalistic observational studies, sampling is almost always haphazard (based simply on who happens to walk by), making it problematic to generalize experimental findings to people other than those actually observed. Nonetheless, naturalistic observational studies can reveal much about human behavior.

Returning to the area of proxemics, a naturalistic observational study could possibly observe pairs of individuals in conversation (standing position) and note the average toe-to-toe distance that they maintain over a 30-second observational period. The researcher would use a recording form to note information such as the type of interacting pair (male/male, male/female, female/female) and age and status differences (teacher/student, parent/child, employer/employee, peer/peer) between the two. Such studies involve few variables, so it is possible to analyze them without the help of a computer.

Many daily activities can be observed and recorded without making subjects aware that their behavior is being monitored. Examples of this type of study are included in Box 7.4.

2. Steps in Conducting a Naturalistic Observational Study

Suppose, for example, that you were doing the "use of seat belt" study and you wished to relate seat belt use to the independent variables of the driver's gender, age, and whether he or she is alone or with others. Let us go through the steps that would be involved in such a study, examining in greater detail how each step would be carried out.

BOX 7.4 *Student Researchers at Work*

STUDENT NATURALISTIC OBSERVATIONAL STUDIES*

Project	Student or Students	Brief
Dressing Appropriately for the Winter	Tracey MacMillan (1995)	This project recorded weather appropriateness of outdoor clothing worn by teenagers during winter conditions.
Male and Female Food Preferences	Tracey Pye (1995)	Observed the differences in food selections of males and females in a university cafeteria.
Parking Violations	Steven Hawley (1995)	This study compared recorded differences (age category, gender, and group status) between people who parked illegally and those who did not.
Gender and Smoking	Robyn MacDonald (1995)	This study recorded the smoking behavior (yes/no) of subjects in various public settings in a small community. Gender, age category, and number in group were related to whether or not the target subject was smoking.
The Effects Professor's Gender on Class Participation	Jeanne Doiron (1995)	A number of class situations were observed and a comparison made on the over- or underrepresentation of "speaking up in class" by gender of student as related to the gender of the professor.
Seat Belt Compliance	Lori Kiley (1995)	Motorists were observed as to whether or not they were wearing their seat belts. Age categories, gender or driver, and number in the car were noted.
Speeding in a Small Town	Gordon Barker (1995)	Using a radar device borrowed from the local RCMP detachments, student researchers noted the speed, gender of driver, age category, and number in the car on a small town thoroughfare.

continued on next page

BOX 7.4 *Student Researchers at Work (Continued)*

STUDENT NATURALISTIC OBSERVATIONAL STUDIES*

Project	Student or Students	Brief
Who Purchases "Healthy" Foods at the Supermarket	Stephanie Power (1996)	Patrons' purchases going through the checkout at a local supermarket were observed for the amount of junk food included in the cart.
Bank Machine Behavior	Kirk D. Bailey (1996)	Observers noted whether users of automatic teller machines checked the printed information provided at the machine and counted the cash before leaving the machine.
Nonverbal Cues Used to Terminate a One-on-One Conversation.	Stacey Desmond (1996)	Interacting pairs were observed in a mall and the nonverbal termination cues were noted and related to age category and gender combinations.
Drinking Patterns	Anne Simpson (1996)	Type of alcohol consumed was observed and related to gender, gender composition of drinking group, and the age of people at local taverns.
Smoking Behavior in 11 to 19 Year Old Students	Jacques Boudreau (1997)	Junior high and high school students were observed as they left school. Smoking (yes/no) was noted along with the gender, age, and number walking together.
Conformity to Stop Sign Rule	Judith Finn (1997); Patricia Mbowe (1997)	Cars were observed as they approached stop signs and the age, gender, and whether the driver was alone in the car were noted by the student researchers.

*The above studies involved observations of public behaviors that were not staged; therefore, informed consent was not required.

Step 1: Restrictions on Observations

Because this study concerns the use or nonuse of seat belts, we would need to restrict observations to those cases in which we can detect whether the driver and passengers in a passing vehicle are wearing seat belts. The first restriction, then, would be to limit the observations to recent models of automobiles because trucks or older cars may use lap belts that could not be seen as a vehicle passes by. Second, we would do the observations in a place in which vehicles are moving fairly slowly so that the observer has time both to see and record the information. Finally, a decision would have to be made as to whether observations will be limited to the driver (this will be easiest) or include other front seat passengers as well.

Step 2: Review of Literature

At this point, a review should be undertaken of the literature to find out what studies, if any, have been done on seat belt use. Furthermore, if the failure to use a seat belt is viewed as a form of risk-taking behavior, the literature on risk taking could be reviewed to find out about the variables that are related to risk taking. For example, a researcher could check the literature to see if adolescents show higher levels of risk taking for this minor infraction. If use of a seat belt is viewed as a form of health-promoting behavior, a review could be done on the health promotion literature to see what other researchers have found.

Step 3: Developing Hypotheses

At this stage, the researcher attempts to make predictions about expected outcomes. Such hypotheses may be derived from common sense, what other researchers have found, or by relating the specific behavior (seat belt use) to its general class (risk taking) and then making predictions.

The following three hypotheses may be appropriate to the seat belt study:

1. Female drivers are more likely to use seat belts than male drivers.
2. Older drivers are more likely to use seat belts than younger drivers.
3. Drivers with others in the car are more likely to use seat belts than drivers alone in a car.

By formulating hypotheses before collecting data, one ensures that one is not inventing the hypotheses after the analysis has been done.

Step 4: Defining Terms

Before collecting the data, a careful definition of each of the variables is required. Seat belt use (or nonuse) refers to the apparent use (or nonuse) of a shoulder seat belt by the driver (or others, if they are included in the study). The observer also records the gender and age (in categories such as under age 25 years, age 25 to 49 years, and 50 years and over) of the driver. The category "alone or with others" is added to classify drivers who are alone and those who are accompanied by one or more people.

Step 5: Develop a Tally Sheet

A **tally sheet** should be developed to record the observations. The first variable listed is usually the dependent variable (wearing or not wearing a seat belt), followed by the independent variables, gender, age, and alone or with others. The sheet may look like the one displayed in Figure 7.1. The tally sheet should be designed so that the observer can quickly tick off the categories of each driver. A check mark is easier than writing the estimated age or writing "female" for a female housing complex is to be categorized as appealing would produce less agreement among coders. If you could not get a 0.6 reliability coefficient here, you should review your definition of the different categories to see if they could be refined further.

(iv) How Is Information to Be Recorded?

Before classifying data, a tally sheet should be developed for recording the information. A possible model for such a sheet would be the one used for recording field observations (see Fig. 7.1). There should be space on the form to note all the variables, including the exact location of the item being measured.

(v) How Is the Information to Be Analyzed?

What techniques are to be used in presenting the information in a report? If the researcher is interested in showing what causes variation in the incidence of the phenomena, how is this analysis to be performed? If computer analysis is anticipated, be certain that coding is done so that transfer to the computer will be easy. If analysis without a computer is anticipated, follow the steps outlined in the naturalistic observational section of this chapter and in Chapter 16.

b. Example of Content Analysis

To illustrate content analysis, a study in the general area of gender roles is featured in Box 7.7. This study was completed by undergraduate students who were interested in changes in gender differences exhibited in magazine advertisements from the 1950s to the 1990s. The students examined advertisements in *Time* magazine testing six hypotheses: three for gender portrayal and three for changes over time.

The students found that women were more likely to be shown in "body photos" rather than "face shots" than men and that women were more likely to be shown in "sexy" poses than men. The researchers also noted that the ratio between body and face shots had not changed over the decades nor had the types of products being promoted. Poses, however, had become significantly more sexy over time.

G. CONCLUSION

Table 7.5 summarizes the strengths and weaknesses of field study approaches. Overall, these studies are weak in clarifying causal inferences and in providing samples representative enough for the findings of a study to be generalizable; they are strong in the area of validity and, in the case of participant observation and in-depth interviews, in the ability to probe deeply into the behavior being examined.

I. Advantages of Field Studies

When we consider the strengths of field studies that involve participant observation, in-depth interviews, or focus group studies, there are numerous advantages. Such studies, for example, usually attempt to provide a holistic understanding of the total social system involved in the case. In the case of participant observation studies, because the analysis is done over a period of time, social and other processes can be observed (e.g., how friendships are formed and dissolved). The relationships between individuals and between parts of their social world are of concern to the researcher. Emphasis is placed on obtaining careful, in-depth descriptions that can help to develop hypotheses worth testing with other research strategies. Furthermore, because observations are made of actual, real-life activities, there is increased validity in the measures: the researcher does not rely on artificial settings (as in experiments) or on respondents' abilities to report their behavior (as in sur-

BOX 7.7 *Social Researchers at Work*

FACEISM: GENDER DIFFERENCES IN MAGAZINE ADS

Method

The procedure entailed a content analysis of the ads in *Time* magazine from the 1950s to the 1990s. Ads were analyzed and classified according to facial versus body prominence in ads, sexy versus nonsexy ads. In all cases, differences in the portrayal were noted for each gender. The students were interested in whether there had been changes over time in how men and women were portrayed. The first 3 years of 3 decades were used in the analysis: 1950 to 1952, 1970 to 1972, and 1990 to 1992. The first 15 ads that met the "rules for selection" criteria were chosen for analysis:

1. Ads had to have either a male or a female adult subject; ads with more than one model were not used.
2. Ads had to have a facial or a full-body shot of the person. A facial photo was one defined as one that showed the person only above the chest area; body shots included those that showed the person from head to toe.
3. Ads had to include a product that could be classified as either domestic or nondomestic.
4. Ads had to have a person in either a sexy or nonsexy pose. Sexy poses were defined as "poses of any gender, seductive clothing on any gender, pouty lips in females and piercing

eyes with a straight mouth on males. Nonsexy poses would include fully dressed models, smiling models, and standard poses."

Data Recording

The selected ads were content analyzed and the information was recorded on a tally sheet, recording for each ad the year of the publication, gender of model, type of shot (face versus body), type of product, and type of pose.

Data Analysis

Information from the tally sheets were transferred to a master table and then cross-tabulation tables were created to display the various relationships and to show the tests of significance.

Results

Six tables were presented to test the hypotheses. Two of the tables are shown here. Table 1 indicates the relationship between type of photo and gender. Note that the female models were more likely to be shown with a full body photograph. The difference is noted as statistically significant. Table 2 indicates that there has been a shift to the use of more "sexy" poses when the 1950s are contrasted with the 1970s and 1990s.

Table 1   Type of Photograph by Gender

	Male		Female		Total	
Type of Photograph	N	%	N	%	N	%
Facial photograph	16	57.0	4	23.5	20	44.4
Body photograph	12	43.0	13	76.5	25	55.5
Total	28	100.0	17	100.0	45	99.9

Chi-square = 4.95; degrees of freedom = 1; one-tailed test probability < 0.05; decision: reject null hypothesis.
SOURCE: Summarized from Chisholm, W., Waye, M., Murphy, F., and Gillis, R. (1997). Faceism and gender roles. Unpublished research design paper. St. Francis Xavier University, Antigonish, Nova Scotia, Canada.

continued on next page

BOX 7.7 Social Researchers at Work (Continued)

FACEISM: GENDER DIFFERENCES IN MAGAZINE ADS

Table 2   Type of Pose by Decade

Type of Photograph	Decade						Total	
	1950s		1970s		1990s			
	N	%	N	%	N	%	N	%
Sexy	1	57.0	7	23.5	7	44.4	15	33.3
Nonsexy	14	93.0	8	53.3	8	53.3	30	67.7
Total	28	100.0	17	100.0	45	99.9	45	100.0

Chi-square = 7.20; degrees of freedom = 2; one-tailed test probability < 0.05; decision: reject null hypothesis.
SOURCE: Summarized from Chisholm, W., Waye, M., Murphy, F., and Gillis, R. (1997). Faceism and gender roles. Unpublished research design paper. St. Francis Xavier University, Antigonish, Nova Scotia, Canada.

veys) but, instead, records actual behavior. The researcher may also probe deeply into a whole culture in order to come to a full understanding of how its various parts fit together. For anthropologists, the major contribution of such studies is not just their ability to enable us to understand the world from the natives' point of view but also their ability to describe a culture that may quickly be disappearing. Such descriptions are of historic significance because if they are not made now, the phenomena may be lost forever.

As noted in Table 7.5, in-depth interviews have the advantage of flexibility because the interviewer can probe deeply into areas that seem to be particularly relevant. The probes do require much skill on the part of the interviewer and cannot be done easily by inexperienced researchers.

Participant observation studies, focus groups, and in-depth interviews can usually be done quite inexpensively (e.g., using one observer with a pencil and lots of paper and time) or be on the expensive side, with several paid observers, a secretarial transcription service, a crew of coders, statisticians, editorial advisers, and recording devices and computers being placed in the field for extended periods and at considerable cost. Most often, however, field studies are of the less expensive variety. Although direct costs may not be that great, keep in mind, however, that the time commitment is often extensive—often several years.

Field experiments facilitate making causal inferences, are strong on validity, and are often fairly inexpensive to complete. Naturalistic observational studies, similar to field experiments, are inexpensive and have high validity because actual behavior is being observed in a natural setting. In such studies, subjects are not even aware that they are being observed.

2. Limitations of Field Studies

Participant observation, in-depth interviews, and focus group studies have important roles in answering many nursing research questions. Many examples of such research may be found in the nursing literature. But they do have their problems.

Table 7.5   Advantages and Limitations of Alternate Designs

Research Design Category	General	Validity	Causal Inference	Multivariate	Probing
Experimental Designs					
Pre-experimental	−	−	−	−	−
Quasi-experimental	±	−	+	−	−
Survey Designs					
Individual questionnaire	+	−	−	+	−
Group administered	−	−	−	+	−
Phone survey	+	−	−	+	−
Interview	+	−	−	+	+
Comparative analysis	+	−	−	+	−
Secondary data	+	−	−	+	−
Meta analysis	+	−	−	−	−
Qualitative Designs					
Phenomenology	−	+	−	−	+
Grounded theory	−	+	−	−	+
Ethnographic	−	+	−	−	+
Field Designs					
Participant observation	−	+	−	−	+
In-depth interviews	−	+	−	+	+
Field experiments	−	+	+	−	+
Naturalistic observational	−	+	−	−	−

In each category, a + means that this is an advantage of the technique; − means this is a possible limitation; ± means that in some conditions it is a limitation, but in others it is an advantage.
- *General* refers to the extent to which extrapolations to larger populations may be made using each of the design or data collection procedures.
- *Validity* is the extent to which indicators clearly measure what they are intended to measure.
- *Causal inference* refers to the ease with which inferences about causal relations among variables may be made.
- *Multivariate* refers to the ease with which information on many variables is collected, leading to the possibility of multivariate analysis.
- *Probing* refers to the extent to which responses may be probed in depth.

One of the weaknesses of participant observation studies, in-depth interview studies, and focus group studies is their inability to tell whether the patterns that emerge are representative or peculiar to the institution or group being studied. An additional problem is that such studies are impossible to replicate because these studies involve examining a unique combination of individuals interacting with one another at a particular time. Although it would be possible for another observer to go into the same institution at a later time, a number of conditions probably will have changed. Moreover, the observers themselves may have rather different impacts on the organization. Thus, there are many factors that confound an interpretation of any changes observed by different researchers. Making verifiable causal inferences is difficult because only one case is being examined.

In naturalistic observational studies, the subjects are observed unobtrusively and are not aware that they are part of a study. A notable disadvantage of such

There is a growing trend in nursing toward research that empowers participants and leads to improved practice. The ideology of health-care reform, improved health-care delivery, the need for evidence-based practice, and a belief that nursing services should be informed by research into the needs of recipients and shaped by collaboration with them all lead to a quest for new research methodologies and approaches that reflect this ideology (Hart and Bond, 1998). Various researchers have coined terms to describe approaches that do not fit traditional research designs. Labels such as collaborative research (Parahoo, 1997), action activist-oriented research (Denzin and Lincoln, 1994), new generation research (Streubert and Carpenter, 1995, 1999), participatory evaluation (Feurstein, 1988), new paradigm (Meyer, 1993), and community reflective action research (Boutlier, Mason and Rootman, 1997) are terms found in the literature to refer to this new brand of research. In addition, there is a growing interest in feminist research, not only in nursing but in the other social sciences as well. And, similar to the other approaches, feminist research has a concern with issues of social change. We have christened such designs with *new-wave applied research* to reflect their growing popularity and utility within nursing. For purposes of this discussion, we have included four designs in this category:

- Action research
- Health promotion research
- Evaluation research
- Feminist research

What do these four approaches have in common? Why have we grouped them together? These are reasonable questions given the lack of consensus on groupings and classifications of research designs. Our response is that we see them as unique designs with unique purposes that do not fit traditional methods. They share in an iterative process that involves some combination of inquiry, intervention, and evaluation that should lead to some improvement in practice or empowerment of participants. The prime intention of this type of research is to have an impact on policy making, be it at the level of the work unit, the community, or the government. New-wave approaches can use quantitative or qualitative approaches or a combination of the two to achieve their research aims. All of the approaches within this new tradition are described in this chapter.

A. ACTION RESEARCH

The term *action research* can be traced back in the literature to the work of Kurt Lewin (1944), who is generally considered the founder of action research and change theory (Hart and Bond, 1998). Lewin, a Prussian psychologist who immigrated to America in 1933, introduced the term *action research* as a way of studying a social system at the same time as attempting to change it. **Action research** is simply defined today as the systematic collection and analysis of data for the purpose of taking action and making change. It provides practitioners, organizations, or communities with tools to solve their problems.

I. Characteristics

Seven criteria have been identified by Hart and Bond (1998, pp. 37–38) to distinguish action research from other methodologies. "Action research:

- Is educative
- Deals with individuals as members of a social group
- Is problem focused, context specific, and future oriented
- Involves a change intervention
- Aims at improvement and involvement
- Involves a cyclic process in which research, action, and evaluation are interlinked

• Is founded on a research relationship in which those involved are participants in the change process."

The aim of all action research is the generation of practical knowledge that has the potential to improve a specific situation or practice. It does not aim to generalize solutions to problems that apply across a range of settings because the solutions are designed for the particular setting in which the research is conducted. In nursing situations, an action researcher would attempt to find a solution for a particular problem by implementing changes in practice and then closely monitor and evaluate the changes during implementation. For example, Gale and associates (1998) describe an ongoing action research project designed to explore, develop, implement, and evaluate the role of the generic health-care support worker in a high-dependency unit for people with complex physical and psychological needs. The introduction of the generic health-care worker has potential to create a number of problems related to professional role boundaries and balance of skill mix in practice settings. The project is funded by the Department of Health, United Kingdom, and consists of three phases. Phase 1 includes an exploration of the new role and the identification of problems and difficulties created by its implementation. Phase 2 is the implementation phase and involves the establishment of a Practice Development Unit to manage and develop the new role. Phase 3 is the evaluation of the impact of the project with data collected from providers and users of the service. Practicing nurses will watch with interest as this project unfolds. It has the potential to teach us a great deal about use of this new role in health-care delivery.

Participatory action research (PAR) is a subset of action research. It consists of three elements: research, adult education, and sociopolitical action (Parahoo, 1997). It emphasizes both research for the

purpose of bringing about *change* and *participation* by community members (either geographic community or people with common interests and shared experiences). PAR places great emphasis on collaboration with research participants by considering them as co-investigators throughout the entire process. Through the process of participation, community members become empowered to define their own problems and find solutions. PAR increases the participants' understanding of the issue they are working on. The research element provides an opportunity for them to test assumptions so that they can be more confident of their ground as they go forward to implement change. The process of participating enables members to build skills, confidence, and knowledge (Barnsley and Ellis, 1992).

2. Steps in the Action Research Process

Action research proceeds in cyclical stages that involve planning, implementing, reflecting, and evaluating and involves collaboration between researchers and participants throughout the entire process. It is an iterative process that parallels the nursing process; this may explain its increasing popularity with nurses. It is a particularly useful research approach in today's rapidly changing health-care environment because it allows nurses to implement changes in practice and simultaneously evaluate the impact of such change. Below is a list of some of the steps that are necessary in most action research studies, including participatory action research projects. Action research is described here as if it were a linear process, but in truth it does not follow a series of stages. Rather it is a dynamic process with a spiral of cycles in which research, action, and evaluation interact with each other at various phases (Waterman et al., 1995).

Step 1: Entry into the Community and Development of a Collaborative Relationship

In action research, the community may represent an actual geographic community; an institution or agency such as a school, health-care facility, or government department; or a grassroots group of people with similar interests and issues. Action research aims to create an equal partnership between the researcher and the researched in which representatives from both come together and form a research team. The extent of the collaboration between the researchers and those researched may vary from review of the problem and diagnosis to full collaboration in all stages of the process. Action researchers who facilitate collaboration at all stages believe they are able to find the most practical solutions to identified problems (Whyte, 1991).

Step 2: Assessment of the Situation and Identification of Issue

This step involves gathering as much data as possible from a variety of sources to identify the problem or issue. At this step, you are interested in getting detailed data about the situation as it exists before a change is implemented. Data generation continues throughout the entire process and involves a wide range of approaches, both qualitative and quantitative. Data collection is usually a collaborative process involving both researchers and participants as members of the research team. At this point, steering groups or planning committees may be formed to inform the process. You are concerned with identifying a problem (something that needs changing).

Step 3: Planning for Research and Action

Planning begins with a detailed analysis of the present situation. Researchers and participants decide which data collection methods are most appropriate to the specific situation. Usually triangulated data generation is recommended with at least three methods selected to transcend the limitations of each other and lead to more effective problem solving (Streubert and Carpenter, 1999). Participant observation, interviews, focus groups, diaries, questionnaires, and surveys are valuable methods of data generation. At the heart of the planning stage is the development of an action plan that will lead to problem resolution. The action plan emerges after data analysis.

Analysis varies depending on the data generation techniques used. Quantitative data are analyzed in traditional ways using statistical methods and qualitative data using qualitative methods. Researchers and participants work together collaboratively on the data analysis, but researchers often take the lead in this step because of their prerequisite knowledge and expertise required for analysis. It is critical, however, to involve participants to make sure that the interpretations of the data fit the reality of the situation. Depending on the analysis produced, an action plan is developed by the co-researchers. The action plan details the planned change intervention, the implementation process, the plan for facilitating reflection, and evaluation plan (Streubert and Carpenter, 1999). This stage requires a number of meetings with the co-researchers to discuss and plan the details. Records and detailed notes are made of all meetings and decisions by the researchers and used in the writing of the final plan.

Step 4: Implementation of the Action Plan and Reflection

This stage involves the actual implementation of the planned change. The implementation usually occurs over a specified period of time. At this point, the researchers may move into a more peripheral role and community members may be more involved in the actual implementation of change. Researchers remain present, however, to guide and facilitate the reflection that occurs with the implementation (Streubert and Carpenter, 1999).

Reflection is the process of thinking about the implementation of the new change and its impact on the key players. It occurs simultaneously with implementation. Reflection is promoted through group meetings and observation periods during which the participants and co-researchers may record their thoughts and experiences with the planned change. Two aids to reflection are dialectic and reflexive critique. **Reflexive critique** is a process that enables participants and researchers to make explicit, alternative explanations for events or experiences. It facilitates discussion between the researchers and participants and leads to greater insights and acceptance of multiple explanations for events. **Dialectic critique,** in contrast, makes explicit, internal contradictions in the data rather than complementary explanations. By exposing the contradictory nature of phenomena in the change situation, the researchers and participants come to a clearer understanding of the change process (Streubert and Carpenter, 1999).

For example, a new method of recording nursing notes is introduced in the maternal and child nursing unit. The new method is evaluated by interviewing nurses working on that unit about their satisfaction with the method. Most nurses interviewed are dissatisfied with the new method, stating that it is time consuming and inefficient. Participants are engaged in reflexive critique by the researcher, who queries further about the source of their discontent. Some nurses reply the charting time is longer because they do not know what sheets to record specific information on and subsequently must reread instructions. Others complain that the new method requires nurses to provide objective and subjective data to support assess-

ments, unlike the old method that simply required nurses to identify the assessment categories. Others complain that the new method takes longer because you have to individualize the notes, unlike the old system that used a generic check-off system. Hence, a number of explanations emerged for nurses' dissatisfaction with the new system based on reflexive critique. Using dialectic critique, the researcher may ask participants to talk about the time element involved in using the new charting system. The researcher would look for conflicting information about time. It may be that new graduates who learned a variety of charting methods in their educational programs say it does not take more time to implement, but older nurses accustomed to the traditional charting system say it is very time consuming. Discussing these two opposite positions would provide insight into the variety of factors influencing implementation of the new charting system.

Step 5: Evaluation of the Implementation

Coresearchers work together to evaluate the implementation according to the action plan. Evaluation can occur at the end of the implementation stage as well as at various points throughout the implementation stage. Evaluation includes data generated during the reflection process as well as additional information on which the team decides. Evaluation data may be similar to data that was collected in the initial assessment phase. Usually evaluation meetings are held with the research team and key stakeholders to discuss the interpretation of the evaluation data and verify conclusions.

Step 6: Report and Reassessment

In action research, a report is written by the research team that incorporates a "plurality of explanations" for events observed as well as questions for future consideration (Streubert and Carpenter, 1999). The report is intended to promote dialogue among participants and stimulate additional courses of action to be taken by participants, with or without the guidance of the researchers. This report on findings and process becomes the initial step in a new cycle of this iterative process.

Step 7: Planning Future Action

Based on the report and evaluation data, planning future action continues. The cycle begins again with implementation, reporting, and reassessment (Deagle and McWilliam, 1992).

3. Challenges in Conducting Action Research

Action research offers many opportunities to nurse researchers. An obvious one is the ability to implement change to improve practice and evaluate the change simultaneously. Another strength is the ability to empower participants through involvement in the research process. Because research produces knowledge, it empowers those who carry it out or commission it. Action research also provides practical knowledge that enables nurses to solve specific problems in their practice setting. Despite these important advantages, action research presents a number of challenges to the researcher, which include:

- **The challenge of involving community members as part of the research team.** Engaging the appropriate stakeholders and maintaining their commitment to the research project over time requires tact, effort, time, and knowledge of the community. The community must first be appropriately defined and then key stakeholders identified. Decisions must be made as to who will be a research participant (i.e., a co-researcher and community member of

the research team) and who will be a research respondent (i.e., member of the broader population who provides data and validates results at various stages). The researcher must be sensitive to the participants' agendas.

- **Diversity of values, perspectives, and abilities among community members and researchers must be valued.** On a practical level, this often presents difficulties based on the different perspectives of researchers, practitioners, community members, and academics. One participant, for example, may be interested in broad social change, but another may be interested only in the improved practice situation that the project should create. This feature of action research complicates the relationships of collaborators and increases the time required to focus the research project and complete action research.

- **Issues of power imbalances and establishment of egalitarian relationships require constant vigilance throughout the research project.** Power balances may shift over the course of the project because various community members may change. Often the commitment to a research project by the community member may not be the same as the commitment of the university-based researcher who participates for the duration of a research grant.

- **All members of the research team must be sensitive and responsive to the need for different forms and types of leadership at different stages of the project** (Lindsey and Stajduhar, 1998). At times, community members will take the lead, particularly during the implementation stage; at other times, the researcher may take the lead, such as in data analysis.

- **Action research is extremely time consuming.** Identifying and mobilizing participants and whole communities to be involved in the research process are time intensive and require a high level of negotiation, tact, energy, and commitment on the part of the research team. Time must be provided to train members to be part of the research team; enable full community participation; and allow the cyclical, iterative process to work as it is intended.

4. Example of Action Research Study

To illustrate action research, let's look at the process of participatory research and community empowerment to reduce nutritional inequities in a group of low-income urban women.

Health education programs have traditionally focused on providing information to individuals as a way of improving their health through lifestyle modification. This method has lacked demonstrated effectiveness for enhancing or improving health status. Travers (1997), following a critique of health education practices, suggests that an alternative orientation is needed in health education. She uses the process of participatory research and community organization to design a project to address the inequities in nutritional practices for a group of low-income urban women. The article highlights the process of social action by monitoring changes associated with the women's experiences. The article is of note because it shows how the participatory research experience can be an empowering educational experience for participants. This article demonstrates how the principles of participatory action research emphasize valuing people's knowledge, deriving questions from the perspective of the people, and helping oppressed people to reflect on their situations. It aims to develop critical consciousness and improve the lives of those involved in the research process. The article also points out the realities and limitations of engaging in this type of research project. Box 8.1 describes the methodology involved in this emancipatory research project and highlights the findings.

B. EVALUATION RESEARCH

The current emphasis on provision of quality care and evidence-based practice and decision-making points to the need for nurses and other health-care professionals to provide evidence that what they are doing works and why it does. Evaluation research provides a mechanism to do this. Evaluation research tends to focus on a particular program, product, method, procedure, event, or policy. An important *distinction* exists between evaluation and evaluation research. Evaluation is a process of assessing the value of something. Practitioners evaluate their performance, their delivery of services, the quality of care provided, and so on by reflecting on what it is that they do and how well they do it. The difference between this and **evaluation research** is that the latter is a systematic appraisal using the methods of social research for the purpose of generating knowledge and understanding that can be used for decision making. It is an applied form of research that provides utilitarian answers to practical questions for decision makers, such as: Who is benefiting from the program or service? Is the program cost effective? Should the intervention or program be continued? Is the program achieving its intended goals? In what areas does the program need to be improved? Another term used to refer to evaluation research is *outcomes research.*

1. Purpose of Evaluation Research

Evaluation research is often classified according to the purpose of the investigative activities. Usually there are three main reasons to engage in evaluation research.

BOX 8.1 *Nurse Researchers at Work*

REDUCING INEQUITIES THROUGH PARTICIPATORY RESEARCH AND COMMUNITY EMPOWERMENT

Background

This study was part of a larger research project with the purpose of initiating nutrition education for social change following an explication of the social organization of nutritional inequities among socially disadvantaged women and their families.

Methodology

Participatory action research was the methodology used in this study with a group of low-income urban women to reduce nutritional inequities for themselves and their families.

Method

Research participants were low-income women who self-selected to attend a coffee group at a local parent center. A total of 33 women actively participated in the group throughout the duration of the study but never all at the same time. Although a sample of convenience, the group appeared representative of the low-income female population in the city in which the research was conducted.

Participant observation was the primary method of data collection. The researcher was a participant observer at the community drop-in parent center in an urban neighborhood in Nova Scotia, Canada. The researcher participated in the life of the center, serving meals in the soup kitchen, unpacking food from the food bank, and preparing and eating meals with the staff and volunteers.

One month after initiation into the parent center, the researcher initiated a series of group interviews with women attending the center to discuss their experiences of feeding themselves and their families. In total, 27 group interviews lasting 2 hours each were conducted over a 16-month period. Semistructured interview guides were used to organize the discussions thematically. Participants also introduced topics through discussion of their relevant experiences. The use of triangulated data collection techniques (participant observation and group interviews) was useful as an internal validity and credibility check because data ob-tained from one source could be checked against data obtained by another.

Qualitative interview data and field notes were analyzed, not so much for interpretation of data but rather to show the process of emancipatory education for the women's group. To do this, data were organized chronologically into chunks that showed the progression of group activities.

Results

Through the process of participatory research, the empowerment of research participants to initiate collective action for social change to reduce nutritional inequities was possible. The results section describes the details of the process by which the participants came to understand their experiences and acted on that understanding to create change.

For the first few months of the group meetings, the discussion was unstructured allowing the women simply to talk about their experiences surrounding the difficulties of trying to feed their families. The women listened to each other's experiences. Suddenly they were not alone. By listening to how others overcame difficulties and similar experiences, they began to learn coping skills from each other and build hope by working together toward solutions. Almost imperceptibly, the group sessions moved from complaining sessions to consciousness-raising sessions. Consciousness raising is a practical process that begins with the experience of oppression. Women come together to talk about their experiences and, in doing so, break the "culture of silence." They begin to see problems not as individual failures but as sources that are rooted in structures affecting the lives of all women alike. The consciousness-raising process mirrored the process of learning experienced by the research participants in this study. They began with their experiences of oppression, by gender, by class, and sometimes by race. They broke the culture of silence by sharing their stories. They came to see the common and political roots of their oppression and thus

continued on next page

BOX 8.1 *Nurse Researchers at Work (Continued)*

REDUCING INEQUITIES THROUGH PARTICIPATORY RESEARCH AND COMMUNITY EMPOWERMENT

were able to shed their self-blame and take on a new way of relating to the social world. This was the beginning.

Exploration of women's food purchasing experiences enabled a process of education leading to community development. At an early meeting, one woman discussed her experiences and perception that food costs more while shopping in low-income neighborhoods. With pricing inequities brought to the group's attention, it was decided to do a comparison of chain stores in low-income and middle-income neighborhoods. The researcher taught the women to do unit pricing to enable them to make in-store price comparisons. The women split into groups to do the unit pricing comparison in four stores: two in the inner city and two in the suburbs. Results revealed that inner-city stores were consistently 5% higher than prices in suburban stores of the same chain. A 10.7% price differential was found between the store most frequently used by the women and the store furthest from their neighborhood. The women learned that cost savings outweighed transportation costs.

In keeping with participatory action research principles, the women decided to take action to address the inequities. First they wrote letters to the stores addressing inequities in pricing, quality, and service. Knowledge of the supermarkets' roles in construction of inequities was the catalyst for community action. They confronted both local supermarket chains with their findings and recommendations for action. Both stores changed buying practices to decrease price inequities between locations. One store introduced a bulk-food section in the inner-city store, a move that eliminated price inequities between neighborhoods. These changes enabled women and socially disadvantaged families to purchase food more affordably. These changes live on long after the research process ended. Because the women were still dependent on commercial outlets for the bulk of their food, the researcher worked with a subgroup of women to secure funding for a grassroots cooperative grocery outlet. It is operated out of the parent center and run by a committee composed of women from the community. This process was an empowering learning experience in a personal, political, and economic sense for the women involved. This is emancipatory health education!

SOURCE: Summarized from Travers, K. (1997). Reducing inequities through participatory research and community empowerment. *Health Education and Behavior, 24*(3), 344–356.

These include needs assessment, formative evaluation, and summative evaluation.

Needs assessment is a form of inquiry that assesses the needs, problems, concerns, or conditions of a group, community, or organization that should be addressed in future planning activities. Needs assessments are usually prompted when one is dissatisfied with the current situation and level of service delivery or quality. The assessment provides valuable information on what is needed to improve the situation for the future. Examples of questions appropriate for this type of evaluation research include:

- What are the perceived needs of new mothers for information on infant care during the postpartum period?
- What are the continuing education needs of RNs moving from acute care to community-based service delivery?
- What is the range of services required to provide comprehensive health promotion services to street youth in urban centers?

- What are the appropriate human resource requirements to staff community-based primary health-care centers serving rural communities?

A needs assessment is useful in setting priorities in health care and allocating scarce resources. Questionnaires, interviews, and focus groups are popular ways of collecting data for needs assessments. Nurse researchers have conducted numerous needs assessments of various client groups. For example, Kulig and Thorpe (1996) studied the teaching and learning needs of culturally diverse post-RN students using both in-depth, semistructured individual interviews and focus groups. McKay and Diem (1995) used a self-report questionnaire to study the health concerns of 1416 adolescent girls attending public schools to identify factors and themes that would help in planning health promotion programs for this population.

Formative evaluation is a form of inquiry that focuses on how well a new service or ongoing program or activity is meeting its objectives. The thrust of formative evaluation research is to identify what is and what is not working currently so that remedial action can be taken to improve the situation at hand. The researcher is interested in determining if, how, and to what extent the goals and objectives of the ongoing program are being met. It yields practical information that can be applied to improve the activity, service, or program. It is similar to action research in that it is focused on making changes for improvement of the present situation (Cormack, 1991).

Summative evaluation is the third category of evaluation research. It is conducted to determine the effectiveness, value, and worth of an innovation. For many evaluation projects, this includes evaluation of the costs as well as the effectiveness of the program or intervention. The results of summative evaluation are useful in determining whether to replicate, discard, modify, or replace an innovation. Unlike formative evaluation research, which produces knowledge that can be used to improve the situation during the actual implementation stage of a project, summative evaluation research produces knowledge that is useful in terms of making decisions about whether the innovation or activity should be continued or discontinued. Its purpose is not to make improvements to the situation during the innovation implementation like in action research or formative evaluation; rather, the purpose of summative evaluation is to make a decision after completion of the implementation of the innovation as to whether or not the innovation made a difference to the group that received it or whether one innovation is better than another. Therefore, what distinguishes evaluation research is not the method used but rather the purpose or intent for which it is done (Cormack, 1991).

Summative evaluation is usually conducted using a comparison procedure. A popular design used for evaluation research is the randomized clinical trial (RCT) or experimental design, which was discussed in Chapter 4 in terms of its limitations and strengths. **Randomized clinical trials** use one or more control groups and experimental groups, depending on the number of interventions. Subjects are randomly allocated to the groups. They are frequently used to test the effectiveness of drugs, therapies, and other interventions. Summative evaluation may also include a comparison of two innovations or activities within the same program.

2. Steps in Evaluation Research

Because evaluation research uses a plurality of approaches, the specific steps in any given evaluation research project vary depending on the design chosen by the investigator and the nature of the evaluation. There is, however, consensus that the traditional approach to evaluation research proceeds through four phases: identification of program objectives, measurement of program objectives, collection of data, and analysis an interpretation of data.

a. Identification of Program Objectives

Objectives are usually developed from the broad statements of program goals. Objectives should be stated in specific behavioral terms that are easily measured. Behavioral terms refer to the specific behavior change the researcher would expect to see in the people to whom the program was delivered. For example, if you are a community health nurse teaching a disease prevention program to school-aged children, your goal may be to have children use proper handwashing techniques. The behavioral objective for this goal might be, "Children will wash their hands before eating meals." It is important that there is consensus between the researcher and program stakeholders about the objectives to be used for evaluation because the objectives set the stage for the other phases.

b. Measurement of Program Objectives

As in any other research project, the investigator now selects a design that will enable him or her to determine whether the behavioral objectives have been attained. A variety of designs are available, depending on the purpose and nature of the project (see the Pluralistic Approaches to Evaluation Research section of this chapter). The researcher must determine how the behavioral objectives will be measured within that design. Will observations of clients' behaviors be measured? Will clients complete self-administered questionnaires? Semistructured interviews? Diaries? Will data be sought from sources other than the clients of the program to determine attainment of objectives? All of these are possibilities.

c. Collection of Data

After the researcher determines how the behaviors of interest will be measured, the process of data collection begins. The amount of time and energy required for this step vary depending on the research design selected in the previous phase. For example, a time series study, a single group before-and-after study, or a randomized experimental study all require two or more data collection periods to get baseline (i.e., before intervention) and comparative data. The researcher collecting evaluation data needs to be sensitive to the dynamics operating in the field. People are often suspicious of evaluators and might feel threatened by the presence of the researcher. This may lead to defensive responses and uncooperative behavior. It is important that the researcher has good interpersonal skills and experience dealing with such situations so that respondents can be put at ease. Participants may also respond the way in which they think the researcher would like them to respond and hence distort their answer. For example, if participants were aware that the researcher was interested in evaluating the positive impact of an early discharge program, they might respond in a way to support the researcher's view.

d. Analysis and Interpretation of Data

This involves taking apart the data that were collected and reorganizing it in a manner that enables the researcher to determine if the objectives have been met. Quantitative data are analyzed using statistical procedures and qualitative data analyzed using a variety of qualitative approaches.

3. Pluralistic Approaches to Evaluation Research

The approach selected for an evaluation research project depends on the purpose of the evaluation. It is important to be clear about the objectives of the evaluation project from the beginning. As previously stated, one approach to evaluation is the classic experiment (or RCT) or methods approximating the classic experiment such as a quasi-experimental design. Recently, however, the value of the experiment has come under attack as a form of evaluation research in nursing. Experiments have been criticized because they cannot provide full explanations of *why* an innovation or program is effective. This is the type of information that is important to the practitioner who wishes to implement the successful innovation in a new setting. There are, however, different opinions on the value of the experiment to evaluation research in nursing. Some believe it is the *sine qua non* of scientific research and they see the RCT as the only way to evaluate health-care interventions (McDonald and Daly, cited in Parahoo, 1997). Proponents of experimental research argue that although a variety of designs can be used to do evaluation research, the experiment, despite its limitations, is the only one that can establish cause and effect.

Those who oppose the use of the RCT for evaluation research in nursing believe it incapable of contributing to the understanding of human experience. Many feminist researchers have argued that women have been victims of experimental evaluation research that is reductionistic in nature. They see physicians imposing medical interventions and treatments on women that have been evaluated using experimental methods that ignore the needs and experiences of the women receiving

them. Others believe the real issues in evaluation research should emerge from intensive onsite knowledge rather than formulating them before data collection. They favor a more qualitative approach that involves inductively constructing explanations about the data rather than developing hypotheses in advance and then collecting data to test them.

The **evaluation case study** is a method that is gaining popularity. These studies are in-depth explorations of phenomena, usually over an extended period of time, using diverse data collection procedures to collect detailed information about an individual, group, organization, program, or social phenomenon. The major advantage to using a case study in evaluation research is the depth of data and the intensive analysis of the situation that can result. Case studies can use both quantitative and qualitative approaches to focus on specific situations. Most case studies yield descriptive data, identify relationships among the variables, and track trends in the data. Case studies are especially helpful in providing descriptive information about the process of program or procedure implementation. A case study approach to evaluation could address such questions as: How is the program or intervention working? What is the impact of the program in the practice setting? Is the program operating the way it was intended? What variables are resources or barriers to successfully implementing the program? What are the strengths and limitations of the program? What are the intended and unintended outcomes of the program or innovation? Case studies yield specific, in-depth, holistic findings. The emphasis is on understanding the specific case (in this case, program or innovation), but it is likely that the findings may be useful in similar situations in which the program may be replicated.

In brief, a mix of designs for purposes of evaluation research is desirable. Each

BOX 8.3 *Nurse Researchers at Work*

COMBINED MOTHER AND BABY CARE: DOES IT MEET THE NEEDS OF FAMILIES?

Combined mother and baby care is thought to be an effective way to prepare a family for the changing roles and added responsibilities that the arrival of a new baby entails, but few studies have evaluated this care delivery system. Therefore, the postpartum staff at Sudbury General Hospital in Sudbury, Ontario, conducted a posttest control group study design with a self-selected sample of postpartum mothers when the unit was changing from traditional to combined mother and baby care. A total of 103 mothers who received traditional care and 102 who had combined mother and baby care completed a questionnaire to assess perceptions of their own competence and satisfaction with the type of care administered. There were no significant differences between the two groups, although there was a positive trend in mothers' competence and satisfaction scores for the primiparous

mothers with combined care but not traditional care; the reverse was true of the multiparous mothers' scores.

Factors that may have confounded the results include insufficient time between institution of the program and its evaluation and the quality of the prenatal education received. Multiparous mothers scored higher on self-care, infant care, and maternal competence than did primiparous mothers regardless of the care delivery system. Future research should take the differences between the primiparous and multiparous mothers into account and focus on the less immediate needs of mothers. Although the results of this study do not statistically support the greater efficacy of combined care over traditional care in meeting the needs of families, evidence suggests that further study may provide more conclusive results in this respect.

SOURCE: Summarized from Bailey, P., Maciejewski, J., and Koren, I. (1993). Combined mother and baby care: Does it meet the needs of families? *Canadian Journal of Nursing Research, 25*(3), 29–39.

unit of analysis and the unit of intervention for health promotion initiatives by nurses. This is in keeping with the *ethos* of health promotion that asserts that people (e.g., individuals, families, and communities) know what they want and need to be healthy.

1. Characteristics

Although it is difficult and perhaps impossible to reach consensus on a universal definition of health promotion research, some authors (Bunton and Macdonald, 1992; McQueen, 1994; Pederson et al., 1994; Pender, 1996) have offered helpful parameters and characteristics that health promotion research ought to reflect. These include:

- Emphasis on individual, family, community, environmental, or societal wellness

- A concern with the conditions for change and the obstacles and barriers to change
- A focus on patterns for policy making in health, patterns of behaviors, and the antecedents of health in the social contexts of behavior
- Emphasis on diverse methods, multidisciplinary approaches, and collaboration of different sectors of society with different traditions
- Use of multiple indicators (to infer effect of health promotion strategy) and statistical analyses appropriate to the indicators
- Application of findings in the context of action is central to health promotion research
- A tool that helps the community to communicate with policy makers and vice versa

- Involvement of the community of interest in the research
- A set of end users that include policy makers, decision makers, health-care professionals, communities, and individuals

Although some health promotion researchers may add other characteristics to this list, most would agree that this represents a helpful, albeit incomplete, list reflective of key features of health promotion research.

2. Scope of Health Promotion Research

It is important that nurses appreciate the complexity of health promotion and the various levels at which it occurs. Health promotion research within nursing has called for a move from the individualistic approach that predominates in health behavior research and health care to a societal approach in which the responsibility is shifted to society for making available the resources that people require for health. Certainly the 1980s and 1990s witnessed the theme of a community versus individual focus in discussions of health promotion in nursing (Gott and O'Brien, 1990). This theme also needs to be reflected in the field of nursing's health promotion research agenda. Given the field's emphasis on holism and our acceptance of the environment as a core variable integral to health, there remains a need to broaden the focus of health promotion research in nursing to include not only the individual and family but also the community and societal level. Let us consider each of these levels.

a. Individual

A large number of health promotion studies in nursing focus on the individual as the unit of analysis or the unit of inter-

vention. These studies, for the most part, aim to describe health promotion practices of individuals, identify determinants of healthy lifestyle or predictors of health behavior, assess lifestyle practices, implement and evaluate health promotion interventions delivered to individuals, or develop instruments to measure health promotion. They are important in terms of developing the knowledge base for nursing and use a variety of approaches to address the research question. Surveys are particularly popular in studies of this nature. Box 8.4 provides an example of a prospective survey that focuses on the individual as the unit of analysis. The study identifies factors that predict physical activity behavior in rural fifth grade children. The study is of importance to the field of health promotion research because understanding the factors that influence physical activity behavior is important in the design of intervention programs targeted at youth. The trend toward increasing physical inactivity in North American youth is one of the most pressing issues facing health professionals today.

b. Family

Although the family plays an important role in the development of health behaviors, there is very little nursing research on the role of the family in health promotion (Pender, 1996). The family is often considered to be the context within which health behavior is learned, but it is actually much more than that. The family is a unit of analysis in its own right. Progress in this area of health promotion research has been slow because of methodological imprecision and measurement problems when the family is considered the unit of analysis or the unit of intervention. Longitudinal surveys that track family lifestyles and their stability over time, use of small focus groups within the family environment, and case studies are approaches

---

BOX 8.4 *A Prospective Study of Physical Activity in Children*

Methods

A prospective study design was used to identify the predictors of vigorous physical activity (VPA) and moderate and vigorous physical activity (MVPA) among 202 rural, predominately African-American children. Selected social-cognitive determinants of physical activity were assessed via questionnaire in the fifth grade. Participation in VPA and MVPA was assessed via the previous day physical activity recall 1 year later in the sixth grade.

Results

For girls, participation in community sports, self-efficacy in overcoming barriers, enjoyment of school physical education, race (white > black), and perception of mother's activity level (active vs. inactive) were significant predictors of VPA. For MVPA, participation in community sports and self-efficacy in overcoming barriers were significant barriers. For boys, whereas self-efficacy in overcoming barriers was the only significant predictor of VPA, beliefs regarding activity outcomes and participation in community sports were significant predictors of MVPA.

Conclusion

Social-cognitive constructs such as physical activity, self-efficacy, access to community physical activity outlets, and positive beliefs regarding physical activity outcomes are important predictors of future physical activity behavior among rural, predominantly African-American children.

SOURCE: Trost, S., Pate, R., Saunders, R., et al. (1997). A prospective study of the determinants of physical activity in rural fifth-grade children. *Preventive Medicine, 26,* 257–263. Cited with permission. (From *Am J Health Promotion,* 1998, *12*(4))

---

that may be considered in the home context.

The relationship between family health and individual health is multivariate and poorly understood. It is an important area of investigation for nurses, but studies of this nature are scarce in the literature. Gillis (1994) studied the relationship of mothers' and fathers' health promoting lifestyles to adolescent daughters' lifestyles using a survey design. The health promoting lifestyle profile (HPLP) was used to measure lifestyle. Results indicated that both mothers' and fathers' lifestyles were positively correlated with their daughters' lifestyles. This suggests there is some consistency among family health attitudes, behaviors, and practices.

c. Community

Community-based health promotion is an exciting area of investigation for nurses. The idea of changing the behavior of an entire community rather than a family, small group, or individual is a challenge that requires effort and coordination of all involved. It includes a range of activities aimed at creating a health-enhancing environment and healthy behaviors for populations or entire communities (Pender, 1996). Research into community-based health promotion offers nursing a wealth of opportunities to be involved in aspects of needs assessments, intervention studies, evaluation research, participatory action research, and methodological research that focuses on the development of new methodologies and measurement techniques. Research into community-based health promotion initiatives needs to be carefully examined to determine valuable information about what works and what does not work with various populations and why. These are important questions for nurses to answer.

The best examples of research into community-based health promotion are provided by the Healthy Cities initiative in Canada, the United States, and Europe. The World Health Organization (WHO) launched the Healthy Cities Initiative in 1986 as a strategy for achieving health for all. It focused on developing healthy public policy, creating supportive environments, strengthening community action, developing personal skills of community citizens, and reorienting health-care services. Interested readers are directed to the work of Flynn (1992) for a U.S. perspective and Manson-Singer (1994) for a Canadian perspective on these projects.

3. Methods

An interesting debate has continued in the literature for some time over methods for health promotion research. Succinctly stated, the debate is over the use of traditional public health measures versus more nontraditional methods. There are many elements to the debate. One is the quantitative versus qualitative issue discussed in Chapter 1. Another is the rigid adherence to research criteria established by statisticians such as the sacred cows of randomness and significance, even though the likelihood that actual research conducted in health promotion will be in violation of the statistical assumptions underlying classical parametric procedures (see Chapter 12). A central challenge to health promotion research is how to break free legitimately from a rigid orthodoxy that is increasingly inappropriate and inadequate for the special areas of study needed (McQueen, 1994).

We support the use of a multiplicity of methods for health promotion research. The research questions and objectives should guide the design selected. Because the range of questions is so broad in health promotion research, a rich repertoire of approaches is required. For example, you may wish to describe the characteristics of a target population such as the needs for peer support of homeless youth; or explain an outcome from a health promotion intervention such as changes in knowledge, attitudes, and health behaviors after a community-based empower-

ment education program for seniors; or implement and evaluate a school-based health promotion program on healthy diet. The point is that different types of research objectives and questions lead to very different study designs. Surveys, interviews, participant observation studies, focus groups, and experimental designs all have something to contribute to health promotion research. Qualitative and quantitative methodologies are appropriate for different types of studies. Regardless of your position in the methods debate, you must be able to clearly justify your choice of design and method.

4. Future Directions

Health promotion research has developed tremendously over the past few years, from a small area of interest pursued by a few investigators and practitioners to a wider set of activities undertaken by federal, provincial, and state health departments as well as university centers that specialize in health promotion research. Health promotion efforts are increasingly being established in multiple and diverse settings, and new directions in research are being forged, such as those proposed by Pender (1996). Future directions include:

1. Identifying health promotion beliefs and practices in diverse families and communities as a basis for effective programming
2. Developing appropriate indicators of change (consequences) at the community level that reflect the effectiveness of health promotion interventions (treatment)
3. Developing consistent methods for assessing health outcomes across a range of programs and communities
4. Determining the synergistic effect of work site, school, family, and community health promotion efforts on population health outcomes

5. Identifying the characteristics of health strengthening environments in families, schools, work sites, and communities
6. Tracking the outcomes of families and communities receiving care from multiservice nursing centers with major emphasis on health promotion and disease prevention

In summary, the future looks bright for health promotion research in nursing. The field of nursing is forging new frontiers in this area. The good news is that health promotion research is still new enough for all of us to be considered pioneers. The multiple definitions and approaches to health promotion indicate a high level of interest in it. This is healthy for nursing and for health care. As nurses broaden the scope of their research activities to include individual, family, and community health promotion projects, their influence in the social, political, and economic arena will also increase, allowing them to impact factors influencing human health.

D. FEMINIST RESEARCH

Feminist research has gained increasing momentum in nursing over the past decade. Many argue that because nursing is a female-dominated profession that advocates for women and children, as well as men, the relationship between nursing and feminism should be explored. The patriarchal society in which we live is a part of the field of nursing's reality as a professional discipline, as a science, and as an art. Many nurses are now focused on the conditions of oppression that exist for nurses and their clients and have a desire to address the social, class, gender, ethnic, racial, and other biases that are inherent in their world and in their research. Feminist research perspectives offer one possibility for nursing to improve its science in this area.

Feminist research has been defined in many ways. As the context and shape of feminism is shifting, so is the manner in which feminist research is defined. This makes the task of defining feminist research perspectives both challenging and exciting. There are many different faces of feminism. In the early beginnings of the second phase of the women's movement (1960s onward), one could easily classify feminist researchers in terms of their political views (e.g., liberal, radical, or Marxist), their preferred research styles, or their academic discipline; however, these distinctions have become blurred. Political orientations are now blurred by internal divisions in feminist thought; many academic researchers are borrowing from other disciplines, and many are mixing quantitative and qualitative approaches or developing new methods to explore questions of interest (Olesen, 1994). One cannot speak of "feminism;" one can only speak of *feminisms* and define them by their adherence to four basic principles:

1. A valuing of women and their experiences, ideas, and needs
2. A seeing of phenomena from the perspective of women
3. A recognition of the existence of conditions which oppress women
4. A desire to change these conditions through criticisms and political action

Feminist research perspectives use a variety of research methods in their work. Many share the assumptions held by interpretive (qualitative) researchers and those who adopt a critical perspective. As Reinharz (1992) noted, most feminist scholars use a variety of research methods. They value inclusiveness more than orthodoxy and allow for creativity in all aspects of the research process.

Although feminist researchers use a wide range of quantitative and qualitative methods, most emphasis seems to be on qualitative methods, particularly using in-depth interviews. Oral histories, **compar-**

ative studies, and field study methods are also common. Similar to most interpretive perspectives, feminist research stresses personal experience embedded in the lives of the participants and subjectivity. Feminist researchers do not stop here, however; they go on and ask the simple but important question, "*And what about the women?*" Where are the women in any situation being investigated? Why are they not present in many situations? If they are present, what exactly are they doing? How do they experience the situation? What do they contribute to it? What does it mean for them? (Ritzer, 1988).

Harding (1987), a feminist philosopher of science, adds clarity to the discussion surrounding definitions of feminist research by providing some simple criteria. She takes the stance that in defining feminist research, three aspects of the study should be considered: (1) the purpose of the inquiry; (2) the explanatory hypothesis; and (3) the relationship between informant or "subject" and the researcher. These three criteria taken together should distinguish feminist research from nonfeminist research, rather than the methods used to gather data. The purpose of feminist research is to create social change that will benefit women. This is core to any definition of feminist research. Feminist research may also benefit other sectors of society such as children, men, homosexuals, oppressed groups, and others, but it must have value for women. Feminist researchers use a variety of methods to collect data. These data are always analyzed within the context of women's lives and are done in such a way that women are empowered rather than portrayed in ways that stereotype them or reinforce traditional stereotypes. The relationship between the researcher and the participants is a horizontal one in which the participant is a partner in the research process. The participant is a legitimate knower of their experience and is an expert.

Feminist research has been defined by some authors in terms of its characteristics. Duffy and Hedin, cited in Bunting and Campbell (1994), provide a useful list of qualities that they attribute to studies conducted from a feminist perspective. These include:

1. A feminist consciousness rooted in an attitude of equality, thereby replacing hierarchies of traditional research methods with horizontal relationships. In these relationships, the participants in a study are seen as partners in the research process. The investigator works in partnership with the participants to refine the research question, conduct the research, validate the findings, and disperse the results.

2. The aim of feminist research is to include women and study phenomena of practical concern to women. The focus is always based on women's experiences and the validity of women's perceptions as the truth for them. In simple terms, the research should be for women.

3. Feminist perspectives involve "conscious partiality" in which the biases of the researcher are acknowledged and openly discussed. The researcher, as in other qualitative approaches, examines her own values, beliefs, assumptions, and motivations. The researcher's point of view and biases become part of the data. This ensures that the researcher is on a level playing field with the participants.

4. Feminist research uses a variety of perspectives and a multiplicity of methods, including both qualitative and quantitative methods. This reflects the complexity of women's lives that are sufficiently complex and diverse to require multiple perspectives.

5. Feminist research aims to create social change. In this way, it can be considered a subset of critical social theory (see Chapter 1). It is action and change oriented and argues that science should be

used to improve the conditions of oppressed people.

6. Feminist research strives to represent human diversity. It includes ethnicity, class, gender, sexual orientation, and culture in the designing, conducting, and interpreting of research. These are often blind spots in traditional research approaches.

7. Feminist research critiques before scholarship, especially looking for androcentric (male bias) and ethnocentric (race and ethnic) biases.

1. Philosophical Tenets

A philosophical foundation and a defined methodology have not yet been broadly accepted by feminist scholars; however, many believe it has emerged from critical social theory. Both feminist and critical approaches believe that knowledge is socially constructed and acknowledge the oppressive nature of social structures. Both focus on the emancipatory goals of the research, but they differ in that gender is not the central concern of critical theorists. Critical theorists emphasize rationality, write principally for other intellectuals, and maintain power inequalities within their research teams. Feminist researchers place gender centrally within the research, make feminist writing accessible to all, and promote equality within their research team (Webb, 1993).

Feminist researchers claim that one cannot adequately understand human societies without paying attention to the universal role of *patriarchy,* which refers to the domination of social groups by men who have greater power and privilege than women and children. Some feminist researchers have argued that inequalities of the genders emerged because of males' greater physical strength. The control this enabled men to exercise resulted in women playing socially subservient roles and in stereotypes that portrayed women as inferior to men. Sexism is thus fostered and

maintained through the transmission of an ideology justifying male domination (Saunders, 1988, pp. 159–160).

Feminist perspectives stress the idea that inequalities suffered by women stem from an ingrained, systemic patriarchy in societies; this patriarchy pervades many institutions and practices, including, in particular, family socialization. Similar to researchers who subscribe to one or other of the critical perspectives, feminists see science as a tool that has largely been in the hands of male oppressors. Feminists take a strong advocacy position in an effort to eliminate sexism from society.

Feminists display a tendency toward synthesizing various critical concepts, symbolic interactionist ideas, and qualitative research styles. Similar to critical theorists, feminists reject the relativistic stances of positivism and the interpretive approaches. This stance can be explained by their interest in achieving gender equality. Instead, they argue that science should be used to improve the conditions of the oppressed. Feminists wish to help eliminate sexism by understanding and documenting its sources. An emphasis on achieving gender equality is central. Box 8.5 summarizes some of the major propositions of feminist perspectives.

Feminist philosophers believe all women are legitimate knowers and that those experiencing particular complexities are the most knowledgeable about that experience. The world of women deals with the particular, with the concrete experiences of child rearing, mothering, parenting, neighborhood interactions, and so on. Knowledge of that world should start from the experience of women. Similar to phenomenological assumptions, feminist philosophers believe that self-reflection, self-awareness, and purity of language constitutes human nature. If this is true, men experience the world differently in the everyday experience of friendship, love, sexuality, moral-

BOX 8.5 _Key Feminist Ideas_

In major cultural institutions (e.g., universities, media, advertising, the writing of history), men's standpoints are represented as universal (Smith, 1987:19).

As one moves from elementary through to university educational institutions, the proportion of women on the staff declines; the proportion of women in administrative positions declines even more as one moves through the hierarchy of educational institutions.

Women have been systematically excluded from the making of cultural ideology. An adequate social science must be grounded in the everyday experiences of both men and women.

An adequate social science must recognize the universal role of patriarchy—the domination of society by males who have greater power and privilege than women and children.

SOURCE: Dorothy E. Smith, _The Everyday World as Problematic: A Feminist Sociology._ Toronto: University of Toronto Press, 1987.

important distinction between _method_ (a technique for collecting evidence) and _methodology_ (how the methods should be used) in feminist research. She writes that what is important in feminist research is a methodology that is consistent with feminist epistemology (theory of knowledge). This includes a methodology that:

1. Places value on women's subjective experiences. Feminist methodology values women as knowers and seeks to reflect with precision women's experiences as they view them.
2. Values the importance of context in women's lives. Women's experiences are embedded in the context of their everyday lives. It is important that the method chosen provides a rich description of context. This should include a description of the social and political factors as well as other variables that may influence the phenomenon.
3. Values the relationship of the researcher and the participants. This relationship is characterized by respect for the participants. They are viewed as equal partners in the research process, but there is considerable debate as to whether equal power can ever be achieved in the research relationship.
4. Values the inclusion of women from diverse social and ethnic backgrounds in their samples so that perspectives of all women can be exposed and understood.

ity, intellect, conflict, and challenge than do females. Consistent with this point of view, feminist researchers call for research methods that reflect their epistemological beliefs, emphasize concrete experiences, and stress the particular that comprises the world of women (Rothe, 1994).

2. Application of Method and Methodology

Feminist research is not a method but rather a multiplicity of methods. Feminist researchers select a method that is appropriate to answer the research question. Over time, feminist researchers have come to a reasoned examination of how all methods can be used to answer feminist questions. Harding (1991) makes an

a. Developing the Research Question

Research questions appropriate for a feminist inquiry are those that are of interest and concern to women. The purpose of feminist research is to create social change that will enhance the lives of women. The questions will vary in focus and form but they will be distinctive in that (1) the issues are of primary concern to women, (2) the question requires women to report their experiences using their own voices, and (3) the question allows for a structural analysis of the conditions of women's lives and should lead to an improvement of it. Experiences such as accessing the health-care system, women's health, constructing relationships, giving birth, mothering, rape, incest, infertility, poverty, and family violence are topics from which questions, appropriate to feminist methods of inquiry, could be developed. Hartrick (1997), a feminist researcher, used elements of phenomenological research and feminist inquiry to examine the experience of self-definition for women who are mothers. Specifically, the research question she asked was, "What is the experience of defining self for women who are mothers?"

b. Role of the Researcher

One of the defining characteristics of feminist research is the nonhierarchical relationships between the researcher and the participants. Feminist researchers strive for horizontal relationships among members on the research team and participants. The researcher views herself as a partner with the participants and involves them in the generation of the research question, the conduct of the research, and the dissemination of results. Although there is considerable debate as to whether the researcher and the participant ever experience an equal power relationship in the inquiry process (Webb, 1993; Ford-Gilboe and Campbell, 1996), there is agreement that the role of the researcher in feminist inquiry is a vulnerable one because the investigator shares her experiences and emotions with the participant.

Feminist researchers promote intersubjectivity and interaction in their research rather than the one-way communication of traditional methods. To do this, the researcher constantly compares her work with her experience as a woman and a scientist. The researcher then shares this

with those researched, who then add their opinions to the research (Klein, 1983). Oakley (1981) produced a landmark piece of feminist writing that showed the reciprocity that exists between a feminist researcher and her participants. In her study, Oakley asked questions of the participants, and they, in turn, asked questions of her. She found it impossible not to give her own views, answer participants' questions, and give advice based on her own experience as a woman. Oakley's behavior reflects the role of the researcher in feminist inquiry.

As with other qualitative approaches, reflexivity is expected of the researcher. **Reflexivity** is defined as the critical thinking required to examine the interaction between the researcher and the data occurring during analyses. The researcher explores personal feelings that may influence the study and integrates this understanding into the study. The researcher needs to be reflexive about her views so that she can uncover deep-seated views on issues related to the research and provide a full account of her views, thinking, and conduct. This is necessary so that readers of the research report are aware of how the researcher's values, assumptions, and motivations may have influenced the framework, literature review, design, sampling, data collection, and interpretation of findings. Making explicit the participation of the researcher in the generation of knowledge adds to the relevance and accuracy of the results (Webb, 1993).

c. Sample

Sample selection involves choosing women who have experienced the phenomenon of interest and are able and willing to share their perspectives. Feminist researchers embrace the diversity of women's lives and experiences and therefore attempt to include women of diverse social class, race, ethnic groups, cultures, and so on in their sample selection. Feminist scholars are critical of the ethnocentric bias in the sampling procedures of many nursing investigations that fail to report race or ethnicity and make the assumption that a white, Anglo-Saxon perspective of the world is appropriate and universally experienced (Ford-Gilboe and Campbell, 1996).

d. Data Collection

Feminist researchers use a variety of methods to collect data. **Oral history interviewing** is a preferred form of data collection. It is a participant-guided investigation of a lived experience in which few prepared questions are asked (Sandelowski and Pollack, 1986). This method is based on the assumption that meaning comes from life stories expressed by women in their own way, without the use of structured questions.

Multiple in-depth interviews are often used to collect rich narrative stories. Because of the close relationship that develops between the researcher and participants, feminist researchers believe that multiple interviews develop trust among the partners. The researcher shares the transcripts with the participants and invites them to contribute to the analysis and interpretation process. This process is believed to contribute to more accurate and sensitive descriptions of feelings, emotions, thoughts, and processes as they unfold (Rothe, 1994).

Feminists who focus on gender issues in female homogenous and heterogeneous settings conduct participant observation within feminist inquiry. It includes the study of women's private domains, workplaces, and organizations. According to Reinharz (1992), it is conducted to achieve the following goals:

1. View women's behavior as an expression of social contexts that shows their behaviors as being shaped by social context rather than context free.

2. Understand the experience of women from their point of view and correct a bias of traditional participant observation that trivializes female activities and thoughts or interprets them from the male researchers' perspective.
3. Document the lives of women to enable the participant observer to see women as full members of their social, economic, and political worlds.

Feminist participant observation generally values intimacy and empathy. The relationship that emerges between the researcher and those observed is often a nurturing one. Unlike male observers who maintain a "respectful" distance between the researcher and subject, women interact differently in the field. They often act on a "nurturing" impulse, which is reciprocated (Hochschild, 1983). The implication of this point of view is that with topics unique to women, only other women can understand their meaning (Rothe, 1994).

Feminist researchers use techniques such as focus group interviews; structured and semistructured interview guides; and documents such as diaries, letters, journals, photographs, and historical and medical records, to name a few. They also use quantitative instruments such as questionnaires and indexes. Hartrick (1997) used a variety of data collection methods in her feminist investigation of the experience of self-definition of self as mother. The primary means was multiple interviews with participants that were audiotaped and lasted from 1 to 2.5 hours in length; in addition, focus group interviews were used to compare and contrast the experiences of women, and letters and writings by one of the participants that expressed her experiences were collected.

e. Data Analysis

The process of analysis is similar to the quantitative and qualitative procedures in general. Therefore, if a feminist researcher is using phenomenology to explore women's lived experiences or grounded theory to develop a theory of empowerment for women, the methods of analysis previously discussed for these perspectives would be followed. The main *distinction* is that the content is likely to be analyzed in terms of artifacts produced by women (or men), about women, for women. The production and perpetuation of patriarchy and ethnocentric bias are major research themes examined in the analyses. Feminists have been vigilant in analyzing texts for the presence of gender stereotyping that limits the opportunities of women, restricts their autonomy, and inhibits female development (Im, 2000; Rothe, 1994).

Many feminist researchers invite participants to be active partners in the data analysis process. Others have participants "recycle" the analyses and then refine them according to the reactions of participants (Webb, 1993). Not all feminist researchers agree with this latter point. Some believe the researcher has access to additional perspectives beyond the immediate research, and in order to carry out a structural analysis of the research, as opposed to only reporting women's experiences using their words, the researcher is required to go beyond the immediate data (Ribbens, 1989). Ribbens believes the feminist researcher may interpret data differently than participants, particularly if the participants do not see themselves as feminists. When this occurs, researchers must take responsibility for the decisions they make and acknowledge this type of power as a paradox in feminist research.

f. Reporting on the Findings

Reports of feminist inquiry use descriptive, nonsexist language to portray the everyday lives of women. They are user-friendly reports that make them accessible to all, not just intellectuals. The reports are distinctive in that they portray women's voices, provide a structural analysis of the conditions of their lives, and include in the analysis the role and influence of the researchers themselves.

It is as important to feminists to have their findings published in popular women's magazines as in the most prestigious academic journals. Many feminist projects are published in book form as popular literature. This presents a bit of a dilemma for nurse researchers who align themselves with this tradition. Political and prestige issues related to research in academic settings require nurse researchers to modify their writing so that they are acceptable to the academic community that judges the value of knowledge produced through research. Some feminist researchers deal with this dilemma by publishing two different versions of their report; versions reflecting the voices of participants are made available to participants, but more traditional forms of academic writing may be used for submissions to peer-reviewed journals. Such modifications in style increase the likelihood that results will be published in a wide variety of forums.

3. Example of Feminist Research

An account of a feminist inquiry is provided in Box 8.6. The following comments are offered about the study in Box 8.6:

This project drew on elements of interpretive phenomenology and feminist inquiry in developing a methodology to explore the experience of self-definition for women who are mothers. Principles of feminist inquiry promoted sensitivity to the cultural aspects influencing women's development and provided guidance about essential aspects in research with women. Interpretive phenomenology facilitated illumination of the lived experience of mothers with consideration of the complexity of that experience.

BOX 8.6 *Nurse Researchers at Work*

WOMEN WHO ARE MOTHERS: THE EXPERIENCE OF DEFINING SELF

Combining elements of feminist inquiry and phenomenology, this study examined the experience of self-definition for women who are mothers. Feminist poststructuralists maintain that the self develops through the process of social interaction and is created and reconstituted through various discursive practices in which people participate. For mothers, Western culture provides conflicting discourses. Discourses around healthy self-definition stress autonomy, differentiation, and separation of the individual from others throughout the life cycle. Discourses around mothering emphasize women's abnegation of self, selflessness, and self-sacrifice. Hence, women are exposed to conflicting and confusing messages.

The purpose of this study was to explore and describe the experience of self-definition for women who are mothers. Specifically, it explored the question: What is the experience of defining self for women who are mothers? Subquestions the study examined included: How do women who are mothers define and express self when they are influenced by and participate in conflicting discourses? Does the edict for self-sacrifice and abnegation of self hinder a woman's process of defining and expressing self? If the process of self-definition is hindered through the conflicting discourses, what influence does this have on mothers' overall health experience?

Seven participants were recruited using purposive sampling. A flyer was used to advertise the study to women who frequented various agencies and centers. A contact person was identified in each agency to discuss the research project with women and increase awareness. Selection criteria included: (1) participants were mothers who had children between the ages of 3 and 16 years, (2) participants had ex-periential knowledge of self-definition, (3) participants had the ability to be introspective about themselves within the context of their social roles and relationships.

Data collection included in-depth multiple interviews, focus group interviews, and letters and writings of one participant. The interview process included three phases: establishing rapport, engaging in open-ended dialogue for the purpose of gathering data, and successive data gathering in the second set of interviews to enable a more complete illumination of the participants' experiences.

Thematic analysis was used to analyze data from the first and second round of interviews. Focus group data was used to compare and contrast themes and experiences of women. The results revealed three elements within the mothers' process of defining self, including reflective doing, living in the shadows, and reclaiming and discovering self. Within each of these elements, a number of other themes were described. Women described an integral relationship between the process of defining self and their experience of health.

In describing their process of authoring and defining self, the women in this study, in essence, also described their experience of health promotion and empowerment. As the women moved through the process of self-definition, they described becoming more aware of the detrimental effect living out roles was having on their health and well-being. Through the process of self-definition, they became active participants, experiencing a sense of empowerment in their life situations and experiences. Health professionals may want to contemplate how they could support this health promoting, reauthoring process.

SOURCE: Summarized from Hartrick, G.A. (1997). Women who are mothers: The experience of defining self. *Health Care For Women International, 18,* 263–277.

The sample included women from a range of social classes, including the "working poor" to the "upper crust" of society. The contexts of the participants' lives were described in detail. The study focused on the experiences of women in their everyday lives as they sought to define their sense of self.

The data collection reflected the researcher–participant partnership model of feminist research. The interviews were open ended and conversational in nature with the researcher following the participants' lead. The researcher simultaneously listened for and explored central themes and meaningful structures within the women's experiences. The women shared in the identification of themes and in the validation of data analysis.

Feminist inquiry has empowering potential for women. Through this investigation, the women continually alluded to the complementary relationship between their experience of self-definition and their overall experience of health. As the women moved toward discovery, they described feeling more in control of their well being and were beginning to make conscious choices to nurture and care for themselves. It appears that the process of self-definition was a health promoting process whereby women became the authors of their own life experiences. For women in this study, the promotion of self-definition and self-expression simultaneously promoted health. This feminist inquiry revealed how through the process of self-definition, they became active participants, experiencing a sense of empowerment in their lives.

E. ADVANTAGES AND LIMITATIONS OF CONTEMPORARY APPLIED APPROACHES

Table 8.1 summarizes the advantages and limitations of the various research designs we have presented throughout Part 2 of this book. Although it is not possible to generalize about all the studies contained within any one type of design, we can conclude that experimental studies have an advantage over other research designs when we need to make clear causal inferences. Surveys are particularly adept at representing populations with samples, and such studies have become associated with complex multivariate analyses. Field studies' strengths are in the area of validity, cost (in some cases), and in probing for depth. Applied research is important as a means of bringing about change and improvements in practice and empowering subjects through participation. The practical problem-solving nature of action research makes it particularly appealing to a nurse who has identified a problem in practice and sees the merit of investigating it and improving practice. Evaluation research leads to decisions about the effectiveness of current practice. This type of research is important because of the utilitarian nature of its results and the significant role it plays as the cornerstone of policy research at the local and national level. Health promotion studies provide an opportunity for the field of nursing to "soar like an eagle" in redesigning health care and creating new models and systems for promoting the health of individuals, families, and communities.

F. POSTSCRIPT TO PART 2

Although the most common designs used in nursing and health-care research have been reviewed in Chapters 4 through 8, others have been omitted. A discussion of methodological research (e.g., controlled investigations of obtaining, organizing, and analyzing data) is not presented in this book. Case studies are discussed in terms of evaluation research. Various kinds of intervention, polls, and special interest approaches to research have also not been included.

As you get ready to design a study, keep in mind that you should choose a design that is appropriate to the research question you are posing. On occasion, more than one type of design can be used to answer a research question. The question is the key concern. Try to decide precisely what it is you want to accomplish

Table 8.1   Advantages and Limitations of Alternate Designs

Research Design Category	General	Validity	Causal Inference	Multivariate	Probing
Experimental Designs					
Pre-experimental	−	−	−	−	−
Experimental	−	−	+	−	−
Quasi-experimental	±	−	+	−	−
Survey Designs					
Individual questionnaire	+	−	−	+	−
Group administered	−	−	−	+	−
Phone survey	+	−	−	+	−
Interview	+	−	−	+	+
Comparative analysis	+	−	−	+	−
Secondary data	+	−	−	+	−
Meta-analysis	+	−	−	−	−
Qualitative Designs					
Phenomenology	−	+	−	−	+
Grounded theory	−	+	−	−	+
Ethnographic	−	+	−	−	+
Feminist	−	+	−	−	+
Field Designs					
Participant observation	−	+	−	−	+
In-depth interviews	−	+	−	+	+
Field experiments	−	+	+	−	−
Naturalistic observational	−	+	−	−	−
Goal-Directed Designs					
Action research	−	−	−	+	+
Evaluation research	+	±	±	+	±
Health promotion research	+	−	±	+	±
Feminist research	±	±	−	±	±

In each category, a + means that this is an advantage of the technique; − means this is a possible limitation; ± means that in some conditions it is a limitation, but in others it is an advantage.

- *General* refers to the extent to which extrapolations to larger populations may be made using each of the design or data collection procedures.
- *Validity* is the extent to which indicators clearly measure what they are intended to measure.
- *Causal inference* refers to the ease with which inferences about causal relations among variables may be made.
- *Multivariate* refers to the ease with which information on many variables is collected, leading to the possibility of multivariate analysis.
- *Probing* refers to the extent to which responses may be probed in depth.

BOX 8.7 *Nurse Researchers at Work*

IF YOU CALL ME NAMES, I'LL CALL YOU NUMBERS.

"Some of my best friends are qualitative researchers, but. . . . As that classic bigot's phrase came out of my mouth, I realized that my opinion of qualitative research had taken an unmistakable nosedive. I was writing the final report for a project that included both qualitative and quantitative methodologies. The project concerned coping strategies used during smoking cessation. Reviewing the earlier phases of the project reminded me of my misconceptions and frustrations with our attempts to integrate the two methods . . .

It is important to realize that there's the Quantitative Church and the Qualitative Church. Quantitative and qualitative approaches are not merely research methods. They are liturgies, outward and highly revered forms that represent entire value systems. Although the methods appear to have similar goals, that is, the explication of new knowledge, they often disagree on everything else, even the definition of knowledge . . .

The first sign of problems emerged when we were gearing up to begin data collection. The qualitative team believed that it would be better to let the participants freely talk into the tape recorder about their experiences, that they should not be given specific directives about what to say, and that follow-up interviews carried out after each day of data collection should be similarly free-flowing. Although I was cognizant that I should be careful about upsetting our collaboration, I had been funded to study coping strategies, and that's what I wanted to study.

While the qualitative team developed a new taxonomy, the quantitative team used a previously developed categorization scheme to classify each strategy. I had hopes of comparing the two systems to determine which was more effective in terms of completeness of coverage and predicting outcome variables, such as whether the participant smoked during the coping episode. Such a comparison would not be possible. Qualitative researchers, it seems, are loathe to predict anything. In addition, the qualitative method was dynamic. The system that was applied to episodes coded early in the process was different and less elaborate than the one used for episodes coded later. Going back and classifying all episodes using the whole system was also out of the question because that's not the way qualitative researchers do it. You cannot, my qualitative research colleague told me, apply a taxonomy on the data set from which it was generated. Well, you can at my church!

The qualitative researcher you collaborate with may have different opinions than the one I collaborated with. It is nevertheless important to realize that such collaborations involve the intersection of two cultures. A final example was the qualitative team's tendency to call the study participants by their first names, a practice that made me surprisingly uncomfortable. The quantitative team referred to the participants by their assigned numbers, a practice that seemed foreign to the qualitative team. I argued that the practice was necessary to protect confidentiality. But in reality, I must admit that it also made our work seem . . . well, more quantitative. In the end they called them names, we called them numbers, and neither knew what the other was talking about."

SOURCE: O'Connell K. (2000). If you call me names, I'll call you numbers. *Journal of Professional Nursing, 16*(2), 74. Cited with permission.

---

and then figure out the design that is best suited to your needs.

As a postscript to Part 2, Box 8.7 presents Kathleen O'Connell's wry commentary on the dynamic tension between qualitative and quantitative practition-ers. We would do well to recognize the gulf between these traditions and try to build bridges between them. Both have enormous contributions to make to the development of nursing knowledge in the 21st century.

E X E R C I S E S

1. Choose one of the following studies and identify the data sources that you would use. Write a proposal for how you will proceed with the analysis. How might:
   - A nurse scientist study the relationship between the percentage of people with skin cancers and the percentage of immigrants in a regional health district?

   - A health economist compare trends in American and Canadian purchase of health insurance?

   - A nursing student analyze the sexual stereotyping of nurses found in popular literature sources?

   - A health promotion nurse explore how local television news structures the public and policy debate on youth violence?

   - A feminist researcher determine whether American magazines reflect standards of attractiveness for women similar to those found in comparable magazines in Canada, Britain, and France. How could the researcher determine that the identified relationship is always the same?

   - A nursing researcher determine if there is a relationship between physician status and the speed with which patients are admitted to hospital. Would it be possible to conduct such a study using secondary data analysis techniques?

2. Rates of school dropout, motor vehicle accidents, homelessness, marriage breakdown, depression, self-esteem, abortion, or adolescent pregnancy. Using one of these concepts, identify problems that may occur in attempting to compare their values in the United States with those in Canada. Can you recommend ways of minimizing the problems of using them in **comparative studies?**

3. You are a school health nurse interested in evaluating the effectiveness of a violence prevention curriculum among children in elementary school. How would you proceed to conduct an evaluation study if you were doing a summative evaluation? In what way would the process be different if formative evaluation was required?

4. Outline the steps that you would follow as a nurse researcher to help a community identify and address their health priorities, help citizens develop a plan of action, and evaluate both the process and impact of any interven-

tions. Of the research designs discussed in this chapter, which one is best suited to this assignment? Justify your response.

5. What unit of analysis might be appropriate for studying intergenerational transmission of family health beliefs and practices?

RECOMMENDED READINGS

Hart, E., and Bond, M. (1998). *Action Research for Health and Social Care.* Philadelphia: Open University Press. A succinct yet comprehensive handbook on action research for professionals and researchers who are interested in using research to improve practice.

Hilton, A., Thompson, R., and Moore-Dempsey, L. (2000). Evaluation of the AIDS prevention street nurse program: One step at a time. *Canadian Journal of Nursing Research, 32*(1), 17–38. A good example of an evaluation research program conducted to show the impacts and outcome changes as a result of an intervention program.

Im, E. (2000). A feminist critique of research on women's work and health. *Health Care for Women International, 21,* 105–119. This paper is a feminist critique of traditional research into women's work and health. It identifies implications for future research on women's work and health.

Kaviani, N., and Stillwell, Y. (2000). An evaluative study of clinical preceptorship. *Nurse Education Today, 20,* 218–226. This paper uses methods commonly found in evaluation research.

Klostermann, B., Perry, C. and Britto, M. (2000). Quality improvement in a school health program. *Evaluation and the Health Professions, 23*(1), 91–106. This paper reports an outcome and process evaluation of a school health program.

Morris, J., Penrod, J., and Hupcey, J. (2000). Qualitative outcome analysis: Evaluating nursing interventions for complex clinical phenomena. *Journal of Nursing Scholarship, 32*(2), 125–130. This paper presents a particular method for evaluating nursing interventions derived from a qualitative research project.

Pederson, A., O'Neill, M., and Rootman, I. (1994). *Health Promotion in Canada: Provincial, National and International Perspectives.* Philadelphia: W.B. Saunders Canada. This text provides a historical and sociological examination of health promotion in Canada.

Pender, N. (1996). *Health Promotion in Nursing Practice* (3rd ed). Stamford, CT: Appleton and Lange. A valuable resource in health promotion practice and research. Provides an in-depth discussion of the nurse's role in promoting healthy lifestyle and preventing illness.

Part 3

EXPLORING BIAS AND ETHICAL ISSUES IN RESEARCH

P art 3 discusses issues that need to be thought about carefully as you commence a research project: these issues have to do with the problem of bias (Chapter 9) and with ethical questions (Chapter 10). Bias considers how the researcher's experiences, values, and worldview influences the research process. By fully understanding bias, its various sources and its impact on research, one becomes free to challenge research knowledge constructively. Ethics, the moral component of knowledge that helps guide research decisions, is explored in relation to planning, implementing, and reporting research findings.

Chapter 9

Understanding Bias

CHAPTER OUTLINE

KEY TERMS

Androcentricity

Bias

Data massaging

Demand characteristic

Expectancy

Experimenter effect

Familism

Gender insensitivity

Halo effect

Normative bias

Overgeneralization

Overspecificity

Random error

Research bias

Researcher affect

Sexism

Systematic error

Chapter 2 argued that humans like to generalize: we are always trying to come up with rules to understand our behavior. For example, we might hear someone say, "She is weepy these days because she is pregnant. It's the hormones." Or we might read that "unemployment leads to depression" or that "all adolescents engage in risk-taking behaviors." These generalizations set up expectations in us about the clients we serve. If these generalizations are to be relied on in nursing practice, they need to be based on unbiased evidence—that is, evidence uninfluenced by what the researcher would like to find. But the tendency to bias conclusions in the direction of expectations or preferences is a danger in all research. This chapter explores the nature of bias and illustrates that, at all stages of the research process, the danger of bias needs to be recognized. The chapter concludes with some rules for detecting and minimizing bias.

Although bias is omnipresent, we must not allow it to intimidate us as researchers. The need is to be on the alert for it and to minimize it where possible. As Somers Roche has noted, bias, similar to "*anxiety is a thin stream of fear trickling through the mind. If encouraged it cuts a channel into which all other thoughts are drained.*" We need to be careful not to let concerns over bias drain our creative energies and prevent us from posing imaginative questions in conducting our research. This chapter is intended to sensitize you to the many sources of bias inherent in the research designs you have examined in the previous chapters. This chapter provides practical advice on controlling bias as you begin designing your research project.

A. THE NATURE OF BIAS

A **bias** may be thought of as a preference—or predisposition—to favor a particular conclusion. In everyday life, we have our likes and dislikes. Often interpretations of our experiences serve to confirm for us what we already knew or thought. In short, bias helps to organize our interpretation of events and make sense of a complex world (Jackson, 1999). So, when staff nurses on a pediatric unit fail to submit the self-scheduling work plan for the next month to the unit manager, she interprets this as a sign that the staff is under a lot of pressure. In addition, she concludes that recent staff cutbacks have made it difficult for her staff to complete the scheduling on time. In contrast, the vice president of nursing sees this failure to submit the work schedule on time as just another indication that self-scheduling will not work and staff nurses are unable to mutually plan work schedules. The point is that we often find corroborative evidence for our predispositions. Whereas the staff nurses and unit manager find a justification for the nurses' behavior, the vice president of nursing finds yet another reason why self-scheduling should be eliminated. Sometimes it takes quite powerful contrary evidence to change our minds, and when we must change our minds, we do so unwillingly, with much moaning and groaning.

Research bias may be defined as the systematic distortion of research conclusions. Typically these distortions are inadvertent, but they can also be intentional. There is no doubt that they occur in all disciplines in which a set of personal preferences prevents an impartial judgment; nursing is no exception. Bias can influence most phases of a project, from problem selection, to the identification of variables, to developing measurements, to collecting and analyzing data, to interpreting the results of the research. When the chance of bias in a research investigation is not addressed, the reliability of the findings needs to be considered highly suspect.

I. Bias in Quantitative and Qualitative Research

To suggest that there is bias, or distortion, implies that there is an unknown truth waiting to be described accurately by the researcher. Bias represents the gap between the *unknown true value* and the *estimated value* of a particular phenomenon. This is implicit in quantitative designs in which the approach suggests that the researcher "knows" and simply wants to confirm his or her knowledge. For example, structured questionnaires offer the respondent a range of replies, made up by the researcher, from which the respondent must select a response. These responses often reflect the previous knowledge, values, and personal preferences of the researcher (Parahoo, 1997).

Bias can also be a significant problem in qualitative research unless researchers recognize and incorporate it into the structure of the study rather than trying to eliminate it as in quantitative methods (Brockopp and Hastings-Tolsma, 1995). The whole point of qualitative research is to look at phenomena from the perspective of the participant, yet this process is influenced by the researcher's perspective. To minimize bias, it is important to clearly record the researcher's perspective. To do this, the researcher establishes an *audit trail.* This is a clear statement of decisions made with documented rationales so that others reading the audit can follow the decision-making process of the researcher.

An assumption of qualitative research is that researchers are an integral part of the research design and of the experience of the participant's world. This is sometimes referred to as "going native." Accepting this assumption allows the researcher to build in checks such as an audit trail to allow the discovery of knowledge that is not distorted by the researcher's biases. Examples of safeguards that responsible qualitative researchers use to reduce un-necessary bias include selecting participants that are unfamiliar to them; clearly *bracketing* their own biases, personal beliefs, and opinions about the phenomenon under study (see Chapter 6); and selecting a topic that is not too close to the researchers on a personal level.

Qualitative studies are also unfairly criticized for having an *elite bias.* This occurs because most qualitative designs rely on purposive sampling techniques or volunteers who have had experience with the research phenomenon under investigation. Often the volunteers tend to be the most articulate and highest status members of a group. Such an elite bias can be prevented by ensuring that the information you use is representative of the *experiences* rather than *participants* per se that are important in qualitative studies (Norwood, 2000).

2. Triple Biases: Nursing, Science, and Culture

Nurse researchers face at least three key sources of bias: the biases inherent within the domain of nursing, the biases of science itself, and the biases acquired as a member of one's society. Although nursing research systematically challenges our predispositions, we as researchers also take our predispositions with us to our research projects. Furthermore, as nurses, we tend to incorporate certain research findings into our predispositions, making them even more difficult to change. Secondly, nursing is partly a science, and science has a system of values and preferences all its own (see Chapter 1). And finally, as a member of a cultural group, nurse researchers have certain predispositions. In a sense, then, nurse researchers have a triple load of biasing predispositions: one acquired as a member of the nursing profession, one acquired as a participant in an academic discipline with a traditional and rigorous method, and one acquired as a member of society. All sources of bias need to be recognized as potential blinders to a clear understanding of human behavior, unfettered by expectations or preferences.

3. Sexism: A Prevalent Form of Bias

A problem that has plagued nursing, health, and social science research is that of *sexism*. At all stages of research, but especially at the design stage, care must be taken to avoid **sexism** (discrimination on the basis of gender). For example, randomized clinical trials (RCTs) have been criticized by feminist groups as extremely limited in their ability to produce data that can contribute to an understanding of human behavior and experience. Some believe that women, in particular, have been victims of this approach, used by physicians, who are mainly men and tend to see the world from a male perspective, and who study women as objects, ignoring their needs and experiences (Parahoo, 1997). Oakley (1989) points out that "the frequency with which doctors impose on patients experiments of an uncontrolled nature has been one of the strongest objections to professionalized medicine made by the women's health movement over the last twenty years in Europe and North America."

Similarly, it is misleading to suggest that feminist perspectives in research are not without bias. For one thing, there is no "single unitary feminist perspective" that can be applied in a research situation. For example, African-American women, women of color, women of minorities, and women with disabilities have been subsumed and made invisible in writings of women in general. White, middle-class feminists in researching women's perspectives, as opposed to men's, also have been biased in their reporting of women's experiences, failing

to note differences between women in terms of factors such as health status, ethnic origin, and social class (Hart and Bond, 1998).

Eichler's *Nonsexist Research Methods* (1988) identifies several types of sexism in research. The major types the author identifies include androcentricity, overgeneralization, and gender insensitivity.

a. Androcentricity

If a researcher presents the world from a male perspective as if this perspective were universal, that person is guilty of **androcentricity.** Historically, much of the health research conducted in North America seems to have such a bias. Women and ethnic groups have been largely ignored in health intervention studies that have focused on white middle-class male samples conducted in academic centers. In 1990, the Office of Research on Women's Health was established at the National Institutes of Health (NIH) to address historical inequities in research design and allocation of federal resources. In 1994, the NIH mandated that women and members of diverse ethnic groups be included in all NIH-funded projects unless an obvious justification for exclusion was present. However, androcentricity continues to be a problem in much of the health research endeavors funded by other sources.

An androcentric view of the world is congruent with the Western biomedical ethos that is based on individualism, materialism, and competitiveness. This approach is in contrast to the views of women, ethnic groups, and the poor, who usually focus on family concerns rather than themselves. These groups do not often risk putting themselves first before their families to obtain costly treatments or time-consuming research appointments. Thus, they exclude themselves from involvement in clinical trials and procedures that focus on themselves at the expense of their families. An example of androcentric research is the exclusion of women, African-Americans, and Latinos from AIDS studies. AIDS data show that these groups lag behind white males in studies of protease inhibitor therapy, clinical trials, medical services, and preventive programs (CDCP, 1999; Flaskerud and Nyamathi, 2000).

b. Overgeneralization

If a researcher claims to study all people but, in fact, samples only men or only women, we have an example of an **overgeneralization.** Eichler uses the example of a sample of women to study parenting; the author points out that when one uses the term "parents" to refer to mothers, one is guilty of overgeneralization because one is ignoring fathers. A parallel problem is **overspecificity,** when single-gender terms are used to describe situations applicable to both genders (e.g., "the doctor . . . he"; "the nurse . . . she") (Eichler, 1988, p. 6).

c. Gender Insensitivity

To ignore gender as an important variable is to display **gender insensitivity.** Researchers should identify the gender composition of their samples and be sensitive to the different impacts social policies have on men and women (Eichler, 1988, pp. 6–7). For example, much of the bereavement research in nursing is biased in that it tends to overrepresent the views of one gender—females (Cook, 1997). An examination of samples used in bereavement research shows that the majority of participants are women. This means that much of our knowledge about the grief experience is based on the female experience. This had lead to women's grief experience being considered the norm and findings related to male grief being compared with this norm.

Familism is a special case of gender insensitivity and involves treating the family as the unit of analysis when, in fact, it is individuals within the family unit that engage in a particular activity or hold a certain attitude. Familism is also a problem when we assume that a particular phenomenon has an equal impact on all members of the family when, in fact, it may affect different family members in different ways.

The view of women in the development of psychology is an excellent illustration of sexism. Shields (1988) argues that much of 19th and early 20th century psychology was severely limited because it assumed female intellectual inferiority. Research was devoted not to questioning this assumption but rather to various attempts to understand this inferiority. Thus efforts were made to:

1. Identify those parts of the brain that were more poorly developed in women than in men
2. Understand how the greater variability in male skills leads to a higher proportion of male geniuses
3. Understand the role of the maternal instinct in maintaining women in passive, subservient roles

Shields concludes her article by noting:

Graves (1968, p. v) included among the functions of mythologizing that of the justification of existing social systems. This function was clearly operative throughout the evolutionist–functionalist treatment of the psychology of women: the "discovery" of sex differences in brain structure to correspond to "appropriate" sex differences in brain function; the biological justification (via the variability hypothesis) for the enforcement of women's subordinate social status; the Victorian weakness and gentility associated with maternity; and pervading each of these themes, the assumption of an innate emotional, sexless, unimaginative female character that played the perfect foil to the Darwin male. That science played handmaiden to social values cannot be denied. Whether a parallel situation exists in today's study of sex differences is open to question (Shields, 1988, p. 55).

B. HOW BIAS AFFECTS THE RESEARCH PROCESS

Nurse researchers are frequently confronted with "interesting" findings for which an explanation should be offered. Let us recall our example on lifestyle patterns and socioeconomic status (SES) from Chapter 2. In that project, high school students' SES and their lifestyle patterns were examined. Now suppose, during data analysis, that a robust relationship emerges indicating that the higher a student's SES, the greater the likelihood that the student will adopt a health promoting lifestyle. At this stage, the researcher may wonder what explains the pattern that has emerged. Possibilities such as the following might come to mind:

- Peers of students with high SESs have healthful lifestyles themselves and influence their friends in such a way that they adopt similar behaviors and attitudes toward health and health choices.
- The parents of students with high SESs place a high value on health and healthful lifestyles and expect their children to do the same.
- Students with high SESs know that they have the time and financial resources to engage in healthful patterns of lifestyle, such as joining a gym or fitness class, eating nutritiously, and so on, and therefore plan to do so.
- Students with high SESs have been exposed more frequently to role models that engage in health promoting lifestyles and are therefore more likely to model themselves after such individuals.

Unfortunately, the study may not have been designed to test, and possibly to rule out, competing explanations. Readers of the report may be convinced, inappropriately, that the researcher has provided evidence for the particular explanation offered: "After all, look at all the tables that are presented." Although a great deal of data documenting a variety of relationships may have been presented, the researcher may have provided little, if any, evidence for the explanation offered, no matter how reasonable it may seem or how many graphs and charts accompany it. We need to design studies that systematically test a variety of possible explanations for the relationship under examination.

Researcher affect is a term we have coined that refers to the danger of researchers' falling in love with a particular explanation for some relationship or a particular view of the world and inadvertently using procedures that lead to conclusions supporting the preferred explanation or worldview. All stages of the research process may be affected adversely by bias. In this section, we examine how bias can affect the initial selection of the problem to be researched, the sample design, data collection, data analysis, reporting of findings, funding decisions, and the use of research findings.

I. Selection of the Problem

The issue of bias in problem selection is that some phenomena are judged to be more important than others—some are considered worthy of exploration and others are not. Because of this, the choice of subject matter provides a clue as to the values held by the researcher. Within the nursing culture, researchers are more likely to study problems that have a consequence to client care. For example, a nurse researcher is more likely to study the variables that may reduce the incidence of decubitus ulcers in institutional-ized frail elderly patients than the inci-dence of family visitors to them. Whereas the former is viewed as a critical clinical question that may lead to improved client care, the latter is not. The researcher is likely to see the prevention of decubitus ulcers as an issue with significant poten-tial to improve quality of life for clients and increase professional practice knowl-edge and one over which nurses have con-trol in practice. It can be argued that iden-tifying the most effective variables in reducing decubitus ulcers can be done without bias. But there is probably no value-free, culture-independent way of choosing variables for a study. Bias re-sults in the selection of the variables con-ventionally considered important and the exclusion of those conventionally consid-ered unimportant.

2. Sample Selection

Whether one opts for a survey, panel study, field study, or experimental design, there are potential sources of bias in the sample selected for study. For example, by choosing to survey attitudes toward abortion in an urban community contain-ing a free-standing abortion clinic, a re-searcher will probably produce a study that shows fairly high levels of support for abortion on demand. To pursue the ex-ample further, a researcher might do a case study of the attitudes of clinic case workers in an inner city community on public policy issues. Once again, attitudes favoring abortion will probably emerge. Choosing both an inner-city community with a free-standing clinic and case work-ers increases the likelihood that the atti-tudes expressed will favor abortion more than would be the case in rural areas or with many other work groups. The expe-rienced researcher, knowing how differ-ent variables usually work out, could po-tentially select a sample that may bias results.

Selection bias is also problematic in studies in which individuals themselves self-select to participate in an investiga-tion. For example, a nurse researcher wishes to assess if a new weight loss pro-gram contributes to improved weight loss and maintenance. If the program is of-fered to all women who attend a health clinic, it is likely that the women who are more highly motivated to lose weight will participate in the program. The problem is the investigator cannot be sure if the new program increased the number of women who lost weight and maintained the weight loss or if only highly motivated women joined the program. One way to avoid this selection bias is to design the sampling plan so that random assignment of women to the new program and to the control group occurs (see Chapter 4).

3. Data Collection

Extensive literature in psychology deals with the influence the experimenter may have in the data collection phase of a study. In their classic studies, Rosenthal and Fode (1963) did a series of important **experimenter effect** studies in which stu-dent researchers were asked to collect data on the number of trials it took rats to learn a maze. The student researchers were informed that a new breed of labo-ratory rat was being developed and that it had been bred for intelligence; the obser-vations were to see if, in fact, there was any difference between the specially bred "smart" rats and ordinary laboratory rats. And so the students set to work, running the two types of rats through the maze.

It turned out that, indeed, the "smart" rats took fewer trials to learn the maze than the "ordinary" ones. Apparently the breeding program was working. There was just one problem: Rosenthal did not have any smart rats. The rats were simply as-signed randomly to the "smart" and the "ordinary" categories. It was the students who were the "real" subjects of this study.

Somehow their expectations about the outcome of the trials had an impact on the results of the study. If the experimenter expects a rat to learn fast, somehow the data will come out that way. Thus, Rosenthal and Fode's findings indicate that there is a tendency to produce findings that are consistent with the experimenter's expectations. The explanation of the so-called experimenter effect has been more difficult to identify.

Did the students "fudge" the data to please the professor? Did they perceive "errors" differently for the two groups, perhaps being less likely to note an error made by the "smart" rats? Did they handle the rats differently? The generally accepted view is that experimenter effect occurs because of both the influence of behavior by expectations and slight, but systematic recording errors by the observer. But no matter what the explanation, Rosenthal's research is of critical importance to the experimentalist as well as to all nursing researchers.

a. Expectancy

A German mathematics teacher had a horse with unusual talents (Jackson, 1999). The amazing horse, known as Clever Hans, could solve simple mathematical problems by stamping his foot to indicate his answer. At first, skeptics thought that Clever Hans' trainer was signaling to the horse, thus accounting for the horse's unusual ability. However, it turned out that even when the trainer was removed from the room, the horse could still do the trick for other people posing the same questions.

The horse was, indeed, very smart. It turned out that Clever Hans' mathematical skills declined dramatically when the audience did not know the answer or when he was blindfolded. Apparently he was watching the audience. If the answer was three, the audience would gaze intently at the hoof of the horse clumping out the answer; after three stomps, members of the audience would raise their heads slightly, focusing their gaze on the horse's head. The horse simply watched the audience—they cued him when to stop. He was a pretty smart horse who was not very good at mathematics but was a good observer of body language.

How is Clever Hans relevant to the nurse scientist? Or, for that matter, what can we learn from Robert Rosenthal's experiments? Suppose you are conducting an interview, and suppose you have just asked a respondent how often she engages in regular physical exercise. The respondent replies: "I don't engage in physical exercise on a regular basis, I am just too busy to do so." You say, raising your eyebrows slightly, "Oh, so you don't exercise?" In all likelihood, your respondent now feels slightly uncomfortable—your eyebrow movement and your comment have communicated a message. After this, future questions about exercise issues may well encourage the respondent to express more interest in exercise and physical activity than she actually has. It is as if the interviewer is demanding a pro-exercise response. Respondents are often interested in figuring out what the survey is "really" all about. They will, therefore, be looking for cues and may be influenced by them. If a horse like Clever Hans can note a slight raising of heads in the audience, it is probable that most human subjects will be sensitive to a raised eyebrow, a change in voice tone, or a shift in the body position of the interviewer. This sensitivity of research subjects to the researcher's expectations of them is called **expectancy.**

Although it is appropriate for research assistants and study participants to be made aware of the general purpose of the study, given the problem of *expectancy,* the nurse researcher should avoid specifying the precise hypotheses of the study either to the participants or the research assistants. Instead, research assistants should be given an honest explanation but one that does not include the precise outcome expected from the treatment. In some cases in which an ethics review board has approved a project involving limited disclosure of information, it may be required that study participants receive a debriefing upon completion of the study (see Chapter 10). It may also be feasible to use a single-, double- or triple-blind experimental design (as discussed in Chapter 4), provided the study does not infringe upon participants' rights. To review, a *single-blind* design is one in which either the participants or the researchers are unaware of the assignment to groups. A *double-blind* trial is one in which both the participants and the researchers are unaware of assignment to groups. A *triple-blind* design is one in which persons other than the researchers evaluate the response without knowing the group assignments of the participants (Parahoo, 1997).

Sometimes it is difficult, however, to withhold information about expected study outcomes from one's research assistants. As a principal investigator, you want to make them feel that they are a part of the study and, therefore, feel that they should know what the study is "really" about. However, if you tell the research assistants what the hypotheses are, they may inadvertently bias results either toward the hypothesis (if they are friendly) or away from it (if they are hostile).

b. Environmental and Cultural Norms

While collecting data, the researcher needs to be sensitive to the norms of the environment and culture in which the research is being conducted. This may require subtle shifts in dress, speech, mannerisms, or actions. For example, if the researcher is conducting interviews with adolescents in a clinic in a low-income neighborhood, imagine the reactions and responses of the teens to a researcher who shows up in a three-piece Givenchy business suit and using a laptop computer. Similarly, if the researcher is collecting data from a group of Native Americans, it is important to recognize that they speak quite softly and view direct eye contact as rude behavior. Hence, unlike Euro-Americans, who value direct eye contact as a sign of interest and attention, the researcher should not be put off by a lack of eye contact from Native American respondents but rather recognize it as a sign of respect.

c. Demand Characteristics

Questionnaires or interview guides may also provide cues to participants and, unless one is careful, these may distort responses in the direction that the respondent thinks the researcher prefers. Such distortions are labeled **demand characteristics.** In such situations, test results are distorted because people respond in the way they think they are expected to respond. The term *demand characteristic* was coined by psychiatrist Martin T. Orne, who noted that subjects in experiments will sometimes play the role of "helpful subject" and produce the results they think the researcher desires (Jackson, 1999). A nurse researcher may phrase a question in such a way that the respondent is encouraged to answer it in one way rather than another. For example, a biased question on palliative care would be, *"Do you agree with the president of the National Palliative Care Association that provision of palliative care services is directly related to effective coping in terminal clients?"* Reference to a respected nursing figure would no doubt load the question in one direction influencing the respondent's answer.

During the data collection phase, a research director must ensure that when a selected respondent refuses to participate or is unavailable that the replacement is selected on an equal probability basis (see Chapter 15). If this is not done, there is a danger that the data collection personnel will simply choose the most convenient replacement, which will tend to bias the study by overrepresenting those people who spend more time at home. In the words of Smith (1991), researchers often have to work with the people who are available; these may comprise "volunteers, hypochondriacs, scientific do-gooders, those with nothing else to do," and so on. Even with probability sampling, bias is present when certain groups such as those too busy to participate in a mail or telephone survey or those too ill to be included in a clinical study are excluded systematically. Researchers need to acknowledge these possible sources of bias in their study designs and provide readers of their research reports with such information so that they may judge the representativeness of the sample and the generalizability of the findings.

d. Halo Effect

Bias may creep into data collection procedures when rating scales are used. The **halo effect** is a carryover effect in which the researcher's first rating may influence the second and subsequent ratings. The general impressions the researcher has of a particular situation may carry over and influence subsequent ratings of similar situations. This is because the researcher has a tendency to reinforce her or his impressions

The halo effect may also result when the researcher attempts to make ratings consistent. Such bias may be reduced by having different raters rate the participants or phenomenon or by having the same raters do the rating at different times without knowledge that they are rating the same participant or phenomenon as done previously.

4. Data Analysis

During the data analysis stage, bias is most commonly introduced in one of three ways: through coding errors, data massaging, and hunting. Any of these may be intentional or unintentional.

a. Coding Errors

At the beginning of an analysis in surveys, interview studies, and participant observation studies, researchers go through a process of coding the information. What this means is that if data are collected in an open-ended format (questions without fixed-response categories), then the information should be placed into categories before analysis begins. The process of coding is subject to two kinds of error, random and systematic.

Random error refers to inconsistencies that enter into the coding process but that display no systematic pattern. For example, suppose that you are coding people into the following educational categories: (1) 8 or fewer years of formal education, (2) 9 to 12 years of formal education, (3) some postsecondary training, or (4) college or university graduation. If you accidentally coded a person with 5 years of education into category (2), you would have made an accidental or random error. In processing data, one often enters the information twice, comparing the first version with the second in order to locate such random errors. Occasionally, entry errors include values that are not within the range of possible values: in the above example, entering a 6 would be an example of such an error. These errors are easiest to spot because after data analysis begins, an out-of-range value will become apparent as soon as one runs a frequency distribution of the variable. And because these errors simply represent "noise" in one's data, they are not as threatening to the conclusions of a study as systematic errors.

Systematic errors are especially problematic. These errors are in danger of biasing a study because they systematically distort the data in one particular direction. For example, suppose that any person who does not answer the question on education is assigned to the lowest category, the category representing those people with 8 or fewer years of education. In such cases, we would be biasing the data systematically for those who refuse to answer the question by always coding them as if they should fall into the lowest educational category. (Normally those who do not answer a question are assigned a missing value code for the question.) Another kind of systematic error could occur if we discovered, after having developed code categories and starting our work, that another and uncategorized kind of response is occurring halfway through the analysis. For example, if, to save time, we do not go back to the beginning and reexamine all of our cases to see if some of the codings have been inappropriately forced into certain categories, we will have decreased the number of cases that fall into the newly discovered category systematically. This kind of difficulty is likely to pop up in studies that have many open-ended questions. (This is one reason, incidentally, why many researchers avoid using a lot of open-ended questions.)

b. Data Massaging

Particularly in surveys and secondary data analyses, a great amount of information is collected on a large number of variables. This data may be treated in a variety of ways—many of which may be viewed as alternative modes of analysis. The researcher may analyze the data in a number of different ways, discarding the results that are "less interesting" and keeping those that "make the most sense." If cross-tabulations are being done, a variety of cutpoints may be tried; some will be retained, and others will be discarded. (If you had measured respondents' education by years of formal school completed and you now wished to group them into

two categories, low and high education, where would you draw the line between the two groups?) **Data massaging** is working with the data until the analysis produces the strongest association among the variables.

Such data massaging violates the principles of objectivity. Unfortunately, it is practiced in all disciplines. Because every discipline has a range of approved methods of analysis, massaging the data may seem perfectly legitimate. After all, the researcher wants to produce the "best" analysis of the data, and in many disciplines, only statistically significant results are publishable. Even more unfortunately, such data massaging is rarely reported in formal presentations of the research.

c. Hunting

Given the modern computer, it is now possible to run tests for many different relationships. There may be four or five different operationalizations of a concept (e.g., SES) available to the researcher in a data set; perhaps the various hypothesized relationships are run using each of these possibilities. Finally, the one that is most congruent with the researcher's expectations gets reported. A rationale for throwing out some of the results can readily be found by arguing that they represent a "poor measurement" of the relevant variable. Most researchers have, from time to time, engaged in some "selective" use of data. If the researcher "hunts" through a data set long enough, an acceptable—even interesting—finding will surely emerge. At that point, the hunt stops.

In the physical and the social sciences, "hunting" is common. What student in chemistry or a physics laboratory has not checked the results obtained by other students? If unexpected results occur, then the procedure is rerun on the grounds that something must have been done wrong. In short, if anticipated results are not obtained, the results are discarded. Even mature researchers have the tendency to work with the data until the "right" finding is obtained. The search for "reportable" findings is a continuous process in all science, yet few papers acknowledge this search. Reading research papers leaves the impression that most projects are easy and straightforward, but few actually are.

The key issue in discussing bias as it relates to analysis is this: What scientific principle determines when analysis is finished? Do we stop analysis when we get a reportable, respectable finding? If we stop analysis when we get the results we like, the bias will be toward confirming expectations. Although some of the data may be consistent with expectations, some may not be. Frequently, inconsistencies are not reported.

For survey researchers, there is a special problem. Given many variables and observations, it is possible to run any variable against every other variable in a search for "significant findings." If we use the 0.05 level of significance (see Chapter 12), then we would expect one in 20 of the relationships examined to be statistically significant simply on a chance basis. Unless the researcher reports the "hunting" that has occurred, the reader of a report will be in no position to regard the conclusions with the skepticism they deserve.

Finally, it should be pointed out that there is nothing inherently wrong with "exploring" data, looking at relationships that have not been hypothesized. But such analyses should not be reported unless it is made clear that no hypothesis has guided the search. At least then the reader has been cautioned.

5. Reporting of Findings

In 1959, T.D. Sterling published a classic paper that suggested that much of what is being published in learned journals may represent fluke results (Sterling, 1959). His argument is that there are a lot of researchers, and many may be working on a similar problem at any time. If the 0.05 level of significance has been used, an average of one study in 20 will produce a statistically significant relationship purely by chance, and such studies may even get published (journals ordinarily do not publish papers reporting "no relationship" findings). The obvious question is what proportion of journal articles are based on these fluke studies. Although Sterling's point is an interesting one, it may overstate the problem (Jackson, 1999). Nonetheless, the argument needs to be kept in mind as one possible source of bias in published studies. In a recent update of the 1959 research, Sterling and associates (1995) note that little has changed in publication decisions with respect to tests of significance. They note that in a 1958 study of psychology journals, some 97.3 percent of the articles reporting tests of significance rejected the null hypothesis; in 1986 to 1987, the figure stood at 95.6 percent rejecting the null hypothesis. Box 9.1 summarizes some of the points raised in the article by Sterling and associates.

Sterling's argument can be extended into another area. There is a selection process that finds certain findings reportable and others unreportable. Indeed, it is unusual for one's first analysis of the data to make it through to the final report. Although there are many good reasons for analyzing data in different ways, the process of deciding which findings to report may have more to do with aesthetics than science.

In nursing research, the issues of both statistical and clinical significance must be considered in determining the reportability of findings. *Clinical significance,* which is discussed in Chapter 12, refers to the potential for research findings to make a real and important difference in clinical practice, in improving

BOX 9.1 *Bias in Publication Decisions*

The scientific method has traditionally been touted as a model of objectivity, but a team of researchers at Simon Fraser University in British Columbia has revealed a significant bias in the way scientific results are reported.

According to their work, scientists who offer positive findings from their work—such as the verification of a hypothetical experimental outcome—stand a better chance of getting published. Meanwhile, those whose findings indicate the lack of a result—such as the denial of an expected experimental outcome—are unlikely ever to see their conclusions in print.

"You get this idiocy that you don't publish negative results," says computer science professor Ted Sterling, who first noted the trend in a research paper he published in 1959. At that time, he analyzed the contents of a selected group of psychology journals and noted the overwhelming prevalence of articles touting positive outcomes. Dr Sterling says he was disappointed to find out that nothing had changed more than 30 years later.

For this article, Dr Sterling and his colleagues sampled a wider variety of scientific journals, but the prevalence of positive results had not changed. The article even cites a rejection letter written by the editor of a major environment and toxicology journal, which states bluntly, "The negative results translate into a minimal contribution to the field."

The Simon Fraser researchers disagree with that observation, suggesting that alerting scientists to negative findings can prevent others from repeating the same experiment and obtaining the same findings, a process that pro-

motes redundant work because few will be aware of the negative result until they find out about it firsthand.

Moreover, the increasing popularity of a statistical method called meta-analysis makes it all the more important to know about negative results. Meta-analysis pools the results of a number of published studies without bothering to carry out any original research. But this approach assumes all the relevant scientific findings, rather than just the positive ones, will be available in print.

"Because access to study results is typically limited to published studies, the question of whether or not published studies constitute a representative sample of relevant studies is of concern," state the researchers in their *American Statistician* paper.

The solution, according to Sterling, lies with a new strategy for selecting scientific work to publish. He advocates "blind-to-outcome" peer review, which would weigh submitted papers on the basis of the importance and relevance of the work, instead of relying on the nature of the outcome. In light of the fact that little about this aspect of scientific publication appears to have changed in 30 years and because the possibly misleading consequences are becoming more serious, his colleagues and he argue that this sort of drastic modification of editorial policy is necessary.

"In short," their study concludes, "more radical measures than public consciousness raising are needed to curtail the influence of publication bias."

SOURCE: *University Affairs*, January, 1996, p. 16. This report was based on Sterling, T.D., Rosenbaum, W.L., and Weinkam, J.J. (1995). Publication decisions revisited: The effect of the outcome of statistical tests on the decision to publish and vice versa. *The American Statistician*, 49, 108–112. Cited with permission.

health status, or to a problem identified as a priority for the discipline. Traditionally, researchers have relied on statistical significance to imply clinical significance (Jeans, 1992). This has lead to the problem of nursing research being rejected by editors because the studies failed to find significant results. This problem was investigated by Polit and Sherman (1990), who analyzed 62 nursing research studies published in *Nursing Research* and *Research in Nursing and Health* to determine if, similar to the researchers in other disciplines, nurse researchers were at high risk of finding nonsignificant results even when their research hypotheses were correct. Results indicated that many nurse researchers are designing inadequately powered studies in which their hypotheses will fail to be supported, even though the hypotheses are correct. Two reasons explain this. One is that the majority of hypotheses tested by nurses involve effects that are small or small to moderate. This is because nursing phenomena are typically so complex and difficult to measure that no single study can hope to explain a substantial portion of the variance. The second reason is the tendency of nurse researchers to use small samples. Nursing studies typically use samples of fewer than 100 participants (Moody et al., 1988). Because of the small sample sizes, often necessitated by the clinical nature of nursing research, a substantial number of published nursing studies and presumably even more of unpublished studies lack sufficient power to detect real effects. Therefore, Sterling's argument that what is published may represent fluke results can also apply in nursing research, in which many studies fail to detect statistically significant differences that are, however, truly clinically important.

The difficulty is that some nonscientific considerations come into play when reports are submitted for publication or for presentation at professional conferences. Are the findings culturally acceptable? Are the findings acceptable to one's peers? Because pressure exists to keep papers and presentations short, only the "major" finding is reported; this "major" finding, however, may not be representative of the findings of the whole research project.

The point here is that not only does the choice of subject matter reflect values but also the researcher's theoretical predispositions may influence the conclusions of the study as much as any data collected. Many nurse researchers have undergone years of socialization in their discipline and, therefore, have developed a nursing perspective on issues. Conceptual and theoretical models prevalent in the discipline shape these perspectives. All conceptual and theoretical views limit—and, at times, bias—our perspective of the topic under study and influence our reporting of findings. In other words, nurses who support the self-care model of nursing frame their conclusions in relation to self-care, and those who support the stress adaptation model of nursing come to stress adaptation conclusions.

Chapter 2 outlined some types of flawed arguments that may find their way into the final report of a study. Included among these were inappropriate appeals to authority; provincialism; setting up a false dilemma; missing, insufficient, or suppressed evidence; and unwarranted conclusions. Readers should be alert to these flaws in reading a final report on a research project.

In addition to being evident in theoretical predispositions and improper argument, bias can also be reflected by insensitivity to minorities, sexism, or in tendencies to go beyond the limits of one's data when interpreting them. And although scholars are trained to be cautious in their interpretations, it is difficult to avoid suggesting extrapolations beyond those justified by the data. Some of these issues are explored more fully in Chapter 19, which deals with report writing.

Bias is just one of many factors that may influence the outcome of a study. How important bias itself is varies across many conditions. When we fail to replicate a study (i.e., fail to get the same finding as another researcher), we cannot assume that the difference in results is caused by bias alone. Many factors, including bias, may have been responsible.

Projects are rarely as straightforward as the final report on the project implies. Consider sampling, for example. Only rare projects do not run into some sampling difficulties. First, there may be problems with refusals and lost questionnaires. Some of the responses may not be clear; when comparisons between the sample and the known parameters of the population are compared, there may often be uncomfortable disparities. Interviewers may have cut corners in the interest of completing the project (such tactics may range from faking interviews to avoiding the normal random respondent selection process, even going so far as to include whomever happens to be available in a sample). In short, research is inevitably messier than our reports of it.

6. Funding

Granting agencies, although they may claim to fund projects on the basis of merit, are themselves subject to bias. In Canada, for example, a variety of councils and foundations related to health care are funded by the federal government, which may favor projects that support legislative agendas. Similarly, in the United States, the National Institute of Nursing Research (NINR) in planning future research for the next 5 years (2000 to 2004) has selected seven key areas that will dominate the institute's research portfolio and be funding priorities. These include chronic illness, health promotion and disease prevention, quality and cost effectiveness of care, management of symptoms, adaptation to new technologies, health disparities, and palliative care.

If external funding has been provided, it is important to determine who the sponsors of a research project are because the findings may be biased in the direction of their interests. For example, nursing studies are often sponsored by drug companies or medical supply companies who wish to sell a product. In these situations, nurses and readers of such research reports need to be cognizant of the potential for bias in the re-

porting of the results. Otherwise, the cost of biased results may be very expensive for the client and the health-care system, both financially and emotionally.

The value society places on different kinds of research is also reflected in the relative amounts of research funds made available. Traditionally, medical research that targets the diagnosis and cure of diseases has received most of the federal health dollars targeted for research in both Canada and the United States. Nursing research continues to be underfunded when compared with other professional disciplines. Jeans (1990, p. 2) raises the question: *Why is it that when legislators clearly place priorities for health research on areas that are the very substance of nursing research, these recommendations do not translate into the actual funding of health research? Who is passing the buck or not passing the bucks, as the case seems to be?* Some nurse researchers suggest it is the entrenchment of a system by a dominant group (medical researchers) that prevents changes in patterns of research funding and, therefore, influences the type of research that is conducted.

In addition, scholars in the traditional disciplines such as medicine and the natural sciences are more readily funded than those in newer areas such as nursing, allied health professions, or interdisciplinary research in health promotion. Indeed, in recent years, some funding agencies have set up special committees to deal with applications for people working in newly developing areas. The establishment of the new review committees is a response to the perception that scholars in these areas are at a disadvantage when competing with scholars in traditional disciplines.

Within the university system, peer-review committees typically adjudicate project-funding decisions. These committees usually face a high demand for funds and severely limited resources. In their funding decisions, they usually select studies that reflect current research trends and that will advance their discipline. In summary, nursing research operates in a social context. Researchers are constrained by peers and granting agencies to not engage in "trivial" research and instead focus on issues that are considered "important." What is considered "important" in one generation may be considered as "trivial" by the next one.

7. The Use of Findings

Given the enormous confidence that Western culture has in science, it is no surprise that the findings of science are powerful tools. Courts, politicians, the media, and the general public seem to respect science. Nurse researchers are increasingly interviewed on radio and television, appear as expert witnesses in courts, and, indeed, provide evidence taken into account when legal and public policy decisions related to health matters are made. Scientific evidence is taken seriously.

Unfortunately, the research literature is easily misrepresented. The research literature contains many findings, some of which support a particular view and others that do not. Researchers who are committed to some social cause, health issue, or a particular theoretical perspective may select evidence that helps establish a particular position—similar to a debater seeking support for a particular conclusion. Because of a desire to support a particular position, the debater is not interested in contrary evidence; only preferred evidence is reported. The problem with using the debater's approach is that many people may think that the findings are objective and impartial and that they reflect dispassionate scientific views. But they may simply be a conclusion seeking corroborating evidence. Debaters enjoy the credibility of science while violating the principle of impartiality.

When researchers slip inadvertently into advocacy roles, they compromise their credibility as "impartial scientists." Readers should note an important distinction between the advocacy role, which is viewed as pejorative in relation to research, and the patient advocacy role, which nurses assume in relation to their practice. The latter is a covenantal professional relationship that grows out of a moral principle of fidelity to the client and a commitment to protecting those at vulnerable points in their lives (Deloughery, 1995). In this role, the nurse and client work together to reach decisions that fit with the unique needs and values of the client. It should not be confused with the citizen–advocate role in which one produces scientific evidence to support a particular position or cause. Nor should the nurse researcher role be confused with either the nurse advocate role or the citizen–advocate role. Nurse researchers must maintain objectivity and a search for truth that is unbiased and impartial if their work is to be taken seriously and if nursing is to be considered a respected, scholarly discipline that contributes to improved practice.

An impartial approach would try to disconfirm a theory, try to rule out alternatives, and continually press any given theory hard in an effort to discover the limits under which it is applicable. Although this can never be achieved perfectly, those who attempt to follow this approach are, nonetheless, trying to eliminate as much bias as possible in their research or in their reviews.

Peter W. Huber has explored the problem of the scientist-for-hire as it relates to the American court system in his book *Galileo's Revenge: Junk Science in the Courtroom* (1991). Numerous court cases in which huge sums of money are at stake involve the use of expert scientific witnesses. Huber argues that the system is at fault because it seems unable to distinguish good scientific testimony from that

of the science charlatans who make careers out of court appearances. American
courts are faulted for setting insufficient
standards as to who may testify. Frequently lawyers consider many scientists, settling finally on the ones who are
willing to make "appropriate" testimony
and to be coached. As personal injury
lawyer, Dennis Roberts notes:

> You get a professor who earns $60,000
> a year and give him the opportunity to
> make a couple of hundred thousand
> dollars in his spare time and he will
> jump at the chance . . . (quoted in Hu-
> ber, 1991, p. 19).

Huber argues that courts would do
well to pay more attention to establishing
the consensus on a topic in the research
community and rely less on the personal
opinion of an expert who has been selected and groomed by a lawyer who is
seeking a favorable outcome. As long as
lawyers are doing the hiring, they are
likely to stack the deck to improve their
chances of winning their cases. This practice fails to represent the findings of science objectively and, therefore, may
compromise the ability of the courts to
come to reasonable conclusions.

The role of the investigator in introducing bias can affect every stage of the
research process. Investigator bias needs
to be acknowledged and made explicit so
that it does not undermine the quality of
research. Cook identifies four areas of investigator bias that may compromise research conclusions: emotional, normative, cultural, and professional bias. Box
9.2 delineates these four areas.

In summary, researchers should be
aware of the way in which bias may affect
the research process as well as the conclusions, reporting, and use of a research
report. The danger of becoming overly
concerned about bias, however, is that researchers may spend far too much time
contemplating the difficulties of research,
and, as a result, not get the job done.

C. ADVOCACY VERSUS PURE RESEARCH

In our exploration of sources of bias in
the various stages of research, we have
noted how the outcomes of research may
be inadvertently distorted. Findings tend
to move in the direction of the culturally
acceptable, in the direction of our expectations, and in the direction of our preferences. And if the pervasive attitudes of
both the relevant scholarly disciplines
and the larger society are liberal, inclusive, and emphasize tolerance, then the
research outcomes will tend to reflect
these views. On the other hand, a more
conservative, exclusive, and intolerant
society will encourage research outcomes that are supportive of these views.
Funding agencies and their selection
processes will particularly encourage
"mainstream" researchers—those whom
referees think meet the standards governing "good" research. A similar argument can be advanced about the publication decisions of journal editors.

In recent decades, a blurring of the line
between *advocacy research* on the one
hand and *pure or descriptive research* on
the other seems to have occurred. One
possible explanation is that practitioners
in nursing, health-related, and social science disciplines have become increasingly aware that all research carries with
it cultural baggage. So, whether we talk of
research design bias, funding decisions,
data collection, analysis, interpretation,
or publication decisions, research tends
to reflect its sociocultural milieu. This re-
alization perhaps helped to legitimize the
use of research to advocate changes or
advance the personal or collective agendas of its practitioners.

The degree of bias reflected in research
reports ranges across a continuum. On the
one hand, there are research reports
specifically designed to study bias (Cook,
1997; Flaskerud and Nyanathi, 2000); the
psychology experiments exploring experi-

predisposed to generate results favoring your personal preferences. By setting aside personal preferences and beliefs surrounding phenomenon under investigation, the investigator prevents the information from biasing or interfering with the recovery of pure description of phenomenon of interest. Sensitivity to one's preferences and values must be constant and ongoing in both quantitative and qualitative investigations so that the purest form of research findings emerge.

Guideline 13: Do not disclose hypotheses to subjects or assistants. Do not reveal specific hypotheses to research subjects or assistants. It seems safest to follow this guideline if expectancy bias is to be reduced. It may, however, be necessary to provide some general idea of what the study is about, but it is best not to provide either research assistants or subjects with the details.

Guideline 14: Cover the attitudinal continuum. When possible, avoid showing your hand by presenting a variety of views. This will give the respondent a sense that all responses are acceptable. Be certain to offer a full range of attitudinal response categories so that no respondent is always forced to the extreme of the continuum.

Guideline 15: Be accepting of all responses. Interviewers must be trained to appear to ask questions neutrally and to respond in the same way to all respondents' answers. Ideally, the interviewer should convey an impression of neutrality yet have a keen interest in respondents' answers. Interviewers should avoid coaching responses.

Guideline 16: Specify data analysis procedures in advance. In quantitative research, hypotheses must be specified in advance as must data analysis procedures to avoid the bias of playing with the data. Analytical procedures must be specified in advance of data collection. Although this may be viewed as a restrictive guideline, if followed, it prevents unwarranted massaging of the data.

In qualitative studies, awareness of researcher bias about the topic helps investigators identify a particular frame of reference that may limit or direct the data interpretation. Self-awareness through the process of *bracketing* promotes honesty in finding the truth and decreases the influence of bias in data interpretation (Streubert and Carpenter, 1999).

Guideline 17: Check for random and systematic errors. Researchers need to be aware of both random and systematic errors and put into place procedures to minimize both types of errors.

Guideline 18: Report extent of data massaging. Report the number of relationships that have been explored in the course of data analysis. Researchers should clarify the number of relationships that have been examined and the reasons why certain findings have not been reported.

The guidelines section is intended to suggest that we need to be more sensitive to bias and to its role in both different types of research projects and different phases of a research project. Predispositions to favor certain outcomes will always be present in human activities, including nursing research. To appreciate that simple idea is a good start.

E. CONCLUSION: THE GAP BETWEEN MYTH AND REALITY

We take the predispositions, or biases, of our culture into our research. We also take the biases acquired as members of the nursing research community to our research. So, regardless of whether we are positivist, interpretive, or critical, (see Chapter 1) in our basic perspective, we bring a set of assumptions, beliefs, theoretical orientations, and expectations to our research. Indeed, a text on methods provides sets of techniques for conducting research and attempts to socialize the student into an understanding and acceptance of the latest approaches to research. In their education, research methods students are provided with a set of dispositions, a set of rules not only for doing research but also for judging the work of other scholars. In short, the norms of research are being communicated.

But the ideas conveyed in a nursing methods text focus on the formal system of science. You learn how to do research "properly." You learn what techniques are appropriate in any given circumstance. And most methods texts urge you not to fall prey to bias, urge you to be fair and objective, and urge you to exercise great care so that you will do *good,* impartial research. Are there any problems with this?

The problem is that an important part of nursing research is missed. Although most presentations of research sound straightforward, there is much that happens in the course of the research process that never gets reported. In short, the research act itself can be the subject of research. A careful examination of most nursing research projects would reveal how bias inadvertently plays a role in research outcomes. There is, then, a formal system of science—somewhat mythical—and there is the real world of nursing science. The gap between myth and reality exists in all academic disciplines.

Research is social behavior. There are expectations of others to be met, norms of behavior to be followed, and findings that are anticipated. This social component of

Table 9.1   Myths and Realities of Nursing Research

Category	Nursing Research Myths	Nursing Research Realities
Value free	Research is objective and value neutral	There are significant subjective elements in all research
Stereotype of nursing	Nurses primarily use experimental data and follow the biomedical model of research	They also do field studies, surveys, social action research, and evaluation research
Sampling	Most studies involve representative samples	Most studies are based on nonrepresentative samples
Refusals	Most people are willing to participate in studies	Refusals run from 0% to 95%; commercial market researchers have the highest nonparticipation rates
Funding	Open to all; based on peer review and an evaluation of the quality of the proposal and the research record of the applicant	Researchers who are not part of the university system or a health research unit have little chance of receiving funding; there are fads in what kinds of projects are funded
Measurement	There is agreement on appropriate way to measure most variables	Little standardization or agreement on measures exist
Report writing	Final reports summarize the results of the observations	Evidence is selectively reported; some facts ignored or not reported
Tests of significance	They assess the extent to which results may be the result of chance sampling fluctuations	They are often inappropriately used when nonprobability sampling is used or when a whole populations studied

science is frequently at odds with the fundamental canons of science. Science as practiced is neither value free nor wholly objective. If actual research practices are observed, a whole host of nonscientific factors enter the picture. Although the achievements of science have, indeed, been impressive, it is nonetheless true that there is a gap between the ideal and actual practices of science. An awareness of this gap and of the sources of bias in research can only benefit beginning research methods students. Just as a good scientist is portrayed as a skeptic, so should we be skeptical of the methods of nursing science itself. Table 9.1 provides a few examples of gaps between actual and ideal practices in nursing science.

E X E R C I S E S

1. What is meant by "researcher affect," and how might it influence the conclusions of a study?

2. What are the fundamental differences between a debater approach to research and an impartial approach? What cues might alert the student to the type of researcher being encountered?

3. Identify a research problem that interests you. Describe the problem briefly. List a minimum of five predispositions that you have concerning this research problem, indicating your expectations in each case. Propose a way of managing your expectations so as to minimize their effect on your research.

4. A nurse researcher is designing a qualitative study to assess the impact of family caregiving for persons with AIDS on the children of primary caregivers. The nurse researcher (a mother of two preschooler children) has recently accepted responsibility to provide home care for her brother who has AIDS. She is exhausted and resentful of this situation. What type of bias might the nurse researcher potentially introduce to this research study? What safeguards could you build into the study design to minimize unnecessary bias?

5. Reflect on your own nursing experience and identify a topic that would be difficult for you to study in an impartial manner. How would you deal with this in a responsible manner?

6. You wish to evaluate a new health promotion program designed to increase the frequency of participation of young women in regular physical exercise. The program is offered to all women attending the local university. You hope to use the findings to advocate for additional health promotion programs on campus. In regards to this situation, answer the following: (1) What role would selection bias play in this study? (2) Why is assessment of the effectiveness of this program problematic? (3) How could selection bias be avoided? (4) What

would determine if this were advocacy research or evaluation research?

7. Examine the following questionnaire items for demand characteristics. Circle wording that you think is problematic (if any). Reword items that might cue the participants to respond in a manner that would distort responses.
- How often do you drink and drive in a typical week?

- Do you prefer to do aerobic or isometric exercises?

- Do you support the president's position on advanced nursing practice?

- Many experienced and expert nurses believe they are overworked in today's health-care environment. Do you agree?

RECOMMENDED READINGS

Cook, A.S. (1997). Investigator bias in bereavement research: Ethical and methodological implications. *Canadian Journal of Nursing Research, 29*(4), 87–93. An interesting discussion of investigator bias as it relates to the research process.

Crookes, S., and Davies, S. (1998). *Research Into Practice.* Edinburgh, Scotland: Balliere Tindall. An excellent discussion of the application of research findings to develop good practice. It integrates a discussion of bias and steps to minimize bias into several chapters in the text.

Flaskerud, J., and Nyamathi, A. (2000). Attaining gender and ethnic diversity in health intervention research: Cultural responsiveness versus resource provision. *Advances in Nursing Science, 22*(4), 1–15. An overview of gender and ethnic bias in health intervention research with practical suggestions for inclusion of women and diverse ethnic groups in such projects.

Rosenthal, R. and Rosnow, R.L. (1991). *Essentials of Behavioral Research* (2nd ed). New York: McGraw-Hill. Chapter 6 of this book is an excellent discussion of experimenter effect bias as well as proposed ways of minimizing the effect.

Sterling, T.D., Rosenbaum, W.L., and Weinkam, J.J. (1995). Publication decisions revisited: The effect of the outcome of statistical tests on the decision to publish and vice versa. *The American Statistician, 49*, 108–112. This article is a follow up to Sterling's paper published in 1959 and shows that little has changed in publication decisions over the past 30 years.

Chapter 10

Ethical Issues in Nursing Research

CHAPTER OUTLINE

KEY TERMS

Beneficence

Confidentiality

Debrief

Declaration of Helsinki

Deontological

Ethics

Ethics review board

Informed consent

Institutional review board

Justice

Nonmaleficence

Nuremberg Code

Process consent

Utilitarian perspective

At every stage of the research process, there are ethical considerations for nurse researchers to consider. For example, research questions such as the following are riddled with ethical challenges: How do I study mentally impaired subjects who may not be able to give informed and voluntary consent? How can I ethically withhold a treatment from subjects that might relieve their suffering? How can I assess pain levels in children who are noncommunicative? Even the decision as to whether a problem should be studied or not has ethical implications for investigators. Because research is central to the evolution of nursing care, the avoidance of conducting nursing research may be considered unethical. Similarly, the failure to engage in evidence-based practice—in other words, to base practice decisions solely on tradition or intuition rather than on empirical findings—denies clients access to the best available care and thus may also be considered unethical.

As more and more nurses participate in research activities, it is important that the profession operate from a sound ethical knowledge base. This chapter provides nurse researchers with guidelines to apply to ethical issues and problems in health research. Let us begin by exploring what ethics is and what ethical decision making in nursing research involves. The chapter then describes several research studies that illustrate ethical dilemmas faced by nurse researchers. Finally, the chapter provides a series of rules to guide nurse researchers in resolving ethical problems.

A. WHAT IS ETHICS?

The term *ethics* has a variety of meanings and associations. The Oxford American Dictionary defines **ethics** as the study of moral principles. It is concerned with the goodness and badness of human actions or with the principles of what is right and wrong in conduct. The intent of ethics is to develop methods for clarifying confusing questions even if final solutions remain elusive. Deloughery (1995) refers to ethics as a study of the "why?" of the moral principles by which a society lives. She elaborates that ethics deals with our concern for good behavior among people and our struggle to resolve ethical differences among members of society.

The authors of this text believe ethics is equally pertinent to all health-care practitioners regardless of their professional designation as nurses, physicians, social workers, dietitians, and so on. However, in this chapter, we focus on efforts to distinguish right from wrong in the process of conducting *nursing* research.

The terms *ethics* and *morals* are often used interchangeably. Downie and Calman (1987) identify three distinct meanings of ethics in the health-care literature. These include ethics as *moral philosophy,* ethics as *ordinary morality,* and ethics as *codes of professional conduct.* In the sense of *moral philosophy, ethics* refers to the branch of philosophy that is concerned with the study of principles that govern human behavior in our social world. It is a theoretical exploration of practical morality. Its aim is to provide an intellectual analysis and understanding of the fundamental principles of everyday morality. In the health-care environment, however, our goal is more than just an understanding of ethics. We hope to bring about an improved state of health through ethical action. This is true whether the action be research or the provision of care.

This leads us to a discussion of the second usage of *ethics* as *ordinary morality.* From this perspective, it relates to the problems of everyday life. As health professionals, the ethical challenges we encounter in practice are often an extension of the moral problems of everyday life. To be useful to problem solving, ethics in this sense must be viewed broadly as including the spectrum of value judgments about what is good and harmful in the world. Such judgments are all pervasive and consider a diverse range of factors, including the health-care professional's own values. Nurses bring with them their own sets of values to professional life. Nurses need to be aware of what these values are and be ready to examine them in light of a changing health-care environment.

In the third sense, *ethics* is defined narrowly as a list of "do's" and "don'ts" often set out in a *code of conduct*. The nursing profession has several traditional codes that guide decision making around ethical dilemmas, many of which are provided later in this chapter. Codes are useful in outlining basic moral principles to direct professional behavior, but they are limited in that they cannot address the full range of moral complexities confronting nurses and other health-care professionals today.

B. ETHICAL DECISION MAKING

Health-care research, in general, and nursing research, in particular, is considered by most to yield positive benefits to society. However, the history of health-care research teaches us that the pursuit of such a "good" has been abused by some researchers over the years. Beecher (1966) and Pence (1990) illustrate the abuses that can result from unscrupulous and overzealous researchers such as in the Tuskegee and Willowbrook studies discussed later in this chapter. Nurses are involved in a variety of research efforts, including research specific to nursing, multidisciplinary research, and research that is conducted by other disciplines on clients receiving nursing care. In all of these situations, nurses are expected to engage in ethical research behavior. Questions for ethical decision making abound: "What criteria can be used to judge the ethical ac-

ceptability of a study?" "How do I make an ethical decision?" "What are the characteristics of ethical research?" "What are the rights of those who participate in my study, and how do I protect those rights?" This section begins to explore some answers.

1. Perspectives for Assessing Ethical Acceptability

Two ethical perspectives have been proposed in western society to assess ethical acceptability of a research project: the *utilitarian* and the *deontological* perspectives. Each of these general perspectives articulates ethical norms that transcend disciplinary boundaries. They may prove helpful to nurse researchers in reflecting on ethical issues in research situations.

a. The Utilitarian View

The **utilitarian perspective** suggests that ethical judgments about a research project should be made by evaluating its consequences for the participants, for society, and for the academic discipline. This view entails the belief that the good of a research project is defined by the consequences of the results. Classical utilitarianism was advocated by the well-known philosopher John Stewart Mill (1806–1873). He proposed that actions should be taken to promote "the greatest good for the greatest number." An obvious problem with the utilitarian perspective is that of how to define "good." The utilitarian perspective considers that the end justifies the means. Based on this perspective, a research project is judged to be ethical if it produces the greatest good for the greatest number.

Small-scale studies with little ability for generalization of findings to the larger society may be judged from a utilitarian perspective to be unethical. For example, research into liver transplantation that has potential to influence quality of life for a small number of participants who receive this costly medical intervention may not be considered ethical unless it can be shown that the results can benefit a large number of people in the long term. In contrast, research into the prevention of liver disease by lifestyle change is justifiable from a utilitarian perspective because lifestyle change is more likely to benefit many more people than will costly surgical procedures available to only a few. In this perspective, one is left with the ethical dilemma of whether to provide the costly surgical procedure to a patient if that is all that is possible. Would it be ethical to deny that person the surgery in this case?

The utilitarian view emphasizes anticipating the possibly unfortunate consequences of the research. Thus, one wants to assess the possible dangers to the participants. Will participation in the study be in any way degrading, dangerous, or expose the participants to undue levels of harm or stress? Can these adverse experiences be justified by the study's contributions to our knowledge of health and human behavior? Are we in any way trapping individuals so that they do things that they otherwise might not do? Are we forcing them to take a position on an issue that they have never thought about? Would participants' involvement in the study reveal unpleasant, unsavory things about them that might otherwise remain hidden? Should research impose unpleasant and perhaps unwanted treatments, experiences, or self-knowledge on participants? And if this is sometimes the consequence, can it be justified by other pay-offs? The utilitarian view permits projects as long as reasonable precautions are taken and subjects are debriefed so that no long-term negative consequences result.

In the biomedical area, permission to use unproven therapies on dying patients is now more readily available. There is pressure to permit the use of unproven drugs or therapies on such patients. In the area of AIDS and cancer treatments, we now permit the use of experimental therapies because of the imminent death of the patient. In one situation, use of such treatments may be viewed as a blessing leading to a remission in the disease process, yet in another situation it may have no beneficial effect on the disease prognosis.

It needs to be recognized that each researcher may have a different definition of what is good. For example, a "cardiac cripple" awaiting a heart transplant has a perspective on the value and use of cardiac transplant research that is quite different from the perspective of a health education student doing lifestyle teaching with disadvantaged women who smoke. Similarly, a cardiac surgeon who heads a transplant research team may have a different perspective on what constitutes good resulting from expensive cardiac surgery research than a hospital administrator who is balancing the bottom line.

b. The Deontological View

The **deontological** approach to research ethics proposes absolute moral imperatives that must never be violated. Someone taking the deontological view might propose absolutes such as never using deception, always masking the identity of participants, and never putting any pressure on respondents to participate in a study. Rather than assessing the consequences of a given research procedure, the deontological approach may propose, in its most extreme form, that deception in experiments is never justified, no matter what the positive contributions to our knowledge might be.

Immanuel Kant (1724–1804) was a well-known deontologist who supported the *categorical imperative;* that is, basic laws apply without exception. For example, telling an untruth is always wrong, regardless of the consequences, or the welfare of the patient must always be placed above the integrity of the research if a conflict exists. Some deotologists take a more flexible view than Kant, accepting more than one basic law and considering context and circumstances in determining priority. Alasdair MacIntyre (cited by Holden, 1979, p. 538) argued that one can distinguish between types of harm to participants. He distinguishes between:

- Harm to a participant's interests (e.g., reporting a case of venereal disease)
- Wrongdoing (e.g., lying to someone, which may not cause any damage)
- A moral harm (e.g., doing something to make the participant less good, such as encouraging the person to tell a lie)

MacIntyre argues that whereas harms can be compensated for, wrongs cannot be; hence, the argument is that if doing a wrong is essential to conducting a research project, then the project should be banned (cited in Holden, 1979, p. 538). For example, if participant recruitment into a study requires deception of participants, then the study should be banned no matter what the benefit to society in terms of knowledge development. The Tuskegee syphilis study discussed in Box 10.6 powerfully demonstrates the serious damage that can result when a degree of deception is accepted in research.

2. Codes and Guidelines for Ethical Decision Making

Throughout its history, the field of nursing has been sensitive to the ethical dimension of doing nursing research. Thus, many professional nursing organizations have developed codes of ethics to guide nurses in their research endeavors. Although these codes are not totally inclusive of every ethical concern a nurse researcher may encounter, they clearly articulate the level of ethical behavior expected of nurse researchers and provide a standard for nurses working through ethical conflicts that may arise in research. They also provide guidance on ethical decision making in clinical practice, education, and administration. In the 1950s, nurses in many countries adopted the *International Council of Nurses Code* as their first code and then went on to develop unique codes reflective of practice in their own countries. Boxes 10.1, 10.2, and 10.3 describe the Codes of Ethics of the American Nursing Association (ANA), Canadian Nursing Association (CNA), and United Kingdom Nursing Association (UKNA), respectively.

In addition to these codes, nurses and others have developed professional guidelines for the protection of human subjects while conducting research. Because most nursing studies deal with human subjects, the protection of participants from harm as a result of research participation is a major responsibility of nurse researchers. For example, the CNA published *Ethical Guidelines for Nurses in Research Involving Human Participants* (1994). This document provides nurses in all domains of practice with guidelines that are relevant to the current and complex reality of research. The guidelines are based on the relevant value statements from the CNA Code of Ethics, such as the respect for client choice and confidentiality, protection of clients from incompetence, and so on.

The ANA has produced two documents that provide guidelines for nurses engaged in research: The *Guidelines for the Investigative Function of Nurses* is summarized in Chapter 1. The *Human Rights Guidelines for Nurses in Clinical and Other Research* (1985) focuses on the rights of human subjects involved in research and the ethical responsibilities of nurses in research settings. The key points of this document are listed in Box 10.4.

The **Nuremberg Code** (1949) was formulated as a result of unethical medical research experiments conducted by Nazi

BOX 10.1 *American Nurses Association (ANA) Code of Ethics*

1. The nurse provides services with respect for human dignity and the uniqueness of the client, unrestricted by considerations of social or economic status, personal attributes, or the nature of health problems.
2. The nurse safeguards the client's right to privacy by judiciously protecting information of a confidential nature.
3. The nurse acts to safeguard the client and the public when health care and safety are affected by the incompetent, unethical, or illegal practice of any person.
4. The nurse assumes responsibility and accountability for individual nursing judgments and actions.
5. The nurse maintains competence in nursing.
6. The nurse exercises informed judgment and uses individual competence and qualifications as criteria in seeking consultation, accepting responsibilities, and delegating nursing activities to others.
7. The nurse participates in activities that contribute to the ongoing development of the profession's body of knowledge.
8. The nurse participates in the profession's efforts to implement and improve standards of nursing.
9. The nurse participates in the profession's efforts to establish and maintain conditions of employment conducive to high quality nursing care.
10. The nurse participates in the profession's efforts to protect the public from misinformation and misrepresentation and to maintain the integrity of nursing.
11. The nurse collaborates with members of the health professions and other citizens in promoting community and national efforts to meet the health needs of the public.

SOURCE: Reprinted with permission from Code for Nurses with Interpretive Statements, ©1985. American Nurses Publishing, American Nurses Foundation/American Nurses Association, Washinton, DC.

BOX 10.2 *Values: Code of Ethics for Registered Nurses (CNA)*

Health and Well-being

Nurses value health and well-being and assist persons to achieve their optimum level of health in situations of normal health, illness, injury, or in the process of dying.

Choice

Nurses respect and promote the autonomy of clients and help them to express their health needs and values, and to obtain appropriate information and services.

Dignity

Nurses value and advocate the dignity and self-respect of human clients.

Confidentiality

Nurses safeguard the trust of clients that information learned in the context of a professional relationship is shared outside the health care team only with the client's permission or as legally required.

Fairness

Nurses apply and promote principles of equity and fairness to assist clients in receiving unbiased treatment and a share of health services and resources appropriate to their needs.

Accountability

Nurses act in a manner consistent with their professional responsibilities and standards of practice.

Practice Environments Conducive to Safe, Competent, and Ethical Care

Nurses advocate practice environments, that have the organizational and human support systems, and the resource allocations necessary for safe, competent and ethical nursing care.

SOURCE: Canadian Nurses Association (1997). *Code of Ethics for Registered Nurses.* Ottawa: Canadian Nurses Association. Cited with permission.

> **BOX 10.3** *Code of Professional Conduct for the Nurse, Midwife, and Health Visitor (UKCC)*
>
> Each registered nurse, midwife, and health visitor shall act, at all times, in such a manner as to justify public trust and confidence, to uphold and enhance the good standing and reputation of the profession, to serve the interests of society, and above all to safeguard the interests of individual clients and patients.
>
> Each registered nurse, midwife, and health visitor is accountable for his/her practice, and, in the exercise of professional accountability shall:
>
> 1. Act always in such a way as to promote and safeguard the well-being and interests of clients.
> 2. Ensure that no action or omission on his/her part is detrimental to the condition or safety of the client.
> 3. Take every reasonable opportunity to maintain and improve professional knowledge and competence.
> 4. Acknowledge any limitations of competence and refuse to accept any delegated functions without first having received instruction in regard to those functions and having been assessed as competent.
> 5. Work in a collaborative and co-operative manner with other health care professionals and recognize and respect their contributions within the health care team.
> 6. Take account of the customs, values, and spiritual beliefs of clients.
> 7. Make known to an appropriate person or authority any conscientious objection that may be relevant to professional practice.
> 8. Avoid any abuse of the privileged relationship that exists with patients/clients and of the privileged access allowed to their property, residence, or workplace.
> 9. Respect confidential information obtained in the course of professional practice and refrain from disclosing such information without the consent of the client, or a person entitled to act on his/her behalf, except where disclosure is required by law or order of a court or is necessary in the public interest.
> 10. Have regard to the environment of care and its physical, psychological, and social effects on clients, and also to the adequacy of resources, and make known to appropriate persons any circumstances that could place clients in jeopardy or which mitigate against safe standards of practice.
> 11. Have regard to the workload of and the pressures of colleagues and subordinates and take appropriate action if these are seen to be such as to constitute abuse of the individual practitioner and to jeopardize safe standards of practice.
> 12. In the context of the individual's own knowledge, experience, and sphere of authority, assist peers and subordinates to develop professional competence in accordance with their needs.
> 13. Refuse to accept any gift, favor, or hospitality that might be interpreted as seeking to exert influence to obtain preferential consideration.
> 14. Avoid the use of professional qualifications in the promotion of commercial products in order not to compromise the independence of professional judgement on which clients rely.
>
> SOURCE: UKCC (1993). *Code of Professional Conduct for the Nurse, Midwife And Health Visitor.* London: United Kingdom Central Council. Cited with permission.

scientists predominantly on inmates of concentration camps before and during World War II. This code is appropriate to researchers in disciplines such as nursing, sociology, psychology, and education, as well as those in biomedical research. The Nuremberg Code addresses issues of informed consent, protection of subjects from risk or harm, the right of participants to withdraw from experimentation, and adequate qualifications of those conducting research. Box 10.5 lists the key points of the Nuremberg Code.

The **Declaration of Helsinki** (1986)

BOX 10.4 *Summary of the American Nurses Association's Guidelines for Protecting Human Subjects*

If research is a condition of employment, nurses must be informed in writing of the nature of the research. If this is not done, nurses must be given the opportunity of not participating in research.

1. Researchers must assess the risks and benefits involved and inform participants of any potential physical or mental risks or benefits and activities or procedures that go beyond personal need. Nurses must monitor sources of potential risk of injury and protect subjects who are vulnerable because of illness or are members of captive groups (e.g., prisoners, students, patients, and the poor).

2. All proposals, instruments, and procedures used in the research study must be discussed with the participants and others involved in the project so that individuals may make an

informed choice as to whether or not to participate.

3. The methods that protect the identities of subjects and protect the privileged information collected from participants must be described by the researcher to potential subjects.

4. Guidelines for protecting human subjects apply to all individuals involved in research projects.

5. Nurses have the responsibility to protect human rights and a professional responsibility to support research that broadens the scientific knowledge base of nursing.

6. Voluntary informed consent must be obtained from all participants or their legal representatives before initiation of a research project.

7. Nurses have the obligation to participate on institutional review boards to review the ethical implications of research proposals.

SOURCE: American Nurses Association (1985). *Human Rights Guidelines for Nurses in Clinical and Other Research.* Kansas City, MO: ANA. Cited with permission.

BOX 10.5 *Highlights of the Nuremberg Code*

1. The voluntary consent of human subjects is absolutely essential.

2. The experiment shall be such as to yield fruitful results for the good of society, unprocurable by other methods, and not random or unnecessary in nature.

3. The experiment should be based on the results of animal experimentation and a knowledge of the natural history of the disease or other problem under study that the anticipated results will justify the performance of the experiment.

4. The experiment should be conducted to avoid all unnecessary physical and mental harm or suffering.

5. No experiment should be conducted where there is an a priori reason to believe that death or disabling injury will occur; an

exception would be where the experimental physicians also serve as subjects.

6. The degree of risk should never exceed the importance of the problem to be solved.

7. Proper preparations should be made to protect subjects against even remote possibilities of injury, disability or death.

8. Only scientifically qualified persons should conduct the experiment.

9. During the course of the experiment, the subject should be able to bring the experiment to an end if he or she wishes.

10. During the course of the experiment, the researcher must be prepared to bring the experiment to an end if he or she believes continuation . . . is likely to result in injury, disability, or death to an experimental subject.

SOURCE: Nuremberg Code (1949). In J. Levine (Ed.). (1986). *Ethics and Regulation of Clinical Research* (2nd ed., pp.425–426). Baltimore: Urban & Schwarzenberg.

was strongly guided in its development by the Nuremberg Code. This declaration differentiates between *therapeutic research* and *nontherapeutic research*. *Therapeutic research* is research that provides participants with an opportunity to benefit from an experimental treatment. *Nontherapeutic research* is research that generates new knowledge that will bring future benefits to society, but those acting as participants most likely will not benefit from their participation in the research. The Helsinki Declaration provides three general rules to guide investigators in conducting nontherapeutic research:

1. Greater care must be taken to protect subjects from harm in nontherapeutic research studies.
2. The investigator must protect the life and health of the participants.
3. Independent justification is required to subject a healthy volunteer to risk of harm just to gain new empirical knowledge.

A code of ethics applied to social, medical, and health-care research in Canada is the *Tri-Council Policy Statement on Ethical Conduct for Research Involving Humans* (1998). The Medical Research Council (MRC), the Natural Sciences and Engineering Research Council (NSERC), and the Social Sciences and Humanities Research Council (SSHRC) have jointly adopted this new document, which provides standards and procedures for governing research involving human subjects.

In the new millennium, we see that most professional associations; all universities, colleges, and hospitals; and most government agencies will have in place codes of ethics to guide researchers. You should familiarize yourself with the applicable code for your discipline or place of work. Despite these codes and documents, unethical research still continues, as you will read in Box 10.6.

3. Principles of Ethical Research

At times, ethical theories such as deontology or utilitarianism may not be adequate to guide nurses in ethical decision making. In these situations, ethical principles rather than theories may prove more helpful. The CNA (1994) identifies three main principles on which to base ethical decisions in research situations involving human subjects. These include respect for persons, beneficence, and justice. Each of these principles warrants discussion.

a. Respect for Persons

Inherent in the ethical principle of respect for persons are the concepts of autonomy, dignity, uniqueness, freedom, and choice. This principle forms the foundation of the participant's rights to informed consent, privacy, and confidentiality. This principle involves respecting people's autonomy or right to choose freely for themselves. Participants have a right to make choices based on their own values and beliefs and be free from undue pressure or coercion by others. Autonomous decisions imply that participants have enough information to make informed choices and they comprehend the implications of the choices they make. Participants must be made fully aware of any risks or benefits anticipated from participation in a study. Autonomy may also be influenced adversely by unequal power relationships between the participant and the researcher. The principle of respect for persons requires that participants' **confidentiality** and anonymity must be safeguarded. The researcher's responsibilities related to these rights are discussed in the rules at the end of this chapter.

b. Beneficence

Two concepts are inherent in this principle: **nonmaleficence,** or the duty to not

BOX 10.6 *What Happened in the Tuskegee Study?*

In 1929, the USPHS conducted studies in the rural U.S. South to determine the prevalence of syphilis among blacks and explore the possibilities for treatment. Macon County, Alabama, in which the town of Tuskegee is located, was found to have the highest incidence among six counties tested. The study concluded that mass treatment could be successfully implemented among black Southerners. With the economic collapse of 1929, the findings were ignored.

Three years later, in 1932, the conditions in Macon County were given renewed attention. The Chief of the USPHS Venereal Disease Division decided the high prevalence of syphilis disease offered an unprecedented opportunity to study the disease in nature. He reasoned that because most blacks went untreated throughout life, it seemed natural to observe the consequences. This was in the face of contradictory findings in every major textbook of the day that clearly advocated treating patients with syphilis even in the disease's latent stages.

The study design called for the selection of black men with syphilis who were between the ages of 25 and 60 years. A physical examination (including radiographs) and a spinal tap were done to determine the incidence of neurosyphilis. The researchers had no intention of providing any treatment to the infected study participants. The research subjects were divided into two groups: 400 men with untreated syphilis and 200 men without syphilis who served as a control group.

Difficulties arose in recruiting subjects to the study. Consequently, the men were told they were ill and were offered free treatment. The offer of treatment appeared to secure the cooperation of participants. The USPHS did not inform participants that they were part of a research study on syphilis. On the contrary, they were told that they were being treated for "bad blood"—a colloquialism for syphilis. Subjects were given mercurial ointment, a noneffective drug, to maintain their interest in the study. The final procedure of the study was a spinal tap to test for neurosyphilis. To secure participants' participation for the potentially painful spinal tap, a letter was sent to them suggesting that the final examination they were now to receive was a very special one and after it was finished they would be given a special treatment if their condition warranted it. Hence, participants continued in the study under the guise of treatment.

In 1933, the USPHS decided to continue with the study despite the fact that their assumption regarding African-Americans' attitudes toward treatment of the disease proved wrong. There is no indication that treatment was ever considered an option for the study participants. At this point, it was concluded that only autopsies could scientifically confirm the findings of the study. Hence, a further series of deceptions and inducements were planned to maintain the men in the study so that autopsies could be performed at a later date. To secure continued cooperation of the men, a black nurse was hired to assess their health and secure approval for autopsies. The nurse offered noneffective medications (i.e., aspirin and tonic) and provided hot meals and transportation on the day of their examinations. When it became difficult to convince the men to come to the hospital as their illness progressed, the USPHS promised to cover the burial expenses of the men. This was a strong incentive because funerals were an important part of the cultural fabric of rural black communities in the South.

By 1936, the first reports of the study appeared in the medical press. It was apparent at this time that the men with syphilis developed many more complications than did the control group. By 1946, the death rate for the men with untreated syphilis was twice as high as it was for the control group. In 1955, it was reported that more than 30% of the test group autopsied died directly from advanced syphilitic lesions of the cardiovascular or central nervous system. In 1950, it was concluded, "We now know, where we could only surmise before, that we have contributed to their ailments and shortened their lives." A black physician, Vernal Cave, later wrote, "They proved a point, then proved a point, then proved a point."

For 40 years, the USPHS denied subjects treatment and took deliberate steps to see that participants did not receive treatment from

continued on next page

> **BOX 10.6** *What Happened in the Tuskegee Study? (Continued)*
>
> other sources. For example, in 1934, local black physicians were sent a list of subjects and letters requesting them to refer any black man on the list back to the USPHS if he sought treatment. In 1941, the army drafted a number of subjects and began treatment immediately. The USPHS supplied the draft board with a list of 256 names they wished to have excluded from treatment. The draft board cooperated. Most men in the study thought they were under the care of government doctors already and, therefore, saw no need to seek additional treatment.
>
> In 1969, the CDC reviewed the study and recommended that it should continue. Only one physician argued that the study should be stopped and the men treated. In July 1972, when the study was first published in the national press and provoked public outrage, data were still being collected and autopsies performed.
>
> SOURCE: Adapted from A.M. Brandt (1978). Racism and research: The case of the Tuskegee Syphilis Study. *Hastings Center Report, 8*(6), 21–29.

inflict harm, either emotional or physical; and **beneficence,** or the duty to promote or do good. To apply the concepts of nonmaleficence and beneficence, a standard of care must be provided by researchers. Standards of due care are usually established by society and by professional role expectations. Nurses' duties to act as a client advocate requires that nurses intervene if a research intervention produces more harm than benefit to a client. It is the researcher's responsibility to minimize risks and maximize benefits to participants; not doing so would contravene the ethical principle of beneficence.

When a nurse researcher is a care provider, the potential for conflict between the *duty to care* and the *duty to advance knowledge* may be imminent. Munhall (1988) and Smith (1997) refer to this as the *research imperative* (i.e., advancement of knowledge) versus the *therapeutic imperative* (i.e., duty to care). Sometimes it is challenging to determine at what point the therapeutic imperative is being compromised by the research imperative. Often good and harm are not easily separated. For example, a nurse researcher who is studying recovery patterns in frail elderly patients after hip replacement surgery may achieve a good outcome through early mobilization of clients (prevention of complications) but in the process may inflict pain and extreme discomfort (bad outcome). In these situations, the researcher must always try to maximize good (early recovery) and minimize harm and discomfort by providing good pain assessment and appropriate medication administration. Munhall suggests that when doubt is evident, the therapeutic imperative must take precedence over the research imperative for the nurse as caregiver. This is because nurses always have the responsibility to act as advocates for clients. The principles of respect for persons and beneficence, as well as the deontological perspective, support this decision.

c. Justice

The principle of **justice** requires that people be treated fairly. The protection of participants from incompetence and the right to receive research treatments are expectations of the justice principle. Justice is an important principle to follow in the selection of subjects for research studies, particularly in expensive biomedical experiments. The risks and benefits of a study should be fairly distributed among participants based on the subjects' efforts, needs, and rights. If possible, random selection of participants avoids potential sources of bias and unfairness in sample selection.

Nurses involved in any aspect of the research process have a responsibility to see that research complies with the principles of respect for persons, beneficence, and justice. This is true for nurses' own research as well as for research conducted by others that affects their clients.

4. Methods of Protecting Human Subjects

Two methods of protecting human subjects have been developed over the past three decades. These include the obtaining of informed consent and the review of research proposals by an ethics committee or institutional review board.

a. Informed Consent

Informed consent is based on the principle of respect for persons and incorporates the ethical concept of autonomy or the client's right to self-determine if he or she wishes to participate in a research study or not. The key elements of informed consent include disclosure of sufficient and appropriate information, understanding of information, and voluntary participation.

Sufficient and appropriate information implies that the researcher must produce a written consent form that ensures that subjects know they are participating in a research study as opposed to a normal treatment procedure. Subjects must be 18 years of age or older and fully understand the information given to them. The researcher should inform the participants in writing as well as verbally what the research protocol entails and what criteria were used to select the sample. The research consent form is signed, witnessed, and dated.

Fain (1999), Jackson (1999), and Martof (2000) are among researchers who sug-

gest that the following information be provided to potential participants in a research study:

1. Title of the study
2. Personnel engaged in the study
3. *Invitation* to participate in a study as opposed to a *request* to participate
4. Reason the individual is being asked to participate
5. Clear statement about the study's purpose
6. Detailed description of study's procedures (e.g., what exactly is required of the participants in terms of time, procedures, information requested)
7. Potential risks (e.g., physical, psychological, emotional) to participants and the steps that will be taken by the researcher to protect against the risks
8. Potential benefits of the study to the participants, society in general, and whether or not there are direct subject benefits
9. Any economic expenses or considerations that may result to subjects from participation in research
10. Steps that will be taken to ensure the confidentiality of data provided by participants
11. Freedom of participants to ask questions and to withdraw from the study at any time without penalty
12. The study will be discontinued if better treatments become available during the study or if it is evident that the study treatment is harmful to the participants or the subjects.
13. The institutional review board and participants will be informed of any new information that may impact on participant safety.
14. Subjects refusal to participate in the study will in no way jeopardize their treatment or otherwise harm them or detract from their rights in any way.

The sample consent form in Figure 10.1 addresses most of the above points. Children younger than age 18 years re-

TITLE

The Relationship of Definition of Health, Perceived Health Status, Self-Efficacy, and Parental Health-Promoting Lifestyle to Health-Promoting Lifestyle in Adolescent Females.
Principal Investigator: Angela Gillis, Ph.D., RN

PURPOSE

You and your daughter are invited to participate in a study of adolescent health-promoting lifestyles. The main objective of the study is to learn about the health-promoting lifestyles of adolescent girls and the factors that influence them to make healthy choices. You were selected as a possible participant because you have an adolescent daughter attending either senior or junior high school in the (name of school district). There will be approximately 175 adolescent females and their parents who will participate in the study.

PROCEDURES

If you decide to participate, each parent will be asked to complete individually a ten-minute questionnaire about his/her health behaviors and lifestyle activities. Each adolescent will complete a booklet of five questionnaires that will take a total of 45 minutes to complete. The questionnaires will ask information about the adolescents' health beliefs, health behaviors, and health-promoting lifestyle practices.

BENEFITS AND RISKS

You and your daughter may benefit from participation in this study by becoming more aware of your health-promoting lifestyle patterns, and by knowing you have contributed information that may help to improve the health of adolescent females. There is no physical risk involved in your participation and any psychological risk is minimal. The major inconvenience will be the time it will take to complete the questionnaires.

COSTS

There is no cost for participating in this study and no compensation will be made to study participants.

CONFIDENTIALITY

Your name will not appear on any questionnaires. Only a confidential code number will appear on the questionnaires. The number will be assigned by me and known only to me. The purpose of assigning the number is to keep parents' and daughters' questionnaires together. Study participants will not be identified in any way in the report of this study. Information will be kept confidential except if the information indicates illegal activity or information that is subject to mandatory reporting requirements or if it is information that represents immediate risk to the health and welfare of the adolescent.

You decision whether or not to participate in this study will not prejudice you or your daughter's future with (Name of school district). If you decide that you and your daughter may participate, you are free to withdraw from the study at any time without penalty.

Figure 10.1   Sample consent form. (*Continued on next page*)

quire a parent or legal guardian to give written informed consent on their behalf. Children age 7 years or older may give assent to participate. Figure 10.2 is a sample assent form.

Comprehension of information is essential to informed consent. The researcher must determine that the participants un-

derstand the information provided to them. It is incumbent on the researcher to make sure the participants understand both the risks involved as well as the benefits. They must also be fully informed about the research protocols so that they can make informed choices.

Voluntary participation implies that par-

Please feel free to ask any questions you may have about the study or your rights as a research participant. If other questions occur to you later you may contact Angela Gillis, Ph.D., RN, Principal Investigator at 902 856-6798.

A copy of this form is attached for you to keep for your records if you so desire. You are making a decision whether or not you and your daughter will participate in the study. Your signature indicates that you have read the information provided, understand it, and have decided that you and your daughter will participate. You and your daughter may withdraw at any time without prejudice after signing this form, should you choose to discontinue participation in the study.

Signature of Mother_____ Date_____

Signature of Father _____ Date _____

Signature of Adolescent _____ Date _____

Signature of Investigator _____ Date _____

Figure 10.1   (*Continued*)

ticipants agree to be part of a study of their own free will without coercion of any kind. The relationship between the participant and the researcher is integral to voluntary participation. At times, the participant may feel psychologically pressured to participate because of the closeness of the relationship that has developed between the two. Participants may not want to disappoint the researcher or may be eager to support the work of the researcher. In other situations, the participants may believe participation is their only option to receive a particular new therapy or drug. In all these situations, the researcher needs to be clear that an *invitation* rather than a *request* or *expectation* has been extended to participants to be part of the study. The researcher should provide clearly stated criteria and the rationale for subject selection. This step will protect the researcher and the participants. It enables

----

TITLE: The Relationship of Definition of Health, Perceived Health Status, Self-Efficacy, and Parental Health-Promoting Lifestyle to Health-Promoting Lifestyle in Adolescent Females.

Principal Investigator: Angela Gillis, Ph.D., RN

Assent: My parent/ legal guardian has explained this study to me. We have Dr. Gillis' telephone number and can call at any time if we have further questions. I have decided to participate in this study even though I know I do not have to do so.

Signature of adolescent or child: _____ Date: _____

Note: Assent is sought in children seven years of age or older. Older adolescents (18 years plus) may sign the informed consent document.

Figure 10.2   Sample assent form.

the researcher to demonstrate that participants have been fairly selected and the principle of justice enacted.

In qualitative investigations, the idea of **process consent** is suggested rather than traditional consent, which is signed at the beginning of a study and not reconsidered unless participants raise a concern about continued participation (Munhall, 1988). In process consent, the researcher renegotiates the consent with the participants as unforeseen circumstances arise. This allows the participants to be part of the decision making as the study unfolds.

b. Institutional Review Boards

Research involving humans should be subjected to approval by an ethics committee commonly referred to as an **institutional review board** (IRB) or an **ethics review board** (ERB). The purpose of the review is to ensure that ethical principles are appropriately applied to research involving human subjects. Most IRBs reviewing biomedical research operate under the guidelines of the Declaration of Helsinki.

Most institutions, hospitals, government agencies, and universities in which research involving human subjects is carried out require specific information to make informed and responsible decisions regarding the ethical acceptability of a proposal. The CNA (1997) and the ANA (1985) suggest that the following type of information should be included in a submission to an IRB:

- The purpose of the study and its significance to health research
- The study design and methodology
- Potential research participants and a description of the selection process
- Risks and benefits to the participants
- Steps to ensure participant choice, confidentiality, and anonymity protection
- Areas of potential conflict of interest

Most IRBs are mandated to approve, reject, or propose modifications to a proposal or to terminate unethical studies in progress. Membership in IRBs is usually multidisciplinary and designed to ensure expertise and independence essential to competent reviews. Hospital IRBs may be dominated at times by physicians who predominantly operate from a quantitative research perspective. This presents a unique challenge to nursing proposals that use qualitative methodologies and may not be well understood by all members of the IRB. Nurses have a professional responsibility to be members of IRBs and educate members about nursing approaches to research. Their main role is to make sure that the rights of human subjects are not violated.

In developing a timeline for the project, the researcher needs to consider the time it will take to obtain ethical approval for a study so that delays can be avoided. Most review boards have regularly scheduled meeting dates that are published in research newsletters. Researchers should inquire as to what deadline date their submission requires in order to meet their anticipated start date. Some projects may qualify for an expedited review that significantly reduces the time requirement. In an expedited review, the chairperson and at least one member of the IRB must read and approve the proposal. Examples of projects that may receive an expedited review include interviews, surveys, studies of existing records in which the data sought are not of a sensitive nature, and situations in which the use of noninvasive procedures are routine.

C. STUDIES ILLUSTRATING ETHICAL DILEMMAS

This section describes three studies that illustrate some of the ethical dilemmas faced by researchers despite the existence of methods of protecting human subjects and of guidelines such as professional codes of ethics, the Helsinki

Declaration, and the Nuremberg Code. After this review, a series of rules is presented to guide researchers in resolving ethical problems that may emerge.

There are a number of studies that have become landmarks in the discussion of research ethics. Two of these studies came to light in the 1970s and have become classic examples of unethical research. The first is the Tuskegee Syphilis Study, which began in 1932 and continued until 1972 when an account of the project in the *Washington Star* provoked public outrage. The project followed the natural course of syphilis in 400 black men who were untreated and remained so over the course of the study, even after the efficacy of penicillin to treat the condition was well established. The second study is the Willowbrook study (1950s–1970s) in which mentally challenged children institutionalized at the Willowbrook Institution were deliberately infected with the hepatitis virus. More recently, AIDS research denying azidothymidine (AZT) to women in African, Asian, and Caribbean nations (1997) has raised concern about the ethical acceptability of research funded by the National Institutes of Health (NIH) and the Centers for Disease Control and Prevention (CDC).

The Tuskegee and Willowbrook studies had substantial impact on the development of regulations governing biomedical and behavioral research. In 1973, the U.S. Department of Health, Education, and Welfare (DHEW) published its first set of regulations on the protection of human research subjects as a result of the Tuskegee atrocities. They also published additional guidelines to protect vulnerable participants such as mentally challenged, ill, and dying individuals. In 1978, the National Commission for the Protection of Human Subjects of Biomedical and Behavioral Research was established to develop ethical principles to underlie research on human subjects and formulate guidelines based on these principles. Its

findings are summarized in the Belmont Report.

In 1980, the Department of Health and Human Services (DHHS) developed a set of regulations based on the commission's recommendations. These regulations are regularly revised to keep pace with the changing health-care and research environment. They currently include:

1. Requirements for and documentation of informed consent
2. Membership of IRBs
3. Criteria for IRB approval of research and exempt and expedited review procedures for certain kinds of research

Although many studies do not pose serious ethical dilemmas for nurse researchers, it is important for beginning researchers to understand the impetus behind the development of the codes of ethics and research guidelines adopted by various professional and governmental agencies.

I. The Tuskegee Syphilis Study

We begin this section by examining a study that raises important ethical issues. In 1932, the U.S. Public Health Service (USPHS) began an experiment in Tuskegee, Alabama, to determine the natural course of untreated, latent syphilis in African-American males. The study included 400 men with syphilis and 200 uninfected men who served as control subjects. The study is now commonly referred to as the Tuskegee Syphilis Study. The study continued for approximately 40 years, through World War II, when a number of men were called up for the draft and would have been treated for syphilis except that they were study participants, and through the 1950s, even after the effectiveness of penicillin treatment was confirmed. The study survived the 1960s and was untouched by the Nuremberg Code, the Declaration of Helsinki, the Civil Rights Movement, and the USPHS Code of Research Ethics. This research begs the question of how could such a seemingly unethical investigation be approved, funded, and allowed to continue for so long at such cost to participants and society? A summarized excerpt from the Hastings Center Report of the Tuskegee Syphilis Study is included in Box 10.6.

Published accounts of the Tuskegee study in the national press in 1972 provoked both critical comment and support from members of the scientific community. Many have opposed the research on ethical grounds; the statements of Brandt (1978), Rothman (1982), and Caplan and colleagues, (1992) are particularly incisive. The following quotation from Brandt provides a sense of his position:

> . . . The Tuskegee Syphilis Study Ad Hoc Advisory Panel Report ignores many of the essential ethical issues which the study poses. The Tuskegee study reveals the persistence of beliefs within the medical profession about the nature of blacks, sex, and disease-beliefs that had tragic repercussions long after their alleged scientific bases was known to be incorrect. Most strikingly, the entire health of a community was jeopardized by leaving a communicable disease untreated. There can be little doubt that the Tuskegee researchers regarded their subjects as less than human. As a result the ethical canons of experimenting on human subjects were completely disregarded.
>   . . . The injustice committed by the experiment went well beyond the facts outlined in the national press or the HEW Final Report. The degree of deception and damages have been seriously underestimated.

Brandt goes on to argue that the final report betrayed a basic misunderstanding of the experiment's purposes and design by focusing on the issues of penicillin therapy and informed consent. The report failed to recognize that the entire study had been predicated on nontreatment. Administration of medication would have violated the rationale of the experiment—to study the natural course of the disease until death. The report also failed to expose the critical fact that not only was voluntary and informed consent not obtained but rather, the men were told and they believed that they were getting free treatment from expert government doctors. According to Brandt, the failure of the report to expose this critical fact calls into question the credibility of the investigation.

Kampmeier, cited by Brandt (1978), wrote a spirited defense of the Tuskegee study in the *Southern Medical Journal* in response to the HEW Final Report. His argument centered on the limited knowledge of effective therapy for latent syphilis when the experiment began. He argues that by 1950, penicillin would have been of no value to these men and suggests that the men were fortunate to have been spared the highly toxic treatments of earlier periods. The USPHS maintained that the study was ethical on the grounds that it constituted " a study of nature." The USPHS insisted that Macon County was "a ready-made laboratory" and the researchers would only be watching the inevitable. They assumed subjects were not going to obtain treatment anyway and there was, therefore, no reason to miss the opportunity to trace the effects of their disease process.

The Department of Health, Education, and Welfare (HEW) Final Report (1973) focused on two ethical objections to the Tuskegee study. These include:

1. The study violated the ethical rule that a person should not be subjected to avoidable risk of death or harm unless he or she freely consents in an informed manner.
2. The study was scientifically unsound and its results meager in comparison

with the known risks it imposed on the subjects involved.

There appear to be five key points in the Tuskegee study that raise ethical issues:

1. The researchers did not obtain informed consent from the participants.
2. The researchers deliberately withheld information from participants about their involvement in a research study and deceived them into thinking they were receiving effective treatment for "bad blood."
3. Unknown to the participants, the researchers denied them penicillin when it became available in the 1940s as an effective treatment and took deliberate steps to prevent them from getting treatment from other sources.
4. Their names were circulated on a list to various physicians, treatment sources, and the U.S. draft board; therefore, participants' rights to confidentiality and anonymity were violated.
5. Participants did not voluntarily participate but rather were coerced under the guise of free medical treatment, assessment by expert government doctors, free hospitalization, and provision of burial services.

The exposure of the Tuskegee study by the national press had a positive influence on the development of guidelines to protect the rights of human subjects in biomedical and behavioral research through the establishment of the National Commission for the Protection of Human Subjects of Biomedical and Behavioral Research. It also raised significant questions about professional self-regulation and scientific bureaucracy. It pointed out the need for greater vigilance in assessing the specific ways in which social values and attitudes affect professional behavior and raised awareness of how groups already disadvantaged in society need to be protected from such unethical investigations as well as included in clinical trials that

may benefit them. Nonetheless, the study raised many agonizing ethical questions that still remain unanswered.

2. The Willowbrook Study

For a period of approximately 20 years (1950s–1970s), mentally challenged children at the Willowbrook Institution in Staten Island, New York, were participants in an unethical research investigation designed to improve the understanding of hepatitis. The study was directed toward determining the period of infectivity of infectious hepatitis. All of the subjects were mentally handicapped children who were given either intramuscular or oral doses of the hepatitis virus. Saul Krugman of New York University was the head of the research team. His team systematically infected new child residents with the hepatitis viruses over the 20-year period of the study. Parents were forced to give permission for their children to be study participants if they wished to gain their child's admission to the institution. Parents gave consent for the administration of the virus, but they were not told the appreciable hazards involved. Parents were told that their children would be placed on the "Krugman" ward that was cleaner, better supervised, and had a higher nurse-to-patient ratio than the general wards. They were not told of the debilitating flulike symptoms, skin rashes, liver damage, and resulting morbidity and mortality patterns that many of the children eventually experienced. During the 20-year investigation, the Willowbrook Institution closed its door to new admissions because of overcrowding, yet the research ward continued to admit new residents. The institute denies this claim, referring to documentation of new admissions on the research unit as administrative errors.

This experiment and the study protocol were well publicized in medical literature. The study was documented among the 22 examples of unethical investigations published by Beecher (1966) in the *New England Journal of Medicine*. Nevertheless, this investigation was allowed to continue for 20 years, even after the efficacy of gamma globulin to weaken (if not prevent) an attack of hepatitis had been established. The Krugman team defended the investigation as a "natural experiment." They argued that residents would most likely contract the disease naturally within a few weeks of admission because of the substandard hygienic conditions and staff shortages that made contagion probable. Furthermore, they believed the study would bring immediate advantages to the participants such as provision of care on a cleaner, better supervised treatment ward, a higher nurse-to-patient ratio, and closer supervision of their condition with fewer opportunities for complications.

Although there is a valid category of research called "natural experiments" in the health sciences, the question remains: Was the Willowbrook experiment an ethical "study in nature?" Rothman (1982) answers this question succinctly. He explains that when no cure or treatment exists for a disease, then observing its course with the informed consent of participants is a *study in nature*. In his opinion, the Willowbrook experiment does *not* belong in this category of research because there is an essential difference between taking advantage of *social*, as opposed to *biological*, conditions. "Poverty, ignorance, filth, and institutional miseries are not in any way comparable to the inevitable course of a mysterious disease or the unknown risks posed by carriers. Indeed, the Tuskegee and Willowbrook experiments offer both practical and principled support for maintaining as rigid a distinction between social deprivation and biological conditions as possible" (Rothman, 1982, p. 6).

The ethical issues raised by this investigation warrant comment. They include:

1. The informed consent process was suspect on two levels, namely, the manipulation of the parents to secure consent of the subjects if they wished to have their child admitted to the Willowbrook Institution and the withholding of vital information about the appreciable hazards of the experiment. Parents were not fully informed about the potential consequences of the inoculation or the types of harm that could come to their children as a result of the disease process. It was apparent that the rights of the subjects' guardians to informed consent were flagrantly disregarded.

2. In the Willowbrook investigation, the research team continued with the study even after the discovery of gamma globulin to weaken or prevent an attack of hepatitis was publicized. This action clearly violates the resolution adopted by the World Medical Association, which states: "Under no circumstances is a doctor permitted to do anything which would weaken the physical or mental resistance of a human being except from strictly therapeutic or prophylactic indications imposed in the interest of the patient." The risk to the participants was clearly too high and not outweighed by benefits for the participants or society. Clearly the dictum that one must not inflict harm on one group for the advantage of another was violated by this study. Social deprivation and continued predictions of it (i.e., that Willowbrook residents would contract hepatitis "naturally" anyway) became a self-fulfilling prophecy in this situation.

3. Unethical AIDS Research

More recently, there has been controversy raised by Public Citizen (1997), a consumer group affiliated with Ralph Nader, that has criticized U.S. AIDS research as being "dangerously flawed." It has claimed that the United States is conducting unethical research that has caused the deaths of approximately 1000 children overseas. At issue are nine studies involving approximately 9000 women from African, Asian, and Caribbean nations that are involved in AIDS research trials in which some of the women are being denied access to AZT; instead, they are being given placebos.

The studies are underwritten by either the NIH or the CDC. Based on federal government documents, the Public Citizen claims that the U.S. government is deliberately denying AIDS-infected women access to AZT, a drug that U.S. studies have shown clearly reduces the transmission of the AIDS virus from pregnant women to their unborn babies by two-thirds. Similar studies involving U.S. women offer effective anti-HIV therapy to all participants. Sidney Wolfe, Director of Public Citizen, claims, "It is Tuskegee part two." Dr. Peter Lurie of Public Citizen states, "It's certainly as bad as anything that has occurred since World War II in terms of the violations of the basics of medical ethics." He goes on to comment, "It is a clear-cut double standard, and for the babies involved it will be lethal. We are demanding today that the federal government provide AZT or similar drugs to all of the women in these studies."

The claims of the Public Citizen sparked debate by U.S. officials. In defense of their work, U.S. researchers claim it is not feasible or scientifically proper to give AZT to all patients involved with the research. Philip Nieburg, an AIDS researcher with the CDC, claims that AZT is unavailable and unaffordable in developing countries. He stresses the importance of comparing new treatments with the existing "standard of care" in a particular country and concludes that AZT is not the standard of care in developing countries. The government insists a placebo comparison is the only way to prove potential new therapies are better than no treatment. Helen Gayle of the CDC defends the study, stating that in the countries involved, the health-care expenditure on women is about $10 per year, and so it is important that any results of this investigation be relevant and affordable.

This investigation raises ethical concerns because of parallels with the Tuskegee and the Willowbrook studies. It reinforces the important need for institutional review boards to review studies conscientiously and for researchers to act ethically. Researchers need to be cautious that they do not place themselves in ethically untenable positions by engaging in research that builds on social deprivation of others. Rothman (1982) cautions that as soon as researchers attempt to take advantage of the social predicament in which participants are found, they become accomplices to the problem, not observers of it. This is because researchers usually have the ability to alter the social deprivation of the study participants, although not the larger class that they represent. Could the research team have administered AZT or a comparable drug to the participants in the study? If researchers approach providing fair and equitable treatment to participants with the same zeal that they pursue their experiments, it may be possible to secure funds or grants to do so. Rothman concludes, "Where the essential cause of a health problem is social deprivation, it is generally within the power of the research team to remedy the situation for their subjects. Hence, they cannot be observers to a plight they can improve" (p. 7).

D. RULES FOR CONDUCTING ETHICAL RESEARCH

The following ethical rules are presented as guidelines and are organized around two themes: (1) nurse researchers' ethical responsibility to participants and (2) nurse researchers' responsibility to the discipline of nursing and society.

I. Rules for the Treatment of Participants

Rule 1. Protect the confidentiality of participants. The researcher's promise to respect the confidentiality of participant responses to a questionnaire or an interview or the identity of a participant in an experiment or field study is to be treated as a sacred trust. It is based on the ethical principal of respect for persons. Most surveys, interviews, experiments, and field studies are completed on the understanding that individual responses and information that would permit the identification of the individual will never be released. Researchers have not only an ethical responsibility to preserve the anonymity of participants but also have a practical interest in doing so: Their ability to collect accurate information would be impaired if the public believed that responses were not kept in confidence.

When it is necessary to identify individual names with particular questionnaires (e.g., as in panel studies) number codes—rather than names— should be used. The questionnaires and a master list listing names and identification numbers can then be stored separately. Such master lists should be destroyed after the study has been completed.

If data are released to other researchers, steps should be taken to mask the individual identities of participants. This can be achieved by removing highly specific identifiers such as area of residence, specific job, or employer identifications.

The Tuskegee study clearly violated the participants' confidentiality. Not only were the identities of participants in the experimental group known, but lists containing their names were deliberately circulated to potential treatment centers and the U.S. draft board to prevent participants from seeking treatment elsewhere.

In qualitative investigations in which sample sizes are limited and the depth of interviewing significant, it becomes challenging to protect the confidentiality of the participants. This is particularly problematic when one is conducting research in areas that require the researcher to probe deeply into the life circumstances of the participants. Direct quotations, rich in detail, are often used to answer the research question. The researcher must be vigilant about not revealing information in the research report or publications that result from it that may reveal the identities of participants. Pseudonyms should be used in both the data collection process and in the transcription of interview tape recordings so that the participants' true identities cannot be associated with the data. The researcher should also periodically remind participants that they are free not to respond to questions or probes that they believe are inappropriate. If someone other than the researcher is transcribing the taped interviews, participants have a right to know this and be assured that their identity will be protected.

Rule 2. Do not place pressure on participants. No pressure should be placed on participants to cooperate in a study. Respondents must feel free to refuse participation, to withdraw at any time, or to refuse to answer any particular question. Researchers should not put pressure on participants or cajole or harass them in an effort to get cooperation with the study. This maxim is based on the principle of respect for person.

Although it is appropriate in mail surveys to follow up with those who do not respond with a phone call, these contacts should provide prospective participants an opportunity to seek additional information about the project to help them decide if they wish to participate.

Participants should not be presented with either excessive rewards or threats of punishment to secure their participation. To do so violates the participant's right to self-determination. The Willowbrook study appeared to place a lot of pressure on parents to consent to have their children inoculated with the hepatitis virus. Indeed, some say it was the only way a resident could be admitted to the overcrowded institution after the general wards were closed. The participants in the Tuskegee study were cajoled over a period of 40 years to cooperate with the syphilis investigation. This included repeated promises of free treatment, supervision by medical experts, free hospitalization, transportation to clinic assessments, and paid burial services. In both these investigations, it appears pressure was intentionally placed on participants to cooperate.

Rule 3. Make the subjects' participation painless and free from discomfort and harm. Completing a questionnaire or interview or participating as a subject in an experiment should be a safe and painless experience for the participant. Researchers must not expose participants to needlessly long experimental trials or questionnaires or ask questions that pry unnecessarily into personal matters. This constraint is not meant to suggest that researchers should not examine certain areas of human behavior but suggests that only relevant information be collected. (Often when people are working on their first project, they suggest many variables; however, when asked what they would do with the information, they are unable to articulate a meaningful analysis.) Moreover, consideration should be given to using alternate, or indirect, indicators for the questions that may offend participants.

Maintaining the safety, comfort, and self-esteem of the participants should be a central concern of researchers. It is based on the principle of beneficence, which requires that one should do good and, above all, do no harm. This requires the researcher to create a situation in which the benefits to the respondents outweigh the risks or harm that may result from the study. Harm can take many forms such as physical, emotional, social, spiritual, or financial forms.

The Willowbrook study has been faulted for its adverse effects on the participants' health state. Should the investigators have injected a virus into the bodies of children that would no doubt produce hepatitis and other adverse reactions in the participants? Should the experiment have been aborted after the efficacy of gamma globulin to weaken, if not prevent, an attack of hepatitis was confirmed? The same question must be asked of the Tuskegee study after the efficacy of penicillin as a treatment for syphilis was established. Other researchers have decided to abort projects when it was clear that the study had potential dangers to participants.

Piliavin and Piliavin (1972), for example, aborted trials on the bystander intervention studies after it was clear that there were dangers involved in staging phony emergencies. The researchers stopped one study when it was observed that bystanders, seeing a person fall with blood trickling from his mouth, activated an emergency stop alarm. It was simply too dangerous and disruptive to continue.

Professor C. Boeck, Chief of the Oslo Venereal Clinic between 1890 to 1910, when the famous Oslo study of untreated patients with syphilis was ongoing, is another scientist who abandoned a study in progress. As lead researcher in the world famous Oslo Study of untreated patients with syphilis, Boeck had withheld treatment to nearly 2000 patients infected with syphilis. He was convinced that current treatments with mercurial ointment were of no value. After arsenic therapy was discovered and made widely available in 1910, he abandoned the study (Clark and Danbolt, 1955).

Rule 4. Identify sponsors. There should be no deception concerning the sponsorship of a project. Participants must be informed about who is doing the study. On this basis alone, they may choose not to participate in the study.

Many people have opened their doors to a person claiming to be doing a survey on satisfaction with delivery of health-care services, only to discover that they are not dealing with a reputable scientist but rather with a door-to-door health insurance salesperson. Feel free to encourage the "researcher" to leave rapidly! Similarly, an individual may choose to not participate in a study conducted by an organization whose aims and objectives are unacceptable to him or her.

Rule 5. Disclose the basis on which participants have been selected. The consensus in the nursing research community is that participants have the right to know how they were selected for participation in a study. In the past, unfair sample selection resulted because of social biases or biases on the part of the researcher or funding source. Biases take many forms in sample selection. They may include treating subjects poorly with little regard for their safety or providing benefits unfairly to subjects that could offer power or money to researchers. The Tuskegee Syphilis Study is an example of how racial and social biases played a role in unfair sample selection.

The prospective participant should be given a reasonable amount of information about the selection process on which a decision to participate can be made. For example, respondents need to know if the selection was made by means of a probability sampling procedure or if it was based on special characteristics (e.g., age group, health status, medical diagnosis, membership in a particular organization, the job one has) related to the research problem or phenomenon under investigation. Random selection can eliminate some of the researcher bias that may influence subject selection. Fair selection of participants is based on the ethical principle of justice, which states that every person should be treated fairly and given what they are due.

Rule 6. Place no hidden identification codes on questionnaires. Researchers should not use hidden codes on questionnaires to assist in the identification of those who have or have not returned questionnaires. Such codes are sometimes used to enable researchers to find out who has not returned a questionnaire; such subjects may be sent another request. Although such codes may save the researcher much time and money, they are unethical. If individuals are to be identified, this information should be placed directly on the questionnaire itself (not hidden) and discussed in a cover letter. For example, a questionnaire may contain an identification code number such as 001. The participant must be informed that this number is used only by the researcher to associate that particular questionnaire with a specific individual. The identification codes and corresponding participant names should be kept in a secure area to protect the identity of participants. Only the researcher should have access to this information.

Rule 7. Honor promises to provide participants with research reports. When an offer to provide a research report to respondents has been given, the promise must be fulfilled. The relationship between the researcher and participants or respondents should be reciprocal. In practice, it is to the advantage of the researcher to fulfill such obligations because doing so will encourage the continued cooperation of participants in long-term projects.

When individuals are offered the opportunity of receiving a report on the study, a separate stamped envelope and request form should be provided for the respondent. The separate return envelope not only keeps the respondent's name disassociated from the questionnaire but also conveys to the respondent that the researcher takes a promise of confidentiality seriously.

Although there may be no ethical responsibility to pay participants who volunteer their cooperation, such payments are encouraged in order to reinforce the idea of a reciprocal contract between researchers and participants. Participant observation studies frequently involve rather long periods of observation, and it is particularly important to reciprocate by providing a payment or a report on the research project.

Rule 8. Informed consent is a key concern. In dealing with competent adults, participation should be based on informed consent—that is, potential participants must be informed about the nature of the study, what kinds of issues will be explored, how participants were selected, what the risks and benefits to the participants are, and who is sponsoring the research. Moreover, prospective participants should be informed about confidentiality and anonymity and they should feel free to withdraw from the study at any time without prejudice if they wish to do so. In surveys, respondents should be told to feel free to skip any questions that they consider inappropriate or ignore interview questions that make them uncomfortable.

Implicit in informed consent is the participant's ability to comprehend the implications of participating in a research study. It is not enough to provide appropriate and sufficient information; the researcher must also ensure that participants understand the information and know they have the freedom to participate or refuse to participate in the study. The concepts of self-determination and autonomy are central to the principle of respect for person. This principle forms the foundation for informed consent.

With studies involving children, ill patients, or incompetent adults, the organization or individual responsible for the prospective participants should provide consent in writing. In addition, children age 7 years or older should give *assent* to participate. Assent means a child has voluntarily agreed to be a participant in a research study. By age 7 years, children are capable of concrete operational thought and, therefore, can provide meaningful assent to participate. As children age, they should be given more responsibility in the consent process.

The issue of informed consent may be a problem for researchers doing participant observation studies. It would not be reasonable to insist that all members being observed would have to consent to being observed. The test in such cases perhaps should be (1) whether sufficient steps are taken to protect the anonymity of those who are observed and (2) that no negative consequences could reasonably be seen to result from the activity of the research project.

To put a blanket prohibition on such studies would mean that works such as Erving Goffman's *Asylums,* Margaret Mead's *Sex and Temperament in Three Primitive Societies,* or Madeleine Leininger's *Transcultural Theory of Caring* could not have been done and the benefit derived from such work would have been lost to society.

Naturalistic observational studies, such as those observing whether the drivers of automobiles have their seat belts fastened, can be performed as long as there is no apparent danger to the subject being observed or to the observer. In such cases, it is not possible to gain the permission of the person being observed. When deciding if the study should be undertaken, the best test the researcher can make is an attempt to balance any good that may come out of the project against its potentially negative consequences.

Some researchers believe covert methods are sometimes appropriate in social science research (Warwick and Douglas; cited in Punch, 1986, p. 29). In some situations, the job of the researcher is to expose the powerful who prey on weaker members of society. This occurs, at times, in research with AIDS patients and victims of violence, child abuse, drug addictions, and various forms of deviant behavior. However, researchers traditionally have been harshly criticized for acting as undeclared participant observers. Laud Humphreys' (1970) study of male homosexual behavior in which he infiltrated the gay community as a covert observer is an example of such deception.

In experimental studies, particularly those involving some deception, there is a problem concerning informed consent. If the experimental manipulation requires deception, it is not possible to inform the subject fully, in advance, of the deception: to do so would spoil the study. In such cases, Rule 9 needs to be applied.

In randomized clinical trials (RCTs), it is not necessary to inform participants if they have been assigned to a treatment or control group; however, it is necessary to inform participants that the research involves use of a placebo or nontreatment group. There is also

no justification for failing to inform participants of how they will be assigned to groups. Such information is essential to informed consent to participate in the study (Neuberger, 1992).

Anytime selective nondisclosure of information or deception is used in a research study, the researcher must question how acceptable it is to do so. With deception, the risks to the participants should be minimal and outweighed by the benefits. Beauchamp and Childress (1989) identify four conditions under which deception may be considered justifiable in research:

1. Deception is essential to obtain important information.
2. No other substantial risk is involved to participants.
3. Other ethical principles are not violated such as beneficence or nonmaleficence.
4. Subjects are informed that deception is part of the study before they consent to participate.

Rule 9. Debrief subjects. When experiments or field studies involve deception, subjects should have the study explained to them after the session. The researcher should note what deception was used and why it was necessary, and the subjects should be reassured that their participation was appreciated and helpful.

2. Rules for Socially Responsible Nursing Research

Nurse researchers have ethical responsibilities not only to the participants in a project but also to society at large and to the nursing discipline. Research-minded practitioners, educators, administrators, nursing students, and other health-care professionals expect nurse researchers to do ethical research. They depend on the results of nursing studies to shape their practice and promote excellence in nursing care. This situation places a considerable ethical responsibility on nurse researchers to conduct unbiased studies and report results in trustworthy manners.

Rule 10. Researchers should distinguish between science and advocacy. In your role as a nurse scientist, do not work on projects in which you are asked to develop a "scientific case" for a conclusion. Given the legitimacy of science in Western culture, it should be no surprise that both scientists and nonscientists are tempted to use this legitimacy to achieve personal or group goals. Evidence that is viewed as scientific carries a lot of weight in argument; therefore, when a presentation is being prepared, collecting or referring to scientific evidence is tempting and sensible.

If you are hired to "develop a scientific case for . . . " then you have an ethical problem. You are being asked to provide scientific evidence to convince others of a particular position. You are, in this case, being asked to make others believe that you have scientific evidence for the particular position. Such research should not be presented as science; to do so would be unethical.

As a citizen–advocate, it is perfectly legitimate to comment on the evidence of others and to produce evidence that is appropriate to the issue under dispute. It should be noted, however, that the information is being presented from the perspective of a citizen–advocate, not from that of an expert nurse scientist. We would be well advised to maintain a distinction between citizen–advocate roles and researcher roles. Too often the line between them is blurred.

Rule 11. Do not hunt through data looking for pleasing findings. The surest way to be guilty of misrepresentation is to search for support for your own views. To do so would be both bad science and unethical behavior. If data are

being scanned for interesting findings, these cannot be reported unless the process by which they have emerged is made absolutely clear.

Rule 12. Be aware of potential sources of bias. Becoming aware of the sources of bias may help you avoid bias in your own work and spot it in the research reports of others. Researchers have an ethical responsibility to report their work fairly, attempting to avoid bias as much as possible. Review the discussion of sources of bias in Chapter 9.

Rule 13. Represent research literature fairly. In the interest of objectivity and ethics, researchers must attempt to accurately portray the body of literature in their area of research. Reporting findings selectively is not acceptable.

Rule 14. Do the best research you can. Research must strive to be competent and impartial, and its results must be reported objectively. Use qualified personnel and consultants. Keep up with developments in your field and use the best techniques of data collection and analysis. Always seek to do the best research you can; do research with care.

Rule 15. Acknowledge all your sources. Acknowledge people who have played a role in your research and acknowledge all literature sources that have directly influenced your study. Excluding the respondents (who have been assured of anonymity), all other people who have assisted in the project should be acknowledged by way of footnotes in your report. Similarly, when literature has been used in developing the project, each source should be cited.

Rule 16. Seek advice on ethical issues. If ethical issues arise, seek the advice of appropriate professional bodies or institutions involved in the project. Most studies do not pose difficult ethical issues; however, when the research team identifies an ethical dilemma, outside consultations are appropriate. Such consultations weigh the benefits of the

B. DESCRIBING AN INDIVIDUAL VARIABLE

In this section, we consider how individual variables may be described. We look at data distributions, measures of central tendency, how variation within a variable is measured, approaches to standardizing variables, and the characteristics of a *normal* distribution.

I. Data Distributions

Quantitative researchers need to simplify the complexity of their data to communicate their results effectively. Many tools are available to researchers to help in this endeavor. Data may be displayed in graphs, summarized by showing how many cases fall in each category, or described using any number of descriptive statistics.

A **data distribution** simply refers to a listing of all the values for any one variable. However, to simply provide a list of the data would not be terribly helpful to the reader of a report. Usually there are simply too many numbers and it is difficult to make much sense out of a listing of raw data. For example, Table 11.1 shows the scores that nursing students received

in two tests. Examine the grades. If you were asked to indicate the test on which the nursing students did best, what would you say? The task is a frustrating one because the mass of detail is overwhelming. The need for some method of summarizing the grades quickly becomes apparent. It is inefficient to read an unordered listing of numbers.

The challenge for the researcher is to find ways to characterize a distribution in a simple way. One of the most basic techniques for simplifying a large data set is to create a **frequency distribution table.** This is a systematic listing of all the values on a variable from the lowest to the highest with the number of times (frequency) each value was observed. Suppose the researcher has recorded the weight, size of home community, and gender of subjects. The researcher may show a frequency distribution in each category of gender (appropriate for nominal and ordinal data), use a bar graph to show how many respondents came from communities of different sizes (also appropriate for nominal and ordinal data), or use plots of the data to describe the distribution of egalitarianism scores among the respondents (appropriate for ratio variables). Table 11.2 shows a frequency distribution and a bar

Table 11.1   Two Sets of Nursing Grades for a First-Year Class

Test A. Results

60	60	82	71	60	58	64	81	58	58	70	57	56
56	69	58	55	82	46	54	62	61	77	70	59	74
87	47	57	63	37	67	55	59	63	59	55	52	58
63	72	54	54	62	69	66	58	53	73	57	68	52
75	47	52	73	72	65	64	63	59	57			

Test B. Results

53	64	83	60	61	61	61	83	54	58	68	55	49
60	59	55	53	69	44	56	48	54	74	71	49	54
86	51	67	63	59	63	55	40	65	63	62	55	49
53	72	59	59	54	69	73	57	59	72	26	65	70
60	45	60	69	66	63	51	59	63	63			

Table 11.2   Frequency Distribution and Bar Chart for Size of Home Community

Size of Home Community	Frequency	Percent	Valid Percent	Cumulative Percent
Under 1,000	18	9.7	10.3	10.3
1,000 to 4,999	20	10.8	11.5	21.8
5,000 to 9,999	17	9.1	9.8	31.6
10,000 to 19,000	15	8.1	8.6	40.2
20,000 to 49,999	29	15.6	16.7	56.9
50,000 to 99,999	21	11.3	12.1	69.0
100,000 to 499,999	10	5.4	5.7	74.7
500,000 to 99,999	7	3.8	4.0	78.7
1,000,000 and over	37	19.9	21.3	100.00
Total	174	93.5	100.00	
Missing	12	6.5		
Total	186	100.0		

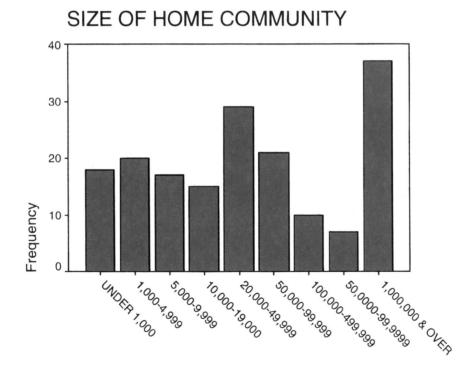

SIZE OF HOME COMMUNITY

graph for the size of home communities for respondents in a study.

The egalitarianism scores (Fig. 11.1) could also be plotted, but this time we will also include a distribution curve line on this plot. Note how the plot line indicates few low scores, many more in the middle, with a tapering off at the high score end. This distribution is described as a *normal distribution*. Normal distributions are de-

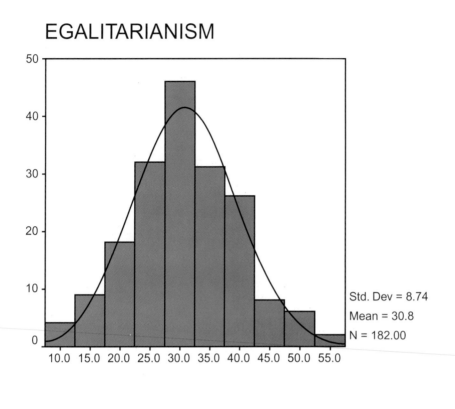

Figure 11.1   Frequency distribution with a normal curve, egalitarianism scores.

scribed in detail later in this chapter; for now, simply note how the distribution roughly forms a bell-shaped curve.

But there are other distribution curves. Not all variables are normally distributed. If, for example, we were to plot the weights of freshman students, we would almost certainly find that the result would be a **bimodal distribution.** The reason for this is that female students have lower average weights than the males. Essentially we would end up combining two normally distributed plots, one for women and one for men, and one that would have two peaks and considerable overlap between the male and female weights (Fig. 11.2.)

If a set of values has little variability, then the distribution is *peaked* and it is said to be **leptokurtic;** on the other hand, if the distribution has a great deal of vari-

ability, the distribution curve tends to be *flat and wide* and is called a **platykurtic** distribution. An example of these two plots is shown in Figure 11.2. The recognition that distributions can be quite different from one another will be important when the time comes to learn about sampling (Chapter 15) and tests of significance (Chapter 12).

Besides plotting the data distribution or showing the frequency distribution, there are other standard ways in which data distributions are described. A variety of conventions are used to describe the central tendency, the variation in or dispersion of a variable, as well as commonly used methods used to standardize variables to facilitate comparisons. We first explore the main tools used to describe a variable's central tendency.

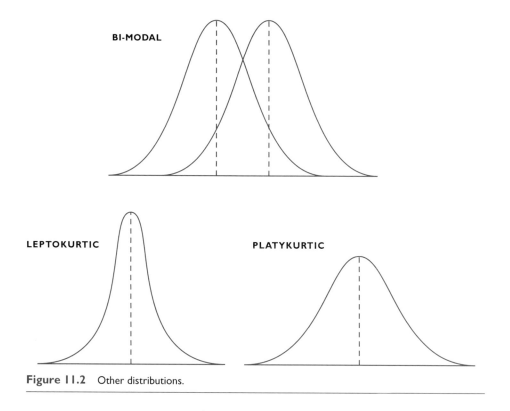

Figure 11.2 Other distributions.

2. Measures of Central Tendency

A **measure of central tendency** is a single numeric value that summarizes the data set in terms of its "average" value. Just as baseball fans cite the batting average to summarize a player's hitting ability, nurse researchers may use the value of 98.6°F (or 37°C) to describe the average adult body temperature. Three measures of central tendency are commonly used: the mode, the median, and the mean.

a. The Mode

The **mode** is the category or value of a *nominal variable* with the most cases in a distribution of values. If one wishes, for example, to describe "average" respondents in terms of their country of origin, then the mode would be the appropriate statistic. In the case of country of origin, it may be Canada. This would simply mean that

Canada was the most frequently occurring response to the question asking respondents to indicate their country. Table 11.3 presents a frequency distribution (simply reports the number of respondents who fall into each category) of respondents who report themselves to be from each of the five countries listed. From Table 11.3, one can identify the modal category by looking at the "Number" column, and pick-

Table 11.3 Distribution of Respondents by Country

Country	Number	Percent
Australia	63	15.5
Canada	165*	40.5
New Zealand	58	14.3
United Kingdom	43	10.6
United States	78	19.2
Total	407	100.1

*Mode.

ing out the category that has the highest frequency; in this case, the category is "Canada."

For nominal or ordinal variables, it is appropriate to determine the mode and the median values as well as the frequency distribution of the variable.

b. The Median

The **median** represents the midpoint of a distribution. One half the cases fall above the median value and one half below it. The median is normally used for *ordinal level variables* or in cases where the use of a mean would be problematic because a few extreme values would give an inappropriate impression of the typical case. The steps in determining the median are:

- Arrange the cases in order from highest to lowest or lowest to highest values.
- Number the values (ignoring no response or missing data).
- If there is an odd number of cases, then the middle value is identified and that value is the median for the distribution.
- If, however, there is an even number of cases, then the mean of the middle two is calculated and that value represents the median.

Table 11.4 illustrates a situation in which a median would be a better description of a sample than would a mean. Here the data list the annual incomes of 15 graduate students enrolled in nurse midwifery programs in California. When we compare the extremely high salary of $580,000 with the much more modest incomes of the other nursing students surveyed, we realize that citing the mean would give the false impression that the incomes of graduate students are quite high. The median value of $18,300 is a much better description of the income distribution than the mean of $54,213. When atypical values are present, the median may provide a better description of the data.

Table 11.4   Median for Nurse Graduate Students: An Extreme Value Problem

Case Number	Income, dollars
1	5,400
2	6,600
3	7,700
4	10,200
5	13,400
6	16,400
7	16,700
8	18,300*
9	19,000
10	20,000
11	20,500
12	22,900
13	24,600
14	31,500**
15	580,000

*Median value is $18,300
**Mean value is $54,213

c. The Mean

The *mean* is a measure of central tendency that typifies a set of observations with a single value. Recall the grades in the two first-year tests shown in Table 11.1. Earlier you were asked to indicate the test on which the nursing students did best. The task is a frustrating one because the mass of detail is overwhelming. The need for some method of summarizing the grades quickly becomes apparent. It is inefficient to read an unordered listing of numbers.

Computing means may be a first step in comparing the grades in the two sections. The **mean** (more formally known as the *arithmetic mean* and less formally as the *average*) is computed by summing the values of a variable and dividing the result by the total number of cases. A mean is used on *ratio level* data. To find the mean grade in each test, we would simply sum the grades and then divide by the number of students. This would result in a mean grade for each section of the course. Table 11.5 reports the means, showing that the average performance was somewhat higher in test A. Students scored 2.0 points higher on the first test than on the second one. That difference is not easily apparent in looking at the raw scores.

3. Measures of Dispersion

Besides describing a variable in terms of central tendency, it is helpful to know something about the extent of the variability, or dispersion, of the values. Are most of the values close to one another, or are they spread out? To illustrate, suppose we have two students, Mary and Beth. Their grades are indicated in Table 11.6. Although both students have an identical 82 percent average, the distributions are quite different. Mary's grades vary little, but Beth's vary considerably. We will explore three **measures of dispersion** in the two students' grades: range, standard deviation, and variance.

a. Range

The **range** is a measure of the gap between the lowest and highest value in a distribution. It is computed by subtracting the lowest value from the highest one. Although the range is a simple one to calculate by using only the extreme scores, it fails to reflect variations between the other scores. It tends also to be rather un-

stable when different samples are drawn from the same population. Table 11.6 indicates that the range of Beth's grades is 28, but Mary's is 10, indicating much less variability in Mary's grades compared with Beth's.

b. Standard Deviation

Researchers rely heavily on the **standard deviation** to give them a sense of how much dispersion there is in a distribution of scores. The standard deviation is used with ratio level data, considers all the values in the data set, and reflects the average amount that each value in the distribution varies from the mean. The higher the standard deviation, the more variability in the distribution; low standard deviations reflect greater homogeneity in the data set. The standard deviation formula is:

$$sd = \sqrt{\frac{\Sigma(X - \bar{X})^2}{N - 1}}$$

Table 11.7 shows how the standard deviation for Beth's grades could be computed. An examination of the table reveals that the standard deviation of Mary's grades is 3.7, considerably less than Beth's 12.2. An examination of the actual grades indicates that, indeed, there is much more variability in Beth's than in Mary's grades. The standard deviation reflects the variability in a set of values.

Beginning researchers should be familiar with how standard deviations are computed. This statistic is an important one. It plays a role in computations such as determining sample size and in doing various

Table 11.5 Summary Statistics for Nursing Grades

Summary Statistics	Test A Grades	Test B Grades
Mean	62.02	60.02
Median	58.00	59.00
Mode	60.00	60.00
Cases, *n*	62	62

Table 11.6   Two Grade Distributions

Subject	Mary	Beth
Sociology	78	66
Psychology	80	72
Nursing	82	88
Anthropology	82	90
Philosophy	88	94
Summary Statistics		
Mean*	82	82
Range†	10	28
Standard Deviation‡	3.74	12.25
Variance§	14.0	150.0

*Mean = Sum of values divided by number of cases.
†Range = Highest value minus lowest value.
‡Standard deviation (see computation in Table 11.7).
§Variance = sd².

tests of statistical significance. In addition, the standard deviation is an element in most advanced statistical techniques. After data have been entered into the computer, it will not be necessary to hand compute standard deviations; nonetheless, it is crucial to understand what they measure.

c. Variance

The third measure of dispersion is **variance.** Similar to other measures of dispersion, it provides a sense of the variability in the data. Similar to the standard deviation, variance reflects the average amount of deviation from the average value in the distribution. Indeed, computationally it is simply the standard deviation squared. The term *variance* will be encountered in later chapters dealing with explained variance and in analysis of variance, a statistical test discussed in Chapter 12. The computation for variance is:

$$\text{Variance} = sd^2 = \frac{\Sigma(X - \bar{X})^2}{N - 1}$$

In the illustration using Mary's and Beth's grades, the variances are 14.0 and 150.0, respectively (see Table 11.6).

Table 11.8 summarizes the single variable statistics that have been presented in this text. Note that it is possible to use all of the summarizing statistics when a ratio level of measurement has been achieved. Indeed, when there are unusual features in the data, such as a few extreme values or a lot of identical scores, it sometimes makes sense to use a summary statistic other than the one highlighted in the table.

4. Standardizing Data

To standardize data is to report data in a way that comparisons between units of different size may be made; data may also be standardized to create variables that have similar variability in them (these are called Z scores; they are introduced later in this chapter).

a. Proportions

A **proportion** may be calculated to show, for example, how many females there are in a population compared to the total population. Suppose we wished to compute the proportion of females in a community with a total of 58,520 persons:

$$\text{Proportion female} = \frac{\text{Number females}}{\text{Total persons}}$$

$$\text{Proportion female} = \frac{31,216}{58,520}$$

$$\text{Proportion female} = 0.533$$

The females represent 0.53 of the population. In other words, there are 0.53 women and girls for every one person in the community.

b. Percentages

If we wished to represent a proportion as a **percentage,** we would simply multiply the

Table 11.7   Computation of Standard Deviation, Beth's Grades

Subject	Step 1 Grade	Step 2 $X - \bar{X}$	Step 3 $(X - \bar{X})^2$
Sociology	66	$66 - 82 = -16$	256
Psychology	72	$72 - 82 = -10$	100
Nursing	88	$88 - 82 =\ \ \ 6$	36
Anthropology	90	$90 - 82 =\ \ \ 8$	64
Philosophy	94	$94 - 82 =\ \ 12$	144
Mean	82.0	Total	600

Step 1: Compute the mean for the scores by summing the scores and dividing by the number of observations.
Step 2: Calculate the deviation from the mean for each observation.
Step 3: Square each deviation score and sum them.
Step 4: Using the formula below, calculate the standard deviation.

$$sd = \frac{(X - \bar{X})^2}{N - 1}$$

$$sd = \sqrt{\frac{600}{4}}$$

$$sd = 12.25$$

Some notational conventions that are used in this text are: $\square$ is a summation symbol; $\bar{X}$ with a bar over it indicates that it is the mean value; N = number of cases; sd = standard deviation.

proportion by 100. In the example just given, we note that females constitute 53.3 *percent* of the population. For a more complex example, Table 11.9 presents the relationship between size of home community and whether the respondent plans to attend university. It is not adequate simply to say that 69 rural students, 44 students from small towns, and 102 students from larger towns plan on attending university.

We report percentages to adjust for the fact that there are different numbers of students involved in each of the categories. By computing the percentages, we are able to say that for every 100 rural students, 52.3 are planning to attend a university compared with 48.9 of every 100 students from the small town category and 73.9 of every 100 high school students from towns with populations of more than 5000.

Table 11.8   Summary Statistics for Single Variables*

Level of Measurement	Measures of Central Tendency	Measures of Dispersion	SPSS Procedure
Nominal	**Mode**		FREQUENCIES
Ordinal	Mode	**Range**	FREQUENCIES
	Median		
Ratio	Mode	Range	DESCRIPTIVES
	Median	**Standard deviation**	
	Mean	**Variance**	

*Bold indicates the statistic used under normal circumstances.

Table 11.9   Plans to Attend University by Size of Home Community*

University Plans?	Rural N	Rural %	Town up to 5000 Population N	Town up to 5000 Population %	Town over 5000 Population N	Town over 5000 Population %	Total N	Total %
Plans	69	52.3	44	48.9	102	73.9	215	59.7
No plans	63	47.7	46	51.1	36	26.1	145	40.3
Total	132	100.0	90	100.0	138	100.0	360	100.0

*If appropriate, test of significance values are entered.

c. Percentage Change

Often nurse researchers compare numbers at one time to those at another time. For example, they may want to measure the percentage increase in the number of teen pregnancies from one period to the next. Table 11.10 illustrates a problem in which nurse scientists may wish to calculate the percentage change between 1990 and 2000 in the number of teen pregnancies. The general form of the equation for calculating **percentage change** would be:

$$\text{Percentage Change} = \frac{\text{Time 2 number} - \text{Time 1 number}}{\text{Time 1 number}} \times 100$$

To calculate the percentage change use the following steps:

- Using the general equation, subtract the time 1 number from the time 2 number.
- Divide the above total by the number at time 1.
- Multiply the above total by 100.

d. Rates

The incidence of a social phenomenon is often presented in the form of a *rate*. A **rate** indicates the frequency of some phenomenon for a standard-sized unit (such as incidence per 1000 or per 100,000). This allows us to easily compare the incidence of a phenomenon in units of different size. To know, for example, that there were 27 suicides in a city of 250,000 (Middle City) in one year and 13 suicides in another city of 110,000 (Small City) does not allow quick comparison unless we compute a suicide rate. A suicide rate may be computed in the following manner:

Table 11.10   Calculating Percentage Change: Percentage Change in Number of Teen Pregnancies between 1990 and 2000, Canada and United States

Country	Number per 1000 Teen Women, 1990 (Time 1)	Number per 1000 Teen Women, 2000 (Time 2)	Percent Change, 1990 to 2000
Canada	41.6	39.5	−5.05
United States	85.0	82.1	−3.41

Note the method of calculating percent change:

$$\text{Percent change} = \frac{\text{Time 2 number} - \text{Time 1 number}}{\text{Time 1 number}} \times 100$$

In the case of the United States in the above table, the calculation would be:

$$\text{Percent change} = \frac{82.1 - 85.0}{85.0} \times 100$$

$$\text{Percent change} = -3.41$$

Suicide rate

$$= \frac{\text{Number suicides per year}}{\text{Mid-year population}}$$

$$\times \ 100,000$$

When calculated, we find that the suicide rate for Middle City is 10.8; for Small City, the rate is 11.10. This means that Middle City has 10.8 suicides in the year for every 100,000 people in the city; in Small City the rate is 11.8 per 100,000. In this case, we see that Small City has a slightly higher suicide rate. Rates can also be computed for specific age categories or on other bases; the only adjustment required is that we use the number of suicides in the category compared with its total size. Rates are computed for many things, including births, marriages, divorces, deaths, and crime.

Table 11.11 presents suicide rates for five fictitious cities. Note that rates permit easy comparisons between units of unequal size. The data are standardized, permitting comparison between the units. If the absolute number of suicides were presented, this would create the impression that suicide is a much more serious problem in the larger jurisdictions. This may not be the case. The rates adjust for the differences in size.

e. Ratios

Ratios are used to compare rates or other measures across categories. For example, suppose one wished to compare the suicide rate of black male teens and white male teens in the United States. Whereas the suicide rate in the United States is 12.2 in black males 15 to 19 years old (per 100,000), the comparable rate in young white males is 19.1. The American white-to-black male suicide ratio for 15 to 19 years old could be represented as:

U.S. white/black male suicide ratio

$$= \frac{\text{White male suicide rate}}{\text{Black male suicide rate}}$$

U.S. white/black male suicide ratio $= \dfrac{19.1}{12.2}$

U.S. white/black male suicide ratio $= 1.56$

This ratio suggests that the white male youth suicide rate is 1.56 times higher than the comparable black male youth rate. Many ratios can be computed that, like rates, facilitate comparison between categories.

Table 11.12 presents the ratio between male and female suicide rates for black and white ethnic groups in the United States. Note that, nationally, men commit suicide 5.79 times more frequently than do women.

Table 11.11   Suicide Rates for Five Cities

	Number of Suicides	Population	Suicide Rate*
City A	49	581,257	8.43
City B	16	134,567	11.89
City C	97	933,590	10.39
City D	1263	7287,940	17.33
City E	1083	10,939,394	9.90

*In the case of City A, the computation would be as follows:

Suicide rate $= \dfrac{\text{Number of suicides in the year}}{\text{Mid-year population}} \times 100,000$

Suicide rate $= \dfrac{49}{581,252} \times 100,000$

Suicide rate $= 8.43$

Table 11.12   Male and Female Suicide Ratios, by Group, Youth 15 to 19 Years of Age, United States*

Group	Suicide Rate, Males	Suicide Rate, Females	Ratio, Male/Female Suicides
Black	12.2	1.9	6.42
White	19.1	4.2	4.54
United States	22	3.8	5.79

*In this table, the male/female suicide ratio is computed for each group by dividing the male suicide rate by the female rate. The result indicates how many male suicides there are for every female suicide.
SOURCE: *Statistical Abstract of the United States,* 1994. Washington, D.C.: U.S. Government Printing Office, p. 101.

In some cases, ratios are reported so that they are standardized to a base of 100. For example, if we had a community with 27,304 males and 31,216 females, we might compute a sex ratio. The ratio for the community could be calculated as follows:

$$\text{Gender ratio} = \frac{\text{Number of males}}{\text{Number of females}} \times 100$$

$$\text{Gender ratio} = \frac{27,304}{31,216} \times 100$$

$$\text{Gender ratio} = 87.5$$

This gender ratio would indicate that there are 87.5 males in the community for every 100 females. Such a ratio allows us to quickly compare the sex ratios of communities, nations, age groups, or any other category.

5. The Normal Distribution

The normal distribution is another key concept used by researchers. Many of the observations we make on individual or group characteristics approximate what is referred to as a **normal distribution.** What does this mean? Many phenomena in the social and physical world are normally distributed. A normal distribution is a theoretical representation of the frequency of scores on a variable. When the scores are plotted, values cluster around the midpoint with a falling off toward the extremes, resulting in a bell-shaped curve (see Fig. 11.3). A variable that is normally distributed has the following characteristics when plotted:

- It forms a symmetrical, bell-shaped curve.
- It has the same mean, mode, and median values, with half the cases falling below the mean and the other half above the mean.
- It becomes smoother as the number of observations and the number of measurement units become finer.

If a plot is made showing the distribution, for example, of the weight of male university students, it would approximate a bell-shaped curve. There will be few cases on the extremes—the very light and the very heavy; most of the cases will be found clustered toward the middle of the distribution.

Another example of a normal distribution is a plot of the outcomes of a series of 10 coin flips. Suppose we flip a coin 10 times, record the number of heads, repeat this operation 1024 times, and then plot

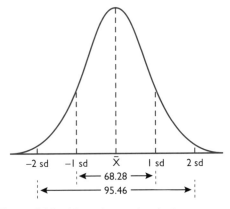

Figure 11.3   Normal curve distribution.

the number of times we got 0, 1, 2, . . . 10 heads in the trials. The outcome will approximate that shown in Figure 11.4, which is a graph of the theoretical probabilities of getting each of the 11 possible outcomes (i.e., 0 through 10 heads). The result approximates that of a normal distribution.

An interesting characteristic of the normal distribution is its connection to the standard deviation. By definition, a fixed proportion of cases in a normal distribution will fall within a given number of standard deviation units of the mean (see Fig. 11.3). About two thirds of the cases will fall within one standard deviation of the mean; just over 95 percent of the cases will fall within two standard deviations of the mean. More precisely:

- 68.28 percent of the observations will be divided equally between the mean and one standard deviation to the right of the mean (34.14) and one standard deviation to the left of the mean (34.14).
- 95.46 percent of the observations will fall ± two standard deviations from the mean.
- 95 percent of the cases fall ± 1.96 standard deviation units from the mean.
- 99 percent of the cases fall ± 2.58 standard deviation units from the mean.

a. Z Scores

Z scores measure the distance, in standard deviation units, of any value in a dis-

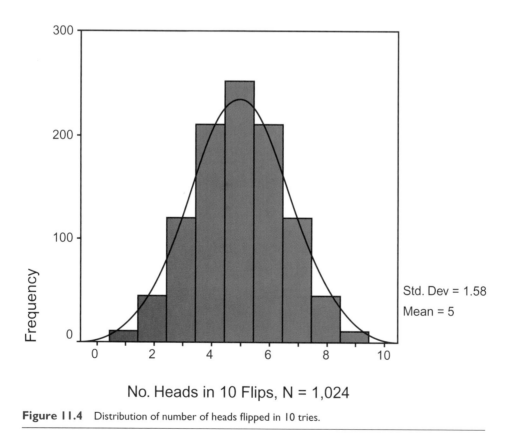

Figure 11.4   Distribution of number of heads flipped in 10 tries.

tribution from the mean. Thus, if some-one's income has a Z score of +1.43, it would indicate that the income is 1.43 standard deviation units above the mean of the distribution. Suppose that the mean income is $65,000 and the standard deviation $22,000; the Z score +1.43 would indicate an income of $96,460. How is this value computed? The formula for Z scores is as follows:

$$Z = \frac{X - \bar{X}}{sd}$$

Where:

X is the observation;

$\bar{X}$ is the mean of the distribution;

sd is the standard deviation of the distribution.

By plugging the values into the equation and solving it, the value $96,460 is obtained, as in:

$$1.43 = \frac{X - 65,000}{22,000}$$

$$X = (1.43 \times 22,000) + 65,000$$

$$X = 96,460$$

One of the consequences of being able to report a value in terms of its Z score is that we now have a powerful comparative tool. Suppose we wanted to compare individuals' relative income positions in two countries; we could simply report the incomes in Z score terms, and this would tell us where each individual stands in terms of his or her country's income distribution. This would permit us to compare a British family's income of £24,000 to an American family's income of $90,000.

Students should recognize that computing Z scores can be used to standardize variables, and the resulting distributions have means of 0 and standard deviations of 1. Thus, instead of just having variables with income scores, educational levels, and occupational prestige, we might have standardized variables containing the Z scores for each variable.

Such standardization can be accomplished easily in SPSS.

To perform this analysis in SPSS, use the DESCRIPTIVES procedure; see Appendix A.

Combining indicators to create an index is a major use of Z scores. Suppose, for example, that we have measures on income and years of education and that we wish to combine them to form a socioeconomic index. It would not make sense simply to add a respondent's years of education to his or her annual income; the reason is that incomes may vary from $5,000 to $500,000 but years of education may vary from 0 to 20. By adding them together, the income component would totally dominate the index. Someone earning $50,000 with 8 years of education would have a score of 50,008, but a person with a BA and $40,000 income would end up with a score of 40,016. Somehow we need to weight the components so that income and education will equally influence the outcome. Using Z scores is an easy way to do this.

Table 11.13 shows the computation of socioeconomic index scores using Z scores. Notice how either a lower-than-average income or a lower-than-average education leads to a reduction in the total socioeconomic score. These indexes can be calculated quickly by a computer and the components weighted in any way the researcher likes. The Z scores, for example, may be added together, resulting in a value that can be taken to represent the relative socioeconomic position of the various respondents, with income and education making equal contributions to the final score. Such computations can be done rapidly within SPSS.

b. Areas Under the Normal Distribution

Another useful property of the normal distribution is that it is possible, with the help of Table 11.14, to calculate the pro-

Table 11.13   **Computing an Index Score Using Z Scores**

	Income	Years of Education
Given population values		
Mean	65,000	11
Standard deviation	22,000	4
Suppose five individuals		
A	55,000	7
B	41,000	12
C	30,000	8
D	64,000	16
E	86,000	9

Compute an index equally weighting income and years of education. The general equation is:

$$Z = \frac{X - \bar{X}}{sd}$$

Case A. Income:	$(55{,}000 - 65{,}000) \div 22{,}000$	=	-0.45
Education:	$(7 - 11) \div 4$	=	$\underline{-1.00}$
	Socioeconomic index score		**-1.45**

Case B. Income:	$(41{,}000 - 65{,}000) \div 22{,}000$	=	-1.09
Education:	$(12 - 11) \div 4$	=	$\underline{0.25}$
	Socioeconomic index score		**-0.84**

Case C. Income:	$(30{,}000 - 65{,}000) \div 22{,}000$	=	-1.59
Education:	$(8 - 11) \div 4$	=	$\underline{-0.75}$
	Socioeconomic index score		**-2.34**

Case D. Income	$(64{,}000 - 65{,}000) \div 22{,}000$	=	-0.05
Education:	$(16 - 11) \div 4$	=	$\underline{1.25}$
	Socioeconomic index score		**1.20**

Case E. Income:	$(86{,}000 - 65{,}000) \div 22{,}000$	=	0.95
Education:	$(9 - 11) \div 4$	=	$\underline{-0.050}$
	Socioeconomic index score		**0.45**

portion of cases that will fall between two values, or above or below a given value.

To illustrate, suppose we wished to know what percentage of incomes would fall above $100,000, given a population standard deviation of $22,000, and a mean of $65,000. The steps followed to solve this problem would be as follows:

Step 1. Draw a normal curve, marking below it the mean and standard deviation values, and drawing a line through the curve at the point where you expect $100,000 to fall. Because the question asks about the percentage above this point, shade the curve to the right of the $100,000 mark.

Step 2. Calculate the Z score to determine how many standard deviation units $100,000 is above the mean, as in:

$$Z = \frac{X - \bar{X}}{sd}$$

$$Z = \frac{100{,}000 - 65{,}000}{22{,}000}$$

$$Z = 1.59$$

Step 3. Look up the value 1.59 in Table 11.14. Move down the Z score column

Table 11.14   Areas Under the Normal Curve

Fractional parts of the total area (10,000) under the normal curve, correspnding to distances between the mean and ordinates which are Z standard-deviation units from the mean.

Z	.00	.01	.02	.03	.04	.05	.06	.07	.08	.09
0.0	0000	0040	0080	0120	0159	0199	0239	0279	0319	0359
0.1	0398	0438	0478	0517	0557	0596	0636	0675	0714	0753
0.2	0793	0832	0871	0910	0948	0987	1026	1064	1103	1141
0.3	1179	1217	1255	1293	1331	1368	1406	1443	1480	1517
0.4	1554	1591	1628	1664	1700	1736	1772	1808	1844	1879
0.5	1915	1950	1985	2019	2054	2088	2123	2157	2190	2224
0.6	2257	2291	2324	2357	2389	2422	2454	2486	2518	2549
0.7	2580	2612	2642	2673	2704	2734	2764	2794	2823	2852
0.8	2881	2910	2939	2967	2995	3023	3051	3078	3106	3133
0.9	3159	3186	3212	3238	3264	3289	3315	3340	3365	3389
1.0	3413	3438	3461	3485	3508	3531	3554	3577	3599	3621
1.1	3643	3665	3686	3718	3729	3749	3770	3790	3810	3830
1.2	3849	3869	3888	3907	3925	3944	3962	3980	3997	4015
1.3	4032	4049	4066	4083	4099	4115	4131	4147	4162	4177
1.4	4192	4207	4222	4236	4251	4265	4279	4292	4306	4319
1.5	4332	4345	4357	4370	4382	4394	4406	4418	4430	4441
1.6	4452	4463	4474	4483	4495	4505	4515	4525	4535	4545
1.7	4554	4564	4573	4582	4591	4599	4608	4616	4625	4635
1.8	4641	4649	4656	4664	4671	4678	4686	4693	4699	4706
1.9	4713	4719	4726	4732	4738	4744	4750	4758	4762	4767
2.0	4773	4778	4783	4788	4793	4798	4803	4808	4812	4817
2.1	4821	4826	4830	4834	4838	4842	4846	4850	4854	4857
2.2	4861	4865	4868	4871	4875	4878	4881	4884	4887	4890
2.3	4893	4896	4898	4901	4904	4906	4909	4911	4913	4916
2.4	4918	4920	4922	4925	4927	4929	4931	4932	4934	4936
2.5	4938	4940	4941	4943	4945	4946	4948	4949	4951	4952
2.6	4953	4955	4956	4957	4959	4960	4961	4962	4963	4964
2.7	4965	4966	4967	4968	4969	4970	4971	4972	4973	4974
2.8	4974	4975	4976	4977	4977	4978	4979	4980	4980	4981
2.9	4981	4982	4983	4984	4984	4984	4985	4985	4986	4986
3.0	4986.5	4987	4987	4988	4988	4988	4989	4989	4989	4990
3.1	4990.5	4991	4991	4991	4992	4992	4992	4992	4993	4993
3.2	4993.129									
3.3	4995.166									
3.4	4996.631									

(continued on next page)

Table 11.14   Areas Under the Normal Curve (*Continued*)

Z	.00	.01	.02	.03	.04	.05	.06	.07	.08	.09
3.5	4997.674									
3.6	4998.409									
3.7	4998.922									
3.8	4999.277									
3.9	4999.519									
4.0	4999.683									
4.5	4999.966									
5.0	4999.997133									

SOURCE: Rugg, H.O. (1945). *Statistical Methods Applied to Education*. Boston: Houghton Mifflin. (Original work published 1917). Cited with permission.

until you come to the value 1.5, then read across to the column headed by 0.09, (this gives you the value for the 9 in the value 1.59) and read the value. You should have found the number 4441. This number should be understood as 0.4441, a proportion.

Step 4. By definition, we know that one half of the cases will fall above the mean. Expressed as a proportion, this would indicate that 0.5 of the cases will fall above the mean. The question we are trying to answer is what proportion of the cases fall above $100,000. Looking at the diagram we made in Step 1, we realize that if the right side of the curve contains 0.5 of all the cases, and, if the value $100,000 is 0.4441 above the mean, then the cases above $100,000 would have to be:

$$0.5000 - 0.4441 = 0.0559$$

Step 5. As a proportion, 0.0559 of the cases will fall above $100,000. Or, another way of expressing the same idea, is to say that 5.6 percent of the cases will fall above $100,000 (multiply the proportion 0.0559 by 100 to get 5.6 percent).

Suppose we wish to determine the proportion of cases that will fall between $40,000 and $70,000, given the same population mean and standard deviation. We

should follow procedures similar to those used in the case above. This time, however, the diagram will show a shaded area between two points on either side of the mean. This time two Z scores will need to be computed, the values looked up in Table 11.14, and the proportions between the mean and each cutpoint will need to be determined, then added together to get the final answer. The computations may be done as follows:

Step 1. Proportion between the mean and $70,000:

$$Z = \frac{X - \bar{X}}{sd}$$

$$Z = \frac{70,000 - 65,000}{22,000}$$

$$Z = 0.23$$

Proportion of normal curve included in Z score of 0.23 = 0.0910.

Step 2. Proportion between $40,000 and the mean:

$$Z = \frac{X - \bar{X}}{sd}$$

$$Z = \frac{40,000 - 65,000}{22,000}$$

$$Z = -1.14$$

Proportion of normal curve included in Z score of $-1.14 = 0.3729$.

Step 3. Adding the proportions together:

$$0.3729 + 0.0910 = 0.4639$$

The computation indicates that just fewer than one half of all the cases, 46.4 percent, fall between the incomes of $40,000 and $70,000. The proportion between the mean and the respective Z scores is shown in Figure 11.5. In this case, the values are added together to determine the proportion of cases that fall between $40,000 and $70,000.

There are other types of normal curve problems that can be solved. Just keep the previous examples in mind, draw a diagram shading in the area you need to determine, and remember that each side of the normal curve contains one half, or 0.5, of the cases. With these things in mind, it should be possible to solve most normal curve problems.

As a review of this first section and before we go on to consider how we analyze relationships between variables, recall that before we begin to analyze any variable, we need to appreciate its level of measurement so that appropriate analyses may be made. The level of measurement attained determines the best ways of summarizing a variable. Note the following:

- To provide a measure of central tendency use the mean (ratio measure-

ment), median (ordinal measurement), or mode (nominal measurement).
- A frequency distribution is used to reflect dispersion with nominal variables; the range is used as a measure of dispersion with ordinal variables; the standard deviation and variance are used to reflect dispersion of ratio level variables.

To perform this analysis in SPSS, use the DESCRIPTIVES for ratio variables and the FREQUENCIES procedures for nominal and ordinal variables; see Appendix A for details.

C. DESCRIBING RELATIONSHIPS BETWEEN VARIABLES

Researchers are concerned with describing the relationships among variables. In dealing with two-variable relationships, one of the variables will be treated as a dependent variable and the other will be treated as an independent variable. (There may not necessarily be evidence to support designating one of them as dependent and the other independent, but to do the analysis we are required to identify one as dependent.) If a control variable is used, it will be an intervening source of spuriousness, or conditional variable.

This section describes some of the major procedures used to examine relationships between variables. Three basic steps must be taken to begin analyzing any relationship:

- The first step is to decide which variable is to be treated as the dependent variable and which one as the independent variable.
- The second step is to determine the level of measurement for each variable.
- The third step is to decide on the appropriate procedure for examining the relationship.
- Finally, the analysis must be performed.

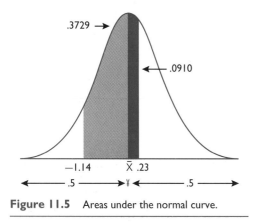

Figure 11.5   Areas under the normal curve.

Because the researcher typically is trying to understand what causes variations in a dependent variable, common sense alone can generally determine which variable should be designated as the dependent variable. However, in other cases, it is not as obvious. For example, suppose you were to examine the relationship between healthy lifestyle choices and perceived health status. In this case, it would not be obvious if positive perception of health status leads to healthy lifestyle choices or if the direction of the relationship is reversed. Hence, it is not clear which variable should be designated as the dependent variable. In such cases, try to decide which variable occurs last in a temporal sequence. It is entirely possible that the two variables mutually influence one another. If this is the case, one will nonetheless have to be designated as the dependent variable.

Having decided which variable is to be treated as the dependent variable, one must next identify the level of measurement of each of the variables. Now, using the information provided in Table 11.15, identify which procedure would be most appropriate for the analysis. Let us explore each of the procedures identified in Table 11.15.

2. Cross-tabulation Tables

Cross-tabulation tables present information so that the relationship between a nominal level dependent variable can be related to an independent variable. Recall that Table 11.9 presented findings on the relationship between the educational plans and the size of the home community for 360 high school students. Let's examine this table again, as it typifies the cross-tabulation table.

A cross-tabulation table classifies cases on two or more variables. In this example, the data are first sorted into categories representing community size; next, each of these categories is sorted into whether the person does or does not plan to attend college. This sorting allows us to see if those from rural areas are more likely to have college plans than their urban counterparts.

a. Rules for Constructing Cross-tabulation Tables

Let us now examine some of the rules for constructing and for interpreting cross-tabulation tables.

Rule 1. In table titles, name the dependent variable first. Tables must be

Table 11.15 SPSS Procedures for Bivariate Analysis by Levels of Measurement

| Dependent | Independent Variable | | |
	Nominal	Ordinal	Ratio
Nominal	CROSSTABS	CROSSTABS	CROSSTABS
			MEANS*
Ordinal	CROSSTABS	CROSSTABS	CROSSTABS
		NONPAR CORRELATION	NONPAR CORRELATION
Ratio	MEANS	MEANS	CORRELATION
	ANOVA	ANOVA	GRAPH
	t Test	t Test	REGRESSION

*In SPSS for this case, run the independent variable as though it were the dependent variable (i.e., name it first); the interpretation of the test of significance would be standard.

numbered and be given a title. In providing a title for a table, the dependent variable is named first, followed by the independent variable, followed by any control variables. In Table 11.9, for example, note that the table title is "Plans to Attend University by Size of Home Community."

Rule 2. Place dependent variable on vertical plane. Label the categories of the dependent variable and arrange these categories on the left-hand side of the table. If the categories involve some cut points, these should be specified (e.g., for income, the first two categories might be "Under 10,000" and "10,000 to 19,999".)

Rule 3. Place independent variable on horizontal plane. Label the categories on the independent variable and arrange them across the top of the table. Again, if there are cut points, be careful to specify these.

Rule 4. Use variable labels that are clear. Avoid the use of computer variable labels that have been designed to meet the space requirements of the statistical program. For example, FAED may have been used to refer to the variable, father's education. Use clear, easily understood labels, as in "Father's Education."

Rule 5. Run percentages toward the independent variable. Percentages should be computed so that each column will total 100 percent. A percentage is computed by dividing the column total into the cell frequency. In the first cell, for example, the computation involves:

$$\text{Cell percentage} = \frac{\text{Cell total}}{\text{Column total}} \times 100$$

$$\text{Cell percentage} = \frac{69}{132} \times 100 = 52.3$$

Rule 6. Report percentages to one decimal point. Percentages should be reported to one significant decimal point.

If the total is 99.9 or 100.1 percent, report it as such.

Rule 7. Report statistical test results below table. Any special information and the results of statistical tests should be reported below the line under the table. (Tests of significance are discussed in Chapter 12.) The preferred method of presenting the probability or significance level is to report the exact value (e.g., $P = 0.0037$).

Rule 8. Interpret the table by comparing categories of the independent variable. Because we are attempting to assess the impact of the independent variable on the dependent variable (in this case, size of community on educational plans), we are interested in the percentage of positive planners for each category of the independent variable. "Although about one half of the rural and small town students (52.3 percent and 48.9 percent, respectively) plan on attending university, some 73.9 percent of those from communities over 5000 have such plans." In short, compare percentages in each column. Usually it is sufficient to use one row (in this case, just the row for those planning to attend college).

Rule 9. Collapse data into fewer categories. When dealing with small samples of fewer than 100 and with variables having multiple categories, it may be necessary to regroup data (i.e., code into fewer categories) before cross-tabular tables are produced. This procedure is necessary to avoid having too few cases in the cells of the table. This recoding may involve both the independent and the dependent variable. For example, if you had a dependent variable dealing with smoking behavior among adolescents (e.g., smoker vs. nonsmoker) and you wished to relate it to a five category variable measuring self-esteem (e.g., very low, low, medium, high, very high), with a small sample, you would need to collapse the independent variable categories into two categories (e.g., high and low).

Rule 10. Minimize categories in a table with a control variable. When control variables are used, it is necessary to minimize the number of categories in the independent and in the control variables. Generally, there should be no more than two or three categories within these variables. There are two major reasons for this limitation. First, the number of cases in each cell will become too small if there are many categories in either the independent or the control variable; second, the interpretation of the table is very difficult if simplicity is not maintained. For example, if you were examining the relationship between gender and smoking behavior in adolescents controlling for the effect of age, you would collapse the age variable (12 to 18 years) into two categories (probably at the midpoint of the distribution). Chapter 17 discusses interpretations of three-variable cross-tabular tables.

b. Lambda

Researchers using cross-tabular analysis are interested in how closely two variables are related. One simple measure is **lambda.** This statistic measures the **proportionate reduction in error** that occurs in estimating a dependent variable, given knowledge of the independent variable. If two variables are strongly associated, then errors in predicting variations in the dependent variable will be considerably reduced if information on the independent variable is taken into account.

The following example shows how lambda is calculated. Suppose we wish to measure the strength of the association between gender and the ability to become pregnant. Table 11.16 reports the result of the appropriate medical examinations on 140 individuals.

If we were asked to guess whether a

Table 11.16   Number of Cases in which Pregnancy Is Possible

Able to Become Pregnant?	Cases, n
Yes	74
No	66
Total	140

person could become pregnant, the best strategy would be to guess the category with the most cases. Each time a case is presented, our best guess is to say, "Yes, can get pregnant." (There are more in the sample who can become pregnant than those who cannot become pregnant.) If we went through all the cases, guessing "yes" each time, we would be right 74 times and in error 66 times.

Table 11.17 supplements the material contained in Table 11.16 by adding information on gender. With this additional information, would we be able to make fewer errors?

This time, instead of using the "Total" column and always guessing yes, we will use the gender information as a basis for our guess: If the case considered is male, we will guess "no, cannot become pregnant." If we do this, we will make zero errors; if the case is female, we will always guess "yes." By following this procedure, we will make a total of 6 errors—the cases of females who are not able to conceive. Given the additional information on gender, we will now only make a total of 6 errors (0 + 6 = 6) in estimating whether a respondent could become pregnant.

Lambda is based on how much error

Table 11.17   Relationship between Ability to become Pregnant and Gender

Able to Become Pregnant?	Gender Male	Female	Cases
Yes	0	74	74
No	60	6	66
Total	60	80	140

reduction occurs with the additional information provided by the independent variable (in this case, gender). Recall that we made 66 errors when we did not have the information on gender. Taking into account the information on gender, we make six errors—60 fewer than we made without the gender information.

$$\text{Lambda} = \frac{\text{Errors not knowing gender} - \text{Errors knowing gender}}{\text{Errors not knowing gender}}$$

$$\text{Lambda} = \frac{66 - 6}{66}$$

$$\text{Lambda} = 0.909$$

In this case, we have reduced the errors in our estimate by 0.909 (proportion) or 90.9 percent. Lambda varies from 0 to 1. The higher the value of lambda, the more closely two variables are associated. A high value on lambda indicates that knowing the additional information about the independent variable (in this case, gender) greatly reduces the number of errors one would make in guessing the value of the dependent variable (in this case, the ability to become pregnant). A value close to 0 would indicate that the additional knowledge of the independent variable leads to a slight proportionate reduction in error. In most cases, the reduction in error will not be as dramatic as that found in the example used above.

c. Gamma

Gamma is a measure of the strength of association used in cross-tabulation analyses of ordinal level variables. This statistic takes advantage of the numerical order of the values and its values fall in the range from −1 to +1. (Later you will find that the correlation coefficient also varies from −1 to +1.) A negative value indicates that the variables are inversely related; the greater X, the less Y. A positive value indicates a relation of the form the greater X, the greater Y. The higher the value, the stronger the association between the variables.

To illustrate the calculation of gamma, Table 11.18 presents data showing the relationship between alcohol and drug use. Note that drug use is taken as the dependent variable and alcohol use is taken as the independent variable.

Is there an association between frequency of alcohol use and frequency of drug use? The data seem to be contrary to our expectations when we look at the category of people who use alcohol more frequently. Only 2 of the 19 frequent alcohol users use drugs once a month or more. Indeed, of the 16 people who report rarely or never using alcohol, 10 of them indicate frequent drug use. If anything, then, there appears to be an inverse relation-

Table 11.18 Frequency of Drug Use by Frequency of Alcohol Use

Frequency of Drug Use	Frequency of Alcohol Use		
	Rarely or Never	Once per Week to Once per Month	Every Few Days
Never	3	8	3
Less than once a month	3	25	14
Monthly or more often	10	15	2
Total	16	48	19

ship between alcohol and drug use. Gamma may be used to measure the strength of this association. Gamma is based on two measures: (1) a measure of a positive trend in the data and (2) a measure of an inverse trend in the data.

A positive trend is one that shows that as one variable increases the other variable increases; an inverse measure shows that as one variable increases, the other variable decreases. The positive trend is reflected by multiplying the number of cases in each cell by a sum of all the cases that are *both below and to the right* of the cell. In the case of Table 11.18, this calculation would be done as follows:

Positive trend measure:

$3(25 + 15 + 14 + 2) =$	168
$8(14 + 2) =$	128
$3(15 + 2) =$	51
$25(2) =$	50
Total positive trend	397

The inverse trend is reflected by multiplying the number of cases in cells by the sum of the cases that are *both below and to the left* of the cell. The calculation would be done as follows:

Inverse trend measure:

$3(25 + 15 + 3 + 10) =$	159
$8(3 + 10) =$	104
$14(15 + 10) =$	350
$25(10) =$	250
Total inverse trend	863

Gamma is calculated according to the following formula:

$$\text{Gamma} = \frac{\text{Positive} - \text{Inverse}}{\text{Positive} + \text{Inverse}}$$

$$\text{Gamma} = \frac{397 - 863}{397 + 863}$$

$$\text{Gamma} = -0.3698$$

Note that the value is negative. The value indicates a modest inverse relation between alcohol use and drug use.

To perform this analysis using SPSS, see the CROSS-TABS procedure in Appendix A.

2. Comparing Means

A nurse researcher may be interested in comparing the responses of two groups of patients to a treatment. For example, you may want to know if touch therapy reduces heart rate in elderly patients with arrhythmias. One way to determine this is to do a comparison of the mean heart rate for those exposed to touch therapy with the mean heart rate of those receiving routine nursing care. Any time one has a ratio level dependent variable (in this case, mean heart rate) and either a nominal or ordinal independent variable, then it is appropriate to compute the mean values of the dependent variable for each category of the independent variable. Table 11.19 presents data that would be appropriate for this kind of analysis. Note that whereas the dependent variable (heart rate) is measured at the ratio level, the independent variable is nominal (treatment group).

a. The MEANS Procedure (SPSS)

In cases in which there are many categories in the independent variable, they will have to be regrouped into two or three categories before the analysis is run. The number of categories created will depend on the following criteria:

- A reasonable number of cases will appear in each category (often we try to have roughly equal numbers in the various categories).
- The categories used must make theoretical sense. We have to exercise caution to ensure that the categories remain as coherent as possible; thus, if we

Table 11.19   Mean Heart Rate by Treatment Group

Treatment Group	Mean Heart Rate	Number of Cases
Touch therapy	74.6	78
Routine treatment	77.1	77
Combined mean	75.8	155

If appropriate, test of significance values are entered here (e.g., $F = 3.514$; df = 2,153; $P = >0.05$).

were recoding religious affiliation from eight categories to three, we would perhaps want to do the grouping so as to reflect the degree to which the religious categories we create either reflect or reject mainstream societal values.

In interpreting the outcome of an analysis, the mean values should be compared. In Table 11.19, for example, the average heart rate of patients in the touch therapy group are compared with those in the routine therapy group.

To perform this analysis using SPSS, see the MEANS procedure in Appendix A.

b. Comparing Means Using the t Test

When you are using samples under 30 and you wish to compare two groups on a ratio level dependent variable, the t test is frequently used. The **t test** is used to determine if the differences in the means may be regarded as statistically significant. Statistical significance indicates only whether observed differences in the mean scores are caused by real differences rather than chance differences. This is discussed in greater detail in Chapter 12.

To perform this analysis in SPSS, use the Independent Samples t TEST procedure; see Appendix A for details.

c. Analysis of Variance

Although used by many researchers, analysis of variance procedures are particularly important to experimenters. The t test is used to compare the means of two groups. When three or more group means

are compared or when the means for two groups are compared at two or more points in time in a single analysis (e.g., a pre–post experimental design), **analysis of variance** is the procedure required to test for statistically significant differences in the mean scores. The procedures involved in doing an *analysis of variance (ANOVA)* require a measurement of two kinds of variation: differences in scores within a group (e.g., differences within the drug group A) and differences of scores between the groups (differences that show up between the drug groups A, B, and C). An analysis of variance involves computing a ratio that compares these two kinds of variability—within-group and between-group variability. In an experimental design, the treatment effect would be tapped in the measure of the between-groups variability.

On examining the data within each column of Table 11.20 (on mean diastolic blood pressure by drug type), note that the variation within each group cannot be explained by a connection with the treatment variable. (In the first column, the drug A data are reported and because all the cases are administered drug A, drug intake cannot explain variations within this column. A similar situation exists within the columns for drugs B and C.) Differences between the three groups, however, may be associated with the treatment variable (type of drug taken) as each group received a different drug.

In Chapter 12, the computations are presented for doing a one-way analysis of variance. In this particular case, the estimates of variance indicate more variation within

Table 11.20   Mean Diastolic Blood Pressure by Drug Type

Drug A	Drug B	Drug C	Total
84	84	80	
87	87	80	
69	80	78	
75	71	68	
86	83	78	
80	78	84	
82	80	90	
95	62	92	
78	82	80	
81	84	86	
Sums 817	791	818	2426
Means 817	791	818	808
Cases, n 10	10	10	30

the groups than between them. Details for the computation and interpretation of ANOVAs are presented in Chapter 12.

To perform this analysis in SPSS, use the ONE-WAY ANOVA procedure; see Appendix A for details.

3. Correlational Analysis

Correlational analysis is a procedure for measuring how closely two variables are related to each other. It is used with variables that are measured at the ratio level. After the fundamentals of this statistical technique are understood, the beginning researcher is in a position to grasp a whole family of related advanced techniques, including partial correlations, multiple correlations, multiple regression, factor analysis, path analysis, and canonical correlations.

A major advantage of using correlational techniques is that many variables can be analyzed simultaneously. Multivariate (many variables) analysis, whose computations have been made easier through the use of computers, relies heavily on

correlational techniques. But the cost of using these powerful statistical tools is that more attention must be paid to measurement. Correlational techniques assume measurement at the ratio level. Although this assumption may be relaxed, the cost of doing so is that the strength of the relationships between variables tend to be underestimated (see Chapter 13 for more on this point).

Given the importance of correlational techniques, it is crucial that beginning researchers understand the fundamentals of these procedures. After they are understood, the more sophisticated procedures are extensions of the simple ones. We have two basic concerns:

- What is the equation that describes the relationship between the variables?
- What is the strength of the relationship between the two variables?

An attempt is made to show how each may be visually estimated; in addition, a simple, intuitively obvious approach to each computation is presented in Boxes 11.1 and 11.2.

a. The Linear Equation: A Visual Estimation Procedure

Our first concern is to determine the equation that describes the relationship between two variables. The general form of the equation is:

$$Y = a + bX$$

The components of the equation are Y, the dependent variable (starting salary to the nearest 10,000 dollars) and X, the independent variable (years of postsecondary education); a is a constant that identifies the point at which the regression line crosses the Y axis; b refers to the slope of the regression line that describes the relationship between the variables. The terms "Y axis" and "regression line" are discussed below.

BOX 11.1 *Calculating a Linear Equation*

Having estimated the equation describing the relation between the variables, let us now compute the actual equation. The table below presents the data and the computations necessary to determine the equation. The following steps are required:

Step 1: Determine the mean value for the X and Y variables. This can be done by summing the values and dividing by the number of cases.

Step 2: Subtract each value of X from the mean of X.

Step 3: Square the values determined in the previous step.

Step 4: Subtract each value of Y from the mean of Y.

Step 5: Multiply the value determined in Step 2 by those determined in Step 4.

Step 6: Sum all columns.

Step 7: To determine the b value: divide the column total determined in Step 5 by the column total in Step 3. As in:

$$b = \frac{\Sigma\,(X - \bar{X})\,(Y - \bar{Y})}{\Sigma\,(X - \bar{X})^2}$$

$$b = 19 \div 26$$

$$b = .73$$

Step 8: Inspect the regression line; if it slopes upward (highest on the right side), then the sign of the b will be positive (+); if it slopes downward (lowest on the right side), then the b value will be negative (−).

Step 9: To determine the a value, apply the formula:

$$a = \bar{Y} - b\bar{X}$$

$$a = 5 - .73(5)$$

$$a = 1.35$$

Step 10: The values may now be applied and the final equation determined. The calculated equation is:

$$Y = 1.35 + .73X$$

Recall that the visual estimation of the formula was:

$$Y = 1.33 + .79X$$

Computing a Linear Equation

Step 1 X Y	Step 2 $X - \bar{X}$	Step 3 $(X - \bar{X})^2$	Step 4 $Y - \bar{Y}$	Step 5 $(X - \bar{X})\,(Y - \bar{Y})$
2 3	−3	9	−2	6
3 4	−2	4	−1	2
5 4	0	0	−1	0
7 6	2	4	1	2
8 8	3	9	3	9
Total	0	26	0	19

$\bar{X} = 5$
$\bar{Y} = 5$
General equation: $Y = a + b(X)$, where:

$$b = \frac{\Sigma\,(X - \bar{X})(Y - \bar{Y})}{\Sigma\,(X - \bar{X})^2} = \frac{19}{26} = .73$$

$a = 5 - 0.73\,(5)$

$a = 1.35$

Hence, $Y = 1.35 + 0.73(X)$

Note: The sign of the b coefficient is determined by inspection; if the slope of the regression line is positive (highest on the right side), then the b coefficient is positive (+); if it is negative (lowest on the right side), then the b coefficient is negative.

BOX 11.2 *Calculating a Correlation: Correlation Coefficient:*
A Simple Computational Procedure

The following table presents the information necessary to hand compute a correlation using a method which parallels the estimation proce- dure outlined above. The steps are simple and can be quickly performed if there are only a few observations.

X	Y	$(Y - \bar{Y})^2$	Y_p	$Y - Y_p$	$(Y - Y_p)^2$
2	3	4	2.81*	0.19	0.0361
3	4	1	3.54	9.46	0.2116
4	5	1	5.00	−1.00	1.0000
7	6	1	6.46	−0.46	0.2116
8	8	9	7.19	0.81	0.6561
Totals		16			Σ 2.1154

*The Y_p value is computed by substituting each value of X into the equation determined in Table 11.1. In the first observation, the computation would be $Y_p = 1.35 + 0.73(2) = 2.81$.

Step 1: The first step is to determine the variation around the regression line. For each observation of X, we will need to compute the predicted value for Y. To do this, we simply go to the equation determined in Section c, plug in the value for X, and solve. The first observation would be done as follows:

$$Y_p = 1.35 + 0.73(X)$$

$$Y_p = 1.35 + 0.73(2)$$

$$Y_p = 2.81$$

The predicted values for Y are determined for each case in the manner described for the first observation.

Step 2: The second step is to compute how much each observation deviates from its **predicted** value. $(Y - Yp)$.

Step 3: The third step is to square the results of the previous step. After this is completed, this column should be summed. $(Y - Yp)^2$.

Step 4: The previous three steps provide us with a measure of the variations around the regression line. To get an estimate of the deviations around the mean of Y, we need only look at the sum for the column:

$$(Y - \bar{Y})^2$$

Step 5: We are now able to plug the values into the formula:

$$r^2 = 1 - \frac{\text{Variations around regression}}{\text{Variations around mean of Y}}$$

$$r^2 = 1 - \frac{\Sigma(Y - Y_p)^2 \div N}{\Sigma(Y - \bar{Y})^2 \div N}$$

$$r^2 = 1 - \frac{.423}{3.2}$$

$$r^2 = 1 - 0.13$$

$$r^2 = 0.87$$

$$r = 0.93$$

Note: If the regression line is highest on the right side, the r value will be positive; if it is lowest on the right side of the plot, the r value will be negative.

For purposes of illustration, we will use the data shown in Table 11.21.

Step 1. The first step in visually estimating the equation that describes the relationship between the variables would be to plot the relationship on graph paper. To have fairly accurate estimates, it is necessary to plot carefully and to ensure that units of measurement of the same size are used on both dimensions of the graph. Figure 11.6 shows what such a graph would look like. Note that the dependent variable (Y) is plotted on the vertical axis and the independent variable (X) is plotted on the horizontal axis.

Step 2. Insert a straight **regression line** so that the vertical deviations of the points above the line are equal to the vertical deviations below the line. There need not be the same number of points above and below the line, nor need any of the points necessarily fall right on the line. The regression line offers the best linear description of the relationship between the two variables. From the regression line, one can estimate how much one has to change the independent variable in order to produce a unit of change in the dependent variable. The following is a hint to locate where the regression line should be drawn. Turn a ruler on its edge; then move the ruler to achieve both minimal deviations from it and equal deviations on both sides of the ruler (Fig. 11.7).

Step 3. Observe where the regression line crosses the Y axis; this point repre-

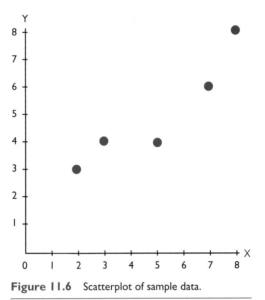

Figure 11.6   Scatterplot of sample data.

sents the constant, or the a value, in the regression equation. Note that in Figure 11.7, we have estimated that it crosses the Y axis at 1.33.

Step 4. Draw a line parallel to the X axis and one parallel to the Y axis to form a right-angled triangle with the regression line, similar to that shown in Figure 11.8. Measure the lines in millimeters. (In Figure 11.8, the vertical measures 72

Table 11.21   Sample Data Set

X	Y
2	3
3	4
5	4
7	6
8	8

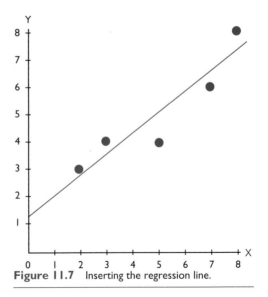

Figure 11.7   Inserting the regression line.

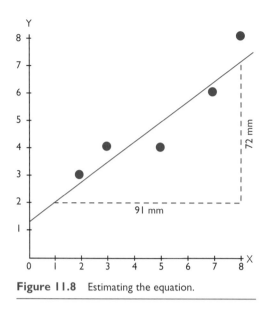

Figure 11.8 Estimating the equation.

mm and the horizontal measures 91 mm.) Divide the horizontal distance into the vertical distance; this computation will provide our estimated *b* value. (In our figure, 72 ÷ 91 = 0.79.)

Step 5. If the slope of the regression line is such that it is lower on the right-hand side, the *b* coefficient is negative, meaning the more *X*, the less *Y.* If the slope is negative, use a minus sign in your equation.

Step 6. The visual estimation of the equation describing the relationship between the variables is determined by simply adding the *a* and *b* values to the general equation:

$$Y = a + bX$$

In our illustration, the values would be as follows:

$$Y = 1.33 + 0.79(X)$$

The above formula is our **visually estimated equation** of the relationship between the two variables. Box 11.2 presents a calculation of the actual equation. After the calculations have been made, we can compare the results with those we got using the visual estimation procedure.

Note that we have come fairly close to the computed figures. In a research project, we would have the computer generate the *a* and the *b* values using the REGRESSION procedure. Estimating equations is a good exercise to become familiar with the different elements involved in regression analysis.

To perform this analysis using SPSS, see the REGRESSION procedure in Appendix A.

In some cases, the *a* value will turn out to be negative; this simply means that the regression line crosses the *Y axis* below the *X axis.* It should be noted as well that as the *b* value increases, the regression line is steeper. In this case, smaller increments in the *X* variable lead to increments in the *Y* variable. A negative value on the *b* indicates a negative slope, a situation in which the data indicate a relationship in which the greater *X*, the less *Y.*

Beginning researchers should recognize that with a linear equation, it is possible to *predict* the value of a dependent variable given a value of the independent variable. When nurse researchers speak of **prediction,** this is often the sense in which they are using the term. Figure 11.9

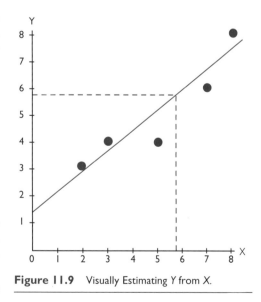

Figure 11.9 Visually Estimating Y from X.

shows how one could visually estimate the predicted value of Y (income), given a value of X (years of postsecondary education). The procedure simply involves locating the X value on the X axis, moving vertically to the regression line, and then moving horizontally to the Y axis. The point at which the Y axis is intersected represents the visual estimate of the Y variable.

A predicted value is computed using an equation in which values of the independent variable (or variables) is (are) plugged into the equation. Suppose, for example, that we attempted to predict the values of Y given X values of 1, 4, and 6. To solve the problem, we would simply use the equation computed above and then determine the predicted values of Y, as in:

Computed equation: $Y = 1.35 + 0.73(X)$

		Y_p
with X value of 1:	$Y = 1.35 + 0.73(1) =$	2.08
with X value of 4:	$Y = 1.35 + 0.73(4) =$	4.27
with X value of 6:	$Y = 1.35 + 0.73(6) =$	5.73

We use the same procedures in situations in which there are multiple independent variables determining the predicted values of a dependent variable, except that there are more values to be plugged into the equation.

b. Correlation Coefficient: A Visual Estimation Procedure

In learning to visually estimate a correlation, it is important to develop some sense of what correlations of different magnitude look like. Figure 11.10 presents graphs of eight relationships. In the first four, the correlation coefficients vary from 0.99 to 0.36. Note that if the correlation dropped below the 0.36 level, it would become difficult to determine where the regression line should be drawn. At the other end of the continuum, note that correlations drop fairly slowly as the scatter around the re-

gression line increases. Plot 5 shows a **curvilinear** relationship in which the plot goes in one direction and then switches to another one. Plot 6 shows a case in which the linear correlation is zero but in which there is a fairly strong association between the variables. Plots 7 and 8 show situations to be wary of—namely, those where a few deviant cases can radically shift the slope of the regression line. The change of two points in the two plots shifts the sign of the correlation from a positive one (plot 7) to a negative one (plot 8).

One reason that it is important to plot out relationships is to permit a visual inspection of the results. If there are extreme values or if the plot indicates a nonlinear relationship, then a linear correlation analysis would be inappropriate.

The **correlation coefficient (r)** is a measure of the strength of association between two variables. The correlation may vary from $+1$ to -1. Perfect correlations are rare, except when a variable is correlated with itself; therefore, almost all of the correlations are represented by values preceded by a decimal point, as in 0.98, 0.37, or -0.56. Negative correlations mean that there is a negative slope in the relationship, meaning the more X the less Y.

Let us now develop an intuitively simple way of estimating the strength of the relationship between two variables. Examine the first four plots shown in Figure 11.10. Note that the closer the plotted points are to the regression line, the higher the correlation. Conversely, the more points diverge from the regression line, the lower the correlation. In estimating the correlation coefficient, there are two kinds of variability that we have to be concerned with: (1) variations around the regression line and (2) variations around the mean of Y.

We can determine the ratio between these two types of variability. In essence, the correlation coefficient (r) reflects this ratio so that the higher the ratio, the higher the correlation. Indeed, we can represent the relationship as follows:

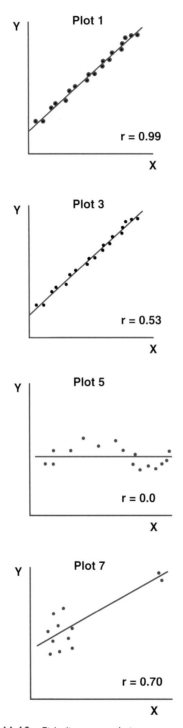
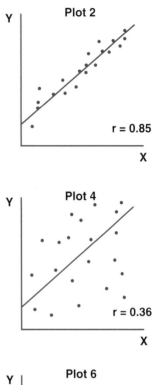
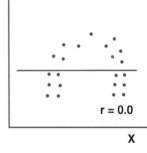
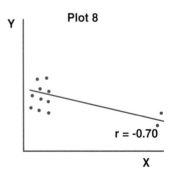

Figure 11.10   Eight linear correlations.

$$r^2 = 1 - \frac{\text{Variations around regression}}{\text{Variations around mean of } Y}$$

As an exercise in trying to visually estimate the strength of a correlation, the following steps may be taken:

Step 1. Plot the data on graph paper and draw in an estimated regression line. Again, remember that the same units of measurement must be used on both dimensions of your graph.

Step 2. Draw in a line parallel to the X axis that will cut through the estimated mean value of Y.

Step 3. To estimate the deviations around the regression line, draw in an additional regression line parallel to the original one for the points on or above the existing regression line. (You may want to cover the points below the regression line to avoid confusion.) Now draw yet another regression line parallel to the other two for the points below the original regression line. Measure and record the perpendicular distance between the two new regression lines.

Step 4. To estimate the deviations around the mean of Y, two additional lines parallel to the mean of Y line must be drawn—the first for those points above the line and the second for those points below the line. Again, the perpendicular distance between these new lines should be measured and recorded.

Step 5. At this point, you should have drawn a graph similar to the one shown in Figure 11.11.

To estimate the correlation, simply enter the values from your graph into the following equation:

$$r^2 = 1 - \frac{\text{Variations around regression}}{\text{Variations around mean of } Y}$$

$$r^2 = 1 - \frac{8}{44}$$

$$r^2 = .82$$

$$r = .91$$

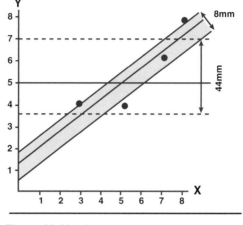

Figure 11.11   Estimating a correlation.

Your estimation is based on the idea that the correlation reflects the ratio of *variations around the regression line* to *variations around the mean of Y*. As the variations around the regression line become relatively smaller, the correlation rises. Conversely, as the two measures of variation approach equality, the correlation approaches zero. Although visually estimated correlations are never reported because they are not exact, the exercise is an excellent one for becoming familiar with the meaning of the correlation coefficient. If you have few cases, it is easy to hand compute the exact correlation using the steps outlined in Box 11.2. However, with more than 15 or 20 cases, you should probably have the computations done by a computer.

Note that the computations in Box 11.2 have led to results roughly similar to those achieved using the visual estimation procedures. (Usually the results will not be so close!) Having done a few visual estimations and a few hand calculations of correlations, you should have a good understanding of simple correlations. There are many statistical techniques that are extensions of correlational techniques. After the basics are understood, then computations may be turned over to a computer.

4. Plotting the Data

It is a good idea to produce a scatterplot of important relationships in your study. A plot will alert you to problems such as:

- A few extreme cases that may be influencing the correlation between the variables (see Fig. 11.10, plots 7 and 8)
- A strong relationship exists, but it is not linear and the correlation does not reflect the true strength of the relationship (see Fig. 11.10, plots 5 and 6)
- There are a lot of data points with the same value; this lack of variation may alert you to a problem in the measurement of one of the ratio variables involved in the plot

Many computer programs, including SPSS, can produce such plots quickly.

5. Computing Spearman Correlations

A nurse researcher may wish to test a relationship between variables that are measured at the ordinal level. For example, the nurse may want to explore the relationship between distance to hospital (under 1 mile, 1 to 5 miles, 5 miles and over) and frequency of visits to emergency departments (low frequency, medium, and high frequency) to identify one of the factors related to emergency department use. **Spearman correlations** are the appropriate measurement of association when the variables are measured at the ordinal level. The details of such computations may be checked in any elementary statistics text and are not presented here. Think of them as being similar to the correlation procedures just discussed.

6. Computing Partial Correlations

A **partial correlation** is a special type of correlation that may be used with ratio level variables. It measures the strength of association between two variables while simultaneously controlling for the effects of one or more additional variables. For example, if a nurse researcher is interested in studying the relationship between perceived health status and the engagement in healthy lifestyles, he or she would probably want to control for the socioeconomic status of the participants. Providing the variables are measured at the ratio level, partial correlations would provide an analytical solution to the problem.

In partial correlations, we adjust the values of the dependent (in this case, engagement in healthy lifestyles) and the independent variable (in this case, perceived health status) in order to take into account the influence of the control variable (in this case, socioeconomic status). The advantage of partial correlations over cross-tabular table analysis is that:

- We make use of all of the data (by not recoding variables into two or three categories as would be done in a cross-tabular analysis (CROSSTABS).
- We can work with fewer cases without running into cell-size problems as happens frequently with cross-tabular table analysis.

Similar to ordinary correlations, partial correlations take on values from $+1.0$ through to -1.0. Partial correlations control one or more independent variables. The number of controls determines the order of the partial. A correlation with one control variable is a *first-order partial correlation;* one with two controls is a *second-order partial correlation,* and so forth. Incidentally, ordinary correlations are sometimes referred to as *zero-order correlations,* which simply means that there are no control variables in the analysis.

The strategy involved in partial correlations is that regression equations can be used to express the relationship between each pair of variables in the equation. For any value of an independent variable, it is possible to predict the value of the dependent variable while adjusting for the influence of the control variables.

The idea of residuals is also useful in understanding partial correlations. In the three-variable case, if the possible combinations (X–Y, Z–Y, and X–Z) are plotted and a regression line is entered for the X–Y relation, we could argue that the deviations from the line are the result of the influence of factor Z plus that of other known and unknown factors. These deviations are *residuals*. They arise when we allow one variable to explain all the variation that it can in another variable; what is left unexplained (deviations from the regression line) are the residuals. By correlating residuals, we can get a measure of the amount of influence a third variable has on the first relationship (X–Y), independent of the second relationship (X–Z).

The notational convention that we use in referring to partial correlations shows the numbers of the two major variables and these are separated from the numbers of the control variables by a "." as in:

$$r_{12.3} = .56$$

In this case, we have a first-order partial correlation reported, with a value of 0.56. This value represents a measure of the strength of association between variables 1 and 2, controlling for variable 3. A third-order partial correlation simply designates three control variables, as in:

$$r_{12.345} = .28$$

Partial correlations will be used in testing causal models in which the variables involved are measured at the ratio level of measurement (see Chapter 17).

Because it is easy to hand-compute a first-order partial, the formula is presented here. It may be used if the researcher has the zero-order correlation matrix.

$$r_{12.3} = \frac{r_{12} - (r_{13})(r_{23})}{\sqrt{1 - r_{13}^2}\sqrt{1 - r_{23}^2}}$$

E X E R C I S E S

1. As an exercise in learning to identify different levels of measurement, go through a sample questionnaire and identify the level of measurement achieved for each question.

2. Calculate the mode, median, mean, range, standard deviations, and variance for the nursing grades in the accompanying table.

Nursing Student Grades for a Mid-term Test	
88	69
72	93
93	92
77	74
94	85
79	87
85	82
66	71
79	74
83	86

3. Using the mean and standard deviation calculated above, use Z scores to estimate the percentage of nursing students you would expect to score 70 percent or below. What percentage would you expect to score over 75 percent? What percentage would you expect to score between 80 and 90 percent?

4. Equally weighting income and education, use Z scores to calculate each person's socioeconomic status from the following data set:

Given the following:	Mean	Standard Deviation
Education	14.0	4.0
Income	$47,000	$13,000

Person A	Education:	12.0 years
	Income:	$88,000
Person B	Education:	16.0 years
	Income:	$105,000
Person C	Education:	11.0 years
	Income:	$44,900
Person D	Education:	18.0 years
	Income:	$92,500
Person E	Education:	13 years
	Income:	$42,500

5. Using the data given here on a respondent's, father's, mother's, and sister's visits to a doctor's office in the past 12 months, plot the data (treating the respondent's number of visits to a doctor's office as dependent) and go through the procedures to visually estimate the correlation and the equation that describe the relationship between the respondent's number of visits to the doctor's office and the number of visits to the doctor's office by the mother.

Sample Data for Visits to the Doctor's Office

Respondent	Father	Mother	Sister
1	3	1	4
2	3	4	3
3	4	3	5
9	7	6	6
10	10	10	8
12	11	9	14
14	13	15	8
5	4	7	2
6	7	5	8
8	8	10	12

6. Compute the r and the equation. How close were your estimates to the actual value?

7. Using the formula computed in question 6, what would you predict the respondent's number of visits to the doctor's office to be if the mother made 1, 6, or 15 yearly visits?

8. Using visual estimation procedures, estimate the correlation between mother's and sister's number of visits.

9. Using visual estimation procedures, estimate the linear equation that describes the relationship between re-

400   A STATISTICS PRIMER

mal distribution curve. As sample sizes become larger, a more peaked (leptokurtic) distribution would result, which means that larger samples require smaller differences in order to reject the null hypothesis. Most times we draw one sample and have no way of knowing if it is a truly representative sample. Perhaps our sample is atypical—we just happened to draw one with a preponderance of red balls and we might, therefore, wrongly conclude that there are more red balls in the container. But because it would take too long to count the thousands of balls in the container, we simply take the chance of being wrong. We can reduce that risk by changing the significance level from 0.05 to 0.01. That would reduce, but not eliminate, the chance of coming to an incorrect conclusion.

b. One Sample Compared with a Regional Distribution: Is There a Relationship Between Family Income and the Use of Alternative Therapy Clinics?

There are situations in which one wishes to compare a cohort of respondents with a known distribution. Table 12.2 reports family incomes of clients attending an alternative therapy clinic that is privately funded along with the income distribution of all families in the vicinity of the clinic. Is there a significant difference between the income distribution of the general population in the area and the income distribution of users of the alternative therapy clinic?

We will follow the six steps in conducting tests of significance:

1. Research hypothesis: Alternative therapy clinic users overrepresent the higher family incomes from the community (note that this implies a one-tailed test). Null hypothesis: There is no difference in the family incomes of alternative therapy clinic users and the family incomes in the community.
2. If the null hypothesis is to be rejected, the result will fall into the tail of the sampling distribution representing high incomes. This is a one-tailed test.
3. We will use the 0.05 significance level in the test, meaning that if the result falls into the 5 percent right tail, we can be 95 percent certain that there is a significant overrepresentation of the wealthier families' using the alternative therapy clinics.
4. Box 12.3 presents a hand calculation of the test statistic.
5. The results reported in Box 12.3 would lead us to *reject the null hypothesis* because the difference observed would occur by chance less than 5 percent of the time. The critical value that must be exceeded in order to reject the null hypothesis is 4.61 (see Table 12.1; note that we look up the value for two *degrees of freedom* using the one-tailed test column because we are predicting the direction of the relationship). Because the calculated chi-square value is 45.61 and this exceeds the critical value of 4.61, we reject the null hypothesis.
6. We can then conclude that there is a statistically significant overrepresen-

Table 12.2 **Alternative Therapy Clinic Users and General Population Family Incomes**

Income, dollars	Clinic Users, n	Sample, %	General Population, %
Over 100,000	30	15.0	7.8
40,000 to 99,999	160	80.0	68.9
Under 40,000	100	5.0	23.3
Total	200	100.0	100.0

BOX 12.3 Computing Chi-Square for Alternative Therapy Clinic Users' Family Income Data

Income Category, dollars	f_o	f_e	$f_o - f_e$	$(f_o - f_e)^2$	$\dfrac{(f_o - f_e)^2}{f_e}$
Over 100,000	30	15.6*	14.4	207.36	13.29
40,000 to 99,999	160	137.8	22.2	492.84	3.57
Under 40,000	10	46.6	-36.6	1339.56	28.75
Totals	200	200			45.61

Chi-square = 45.61; df = 2; probability < 0.05.
*The **expected frequencies** are computed on the presumption that if there is no difference between the general population and the families of clinic users, then the income distribution would have similar proportions in the various categories. In the first cell, where there were 30 clinic users, we would have expected 15.6 ($200 \times .078 = 15.6$). In the general population, 7.8 percent of the families had incomes above $100,000.

Degrees of freedom = 2. Two cells would have to be computed before the final one could be calculated by subtraction, as in f_e cell $c = [200 \times (15.6 + 137.8)]$.

Required critical chi-square value to reject the null hypothesis is 4.61 (one-tailed test, 2 degrees of freedom, at the 0.05 level); see Table 12.1.

Decision: Because the chi-square value is 45.61 and this exceeds the critical value, the null hypothesis is rejected.

tation of the wealthier families' using the alternative therapy clinic. The risk we take in making that conclusion is that we may, by chance, just happen to have overselected wealthier families. A difference of that magnitude, however, would occur in fewer than 5 percent of the samples we draw. Another way to think about it is to say that we can be confident that we will make the correct decision 19 out of 20 times.

c. Calculating a Chi-Square for a Typical Cross-Tabular Analysis: Frequency of Drug Use by Gender

Box 12.4 presents a two-variable cross-tabular table showing the relationship between frequency of drug use by gender. Beneath the table, the computational procedures are presented for the computation of the chi-square.

We will follow the six steps in conducting tests of significance:

1. Research hypothesis: There is a difference in drug use by gender (note that this implies a two-tailed test). Null hypothesis: There is no difference in drug use by gender.
2. If the null hypothesis is to be rejected, the result will fall into either tail of the sampling distribution, this being a two-tailed test.
3. We will use the 0.05 significance level in the test, meaning that if the result falls into the 2.5 percent right tail or the 2.5 percent left tail, we can be 95 percent certain that there is a significant difference in drug use by gender.
4. Box 12.4 presents a hand calculation of the test statistic.

BOX 12.4 *Frequency of Drug Use by Gender*

Frequency of Drug Use in Lifetime	Gender				Total	
	Male		Female			
	N	%	N	%	N	%
No experience	47	34.8	63	49.2	110	41.8
Once or twice	51	37.8	39	30.5	90	34.2
Three or more times	37	27.4	26	20.3	63	24.0
Totals	135	100.0	128	100.0	263	100.0

Chi-square = 5.689; df = 2; probability = > 0.05.

The chi-square could be hand computed in the following manner:

Cell	f_o	f_e	$(f_o - f_e)$	$(f_o - f_e)^2$	$(f_o - f_e)^2/f_e$
a	47	56.5	9.5	90.25	1.597
b	63	53.5	9.5	90.25	1.687
c	51	46.2	4.8	23.06	0.499
d	39	43.8	-4.8	23.06	0.526
e	37	32.3	4.7	21.72	0.673
f	26	30.7	-4.7	21.72	0.707
					Σ 5.689

Required critical value to reject the null hypothesis is 5.99 (two-tailed test, 2 degrees of freedom, at the 0.05 level); see Table 12.1.
Decision: Because the chi-square value is 5.689 and this does not equal or exceed the critical value (5.99), the null hypothesis is accepted.

Further Notes:
Determining **expected frequencies:** The easiest way to calculate the expected frequencies in a cell of a standard cross-tabular table is to multiply the row marginal total by the column marginal total and divide this result by the total number of cases in the table. (Exclude missing cases from the table before calculations are made.) For cell *a*, the calculation would be (110 $\times$ 135)/263 = 56.5. For cell *c*, the calculation would be (90 $\times$ 135)/263 = 46.2. The remaining expected frequencies can be computed in a similar manner or determined by subtracting the calculated cells from the marginal total; cell *e* could be determined by adding together the computed expected frequencies for cells *a* and *c* and this total could be subtracted from the column marginal total, as in 56.5 + 46.2 = 102.7, then 135 - 102.7 = 32.3.

Determining **degrees of freedom:** The easiest method for determining degrees of freedom in standard cross-tabular tables (such as

continued on next page

BOX 12.4 *Frequency of Drug Use by Gender (Continued)*

the one used in this example) is to count the number of rows and columns in the table and use the following formula:

Degrees of freedom = (# rows − 1) × (# columns −1)

Degrees of freedom = (3 − 1) × (2 − 1)

Degrees of freedom = 2

We could also use the slower method of figuring out how many cells we would have to hand calculate the expected frequencies before we could get the rest by subtraction. The answer is 2.

---

5. The results reported in Box 12.4 would lead us to *accept the null hypothesis* because the difference observed would occur by chance more than 5 percent of the time. The critical value that must be exceeded in order to reject the null hypothesis is 5.99 (see Table 12.1; note that we look up the value for two *degrees of freedom* using the two-tailed test column because we are not predicting the direction of the relationship). Because the calculated chi-square value is 5.689 and this does not equal or exceed the critical value of 5.99, we accept the null hypothesis.

6. We can then conclude that there is not a statistically significant relationship between drug use and gender. The differences between the genders observed in drug use may well be the result of random sampling fluctuations; we cannot be 95 percent certain the differences observed reflect a "real" difference in drug use. Note, however, that had we been doing a one-tailed test, we would reject the null hypothesis. In this case, the decision to do a two-tailed test has had a crucial impact on the interpretation of the result.

To perform this analysis using SPSS, see the CROSSTABS procedure in Appendix A.

The next two sections introduce tests that involve the comparison of means between categories. Each test assumes that the dependent variable is measured at the ratio level. We will begin with two versions of the t test.

C. THE t TEST OF STATISTICAL SIGNIFICANCE

The **t test** is a popular test of statistical significance most commonly used in studies requiring the comparison between two groups on a measure or a comparison of measures taken at two different times. Suppose that an experimental control group design has been used to measure the acquisition of psychomotor injection administration skills (measured at the ratio level) and that the study involves the comparison of 20 nursing students, 10 taught in the conventional manner and 10 using a new interactive computer methodology. What test would be appropriate here? We could collapse the psychomotor skill scores into high and low scores and then run a chi-square. But this would not make full use of our data. In effect, we would be throwing out all the variability within the two grade categories. Instead, it would make more sense to compare the means of the psychomotor skills scores of students exposed to the different teaching techniques. And because we have a small sample, a t test would do what we want.

The t test is used most often in cases in which:

- Sample sizes are small (typically under 30).
- The dependent variable is measured at the ratio level.
- Assignment to groups has been done independently and randomly.

- The treatment variable has two levels, presence and absence.
- The population from which the sample was drawn is normally distributed; therefore, the distribution of sample means would be normally distributed.
- The researcher wants to find out if there are statistically significant differences between the groups.

Two commonly used variants of the t test are presented in this section. The first is appropriate for a between-subjects design and the second is appropriate for a within-subject design. The t test represents the ratio between the difference in means between two groups and the standard error of the difference. The **standard error of the difference** reflects the average amount of deviation in the two comparison groups (the formula for it is provided in Box 12.5) The t test formula is as follows:

$$t = \frac{\text{Difference between means}}{\text{Standard error of the difference}}$$

1. Between-Subjects t Test

Box 12.5 shows how one could compute the t score in a **between-subjects** design for differences in blood pressure readings resulting from the administration of touch therapy by nursing students to women subjected to artificially induced stress in a laboratory setting. This was reported in Table 4.2.

We will follow the six steps in conducting tests of significance:

1. Research hypothesis: There is a difference in the change in blood pressure readings for those receiving therapeutic touch therapy versus those receiving casual touch (note that this implies a two-tailed test). Null hypothesis: There is no difference in the change in blood pressure by type of touch therapy.
2. If the null hypothesis is to be rejected, the result will fall into either tail of the sampling distribution, this being a two-tailed test.
3. We will use the 0.05 significance level

in the test, meaning that if the result falls into the 2.5 percent right tail or the 2.5 percent left tail, we can be 95 percent certain that there is a significant change in blood pressure levels by type of touch.

4. Box 12.5 presents a hand calculation of the test statistic.
5. The results reported in Box 12.5 would lead us to *accept the null hypothesis* because the difference observed would occur by chance more than 5 percent of the time. The critical value that must be exceeded in order to reject the null hypothesis is 2.10 (In Table 12.3; note that we look up the value for 18 *degrees of freedom,* using the two-tailed test column because we are not predicting the direction of the relationship). Because the calculated t test value is 1.46 and this does not equal or exceed the critical value of 2.10, we accept the null hypothesis.
6. We conclude that there is not a statistically significant relationship between change in blood pressure readings and type of touch. The differences in outcomes by type of touch may well be the result of random sampling fluctuations—we cannot be 95 percent certain the changes observed reflect a "real" difference in the consequences of the type of touch therapy applied.

Although the *average change* in diastolic blood pressure readings for subjects in the therapeutic touch group is slightly higher, there was a lot of variation within the two groups. The test of significance leads us to accept the null hypothesis: there is simply not enough between-group variation compared to within-group variation to reject the null hypothesis.

2. A Within-Subject t Test

A variation of the t test is available for dependent samples (in which the comparison groups are not selected independently, as in *repeated measures designs* in

BOX 12.5 Between-Subjects t Test for Equal-Sized Groups (From Therapeutic Touch and Blood Pressure Data, Chapter 4)

In Chapter 4, data were reported comparing therapeutic touch with casual touch on blood pressure (BP) readings. The means and standard deviations were reported for diastolic BP using each type of touch. This was a between-subjects design with random assignment to groups and was conducted by student nurses. The data were as follows:

Experiment	Therapeutic Touch		Casual Touch	
	Name	Change in BP	Name	Change in BP
I. Student nurses: Between-subjects design; random assignment to groups	Kathleen	10	Paula	12
	Li	9	Marlies	7
	Danielle	11	Vanny	6
	Kim	8	Paula	6
	Kevin	12	Sandra	11
	Mary	4	Marius	1
	Yvonne	5	Chris	2
	Tara	7	Andrea	4
	Ursula	8	Tony	7
	Holly	10	Carol	8
Mean		8.40		6.40
Standard deviation		2.547		3.502
Mean difference			2.00	

Using the following formula we can quickly compute the t test:

$$t = \frac{\bar{X}_1 - \bar{X}_2}{\text{Standard error of the difference}}$$

The standard error of the difference may be computed using the following formula:

$$\sqrt{\frac{sd_1^2}{N_1} + \frac{sd_2^2}{N_2}}$$

where sd_1^2 is the variance for group 1 and sd_2^2 is the variance for group 2. N_1 refers to the

number of subjects in group 1; N_2 refers to the number of subjects in group 2.

Step 1: Subtract the mean change in BP for the therapeutic touch group from the mean BP change for the casual touch group (8.40–6.40 = 2.00). This is the value we will use in the numerator (the value above the line in the equation).

Step 2: For the denominator (below the line in the equation), we require the variance for each type of touch therapy and because we

continued on next page

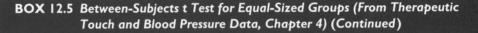

BOX 12.5 *Between-Subjects t Test for Equal-Sized Groups (From Therapeutic Touch and Blood Pressure Data, Chapter 4) (Continued)*

have the standard deviations reported in the table, all we have to do is square the standard deviations to get the variances. Hence:

Variance therapeutic touch:
$$sd^2 = 2.547^2 = 6.487$$
Variance casual touch:
$$sd^2 = 3.502^2 = 12.264$$

Step 3: The *n* (number of cases) for therapeutic touch is 10; the *n* for casual touch is also 10.

Step 4: Calculate the values for the denominator by using the values calculated in Step 2, using the equation given above.

$$\text{Standard error of difference} = \sqrt{\frac{sd_1^2}{N_1} + \frac{sd_2^2}{N_2}}$$

$$\text{Standard error of difference} = \sqrt{\frac{6.487}{10} + \frac{12.264}{10}}$$

Standard error of difference = 1.370

Step 5: Plug the values into the equation for the t test, as in:

$$t \text{ test score} = \frac{2.00}{1.37}$$

t test score = 1.46

Step 6 Determine the degrees of freedom by subtracting number of groups from number of cases (20 − 2 = 18).

Step 7: Decision: Because the t value does not exceed the one shown in Table 12.3, we accept the null hypothesis. The differences in the BP readings may simply be the result of sampling fluctuations.

which we collect data from the same subjects run under each of the treatment conditions; these are known as *paired sample designs*). The steps for hand computing a dependent t test are reported for the **within-subject** design touch therapy data originally reported in Chapter 4 (Box 12.6).

We will follow the six steps in conducting tests of significance:

1. Research hypothesis: There is a difference in the change in blood pressure readings for those receiving therapeutic touch therapy versus those receiving casual touch (note that this implies a two-tailed test). Null hypothesis: There is no difference in the change in blood pressure by type of touch therapy.
2. If the null hypothesis is to be rejected, the result will fall into either tail of the sampling distribution, this being a two-tailed test.
3. We will use the 0.05 significance level

in the test, meaning that if the result falls into the 2.5 percent right tail or the 2.5 percent left tail, we can be 95 percent certain that there is a significant change in blood pressure levels by type of touch.

4. Box 12.6 presents a hand calculation of the test statistic.
5. The results reported in Box 12.6 would lead us to *reject the null hypothesis* because the difference observed would occur by chance less than 5 percent of the time. The critical value that must be exceeded in order to reject the null hypothesis is 2.26 (see Table 12.3; note that we look up the value for 9 *degrees of freedom* using the two-tailed test column because we are not predicting the direction of the relationship). Because the observed t test value is 6.71 and this exceeds the critical value of 2.26, we reject the null hypothesis.
6. We conclude that there is a statisti-

Table 12.3   Critical Values for the *T* Distribution: One- and Two-Tailed Tests*

Degrees of Freedom	0.05 Level of Significance		0.01 Level of Significance	
	One-Tailed	Two-Tailed	One-Tailed	Two-Tailed
1	6.31	12.71	31.82	63.66
2	2.92	4.30	6.96	9.92
3	2.35	3.18	4.54	5.84
4	2.13	2.78	3.75	4.60
5	2.02	2.57	3.36	4.03
6	1.94	2.45	3.14	3.71
7	1.90	2.36	3.00	3.50
8	1.86	2.31	2.90	3.34
9	1.83	2.26	2.82	3.25
10	1.81	2.23	2.76	3.17
11	1.80	2.20	2.72	3.10
12	1.78	2.18	2.68	3.06
13	1.77	2.16	2.65	3.01
14	1.76	2.14	2.62	2.98
15	1.75	2.13	2.60	2.95
16	1.75	2.12	2.58	2.92
17	1.74	2.11	2.57	2.90
18	1.73	2.10	2.55	2.88
19	1.73	2.09	2.54	2.86
20	1.72	2.09	2.53	2.84
25	1.71	2.06	2.48	2.79
30	1.70	2.04	2.46	2.75
40	1.68	2.02	2.42	2.70
60	1.67	2.00	2.39	2.66
120	1.66	1.98	2.36	2.62
∞	1.64	1.96	2.33	2.58

*Please consult the appendix of any statistics text if you require additional degrees of freedom or other levels of significance.

cally significant relationship between change in blood pressure readings and type of touch. The differences in outcomes by type of touch are not likely to be caused by random sampling fluctuations—we can be 95 percent certain the changes observed reflect a "real" difference as a result of the type of touch therapy applied. Note that the differences in the mean change in diastolic blood pressure achieved with the two different types of touch is slight (1.00 U), yet the difference in this case is found to be statistically significant (we reject the null hypothesis). Compared with the student nurses (see Box 12.5), the expert nurse practitioners using the two touch therapies produced much less variation in blood pressure readings (standard deviations of 0.816 and 0.823 compared with 2.547 and 3.502, respectively, for the student nurses).

When a test of significance is required to test the significance of differences between means for a study with a more complex experimental design, such as those with several independent variables or more than two different levels in the treatment or control variable, the researcher typically uses *analysis of variance* techniques. These are introduced next.

D. THE F TEST OF STATISTICAL SIGNFICANCE

A further test of significance associated with comparing two or more group means involves an *analysis of variance*. The distribution associated with this test is the **F distribution** and is used to test whether

---

BOX 12.6 *Testing Touch Therapies: A Within-Subject Design (From Therapeutic Touch and Blood Pressure Data, Chapter 4)*

Experiment	Therapeutic Touch		Casual Touch	
	Name	Change in BP	Name	Change in BP
III. Expert nurses: within-subject design	Jamie	12	Jamie	10
	Petra	11	Petra	10
	Margo	11	Margo	11
	Jill	13	Jill	12
	Sandra	13	Sandra	12
	Dale	12	Dale	11
	Paula	11	Paula	10
	Teresa	11	Teresa	10
	Linda	11	Linda	10
	Melanie	12	Melanie	11
Mean		11.70		10.70
Standard deviation		0.823		0.823
Mean difference			1.00	

continued on next page

BOX 12.6 *Testing Touch Therapies: A Within-Subject Design (From Therapeutic Touch and Blood Pressure Data, Chapter 4) (Continued)*

Calculating a Within-Subject (Dependent Groups) t Test

Subject	Time 1 Therapeutic Touch	Time 2 Casual Touch	Difference Between Time 1 and Time 2 (D) Step 1	Average Difference (AD) Step 2	AD − D Step 3	(AD − D)² Step 4
Jamie	12	10	2	1	−1	1
Petra	11	10	1	1	0	0
Margo	11	11	0	1	1	1
Jill	13	12	1	1	0	0
Sandra	13	12	1	1	0	0
Dale	12	11	1	1	0	0
Paula	11	10	1	1	0	0
Teresa	11	10	1	1	0	0
Linda	11	10	1	1	0	0
Melanie	12	11	1	1	0	0
Totals			10			2

Average Difference = 10 ÷ 10 = 1.0
Variances of differences = 1 ÷ 9 = .111

Step 1: Subtract time 2 measure from time 1 measure to get the difference score (D) (in the case of Jamie, $12 - 10 = 2$).

Step 2: Calculate the average difference score (AD): Sum the values for the 10 subjects ($2 + 1 + 0 + 1 + 1 + 1 + 1 + 1 + 1 + 1 = 10$); divide sum by number of subjects ($10 ÷ 10 = 1$).

Step 3: Subtract the difference score (D), calculated in Step 1, from the average difference score (AD) calculated in Step 2: (in the case of Jamie, $2 - 1 = 1$).

Step 4: Square each value calculated in Step 3.

Step 5: Sum the squared values in Step 4 and divide by the number of subjects minus 1 ($10 - 1 = 9$). The measure of the variance of the differences is $2 ÷ 9 = 0.222$

Step 6: To get the standard deviation of the differences, calculate the square root of the variance of the differences, as in:

Standard deviation of differences
$= \sqrt{0.222} = 0.471$

continued on next page

BOX 12.6 *Testing Touch Therapies: A Within-Subject Design (From Therapeutic Touch and Blood Pressure Data, Chapter 4) (Continued)*

Step 7: Calculate the standard error of the difference by dividing the standard deviation of the differences by the square root of the number of pairs of scores, as in:

Standard error of the differences
$$= 0.471 \div \sqrt{10} = 0.149$$

Step 8: Compute the t ratio by dividing the average difference (AD) by the standard error of the difference, as in:

$$t = 1 \div 0.149$$

$$t = 6.71$$

Step 9. Determine the degrees of freedom by subtracting 1 from the number of pairs of scores ($10 - 1 = 9$). Look up the t value in Table 12.3. The two-tailed value with 9 df = 2.26.

Step 10. Decision: Because the calculated t value (6.71) exceeds the critical value (2.26) in Table 12.3, we reject the null hypothesis.

---

there is a significant difference in the means of various categories. Some of this material will not seem to be new because similar ideas were presented in Chapter 11 when discussing both the chi-square test and correlation analyses. **Analysis of variance** is typically used when:

- The dependent variable is measured at the ratio level.
- The treatment variable has two or more levels.
- In cases in which two or more treatments are used simultaneously.
- It is assumed that the population from which the sample was drawn is normally distributed and, therefore, that the distribution of sample means would be normally distributed.
- The researcher wants to find out if there are statistically significant differences between the groups.
- The researcher wants to check to see if the various treatments may be interacting with one another.

1. One-Way Analysis of Variance

A **one-way analysis of variance** provides a test of significance for the effect of a independent variable on a dependent variable.

To illustrate this procedure, we will examine data on *identity awareness scores* in adolescents. The researcher wishes to examine whether these scores vary significantly for *early, middle, and late adolescence.* Identity is the central developmental task of adolescence. Identity awareness was measured using six items that reflect how adolescents make choices by exploring alternatives and committing to roles. The sample involves a total of 182 respondents from the early (age 10 to 13 years), middle (age 14 to 17 years), and late adolescent (age 18 to 20 years) age groups. Our research hypothesis is that identity awareness scores will vary by age group. The null hypothesis is that there is no difference in identity awareness scores across age groups.

Box 12.7 presents the analysis of our study of identity awareness in adolescents. Various computations are made and the resulting test of significance, the F test, indicates that the null hypothesis should be rejected. The differences in the mean scores on identity awareness (27.35 in early adolescence, 30.60 in middle adolescence, and 34.35 in late adolescence) are more than one would expect from normal sample fluctuations. We conclude, therefore, that there is a statistically sig-

BOX 12.7 One-Way Analysis of Variance of Identity Awareness by Adolescent Age Group Identity Awareness Scores

	Early Adolescence	Middle Adolescence	Late Adolescence	Total
	34	36	37	
	28	49	34	
	24	38	33	
	31	33	24	
	30	27	31	
	30	34	43	
	...	...	...	...
Sums	1989	1559	2061	5609
Means	30.60	27.35	30.82	
Cases, n	65	57	60	182

Steps in Computing a One-Way Analysis of Variance

Three measures of variation are required to compute the analysis of variance. These are total variation, between variation, and within variation:

Total variation = Between variation + Within variation

The *total variation*, which is all the variability in the data, may be computed by summing the squares of all the identity awareness scores and subtracting from that result the square of the sum divided by the total number of cases, as in:

Step 1: $34^2 + 28^2 + \cdots + 43^2 = 186677$
minus
Step 2: $5609^2 \div 182 = 172862$
equals
Step 3: $186677 - 172862 = 13815$
Total variation = 13815

Step 4: The *between variation*, which is the variability resulting from the different treatments (age groups), may be computed by squaring the column totals, dividing this value by the number of cases, then summing the result, and finally subtract the value in step 2 above, as in:

$((1989^2 \div 65) + (1559^2 \div 57) + (2061^2 \div 60)) - 172862 = 1437$

Step 5: The *within variation*, which is the variability resulting from differences among members within each age group, may be determined by simply subtracting the between variation from the total variation, as in:

$13815 - 1437 = 12378$

Step 6: An F ratio table may be computed as follows:

	Sums of Squares	Degrees of Freedom	Mean Squares	F	F Prob.
Total variation	13815	$N - 1 = 181$			
Between variation	1437	$k - 1 = 2$	718.4	10.39	.0001
Within Variation	12378	$N - k = 179$	69.2		

where k = number of categories in the independent variable.

continued on next page

BOX 12.7 One-Way Analysis of Variance of Identity Awareness by Adolescent Age Group Identity Awareness Scores (Continued)

Step 7: To estimate the mean squares (population variance) for the between and within rows, divide the sums of squares for the row by the degrees of freedom for the row, as in:

i) *Between* estimate of mean squares:
   $1437 \div 2 = 718.4$

ii) *Within* estimate of mean squares:
   $12378 \div 179 = 69.2$

Step 8: To calculate the F ratio divide the *within variation* (69.2) into the *between variation* (718.4):

$718.4 \div 69.2 = 10.39$

Step 9: If the probability is not calculated for you (in cases in which the values are hand calculated or when using some software package), you will need to determine the value that has to be exceeded in order to reject the null hypothesis by looking up the value on the F distribution table (see Table 12.4). The F table requires the use of two values for degrees of freedom: the *between variation df* is placed across the top of the table (in the sample case df = 2); the *within variation df* is arranged along the vertical column (in our table, df = 179; see table in Step 6 above for these values). We will test the hypothesis at the 0.05 level. The critical value given in the table is 3.07. The F ratio must equal or exceed this value in order to reject the null hypothesis.

Step 10: Because the F ratio for the sample data is 10.39 (exceeding the critical value), the null hypothesis is rejected. Variability of the magnitude reported in the identity awareness scores is regarded as statistically significant. If the differences between the age groups had been smaller and we were led to accept the null hypothesis, we would argue that the differences observed simply reflect sampling fluctuations and we cannot reasonably conclude that there is a "real" difference in the identity awareness scores of the respondents from each of the three age groups. (In most software packages, the exact probabilities are provided for the researcher, which allows the researcher to skip steps 9 and 10.)

---

nificant difference in identity awareness scores of samples drawn from the three adolescent age groups.

We will follow the six steps in conducting tests of significance:

1. Research hypothesis: Identity awareness scores will vary by age group. The null hypothesis is that there is no difference in identity awareness scores across age groups

2. If the null hypothesis is to be rejected, the result will fall into either tail of the sampling distribution, this being a two-tailed test.

3. We will use the 0.05 significance level in the test, meaning that if the result falls into the 2.5 percent right tail or the 2.5 percent left tail, we can be 95 percent certain that there is a significant change in identity awareness score.

4. Box 12.7 presents a hand calculation of the test statistic.

5. The results reported in Box 12.7 would lead us to *reject the null hypothesis* because the difference observed would occur by chance less than 5 percent of the time. The critical value that must be exceeded in order to reject the null hypothesis is 3.07 (Table 12.4; note that we look up the value for 2 and 179 *degrees of freedom*). Because the observed F value is 10.39 and this exceeds the critical value of 3.07, we reject the null hypothesis.

6. We conclude that there is a statistically significant relationship between identify awareness scores and age of youth.

Table 12.4 Critical Values for the F Distribution: One-Tailed Tests, 0.05 Level of Significance*

df for the Denominator	df for the Numerator				
	1	2	3	4	5
2	18.51	19.00	19.16	19.25	19.30
3	10.13	9.55	9.28	9.12	9.01
4	7.71	6.94	6.59	6.39	6.26
5	6.61	5.79	5.41	5.19	5.05
6	5.99	5.14	4.76	4.53	4.39
7	5.59	4.74	4.35	4.12	3.97
8	5.32	4.46	4.07	3.84	3.69
9	5.12	4.26	3.86	3.63	3.48
10	4.96	4.10	3.71	3.48	3.33
11	4.84	3.98	3.59	3.36	3.20
12	4.75	3.88	3.49	3.26	3.11
13	4.67	3.80	3.41	3.18	3.02
14	4.60	3.74	3.34	3.11	2.96
15	4.54	3.68	3.29	3.06	2.90
16	4.49	3.63	3.24	3.01	2.85
17	4.45	3.59	3.20	2.96	2.81
18	4.41	3.55	3.16	2.93	2.77
19	4.38	3.52	3.13	2.90	2.74
20	4.35	3.49	3.10	2.87	2.71
25	4.42	3.38	2.99	2.76	2.60
30	4.17	3.32	2.92	2.69	2.53
40	4.08	3.23	2.84	2.61	2.45
60	4.00	3.15	2.76	2.52	2.37
120	3.92	3.07	2.68	2.45	2.29
∞	3.84	3.00	2.60	2.37	2.21

*Please consult the appendix of any statistics text if you require additional degrees of freedom or other levels of significance.

The differences in outcomes by age group are not likely to be caused by random sampling fluctuations—we can be 95 percent certain the identity awareness differences observed reflect a "real" difference across the three age group categories.

The test of significance is based on the idea that, when a sample is drawn, there will be fluctuations in the mean identity awareness scores. What the test is doing is assessing the chance, if the true difference between the age groups in identity awareness is zero, of getting a sample fluctuation of the magnitude shown in the sample data. In the case under examination, the differences range from a low of 27.35 in early adolescence to a high of 34.35 in late adolescence on the identity awareness index. The test of significance reveals that the observed fluctuation is greater than a fluctuation that would probably be caused by normal sample variability. In other words, if there were no "real" identity awareness difference between the age groups, a sample would reveal a difference ± 7.0 points less than 5 percent of the time simply because of sampling fluctuations. On the other hand, if the observed difference could occur more than 5 percent of the time, we would accept the null hypothesis and conclude that there are no statistically significant differences in identity awareness in the populations studied.

To repeat—and to emphasize: A statistically significant relationship is one in which the observed difference would occur by chance less than 5 percent of the time. If the test were set at the 1 percent level, it would simply be more difficult to reject the null hypothesis; here, the difference would be statistically significant only if it could occur by chance less than 1 percent of the time.

Similar to the computational procedure involved in determining the correlation between two variables, the procedures for an analysis of variance require a measurement of two kinds of variation: variations within a column (e.g., differences within each age group), and variations between columns (e.g., differences that show up between early, middle, and late adolescence). An analysis of variance involves computing a ratio that compares these two kinds of variability—within-column and between-column variability.

On examining the data within column one (early adolescence data) of Box 12.7, note that age group cannot explain variations *within* this column (all cases are in the early adolescence age group). Differences in identity awareness scores *between* the columns, however, may be explained by the association with the independent variable (age group).

Box 12.7 goes through the computation of a one-way analysis of variance for the sample data. In this particular case, the estimates of variance indicate more variation between the columns than within them; as a result, the F ratio is more than one. After the F ratio is computed and the critical value is looked up in Table 12.4, the decision is made to reject the null hypothesis because the critical value is exceeded.

2. Two-Way Analysis of Variance

Experimental researchers also use a **two-way analysis of variance,** or a multifactor analysis of variance, when their design has two or more independent variables. Theoretically, any number of independent variables is possible, but in practice rarely more than three or four are used because of the large sample size that would be required to run the analysis. The inclusion of additional complexity is relatively simple and provides an opportunity to explore the interaction of treatment variables (in which effects change for different combinations of treatment variables) in influencing the dependent variable. Note that the variations, which are compared in an analysis of variance, are composed of two elements: random error and possible treatment effects. The test that is done compares the ratio of the differences in the following way:

$$F = \frac{\text{Random error} + \text{Possible treatment effects}}{\text{Random error}}$$

The interpretation of the results of an analysis of variance test examines:

- The main effect of treatment variable A
- The main effect of treatment variable B
- An interaction of the treatment variables ($A \times B$)
- An error term (within groups)

Box 12.8 presents the results of a two-way analysis of variance test. To interpret such a table, one normally begins with an examination of the main effects; if there are significant main effects, one would then examine whether there are significant interaction effects.

BOX 12.8 *Sample ANOVA Results*

Suppose we had run an experiment with one dependent variable and two treatments and we wish to test for possible interactions between the treatments. In such a case, we would perform a two-way analysis of variance, with a test for interaction.

The output might be summarized in the following way:

Source of Variance	Sums of Squares	df	Mean Square	F	Sig. of F
Main effect (A)	1449.393	2	724.697	10.421	0.000
Main effect (B)	12.652	1	12.652	0.182	0.607
Interaction (A × B)	125.990	2	62.995	0.906	0.406
Error term-within group	12239.591	176	69.543		
Total	13815.016	181	76.326		

1. **Understanding the Values in the Summary Table**

   i) The **degrees of freedom** are calculated as follows:
   - Main effect (A): df = 1 less than number of levels in that factor. [In this case, 3 − 1 = 2]
   - Main effect (B): df = 1 less than number of levels in that factor. [In this case, 2 − 1 = 1]
   - Interaction effect (A × B): df = product of the dfs making up the interaction. [In this case, 2 × 1 = 2]
   - Error term: df = total number of cases minus the product of number of levels of A and B. [In this case, 182 − (3 × 2) = 176.]
   - Total df = N − 1 [In this case, 182 − 1 = 181]

   ii) To compute the mean square for an effect, divide the sum of squares for the effect by its *df*.

   iii) To compute the F value for each effect, divide the *mean square* by the *mean square error term-within groups*.

2. **Interpreting the Results**

   In inspecting your results, you should examine two issues as you begin to interpret your results. First, you will want to know if your treatment variables had a significant effect; if either or both did, you should see if there is any interaction between the treatments.

   a. **Main Effects**

   To decide if a treatment was statistically significant, you will need to compare the F value to the values found in Table 12.4 using the appropriate degrees of freedom. If the value you obtained is larger than the one reported in Table 12.4, you have a statistically significant effect. To use Table 12.4, you will need values for the required degrees of freedom; use the smaller value across the top of the table and the larger one on the vertical axis.

   b. **Interaction Effects**

   If you have a significant main effect, you will then want to inspect your results for any interactions between the effects. Your job is simple if there is no significant interaction effect; you simply report that none was present. It is more complicated with an interaction; in this case, the effect of a treatment is not independent of the other treatment; it may be that under the high condition of treatment A, we find that treatment B does not enhance the impact on the dependent variable.

   See Figures 18.1, 18.2, and 18.3 in Chapter 18 for an illustration of how plots can be used to show relationships with and without significant interactions.

3. Repeated Measures Analysis of Variance

In a number of nursing situations, a researcher may be interested in studying the effects of an intervention over several points in time or a researcher may expose the same subject to two or more treatment conditions when it is reasonable to assume that one treatment cannot contaminate a second treatment condition. In such situations, **repeated measures analysis of variance** may be used to test for differences among the mean scores of the treatment conditions.

For example, if you are interested in studying adherence to a regular exercise regime after exposure to a 6-week work site health promotion physical activity program for exployees, the researcher would use a pre-post–experimental control group design in which the subjects are randomly assigned to the experimental (health promotion program) and to the control group (regular work site routine).

The researcher would collect data on the frequency of exercise before initiation of the health promotion program (time 1), at the midpoint of the program (time 2), 2 weeks after completion of the program (time 3), and 3 months after completion of the program (time 4). An F statistic would be calculated to determine differences in the mean scores of exercise frequency for both the experimental and control groups. This would be referred to as the *between-subjects effect*.

This statistic would determine if, across all time periods, there was a difference in the frequency of exercise for the experimental and the control groups. A second F statistic would be calculated to determine differences in exercise frequencies across all time periods within each group. This would be known as the *within-subjects effect*. This statistic would determine if, across both the experimental and control groups, the frequency of exercise differed at times 1, 2, 3, and 4. Finally, the *interaction effect* would be examined to determine if there was a differential treatment effect on exercise frequency at different points in time. Repeated measures analysis of variance is a useful tool for the nurse researcher given that nurse researchers often record data for subjects at several points in time.

Analysis of variance is a major analytical tool, used particularly by experimental researchers. Normally, computers will make all such computations. You need not concern yourself with memorizing the calculation formula included in the boxes in this chapter. However, to fully understand what inferential statistics can do for you, you need to be aware of what the statistical test is doing with your data to answer your research question or test your hypotheses. The researcher will encounter F distributions in using the MEANS, ANOVA, MANOVA, and REGRESSION procedures in SPSS.

To perform this analysis using SPSS, see the ANOVA procedure in Appendix A.

E. WHEN TESTS OF STATISTICAL SIGNIFICANCE ARE NOT APPROPRIATE

At the beginning of this chapter, readers were cautioned that although the findings of a study may be statistically significant, they may not be clinically significant. To be clinically significant, the findings must have meaning for patient care in the presence or absence of statistical significance. Whereas statistical significance indicates that the findings are unlikely to result from chance, clinical significance requires the nurse to interpret the findings in terms of their value to nursing. Therefore, statistical significance is not the only criterion of importance, and the practitioners would do well not to be overly impressed by its presence or absence. And sometimes tests of significance are simply inappropriate. Yet they are widely used, often improperly (Munro and Page, 2001; Polit, 1996). Why is this the case?

Performing tests of significance is, no doubt, often motivated by the desire to be scientific—or appear to be scientific. If one's data turn out to be "statistically significant," then that is taken to demonstrate the importance of the finding and to confer scientific legitimacy on one's work. Such tests help to create the impression that the God of science—that independent, unbiased arbiter of truth—has blessed one's research with approval. A second motivation has to do with the fact that such tests are routinely—even if inappropriately—reported in the literature. Hence, to produce a report that meets the standards of the discipline, tests of significance are expected. A third possibility is that some researchers poorly understand tests of significance and these tests are inappropriately used because of such misunderstandings. For a variety of reasons, many studies should not use tests of significance. The following rules indicate when such tests are inappropriate.

Rule 1. Tests of significance are not applicable when total populations are studied. If a study is being done on the wage differences between male and female nursing administrators in one institution and data relating to all the nursing administrators are analyzed, then a test of significance would not be in order. If a $1500 difference is observed after the appropriate controls are introduced, this difference is absolute. The researcher must decide whether the difference is to be characterized as substantial, modest, or trivial. To say that it is statistically significant is simply incorrect! Remember, tests of significance assume that sampling procedures have been followed—they are not applicable when total populations have been studied.

Arguments have been advanced that a study like the one above represents one sample out of a universe of possible samples that might be taken. The problem with this argument is that not all hospitals were given an equal chance to be included; second, if you wish to make the argument that this is but one case among many, then you have shifted the unit of analysis to the institutional level (a hospital) and now have one case represented by one difference. Here you would be left with a difference of $1500, but with no knowledge of what differences are present in other institutions.

Rule 2. Because tests of significance only provide a measure of the probability of a given difference's being the result of sampling fluctuations, assuming that probability sampling procedures have been used, such tests are not appropriate if those methods are not used. If an experimenter asked people to volunteer to be in a treatment group and then wished to compare these individuals with others who agreed to serve as controls, any test of significance on the differences between the groups would be meaningless.

In experimental designs in which volunteers have been sought for participation (convenience sample) but in which subjects have been assigned to treatment and control groups using random sampling techniques, it is appropriate to use tests of significance to compare the treatment and control groups. However, in such instances, the population should be regarded as those who volunteered for participation.

Rule 3. Tests of significance are to be considered suspect when there is a substantial nonparticipation rate. If substantial numbers of respondents have refused to participate (for argument's sake, let's say 40 percent), then tests of significance become problematic because it is difficult to assume that nonparticipants are similar to those who agree to participate in the study. Therefore, the extent to which such data can be considered representative can be called into question.

Rule 4. In *nonexperimental research,* if one is exploring a relationship that has been shown to be statistically significant, it is inappropriate to use a test of significance once again when controls have been applied to test for an intervening variable. The issue in evaluating models is to assess the impact of the control on the original relationship and to observe whether the differences have remained the same or if they have increased, decreased, or disappeared. Frequently, they may change from being statistically significant to being statistically insignificant, but this change may simply represent the fact that the data have been partitioned in order to do the analysis (perhaps cut in half). Therefore, the switch from significance to nonsignificance may simply reflect the fact that fewer cases are being used.

Researchers should note how much the original relationship has shifted, not simply note whether the relationship is still statistically significant. To avoid confusion, do not use tests of significance when causal models are being evaluated beyond the stage of the initial relationship. For example, if the relationship between X and Y is being explored and if sampling and other conditions are appropriate, then a test of significance for the relationship between X and Y is legitimate. However, having established that there is a statistically significant relationship between X and $Y,$ a further test of significance would not be appropriate when one is testing to ensure that the relationship is not spurious because of its connection to some third variable. (This point is discussed in detail in Chapter 17.)

Rule 5. Tests of significance may not be applied to relationships that were not formulated as hypotheses before the collection of data for the study. Researchers routinely collect data on many variables; it is not unusual in a survey, for example, to collect data on 100 or more variables. If we run every variable against every other one, we will not only generate enormous piles of computer output, but we will also generate results for many hundreds of theoretically meaningless relationships. We will also encounter many "statistically significant" relationships. Indeed, one would expect that on a simple chance basis, one in 20 tables will prove to be statistically significant, providing one is using the 0.05 significance level for one's tests. Unfortunately, researchers rarely report how many relationships were analyzed, what confounding data have been discarded, and which causal models were not fully developed before data collection.

An exception to the above rule has to be made for those analyzing secondary data. In such cases, it is impossible to formulate hypotheses before data collection; nonetheless, hypotheses should be formulated before data analysis. Moreover, it should be noted that some researchers find it useful to run tests of significance, even in inappropriate situations, to help shed light on the relationships explored even though they do not report these tests in their articles.

Researchers must use tests of significance only with great care. Above all, beginning researchers must appreciate what such tests really measure. All too often it is not recognized that a finding may be equally important whether the relationship is statistically significant or not. Nurse researchers are in the business of trying to understand and describe phenomena of concern to nursing; therefore, to discover that there is no relationship between A and B is as important as it is to discover that there is a relation between A and

B. Futhermore, if one is testing a theory, it is especially important to find that a predicted relationship does not hold true because this will cast doubt on the theory and, perhaps, lead to a refinement or refutation of it. In short, do not despair if your study does not yield statistically significant results. Science proceeds through disconfirmation, ruling out alternatives, rejecting, modifying, and continually rethinking theoretical formulations.

E X E R C I S E S

1. Test the null hypothesis that there is no difference in the rate of complications for clients with AIDS who are receiving intravenous antibiotics with a heparin lock in place, without changing it, for 48 hours versus 96 hours. Test the hypothesis at the 0.05 level. The data are shown in the following table.

Rate of Complications in Patients with AIDS by Heparin Lock Replacement Time

Complication rate	Heparin Replacement Time Group					
	48 hours, N %		96 hours, N %		Total, N %	
Had complications	31	47.0	21	34.4	52	40.9
No complications	35	53.0	40	65.5	75	59.1
Total	66	100.0	61	99.9	127	100.0

2. You have examined the salaries of all the nursing staff working in a large teaching hospital. What is the appropriate test to determine if there is a statistically significant difference between the salaries of men and women? (Caution: This is a trick question!) The data are shown in the following table.

Income List by Gender, Large Teaching Hospital

Men, dollars	Women, dollars
46,200	46,600
47,300	46,800
38,800	49,100
50,200	48,700
49,600	37,700
48,800	48,600
47,900	57,700
51,100	50,400

Chapter 13

Data Collection and Measurement

CHAPTER OUTLINE

KEY TERMS

Concept
Conceptual hypothesis
Concurrent validity
Construct
Construct validity
Content validity
Credibility
Criterion validity
Cronbach's alpha
Data collection
Elite bias
Equivalence
External validity
Face validity
Index

Internal consistency
Internal validity
Kuder-Richardson coefficient
Likert-based index
Magnitude estimation procedures
Measurement
Measurement error
Nominal measurement
Observational measurement
Operationalization
Operational level
Ordinal measurement
Pilot study
Predictive validity

Questionnaire
Ratio measurement
Reliability
Response set
Scale
Semantic differential
Split-half method
Stability
Summated rating index
Theoretical level
Theoretical substruction
True value
Validity
Visual analogue scale

You have completed the steps outlined in Chapter 3 to get your project started. You have identified the research problem, reviewed the existing literature, selected a theoretical framework to guide the study, and articulated the research problem as an interrogative question, a declarative statement of purpose, or a hypothesis. Now you are ready to translate the research concepts in your problem statement into observable and measurable phenomena. This will enable you to measure the variables of interest in the study. *Measurement* refers to the process of assigning values to observations so as to reflect variables. Then you can proceed to data collection, the process of gathering information from identified participants to answer the research question. Because the quality of a study is often determined by the data collection and measurement methods selected, this chapter focuses on these two vital steps. General measurement principles and concepts are discussed; these include the levels of a research project, validity and reliability issues, measurement levels, measurement error, and steps that can be taken to reduce measurement error. In addition, various means available to nurse researchers for collecting data and measuring nursing phenomena are explored and the process of instrument development discussed.

A. LEVELS OF A RESEARCH PROJECT

Most methods of data collection involve an attempt to measure variables. Measurement takes many forms: from unobtrusively observing nursing clients and recording which of them use the recreation facilities available in the hospital sunroom, to getting information on suicides from public statistics, to observing levels of aggression in psychiatric clients who are frustrated as part of an experiment, to classifying television soap operas according to whether they stereotype health professionals by gender, to having individuals complete questionnaires or undergo personal interviews.

We measure things because we wish to accurately describe objects. We wish, for example, to know how popular a new smoking cessation program is now compared with when it was originally introduced; to describe the program's popularity in various parts of the country; to see if the program's popularity varies with the gender of the person doing the rating, the length of time the person smoked, or the number of smoking cessation programs attended previously by the participant; or to understand what factors explain gender differences in the program ratings. If we pose such questions, we will need to measure the appropriate variables and analyze them. We could guess about the answer, but we would not have much confidence in our answer unless the question is tackled seriously and the data to answer the question are collected objectively and systematically. *Objectively* implies the individual who collects it does not influence the data in any way. *Systematically* refers to a consistent method for collecting the data so that everyone involved follows the same procedures for data collection (LoBiondo-Wood and Haber, 1998).

Measurement is the process of linking abstract concepts to their empirical indicators. Typically, researchers work from the general to the specific: for each general concept, an indicator is identified. To look for a way of reflecting the idea of social support is to ask a measurement question. How might we best measure, or indicate, a person's level of social support? We refer to concepts we intend to measure as *variables.*

Figure 13.1 presents the levels of a research project. To move down the figure is to move from the general to the specific—

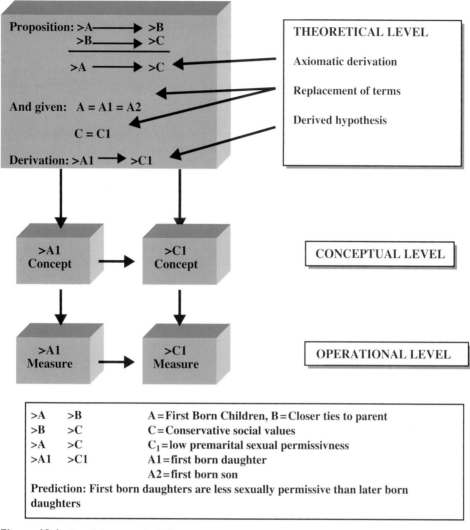

Figure 13.1 Levels in research design.

from the **theoretical level** to the **operational level.** At the theoretical level there are a number of interconnected propositions, assumptions, and statements of relationship between concepts. By employing axiomatic derivations and replacement of terms (see Chapter 2), it is possible to derive *conceptual hypotheses.* Such hypotheses may also be identified by reviewing the research literature, or by an insightful analysis of the problem. A **conceptual hypothesis** is a statement of the relationship between two or more concep-

tual variables or constructs. An example would be: "the greater the integration into campus life, the greater the students' social support during their college years." Having stated the conceptual hypothesis, the researcher would proceed to the operational level, deciding how each of the constructs (integration into campus life and social support) would be measured, and what procedures would be used to collect and analyze the information.

Theoretical substruction is the dynamic thinking process that the researcher engages in to move from the theoretical level of a quantitative study to the operational or measurement level (Wolf and Heinzer, 1999). Through substruction, the researcher identifies the foundational elements of a study, determines the relationships among the elements, and depicts this in a diagram (Dulock and Holzemar, 1991). This process brings clarity to the research process and enables the researcher to better understand the relationship among the theoretical, conceptual, and operational level of the study. It also illustrates the hierarchical order among the major constituents of the study. Figure 13.2 presents a substruction that illustrates the connections from the research question through to the measurement and data analysis process. In Figure 13.2, the theoretical level demonstrates the major concepts of a proposed theory on adolescent identity in cancer survivors and the relationships among the concepts.

The suggested theory states that identity is predicted by the strength of maternal attachment and family coping ability. At the next level, constructs reflective of the concepts are selected. For example, the concept of maternal attachment is reflected in the construct relationship to mother; the concept of family coping is reflected in coping with normative life events and coping with nonnormative life events; and the concept of identity is reflected in three constructs: self-worth, life satisfaction, and general affect. The final step involves selecting an instrument or measurement device to operationalize the constructs. **Operationalization** refers to translating the constructs of interest into observable and measurable phenomena. In our example, we see that relationship to mother is measured by the Maternal Scale of the Inventory of Parent and Peer Attachment (IPPA) instrument, coping with normative and nonnormative life events is measured

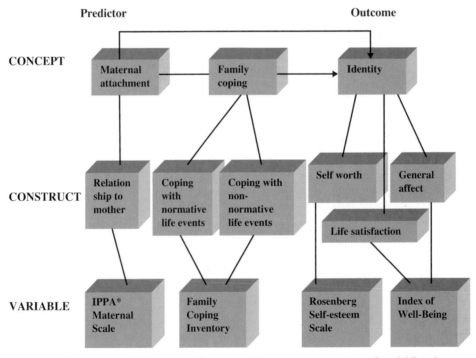

Figure 13.2 Theoretical substructure: Identity in adolescent cancer survivors after childhood diagnosis and its relationship to maternal attachment and family coping. A possible model.

by the Family Coping Inventory (FCI), social worth is measured by the Rosenberg
Self-Esteem Scale, and general affect and
life satisfaction are measured by the Index
of Well-Being. The selection of the data collection instruments ultimately directs the
choice of analytical methods.

In some qualitative approaches, the
process is reversed and, after doing some
observations, the researcher may ask,
"Well, what concept does this reflect?" In
this case, the researcher begins with observations and then tries to link them to
more general ideas. This is the approach
recommended by the grounded theory
method (Strauss and Corbin, 1997). This
approach involves a process of discovery
in which the researcher begins with observations and tries to make sense of them, to
identify the concepts the data seem to reflect. As observations are made, the concepts are continuously identified and refined. Concepts become the basic units of
analysis:

> In grounded theory, representativeness
> of concepts, not of persons, is crucial.
> The aim is ultimately to build a theo-
> retical explanation by specifying phe-
> nomena in terms of conditions that give
> rise to them, how they are expressed
> through action/interaction, the conse-
> quences that result from them, and vari-
> ations of these qualifiers . . . For in-
> stance, one might want to know how
> representative "comfort work" is of the
> total amount of work that nurses do . . .
> Do nurses engage in it all of the time or
> some of the time? What are the condi-
> tions that enable them to do it or pre-
> vent their doing it? (Corbin and Strauss,
> 1990, p. 9).

Measurement refers to the process by
which categories or numbers are used to
reflect or indicate concepts and constructs. A **concept** is a general idea not
directly observable in the real world. A
construct is a concept specified in such
a way that it is observable in the real

world. Making a concept potentially observable facilitates testing of it. Some authors distinguish construct from concept by stating that constructs are
"constructed or invented" by the researcher. A construct refers to an observable characteristic of an individual,
group, or nation. Constructs help us to
organize our thinking about the world.
Nurse scientists use constructs such as
health status, job satisfaction, compliance, and self-care ability. There are
hundreds of such constructs. It is important that the researcher define precisely what is meant by each construct
used. Precision helps to make clear what
is included in the idea and also provides
a guide as to how it should be measured.
The *operational level* of research refers
to the indicators used to reflect the constructs as well as to the procedures used
to collect and analyze data.

The review of the literature is helpful in
showing how other researchers conceptually define and measure variables of interest to the researcher. After variables are
conceptually and operationally defined,
the researcher searches the literature
again to identify instruments that may be
used as is or modified for use in the study.
When instruments are available, the researcher must first seek permission from
the author before implementing their use
in a study (LoBionda-Wood, 1998).

B. LINKAGES BETWEEN LEVELS

Measurement, in essence, refers to the
linkage between the conceptual and the
operational levels of a research project.
There are two key issues in this linkage:
validity and *reliability.*

I. Validity

In Chapter 1, **validity** was defined as the
extent to which a measure reflects a con-

cept, reflecting neither more nor less than what is implied by the conceptual definition. Validity has to do, then, with the congruence of concept and indicator. When an instrument is considered valid, it measures the concept it was intended to measure. There are five types of validity: *face, content, concurrent, predictive,* and *construct validity.* An instrument may be judged to possess one, all, or any combination of these types of validity. Table 13.1 describes the various types of validity, describes how one would test for them, and provides examples of studies that used tests for validity. For a full discussion of each test, interested readers should consult the reference citation. Unlike reliability, there are no simple statistical tests to assess validity, yet beginning researchers should look for evidence that the data collection instrument is a valid measure of the research phenomenon.

Beginning nurse researchers should, at minimum, be aware of the types of validity outlined in Table 13.1 and convinced that selected measures have *face validity.* A measure has **face validity** if, on inspection, it appears to reflect the construct that you wish to measure. **Content validity** refers to the extent to which a measure reflects the dimension (or dimensions) implied by the concept. Typically, content validity requires a more formal assessment, including the use of a panel of experts, corroboration of the measurement with the concept's dimensions noted in the literature review, and with the study's theoretical framework in order to assure that the content of the measures reflect the framework. There are two types of **criterion validity:** *concurrent* and *predictive.* If you were attempting to develop a measure to predict success in nurse registration examinations, you could assess the validity of your measure by correlating it with success rates on registered nurse examinations. A high correlation would indicate high **predictive validity.** In this example,

concurrent validity would be demonstrated if two different tests were given and the scores correlated highly with each other. If a theoretically derived hypothesis turns out as predicted, it would constitute one piece of evidence for the validity of the measures. This latter type of validity is known as **construct validity.** Another way to think about construct validity is to recognize that it is based on inductive evidence. If one finds evidence to support a theoretically derived hypothesis, then it would indicate that one's measures have construct validity.

Experimentalists, in particular, distinguish between internal and external validity (see Chapter 4). **Internal validity** may be taken to mean that the researcher has demonstrated that the treatment, in fact, produced the changes in the dependent variable. **External validity** has to do with the extent to which results may be extrapolated from the particular study to other groups in general.

When the concept to be measured is a concrete one such as age or body weight, the issue of measurement is straightforward. Many times, however, direct measures of concepts relevant to nursing research are not available. Often nurses are interested in exploring abstract ideas such as health, lifestyle, self-esteem, social status, coping, stress, fatigue, pain, or resilience. Rarely are direct measures available for such concepts. This requires the researcher to use *indirect measures* that are measures of the characteristics or attributes of the abstract concept. For example, if you are interested in measuring lifestyle patterns, indicators may include nutrition practices, ability to deal with problems, stress management techniques, rest and relaxation patterns, exercise levels, attitudes, decision-making styles, social support systems, coping patterns, and self-actualization behaviors. It is a challenge to get a valid measure of these aspects through one measurement approach. The researcher would first need to

Table 13.1   Types of Validity and Their Tests

Type	Definition	Test For Validity	Example
Face validity	Upon inspection or face value, the instrument appears to be a good indicator of the concept it is intended to measure.	Expert opinion. Use a panel of experts to determine if the tool measures what it is intended to measure.	Gillis, 1997
Content validity	The instrument items reflect the full range of the attributes of the concept being measured.	Verified by other evidence such as literature review to determine what content should be included; opinion of experts on scope and representativeness of content; use of study's theoretical framework to support the content validity of the tool.	Ewen, 1993
Criterion validity			
1. Concurrent validity	The correlation of one measure with another measure of the same phenomenon.	Test instrument with another instrument that measures the same concept and is known to be valid.	Norbeck et al., 1982
2. Predictive	The instrument can accurately predict a phenomenon. For example, GPAs can predict NCLEX success rate or risk behavior scales are often used to predict the probability of risk-taking acts in adolescents and the agreement of the scales with subsequent risk behaviors gives a measure of their predictive validity.	Tested by using the instrument in a study and then comparing the results with a future outcome.	Norbeck et al., 1982
Construct validity	The measure distinguishes participants who differ on the construct being measured by the instrument.	Establishing construct validity is a complex process involving several approaches. These include: • Hypothesis testing approach • Convergent and divergent approaches • Contrasted group approach • Multitrait-multimethod approach • Factor analysis approach • Causal modeling approach	 Norbeck et al., 1982 Bunn & O'Connor, 1996 Gillis, 1997 Carruth, 1996

clearly define the conceptual definition of lifestyle so it is obvious what aspects of lifestyle the research is dealing with and then operationalize the definition by selecting indicators congruent with the conceptual definition. Does the researcher wish to define lifestyle in terms of actual health behaviors engaged in or attitudes and values toward health behaviors or a combination of behaviors and attitudes? The instrument or tool selected to measure lifestyle would vary depending on the researcher's definition of lifestyle.

a. The Idea of Validity in Quantitative Research

To illustrate, let us examine one possible conceptual definition of socioeconomic status. If socioeconomic status is defined as a "hierarchical continuum of respect and prestige" and we then choose to operationalize the concept by measuring the annual salary of each individual we study, we will most certainly have problems convincing others of the validity of our measure.

On inspection, it becomes clear that annual salary would not adequately reflect an individual's place on a continuum of respect and prestige. Such inspections are generally referred to as *face validity*. The following are reasons why you might doubt the validity of the proposed measures:

- A local drug dealer is making a fortune but enjoys little respect in the community.
- The best poker player in town always seems to have lots of money, takes expensive trips, and many people admire his worldliness even though his salary at the local pub is little above the minimum wage.
- The Protestant minister is looked up to by almost everyone even though his salary is a pittance.
- The widow of a doctor who served the community with dedication for many years has inherited her husband's substantial estate. Although she has no salary, she probably has more prestige than anyone else in the community.

The problem here is that salary does not always capture the concept of social prestige adequately, and even if you could get a measure of annual income rather than salary, you would still not have a valid measure of the concept as defined. (Think of your own home community. Can you think of cases in which annual income might not reflect prestige?)

When measuring socioeconomic status, many nurse researchers rely on occupational rating scales that have been based on either:

- The four-factor index of social status proposed by Hollingshead (1975) that includes education, occupation, gender, and marital status. This index provides a measure of social status reflective of the social system of the United States.
- The average levels of income and education for people in any given occupation in Canada (Blishen and McRoberts, 1976).
- The subjective assessment of the prestige of different occupations (see Pineo and Porter, 1967.

All of the above approaches lead to quite similar rankings of different occupations. A major advantage of using such indexes is that it is quite easy to find out a person's occupation and then simply use the score supplied in one of the above indexes to reflect the socioeconomic status of the individual.

However, one of the problems of using prestige indexes is that such indexes may not reflect the complexity of the organization of the modern household. For example, such indexes traditionally did not produce a prestige score for "housewife" (researchers would assign a missing value code or a separate special code to housewives), and researchers simply tended to use the father's occupational prestige as a measure of the family's socioeconomic level. Given the participation of women in the labor force, this is no longer a satisfactory solution for gauging household socioeconomic status. To avoid the inherent sexism of using the father's occupational prestige rating as a measure of a household's socioeconomic status, in recent years our students have been basing ratings of a household's socioeconomic status on the *higher* of the two occupational prestige scores in households in which parents are living together and both are employed outside the household. When only one of the parents is employed outside the household, the occupational prestige of that person is used. Simply adding the prestige scores together would result in a prestige score that would not be in line with public perceptions. (For example, the combined prestige scores of parents who are both teachers would be about one and a half times that of a single-earner physician household.) It would be possible to add the values together but weight the lower of the two at a reduced level, perhaps using only one quarter of its value or add them together and divide by two, as suggested by the Hollingshead index. These calculations are easily done in the Statistical Package for the Social Sciences (SPSS), but they are a little tricky (because of the housewife problem). An example is shown in Appendix A.

To perform this analysis using SPSS, see the Index Construction section of Appendix A.

Clearly, however, a definition of socioeconomic status that stresses the relative respect and prestige of members of a community begs for a measure that would get at the extent to which different individuals in the community are looked up to. In a community health nursing study, it may be important to get a valid measure of this aspect of socioeconomic status because you

may wish to contact prestigious community members in the future to support a health promotion project for their community. The local drug dealer or poker player who may receive high scores on some indicators of socioeconomic status would not bode well as respectable and prestigious exemplars of the new project. An option would be for the nurse researcher to contact a panel of local informants who could estimate the relative prestige of known members of the community.

When choosing indicators, one should, ideally, not select causes, consequences, or correlates of the variable but, instead, get a direct measure of the phenomenon itself. As annual income may be one of several important causes of variation in prestige, one must not simply measure prestige by income. To do so would be to choose a correlate as one's only measure. Similarly, to measure the prestige of the previously described widow by the success of her children would be to look at a consequence of her position and may not adequately reflect her prestige itself. Again, the resulting measure may be correlated with her prestige but not reflect it adequately.

Researchers must ensure that measures developed to reflect an independent variable are indeed *independent* of those used to reflect the dependent variable. If care is not taken, a researcher may end up with two different measures of the same phenomenon and may inappropriately conclude that there is a strong causal relationship between the two variables; instead, there may only be a correlation between two measures of the same underlying phenomenon. For example, suppose we measured the weight of hospitalized children in pounds; suppose we then weighed the children again, this time in kilograms. We would then have two measures, highly correlated, that reflect the same underlying reality. But we would err if we concluded that the weight in pounds *causes* weight in kilograms. These measures lack independence—they both reflect the same underlying variable (the weights of the children).

The example is a simple one, and few researchers would be in danger of concluding that variation in pounds influ-ences weight in kilograms. But in nursing research, things are not always so easy. Suppose that you were measuring factors that influence healthy lifestyles in adolescents and that you included the following among the measures of healthy lifestyles:

Independent Variables (Causes of Variation in Healthy Lifestyle)	Dependent Variable (Healthy Lifestyle)
Concept of health	Social support
Perceived health status	Nutrition practices
Family support	Physical participation activities
Peer support	Stress management
	Safety practices

Clearly there is some overlap between measures of the independent and dependent variables; note that social support is one of the measures used for dependent variables and that family and peer support are two of the measures used for independent variables. You would need to review these indicators to ensure that they are measuring different variables and not simply reflecting the same underlying reality. If you are not careful, you may inadvertently inflate the relationship and come to an inappropriate conclusion. Thus, we can formulate the following rule: ***Make certain that the indicators of your independent and dependent variables do not overlap.*** This means that researchers must be careful to ensure that the strength of the association between the independent and dependent variable is not inflated by failing to use measures that reflect different concepts.

Another issue, not typically discussed in nursing research texts, is the problem of inflating the apparent validity of a measure by choosing a conceptual definition after considering what the most convenient measure would be. What does this mean? In the discussion so far, we have assumed that the researcher is working down from the theoretical to the conceptual and, finally, to the operational level of research. In fact, much research does not follow such a simple path.

Before researchers offer conceptual definitions of variables, they often have given thought to how they will measure the variable. One way to increase the apparent validity of a measure is to select a conceptual definition that is most congruent with the proposed measure. To go back to the earlier example of measuring socioeconomic status, socioeconomic status was defined as a "hierarchical continuum of respect and prestige." If the design of the study was to be a door-to-door questionnaire in a community, then the researcher might well reconsider the conceptual definition of socioeconomic status because it would be difficult to measure it easily in this way using a questionnaire. It is easier to ask about educational level, occupation, or even income. Knowing this, the researcher might decide that a definition of socioeconomic status along the lines of "differential access to scarce resources" would be more appropriate; now the researcher can achieve greater face validity by using some combination of education, occupation, or income to reflect socioeconomic status.

Ultimately, in quantitative research, analysis proceeds by examining relationships between indicators. And one must be careful when evaluating such research because, even though two studies may examine socioeconomic status, the measures used to determine socioeconomic status may differ enormously. Is this a shell game? To the extent that conceptual definitions are selected to enhance validity, one could argue that something of a slight of hand is going on. Thus, even with clearly defined constructs and an indication of the measures used, the research consumer must always be alert to tautologies lurking beneath the surface of a research report.

b. The Idea of Validity in Qualitative Research

In qualitative research, the issue of external validity may need to be thought about in a slightly different way. Given the small number of cases typically studied in qualitative projects, the issue of validity is perhaps better thought about in terms of **credibility.** As Sandelowski (1986, 1993) has argued, a qualitative study is credible when it presents accurate descriptions or interpretations of a meaningful human experience that the people having that experience would immediately recognize as reflecting their own experiences. A study is also credible when other researchers or readers can recognize the experience when confronted with it after having only read about it in a study.

Traditionally in qualitative studies, the degree to which a description "rings true" to the participants of the study, other readers, or other researchers has been taken as an indication of whether the researcher has, in fact, measured what you wished to measure. Furthermore, it has been argued that the closeness of the researcher and the participant being studied should be encouraged rather than discouraged. Only through such closeness can the researcher truly penetrate and understand the experiences of the participant. More recently, Sandelowski (1993) has argued

that there are dangers in thinking that information previously collected can be subsequently simply checked, corroborated, or corrected. This may be valid for only certain cases. Participants may, for example, find that their recollections of the moment when the original data were collected cannot be decontextualized to constitute a test of validity. Attempts to do this may cause as many problems as they solve.

Sandelowski cautions about the danger of making a fetish of rigor. She warns that trying to model the quantitative standards of rigor, takes us too far from the

> ... *artfulness, versatility, and sensitivity to meaning and context that mark qualitative works of distinction. It is as if, in our quasi-militaristic zeal to neutralize bias and to defend our projects against threats to validity, we were more preoccupied with building fortifications against attack than with creating the evocative, true-to-life, and meaningful portraits, stories, and landscapes of human experiences that constitute the best test of rigor in qualitative work (Sandelowski, 1993, p. 1).*

In terms of external validity, the very act of controlling so many extraneous factors (as in an experiment) actually serves to reduce the generalizability of such studies; in qualitative studies, such artificiality is reduced given that studies are done in natural settings even though the limited sample sizes mitigate against extrapolations to other populations.

In distinguishing qualitative from quantitative research traditions, Sandelowski notes:

> ... *the artistic approach to qualitative inquiry emphasizes the irreplicability of the research process and product. Every human experience is viewed as unique, and truth is viewed as relative. The artistic integrity, rather than the scientific objectivity, of the research is*

achieved when the researcher communicates the richness and diversity of human experience in an engaging and even poetic manner . . . qualitative methods such as historical inquiry may employ the methods of science but the presentation or reporting style of art (Sandelowski, 1986, p. 29).

In order to maximize rigor in qualitative research, several suggestions are relevant:

- **Keep careful records.** Researchers should keep detailed records of all decisions that have been made and how they were made. This establishes an audit trail. Details on how the subject matter was selected, how data were collected, what evidence was deemed unimportant, and the ways in which categories were developed should all be noted. The objective here is to illustrate as clearly as possible the researcher's thought processes that led to the conclusions of the study.
- **Avoid the holistic fallacy.** This fallacy would make the results of the study look more patterned than they actually are; the researcher should attempt to establish how typical the observations of the study are. Be careful not to report only events and behaviors that are patterned and consistent; report the exceptions as well.
- **Guard against an elite bias.** Elite bias is a danger because informants are more likely to be drawn from the more articulate, high-status elements in a society. Hence, unless care is taken, there is a tendency to overrepresent the views of the elite in one's research.
- **Be wary of being taken over by the respondent.** If the researcher identifies completely with the views of a respondent, it may be difficult to maintain a clear distinction between the researcher's experiences and those of the respondent. This may be a problem unless the researcher attempts to record how the respondent and the researcher have mutually influenced one another. If this is done, the report will recognize the reciprocal influence of the respondent on the researcher.

The issue of generalizability (external validity) poses difficulties in many research designs, but it presents special challenges in ethnographic studies. Conventional sampling procedures are usually not relevant to ethnographic studies because such studies depend so extensively on case studies. However, it may be possible to argue that the circumstances studied in a particular ethnographic case study are comparable to other situations and that the conclusions of the study may therefore be applied to them. One solution is to carry out research on numerous sites. However, there are four factors that may influence the credibility of such cross-group comparisons:

1. **Selection effects.** The researcher may select sites in which some factors may not be present. A study based on such a site may, therefore, not allow testing of certain ideas.
2. **Setting effects.** Studying a nursing situation may itself influence the results derived. The impact of the researcher's intrusion may vary from setting to setting, distorting the results more in some settings than in others. Hence, it is difficult to compare the degree to which the researcher influenced the results of different studies conducted at different sites.
3. **History effects.** Each group studied is subject to unique historical influences. When sites are studied at different times, history rather than the interaction of factors within the site may explain some of the variations between the sites.
4. **Construct effects.** Concepts may be regarded differently by both observers in different settings and those being observed.

2. Reliability

Reliability was defined in Chapter 1 as the extent to which, on repeated measures, an instrument yields similar results. Terms such as dependability, consistency, stability, and accuracy are often used interchangeably to refer to reliability. The first three terms refer to the instrument's ability to produce the same results on repeated measures. For example, if a scale were used to weigh a newly admitted hospital client, one would expect the scale to yield the same value if three consecutive readings were taken of that individual's weight. The fourth term, *accuracy,* reflects a different dimension of reliability: the measurement tool's ability to reflect the true value being measured.

True value is the value that would be obtained if the measurement tool were perfect. In other words, the true value is free of random measurement error. Few, if any, instruments or measurement tools are totally free of measurement error. In summary, one would expect a reliable measurement tool to yield similar results on subsequent administrations of the instrument to measure a variable that is relatively constant. Reliability issues emerge in both "single indicator" questions and in those in which a number of indicators are used to reflect a variable.

Reliability is a relative term. It exists in degrees and is usually expressed as a form of correlation coefficient, with 1.00 indicating perfect reliability and 0.00 indicating an absence of reliability. The intended application of the instrument determines what is an acceptable reliability coefficient. For example, if one is using an instrument to make a lifesaving decision related to a medical treatment, one would demand a high reliability coefficient such as 0.90 or above. If, however, the researcher is using the instrument for group comparison on a psychosocial phenomenon, a lower reliability coefficient is acceptable. Nunnally (1978) suggests that reliability coefficients of 0.70 or above for new instruments and 0.80 or above for established instruments are acceptable.

Estimates of reliability need to be determined each time the instrument is used with a different population or sample. Reliability estimates are population dependent, so one must never assume that an established instrument will yield the same high levels of reliability in a diverse population. For example, an instrument designed to measure healthy lifestyle in rural adolescents may yield reliable results when administered to rural adolescents, but low correlations may result when the same instrument is administered to a group of urban adults. It is important to always test the reliability of instruments used in a study before conducting other statistical tests of the data.

a. The Idea of Reliability in Quantitative Research

There are both simple and complex ways of assessing reliability in quantitative investigations, yet no single correct approach exists. The three attributes of reliability should be considered in the assessment of an instrument. These include stability, internal consistency, and equivalence. Table 13.2 outlines the various types, tests for, and examples of research studies that test reliability.

(i) Stability

Stability is concerned with the consistency of the results with repeated measures. Perhaps the easiest way to assess stability is to repeat a question that has been posed. The idea of a *retest procedure* is that if the same question is posed twice and the respondent understands the question identically on both occasions, the response should be identical on both occasions assuming that the variable measured remains the same at the two testing times. This type of reliability is especially important in studies in which an instrument is

Table 13.2   Types of Reliability and Their Tests

Type	Definition	Test For Reliability	Example
Stability	Consistent results are obtained on repeated administration of the measurement.	Test–retest procedure. Administer a questionnaire to the same person on two separate occasions and examine the consistency of their scores. A good correlation suggests good test–retest reliability.	Gillis, 1997
		Parallel form. Same as test–retest procedure except you use two comparable forms of the same instrument	Hoskins, 1988
Internal consistency	Items within the scale or instrument reflect the same variable.	Item-total correlations. This is the correlation between each item and the total scale. Uncorrected item-total correlations above 0.25 are acceptable.	Chalmers et al., 1997
		Kuder-Richardson (KD-20). This correlation is used with instruments that have a dichotomous response format (yes/no).	Sherman, 1996
		Cronbach's alpha. A coefficient measure of reliability that compares each item in a Likert scale with each other simultaneously.	Gillis, 1997
		Split-half procedure. Divide the instrument into two halves to make a comparison. Scores from the two halves are correlated. The Spearman-Brown formula is used to calculate the correlation coefficient.	
Equivalence	Different observers or different forms of an instrument yield the same results.	Interrater reliability. Two or more observers rate a situation and scores are correlated. It is expressed as a correlation coefficient or as a percentage of agreement between scorers. Panel form. See Stability.	Oliver and Redfern, 1991

administered at two or more points in time. For example, in a nursing intervention study, a researcher may administer the instrument at time 1, apply an intervention to an experimental group, and re-administer the same instrument after the intervention at time 2 to measure differences in a dependent variable in both the experimental and control group as a result of the intervention.

Gillis (1997) tested the reliability of the 43-item Adolescent Lifestyle Questionnaire (ALQ) by using the test–retest procedure. She administered the ALQ to 65 school-based adolescents at an interval of 2 weeks. The adolescents ranged in age from 12 to 19 years. The Pearson product-moment correlation coefficient was 0.88 for the total score and ranged from 0.80 to 0.88 for the seven subindexes. This high stability coefficient indicated that scores changed very little between the test and retest time. Hence, the instrument demonstrates high stability and a respectable level of reliability.

A second simple approach, although often not feasible, is to verify the answers independently. Occasionally, for example, it may be possible to compare a student's self-reported grade to that "actually" received by the student. Here the issue is the extent to which students systematically over- or underreport grades.

(ii) Internal Consistency

Internal consistency refers to the ability of the items in an instrument to measure the same variable. *Homogeneity* is often used to refer to the internal consistency of an instrument. A homogenous instrument contains items that are strongly correlated to each other. The higher the intercorrelations among the items, the greater the internal consistency of the instrument. Homogenous instruments are unidimensional; that is, the items taken together measure one construct. Because all the items reflect the same underlying construct, the researcher can sum the in-dividual item scores to get a total score that reflects the construct. Often nursing research deals with phenomena that are multidimensional such as job satisfaction, health motivation, social support, satisfaction with nursing care, or health status. In these situations, the nurse researcher must establish separate internal consistency estimates for each dimension of the construct. For example, Chalmers and associates (1997) developed the Primary Health Care Questionnaire (PHCQ), which includes three dimensions: knowledge about PHC, attitudes toward PHC, and an open-ended section that addresses PHC practices. Separate internal consistency reliability estimates were determined for the 35 knowledge items (Cronbach's alpha of 0.76) and the 34-item attitude index (Cronbach's alpha of 0.85).

Methods available to test the internal consistency of a measure include the ***Kuder-Richardson (KR-20) coefficient,*** *item-total correlations, split-half reliability, and Cronbach's alpha.* A full discussion of these methods is beyond the scope of this text. Interested readers are referred to Table 13.2 for examples of each.

When you are assessing the *reliability of the items* being used to construct an index (an index represents the combination of several items into a single score), you can randomly split the items into two groups, compute the indexes, and then correlate the resulting two scores. Internal reliability is indicated by a high correlation between the two groups of items. This method is known as a **split-half method** and was one of the first methods available for testing reliability (homogeneity). The advantage of this procedure is that it allows researchers to assess test–retest reliability without administering the instrument twice. The Spearman-Brown correlation is usually used in this procedure.

Another procedure to assess homogeneity is to compare an individual item's correlation with the total index score. If an item is consistent with the total score, it will correlate with it. This technique, known as the *internal consistency approach* to reliability is discussed further when index construction is described. The item-total correlations represent a group of correlations between each item and the total score for the instrument. Item-total correlations are useful in instrument development. They are helpful in determining which items to retain and which ones to discard in creating a final index. The item-total correlations should be high enough to indicate internal consistency but low enough to indicate that they are not redundant. Nunnally (1978) suggests that uncorrected item to total correlations above 0.25 and below 0.70 are typically acceptable for item retention when developing a new index.

The most common method used by nurse researchers for assessing internal consistency is **Cronbach's alpha.** This test is based on the strength of the intercorrelations of all the items in the instrument as well as the number of items used (see Appendix A). The alpha value ranges from 0 to 1, with 1 indicating perfect internal consistency and 0 no internal consistency. Because the alpha coefficient is dependent on *both* the number of items used in creating the index and the average interitem correlation, there is no easy answer as to how high a value is required. As a rule of thumb, you need an average interitem correlations above 0.30 and, with five items in the index, that would yield an alpha of 0.682. Normally it seems easiest to judge the adequacy of an index by the average interitem correlation rather than the alpha value itself. Because alpha values increase as a function of the number of items used, one can increase the alpha value simply by adding items. An alpha of 0.700 means one thing if there are five items in the index, but quite another if there are 14

items. Using the "0.30 rule" is recommended to provide greater uniformity in the development and assessment of indexes. Table 13.3 indicates the alpha values that are associated with the number of items and the average interitem correlation.

Gillis (1997) tested the internal consistencies of the total Adolescent Lifestyle Questionnaire and each of the subindexes using Cronbach's alpha. The total instrument was found to have high internal consistency, with an alpha coefficient of 0.91. Alpha coefficients for the seven subindexes ranged from 0.60 to 0.88 (Table 13.4).

(iii) Equivalence

Equivalence refers to the degree of agreement among two or more different observers using the same measurement tool or the agreement between two or more alternate forms of an instrument. Equivalence for parallel versions of an instrument is determined by correlating the two scores with each other. Interrater reliability assesses the extent to which two people consistently agree or disagree on observations. The formula for calculating interrater reliability is provided in Chapter 7 as part of the discussion of content analysis. Refer to that section for a review of the calculations. It should be noted that interrater reliability may be determined several times in a study because factors such as boredom, fatigue, or familiarity may interfere with the rater's ability to accurately rate observations.

No matter what indicators are used, researchers always try to reflect precisely the reality that is being described.

b. The Idea of Reliability in Qualitative Research

When a particular group is studied using qualitative methods, there are problems with replication because the circum-

Table 13.3   Cronbach's Alphas for Various Interitem Correlations and Number of Items*
Mean Interitem Correlation

Items, n	0.10	0.20	0.30	0.40	0.50	0.60	0.70	0.80	0.90
2	0.182	0.333	**0.462**	**0.571**	**0.667**	**0.750**	**0.824**	**0.889**	**0.947**
3	0.250	0.429	**0.562**	**0.667**	**0.750**	**0.818**	**0.875**	**0.923**	**0.964**
4	0.308	0.500	**0.632**	**0.727**	**0.800**	**0.857**	**0.903**	**0.941**	**0.973**
5	0.357	0.556	**0.682**	**0.769**	**0.833**	**0.882**	**0.921**	**0.952**	**0.978**
6	0.400	0.600	**0.720**	**0.800**	**0.857**	**0.900**	**0.933**	**0.960**	**0.982**
7	0.438	0.636	**0.750**	**0.824**	**0.875**	**0.913**	**0.942**	**0.966**	**0.984**
8	0.471	0.667	**0.774**	**0.842**	**0.889**	**0.923**	**0.949**	**0.970**	**0.986**
9	0.500	0.692	**0.794**	**0.857**	**0.900**	**0.931**	**0.955**	**0.973**	**0.988**
10	0.526	0.714	**0.811**	**0.870**	**0.909**	**0.937**	**0.959**	**0.976**	**0.989**
11	0.550	0.733	**0.825**	**0.880**	**0.917**	**0.943**	**0.962**	**0.978**	**0.990**
12	0.571	0.750	**0.837**	**0.889**	**0.923**	**0.947**	**0.966**	**0.980**	**0.991**
13	0.591	0.765	**0.848**	**0.897**	**0.929**	**0.951**	**0.968**	**0.981**	**0.992**
14	0.609	0.778	**0.857**	**0.903**	**0.933**	**0.955**	**0.970**	**0.982**	**0.992**
15	0.625	0.789	**0.865**	**0.909**	**0.938**	**0.957**	**0.972**	**0.984**	**0.993**
16	0.640	0.800	**0.873**	**0.914**	**0.941**	**0.960**	**0.974**	**0.985**	**0.993**

*If we set 0.30 as the minimum average, interitem correlation for an acceptable index, the column headed by 0.30 would constitute the minimum alphas required. Thus, the bolded values represent those that are acceptable. Unbolded values are below the acceptable level. For example, if you had a 12-item index and the mean interitem correlation was 0.20, the alpha value would be 0.750. Because this is in the nonbolded area, the index would not be sufficiently reliable. However, three-item index, with an alpha of 0.562 should be treated as an adequate index.

stances and the individuals can never be the same at some later time.

> . . . *what observers see and report is a function of the position they occupy within participant groups, the status accorded them, and the role behavior expected of them. Direct observer effects may occur when informants become dependent on the ethnographer for status enhancement . . . (LeCompte and Goetz, 1982, p. 46).*

Social settings in which questions are asked can also be important. So unless the qualitative researcher fully reports how and where the observations were made, there is little chance of replicating a study. To increase the chances of repli-cating a study, LeCompte and Goetz (1982) have suggested the use of five strategies:

1. Focus on verbatim reports and stick to the facts.
2. Use multiple researchers because it allows the results of the researchers to be compared.
3. Use participant researchers; this involves training individuals in observational techniques.
4. Use peer examination. When careful descriptions have been made, researchers can check their results against the observations and experiences of fellow researchers.
5. Use mechanical recording devices such as audiotapes and videos to allow oth-

Table 13.4 Internal Consistency of the Adolescent Lifestyle Questionnaire and Its Subindexes

Subindexes	Number of Items	Cronbach Alpha
Identity awareness	9	0.84
Nutrition	8	0.88
Physical participation	4	0.82
Safety	7	0.74
Health awareness	4	0.71
Social support	7	0.80
Stress management	4	0.60
ALQ total	43	0.91

ALQ = adolescent lifestyle questionnaire.
Source: Gillis, A.J. (1997). The adolescent lifestyle questionnaire: Development and psychometric testing. *Canadian Journal of Nursing Research, 29*(1), 29–46. Cited with permission.

ers to check your observations independently at a later date.

Avoiding incorrect conclusions, such as identifying relationships incorrectly, is a challenge for qualitative researchers. There are three issues that must be handled:

1. Qualitative researchers must establish the ordering of events and phenomenon; because qualitative researchers make observations over time, establishing the ordering of events is usually not problematic. Researchers are present on the research site over time and are able to observe actions and reactions.
2. Researchers must establish that the variables are related to one another (vary together); researchers depend, to some degree, on the occurrence of social events that permit her or him to see whether the variables are varying together. In contrast, experimentalists create a situation that systematically varies the intensity of the treatment and observe the reaction to the treatment.
3. Researchers must eliminate rival hypotheses. All researchers who attempt to eliminate rival hypotheses face a challenge because new hypotheses can always be suggested. Qualitative researchers have to test alternative hypotheses continually as observations are being made. Because observations are made over time, there are opportunities to explore such hypotheses as the study unfolds.

C. MEASUREMENT ERROR

Typically, we begin with the assumption that the manifestations of the phenomenon we wish to measure have:

1. Two or more values inherent in them (i.e., we are dealing with a variable, not a constant).
2. That any manifestation has a *true value*.

Measurement error always occurs because our instruments are imperfect, our research participants do not always pay sufficient attention to our instructions, or we are not careful enough in coding data. It exists in both direct and indirect measures of variables.

In essence, **measurement error** is any deviation from the true value. As described previously, a **true value** is the underlying exact quantity of a variable at any given time. In measurement, we attempt to reflect this true value as precisely as we can. By specifying "at any given time," we acknowledge that variables change over time and that any measure will vary from day to day. Just like our weight, such measures vary slightly from one day to the next. And although some variables, such as our gender or religious affiliation, remain quite stable, it is nevertheless possible that a change may occur. Sex change operations and religious conversions are not unknown.

Measures are made up from the following components:

MEASURE = TV ± (SE ± RE)

The above equation contains four elements:

- *MEASURE.* This refers to the value that the researcher assigns to the variable in the process of recording the information.
- *TV.* The *True value* is the underlying exact quantity of the variable.
- *SE. Systematic error* is nonrandom error representing systematic under- or overestimation of the value. In systematic errors, the variation in measurement values is usually in the same direction and is caused by a stable characteristic of the population studied or the measurement tool. For example, a blood pressure machine that measured diastolic blood pressure at four points higher than the true diastolic reading would elevate by four points the systematic error in each person's reading.
- *RE. Random error* is fluctuation around the "true" value, in which higher or lower scores are equally likely (Carmines and Zeller, 1979). With random errors, the direction of the difference between the true value and the measurement value is without pattern. It may be high in one case and low in a subsequent case. Random error usually results from a transient state in the study participants or in the administration of the instrument. For example, anxiety on the part of study participants can affect responses on the instrument.

An example: Suppose a male respondent is asked to indicate his weight on a questionnaire. The respondent writes in "70 kilo." Providing that the information is then correctly transcribed in entering the data into the computer, the MEASURE is recorded as 70.0 kg; suppose the TV, or true value, is 73.367132 kg (rounded!). People usually underreport their weight by 2 kg; this is *SE,* the systematic error; the remaining 1.367132 kilograms is random error *(RE).*

$$\text{MEASURE} = TV \pm (SE \pm RE)$$

or

$$70.0 = 73.367132 - (2.0 + 1.367132)$$

The adequacy of a measure is the extent to which the indicator reflects the true value of the variable. All of the listed components vary over time and through the various stages of data collection in a research project. Usually we think that the subject makes measurement errors, but actually the situation is more complex. First, the *true value* of variables changes over time. If we repeat a measure several times to make certain that we have an accurate reflection of the variable, differences will be caused by variations in the true value, random error, and systematic error. (Respondents may change their attitudes over time, so the true value itself may shift; theoretically, it is fixed only at the time measured.)

Researchers can do several things to reduce random and systematic error. Random error refers to fluctuations that are unsystematic—for example, a respondent who cannot decide whether to rate the quality of lectures in the prenatal course as a 6 or a 7 on a 9-point index and finally decides on a 6, may have made a random choice. Systematic error is error in one direction. For example, if you tell respondents what you expect to find, they may bias their responses to confirm the expectation. When feasible, consider using some of the following ways of reducing error:

Tip 1. Take the average of several measures. Sometimes it is possible to repeat a measure several times and then use the average of these measures to reflect the variable. A subject could be weighed on three different scales and the average used. In this way, the researcher hopes to average out random measurement error.

Tip 2. Use several different indicators. In measuring a variable such as attitudes toward abortion, a researcher would typically pose several questions and then combine the responses to form an index. By combining the responses to several questions, the researcher hopes to minimize the effect of any one question.

Tip 3. Use random sampling procedures. By giving all people an equal chance of being included in your study, it is possible to minimize distortions that occur when people select themselves. If the goal, for example, was to estimate the popularity of a national health-care program, one would want to reflect the views of the whole country, not special groups within it. By reporting on what the average person thinks about the health program, you will minimize the random fluctuations that might occur if you talked to very few, unsystematically selected respondents. By not oversampling those who spend more time at home, you will have avoided systematically biasing the study by overrepresenting the views of people with that characteristic.

Tip 4. Use sensitive measures. In asking questions, provide respondents with as broad a range of response categories as possible so as not to constrain them. In questions used to create indexes, provide many response categories; in asking respondents to estimate the population of their community, provide many categories. By providing many response alternatives (or, indeed, allowing the respondent simply to respond without using any categories at all), the researcher can decrease the amount of random error in measurement. However, you can go overboard in suggesting increased numbers of response categories. If there are too many response categories, a respondent's ability to make distinctions may be exceeded. To ask someone to report their weight to two-decimal point accuracy would be silly; few people know their weight with such accuracy.

Tip 5. Provide clear instructions for how questions are to be answered. Respondents' varied understandings of what is being asked of them are one source of random error. Thus, variation in response may simply be the result of these different understandings. Attempt to develop instructions and questions that are clear and have but

one interpretation. You might say, "In the following items, *circle a number* to indicate the strength of your opinion."

Tip 6. Error checking data. Both systematic and random errors can occur easily. Conducting error checks on the data should eliminate these. If data are being coded (the process of assigning categories to responses) by several people, interrater reliability checks should be carried out in training the individuals to do the work. Only when high levels of interrater reliability are achieved should the coding proceed (see Chapter 6). The use of video recording equipment has permitted those doing observational studies to confirm their data by having other experts examine the work.

Tip 7. Reduce subject and experimenter expectations. As discussed in Chapter 8, subject and experimenter expectations can systematically alter the measures achieved in a research project. Attempt to control these expectations as much as possible.

Precise measurement is, indeed, a challenge. Any time a measurement is taken, errors will occur. The errors may be slight or substantial. Measurement should be seen as a matter of probability; most of the time, a researcher's measurements will fall within a given margin of error. This implies that, some of the time, measurements will not fall within a given (and acceptable) margin of error. Researchers attempt to estimate the amount of error that is likely in their measurements. The specific procedures for doing this are explained in Chapter 11.

Figure 13.3 presents a target-shooting analogy to help show the relationship between reliability, true value, and validity. In measurement, we attempt to consistently (reliability) hit the bull's eye (the true value) and if we do so, we have measured what we intended to (validity).

An inspection of Figure 13.3 shows that a measure may be reliable but lack validity; however, a measure that is valid is

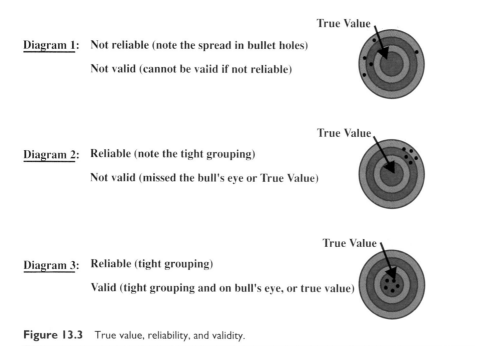

Diagram 1:   Not reliable (note the spread in bullet holes)

Not valid (cannot be valid if not reliable)

Diagram 2:   Reliable (note the tight grouping)

Not valid (missed the bull's eye or True Value)

Diagram 3:   Reliable (tight grouping)

Valid (tight grouping and on bull's eye, or true value)

Figure 13.3   True value, reliability, and validity.

also reliable because measures that hit the bull's eye are closely grouped and, therefore, must be reliable. The three diagrams illustrate the point.

- Diagram 1 depicts measurements that are neither reliable nor valid; the measurements have missed the true value (bull's eye) and produced a lot of scatter.
- Diagram 2 displays a reliable measure but one that lacks validity. Note that the shots are closely grouped together (hence reliable) but that they are not right on the bull's eye, which represents the true value.
- Diagram 3 displays a valid and reliable measure in which the shots are nicely grouped on the bull's eye.

D. LEVELS OF MEASUREMENT

Three levels of measurement were presented in Chapter 11. An understanding of levels of measurement is necessary because the ways in which one should go about analyzing a variable are constrained by the measurement level achieved in data collection. As a general rule, one should attempt to achieve the most precise measurement possible.

One way to begin to understand levels of measurement is to ask if the variable being measured has an underlying continuum (does it vary from low to high and do the categories imply an underlying quantitative dimension?). If there is no underlying continuum, with the variable being made up of a number of discrete categories, then the measurement will be at the nominal level; if the variable has an underlying continuum, then the level of measurement will be either ordinal, interval, or ratio. As discussed in Chapter 11, this text distinguishes three levels of measurement: nominal, ordinal, and ratio.

1. Nominal Measurement

The **nominal level** represents the lowest level of measurement. Examples of **nominal measurement** (those with an arbitrary assignment of numbers to categories) include measurements of such variables as religious affiliation, gender, program of study, political party affiliation, and ethnic origin. Although there may be underlying continua related to religious affiliation (e.g., degree of religious commitment or frequency of church attendance), by itself, the religious organization is a nominal category; it may be Baptist, Buddhist, Hindu, Lutheran, Roman Catholic, or Jewish. When a respondent checks off which (if any) religious affiliations he or she was associated with while growing up, the measurement level attained is nominal. One category is neither higher nor lower than any other—the categories are simply different. For example, Catholics are no higher or lower than Protestants. Nominal measurement involves no underlying continuum and the numerical values assigned are arbitrary and have no arithmetic meaning. Such values cannot be added, subtracted, multiplied, or divided. Additional examples are provided in Table 13.5.

2. Ordinal Measurement

The ordinal level represents the second lowest level of measurement. **Ordinal**

measurement involves an underlying continuum with the numerical values ordered so that small numbers refer to lower levels on the continuum and larger numbers to higher points; however, the distances between the assigned numbers and the underlying continuum are not in a one-to-one relationship with each other. Note the following questionnaire item asking about the size of a respondent's current home community:

Under 5000 ————————1☐
5000 to 19,999 ——————2☐
20,000 to 99,999 —————3☐
100,000 to 999,999 ————4☐
Over 1 million ——————5☐

Note that the numbers assigned by the researcher (1 through 5) are arranged so that higher numbers refer to larger population centers; but note that the intervals between the numbers are not equal (whereas the second category spans a population range of 15,000, the fourth category spans a range of 900,000).

Another frequently used type of question asks respondents to assess their de-

Table 13.5   Examples of Nominal Level Measurement*

Type of Research Design	Variable	Measure
Experiment	Expectancy created?	Subject run under conditions in which the outcome is: Expected - - - - - - - -1☐ Not expected - - - - 2☐
Survey questionnaire	Place of residence	The place where I live now is: Canada - - - - - - - - - -1☐ Mexico- - - - - - - - - - 2☐ United States - - - - 3☐ Other - - - - - - - - - - 4☐
Participant observation	Behavior related to illegal activities	George: Initiates activities - - - - - - - - - - - - 1☐ Supports activities of others - - - - 2☐ Rejects activities of others - - - - - - 3☐
Content analysis	Type of gender role TV character plays	Character X plays a gender role that is: Traditional - - - - - - - - 1☐ Nontraditional - - - - - 2☐

*Nominal measurement involves no underlying continuum; numeric values assigned have no meaning; values cannot be added, subtracted, or multiplied.

gree of agreement with a statement such as the following one:

Nurse practitioners enhance the quality of care in primary health centers.

Strongly disagree 1 2 3 4 5 6 7 8 9 Strongly agree

This kind of item provides ordinal measurement. Although we know that high numbers indicate a greater degree of agreement with the statement, we do not know whether the distances between the values are equal; the distance between 4 and 5 on the scale may not be the same size as the distance between 8 and 9. Ordinal measurement orders values but does not assure equal gaps between the measurement points. Additional examples of ordinal level measurement are provided in Table 13.6.

In conclusion, ordinal measurement involves an underlying continuum; numerical values assigned are ordered but intervals are not equal. When ordinal measures are combined, the values may be added or subtracted but not multiplied or divided because there is no true zero point.

3. Ratio Measurement

Finally, ratio measurement is the highest level. **Ratio measurement** involves an underlying continuum. The numerical values assigned are ordered with equal intervals; the zero point is aligned with true zero; and when different ratio measures are combined, the values may be added, subtracted, multiplied, or divided. Furthermore, it should be readily apparent that a ratio scale has all the qualities of lower levels of measurement (nominal, ordinal, interval), that an interval scale has all the qualities of the nominal and ordinal scales, and so on.

For example, in the case of income, the nature of the variable is such that it is possible to represent income with a number that reflects the income of a person exactly. In this case, it is also possible to use

Table 13.6 Examples of Ordinal Level Measurement*

Type of Research Design	Variable	Measure
Experiment	Expectancy level created	Subject run under conditions of: Low level – 1☐ Medium level – 2☐ High level – 3☐
Survey questionnaire	Size of community	The place where I live now has a population of: Under 5000 – 1☐ 5,000 to 19,999 – 2☐ 20,000 to 99,999 – 3☐ 100,000 to 999,999 – 4☐ More than 1 million – 5☐
Participant observation	Supportive behavior	Support of illegal activity: No support – 1☐ Some support – 2☐ Strong support – 3☐
Content analysis	Degree of traditional gender role	Character X plays a gender role that is: Nontraditional – 1☐ Neutral – 2☐ Traditional – 3☐

*Ordinal measurement involves an underlying continuum; numeric values assigned are ordered but intervals are not equal; values may be added or subtracted but not multiplied.

zero to reflect no income and other numerical values to reflect all other income levels. Here it is correct to say that an income of $50,000 is twice as much as an income of $25,000. With ratio-level measurement, it is possible to add and subtract constants as well as to multiply or divide by them without changing the proportionality among the values.

If a researcher were to have respondents indicate with a check mark which of the magazines on a list that they had scanned or read in the previous month and a total was taken of the number ticked off, the result would be a variable that varies from 0 to the number required if a respondent checked off all the items listed. This number would be a ratio measurement. Note that a 0 in this example refers to no exposure to any of the magazines listed, and other values simply provide a count of the number of the listed magazines that the respondent has scanned or read in the past month. There is a one-to-one relationship between the value assigned by the researcher and the number of listed magazines identified by the respondent.

Similarly, when communities are being studied, measures such as the proportion of visible minorities, the proportion of retired people in the population, and various rates and ratios (e.g., suicide rate, dependency ratio, gender ratio) are all ratio level measures (see Table 13.7 for additional examples).

Some textbooks distinguish *equal interval* as a fourth level of measurement. Box 13.1 explains what happened to the fourth level of measurement frequently distinguished in research texts.

E. THE EFFECTS OF REDUCED LEVELS OF MEASUREMENT

This chapter has encouraged researchers to achieve the most precise measurements that are practical. To explore the consequences of reducing the level of measurement, the authors examined what would happen if a ratio level variable (student's high school average grade) was regrouped using random numbers to establish cutpoints, into 9, 7, 5, and 3 categories. (To regroup the high school average grade into three categories, two random numbers were selected that fell between the lowest and highest value and these established the cutpoints. If the random numbers were 49 and 72, then all grades between 50 and 71 would be coded a 2; grades between 0 and 49 coded as 1; and

Table 13.7   **Examples of Ratio Level Measurement***

Type of Research Design	Variable	Measure
Experiment	Accuracy of recall	Number of correct answers in trial: _____
Survey questionnaire	Weight?	My weight is: ___ pounds or ___ kilos
Participant observation	Community involvement	Number of people at health fair on January 15: ___
Content analysis	Conservative gender portrayals	Ratio of men portrayed in nontraditional gender roles to women portrayed in nontraditional gender roles: ___ : ___

*Ratio measurement involves an underlying continuum; numeric values assigned are ordered with equal intervals, the zero point is aligned with true zero. When different ratio measures are combined, the values may be added, subtracted, multiplied, or divided.

BOX 13.1 *What Ever Happened to Equal Interval Measures?*

The conventional *equal interval* level of measurement (Stevens, 1951) is not presented in this text for the sake of pedagogical simplicity. For analyses that require equal interval or ratio measurement, in most cases the measurement will be ratio level. Many texts in the social sciences use the temperature measures of Celsius versus Fahrenheit as examples of situations in which the intervals between the points are equal but where the zero point is misplaced (absolute zero is about −273°F). The table below shows the traditional measurement levels and their associated properties.

Arguably, most social science measures that meet the equal interval assumption also meet the ratio measurement assumption of a correctly aligned zero point (see Blalock, 1979). Individual variables such as age, weight, height, income, years employed, number of magazines read last week, and the number of dates one had last month all would constitute ratio measures providing the data recorded reflect the characteristic being measured and not placed in some pre-coded set of categories with uneven category sizes.

Similarly, measures reflecting properties of communities or countries (or other groupings) such as the proportion of nonnative-born members, the crime rate, and the number of motor vehicles per person all represent ratio level measures.

Although most textbook authors present the four types of measurement, some do not (see Levin and Fox, 1991; Rosenthal and Rosnow 1991; Jackson, 1999). For the sake of simplicity, equal interval measures are not identified as such in this text. Readers should be aware that the measurement assumptions of various statistics that often call for interval level measurement are stated as ratio level measurement in this presentation. But because virtually all the social science measures that are at this level are ratio level measures, this should rarely prove to be a difficulty.

Table 1 Traditional Levels of Measurement

Measurement Feature	Nominal	Ordinal	Equal Interval	Ratio
Identifies categories?	Yes	Yes	Yes	Yes
Orders observations?	No	Yes	Yes	Yes
Equal intervals between points?	No	No	Yes	Yes
Properly assigned zero point?	No	No	No	Yes

grades 72 and above coded as 3. New versions for each of these variables were created 10 times for the categories 3, 5, 7, and 9.) The new versions of the variables were then correlated with unchanged ratio variables (high school English grade and first-year university grade). As anticipated, the correlations declined further with each succeeding grouping into fewer categories (Box 13.2). It is recommended that readers take time to carefully review the contents of Box 13.2 to appreciate the importance of precise measurement. Although this material is somewhat technical in nature, it illustrates a concrete example of the three principles identified below.

The analysis suggests that when reduced levels of measurement are achieved, the result will underestimate the strength of association between variables. Furthermore, in doing analyses that permit a comparison of the relative effects of indepen-

BOX 13.2 *The Effects of Reduced Levels of Measurement*

An attempt to examine the consequences of reduced levels of measurement was carried out.

1. The hypotheses. The hypotheses that guided this investigation were as follows:
   Hypothesis 1: The greater the number of categories in an ordinal variable, the less reduction there will be in the correlation between the variable and other variables.

2. In doing a regression analysis:
   Hypothesis 2: A ratio variable that is measured using a Likert-type question (ordinal level measurement) will reduce the amount of variation explained in the analysis compared with how much variation would be explained had ratio level measurement been achieved.
   Hypothesis 3: The beta weights of Likert-type items (ordinal level measurement) will

be reduced in comparison to those using raw scores.
Hypothesis 4: The above effects will be greater for those variables having fewer categories.
Hypothesis 5: Beta weights of variables not categorized will be enhanced in comparison to those where categorization has been done.

A data set containing 3617 cases was used in this investigation. The variables included university student's high school average, high school English grade, and average at the end of their first year of university study. Correlations were calculated (see Table 1) for the relation between these variables. The correlation between university average and the English grade high school average was 0.464 and 0.573, respectively; the high school English grade and the average high school grade correlated at 0.662.

Table 1 Correlations Between First-Year University Average, Average High School Grade, and English High School Grade (n = 3617)

Correlations	First-Year University Average	Average High School Grade	English High School Grade
First-year university average	1.000		
Average high school grade	0.573	1.000	
English high school grade	0.464	0.662	1.000

A regression analysis was done taking first-year university average as the dependent variable, using high school English grade and the high school average grade (excluding the English mark) as independent variables. The results of this analysis are shown in Table 2. The R^2 was 0.341 (34.1% of the variance explained); the beta weight for the English grade was 0.152; for high school average it was 0.472. The impact of high school average was about three times as great as the English grade alone.

Table 2 Regression Analysis Predicting First-Year Average Grade (n = 3617)

Variable	b Coefficient	Beta Weight	Percent Explained
High school English grade	0.16290	0.15195	8.30
High school average*	0.54188	0.47203	25.78
		% Explained	34.08
Constant	11.08264		
Multiple R	0.58383		
R square	0.34085		

*The high school average was calculated excluding the high school English grade.

continued on next page

BOX 13.2 *The Effects of Reduced Levels of Measurement*

In an attempt to test the hypotheses, a series of trials was done on the data testing the effect of regrouping the high school average variable. We wished to compare what would happen if it were collapsed into 3, 5, 7, and 9 categories. We also wished to observe the impact of such collapsing on the R^2, and the beta weights. A table of random numbers was used to determine the cutpoints; a total of 40 variables were created in this way (10 for 9 category variables, 10 for 7 category variables, 10 for 5 category variables and 10 for 3 category variables). In all cases, the new variables were used as an independent variable in each trial along with the English grade in all cases using the university average as the dependent variable. The results of the correlational analyses are summarized in Table 3; Table 4 summarizes the results of the 40 regression analyses.

Table 3   Average Change in Correlations Between High School Average Grade and First-Year University Grade When Data Are Grouped into 3, 5, 7, and 9 Categories*

Number of Categories	Average Decline in Correlation	Standard Deviation	Number of Recodings
9	−0.03810	0.03151	10
7	−0.05790	0.03208	10
5	−0.11260	0.09623	10
3	−0.18240	0.16038	10

*The raw data, based on 3617 cases (St. Francis Xavier University), was used for this analysis. The high school average grade was recoded into 9, 7, 5, or 3 categories, 10 recodings for each category. For each, the new variable was then correlated with the first-year university average. The above table summarizes the results. For example, when the data were recoded into three categories, the average drop in correlation (for the 10 randomly determined cutpoints) was 0.18.

Table 4   Summary of Changes in R^2 and Betas When One Variable Is Grouped into 9, 7, 5, and 3 Categories, Regression Analyses

Number of Categories in Recoded Variable	Mean Change in R^2	Mean Change in Beta HS	Mean Change in Beta ENG
9 Categories	−0.025	−0.067	0.059
7 Categories	−0.033	−0.099	0.094
5 Categories	−0.055	−0.162	0.135
3 Categories	−0.069	−0.217	0.179
Probability	0.0059	0.0039	0.0001

HS 5 high school average grade; this is the variable that was recoded.
ENG 5 high school English grade; this variable was left in its raw form for the analysis.
This analysis summarizes the results of 40 separate regression analyses (10 for recoding into 9 categories; 10 for the recoding into 7 categories; 10 for the recoding into 5 categories; and 10 for the recoding into 3 categories). The total n for each analysis is 3617. Table 2 presents the results when the high school average is used in its raw form.

SOURCE: Winston Jackson. The author wishes to thank Dr. Bernard Liengme, registrar, St. Francis Xavier University, for providing the data for the analysis.

dent variables on a dependent variable (see Chapter 18), the effect of an independent variable that has a reduced level of measurement will be underestimated. The research suggests the following general principles:

Principle 1. The greater the reduction of measurement precision, the greater the drop in the correlation between the variables.

Principle 2. In analyses comparing relative effects of variables, the effects of those variables with reduced levels of measurement are *underestimated* by comparison with those whose measurement is more precise.

Principle 3. Conversely, variables whose measurement is more precise will have their effects *overestimated* relative to those whose measurement is less precise.

These three principles suggest that we should attempt to reflect the underlying concepts as precisely as possible. But there are constraints. It is foolish to ask people to give us exact answers when there is little likelihood that they will be in the position to make precise estimates. For example, asking anyone on campus to estimate the weight of a school bus would invite highly variable and inaccurate answers. Furthermore, it is sometimes inappropriate to ask for extremely precise information if a respondent will consider such information too personal. For example, in some populations, asking someone his or her exact annual income would fall into that category. Sometimes, in order to soften a question and to make it less threatening, we reduce its precision. In asking about age, for example, we sometimes ask people to indicate into which age category they fall rather than reveal their exact age. So the rule to be followed is to *achieve as precise measurement as is practical.* Researchers recognize that weaker measurement typically result in underestimating the importance of a poorly measured vari-

able relative to other, more precisely measured variables.

F. PROCEDURES FOR DATA COLLECTION

Data collection is the process of gathering information from identified participants to answer a research question. The amount of time, planning, and energy required for data collection depends upon the specific research question, design, and measurement tools available. In preparation for data collection, the researcher must answer a number of questions, such as:

- What data are to be collected?
- What methods will be used to collect the data?
- From whom will data be collected?
- How will participants be identified and selected?
- Who will collect the data?
- Where will the data be collected?
- When will the data be collected?
- How will consistency of data collection methods be established and monitored?

Each question necessitates an answer by the researcher before data collection commences. The answer varies depending on the nature of the research project. The researcher should detail strategies used to address each question in the writing of the research report. This information is useful in evaluating the study results or planning a replication of the study. Box 13.3 illustrates a description of the data collection procedure as it would appear in a journal article. Note the article describes who the participants were, how they were selected, the sites for data collection, and the measures used to collect the information from participants.

A variety of quantitative and qualitative data collection methods are available to nurse researchers to gather infor-

BOX 13.3 *Nurse Researchers at Work*

STRESS, COPING, AND SOCIAL SUPPORT AMONG HOMELESS YOUTHS

Participants in this study were homeless or potentially homeless youths who were ages 13 through 23 years. Homelessness included living in one of the following places during the past 12 months: street; subway; abandoned car or building; park; beach; car, bus, or van; girlfriend, boyfriend, lover, or friend's house or apartment; foster home; group home; halfway house; treatment center; shelter; mission; motel; hotel; boarding house; or jail.

Procedure

Systematic sampling methods were used to obtain a sample of homeless youth in Los Angeles, California. Sampling occurred through two sampling frames: one fixed or service sites (i.e., shelter or drop-in centers) and one for natural street sites (i.e., street corners) where homeless youth gather.

Fixed sites. Previous research indicated that approximately one half of the Los Angeles homeless youth population could be reached through shelters and drop-in centers. Three shelters and six drop-in centers were selected as fixed primary sampling units (PSUs), and 50 percent of the sampling assignments were at these fixed sites. Interview teams consisting of two to four members were given random assignments to one or more of these fixed sites each day. After reviewing the agency's sign-in roster to determine how many youths were in the agency, they determined the sampling fraction from a sampling fraction table according to the number of potential participants. Using the sampling fraction and a predetermined random start number, youths were selected from the sign-in roster and invited to participate in the study.

Street sites. Street-based sampling occurred along five major boulevards. Along these boulevards, 73 street areas, four parks, and three restaurants were identified as natural PSUs. Interviewer teams were assigned randomly to one of these PSUs, where they determined the number of potentially eligible youths in the area and then determined the sampling fraction. Youths were then counted and selected according to the sampling fraction and the predetermined random start number.

Youths selected for recruitment were asked to answer an eight-item screening instrument to determine whether they were eligible to participate in a 60- to 75-minute structured interview. The interviews were conducted at a nearby coffee shop and fast-food restaurants, permitting the interview to occur in a safe, quiet setting. Compensation for participation included a meal worth $10 and $10 in food vouchers.

SOURCE: Summarized from Unger, J., Kipe, M., Simon, T., et al. (1998). Stress, coping, and social support among homeless youth. *Journal of Adolescent Research, 13*(2), 134–157.

mation. The choice depends on three concerns (Massey, 1995):

1. The identified research problem, question, or hypothesis
2. The research design
3. The amount of information already known about the variables

The main methods used in quantitative research include questionnaires; special scales and indices to measure knowledge, skill, and attitudes; biochemical and physiological measures; projective techniques; and the Delphi technique. Qualitative methods include unstructured interviews, focus groups, observation sessions, and records or historical documents.

In qualitative research, data collection is greatly facilitated by using an organized process. Indeed, Montgomery (2000) has suggested the use of a "qualitative data collection bag" that nurses can use to prepare for successful data collection. The items in the bag include:

- Consent forms
- Participant information sheets
- Pens and paper
- Notebook for thoughts, feelings, mood
- Materials to record the decision trail
- Tape recorder with batteries
- Electricity adapter
- Audio tapes
- Return self-addressed, stamped envelopes (if needed)
- Compensation (monetary and nonmonetary)
- Interview guide

Keeping the well-stocked bag close at hand facilitates timely and efficient data collection, minimizing loss of data collection opportunities.

Consistency in data collection procedures is important in reducing bias that may be introduced if more than one individual is involved in data collection. As much as possible, data should be collected in the same way from each participant. For example, if more than one instrument is administered, they should be given in the same order to all participants, in the same context and setting, and with the same set of directions. When assistants are hired to collect data, they must be trained to do so systematically. Usually a written protocol that outlines the procedures for data collection is provided to research assistants. Interrater reliability needs to be established and monitored throughout the data collection period.

In quantitative designs, data collection methods are predetermined, standardized, and specified in advance so that little is required in terms of input from the investigator after data collection begins. The situation is quite different in qualitative designs in which greater flexibility and less structure are evident in the data collection process. In qualitative designs, the researcher is considered the data collection instrument. The researcher may vary the questions asked of respondents and may eliminate or introduce new ques-

tions depending on the data produced. Not all respondents may be asked the same questions, nor may all respondents be included in all aspects of the investigation. The sample may not be determined in advance of the data collection procedure; rather, it must remain fluid throughout the study as the researcher takes the liberty of adding new participants depending on the emerging findings.

Nursing deals with many complex phenomena. Measurement of such phenomena presents a challenge to nurse researchers. As the discipline of nursing develops, new constructs are emerging and, along with them, so is the need for valid and reliable instruments to measure these constructs. Some phenomena of interest to nurses remain unexplored because no appropriate strategies exist to collect data about them. The situation is changing, however, as more nurse researchers engage in instrument development studies or borrow instruments developed by others and modify them for use in nursing investigations. The most common data collection strategies in nursing research are discussed in this section and include various indexes and scales; physiologic measures; special measurement procedures such as magnitude estimation and visual analogues; and interviews, observations, and questionnaires.

I. Indexes

Combining several indicators into one score results in an **index** or scale. Although these terms are often used interchangeably, when a distinction is made, an *index* refers to the combination of two or more indicators. A **scale** refers to a more complex combination of indicators in which the pattern of the responses is taken into account. The terms are used interchangeably in this text.

Indexes are routinely constructed to reflect psychosocial variables such as social support, socioeconomic status, satisfaction with care, group dynamics, or an attitude toward an issue of concern to the field of nursing. (For details of many classic indexes and scales, see Miller, 1977, or Frank-Stromberg et al., 1997.) Scales and indexes may also reflect self-report measures on various physical sensations such as pain, nausea, appetite, fatigue, sexual satisfaction, and so on. Frequently, a researcher will construct subindexes that may be treated alone or combined with other subindexes to form a composite measure. For example, a researcher measuring attitudes toward abortion might construct a subindex for "soft reasons" (e.g., economically inconvenient, preference for having a baby later) and "hard reasons" (e.g., pregnancy as a result of rape, severely handicapped). These subindexes might also be combined to form an overall index. In each case, however, the researcher will have to ensure that appropriate items are included in each subindex.

a. Item Analysis

It is important that the components of an index discriminate—that is, various elements must discriminate between high scorers and lower scorers. To illustrate, suppose that you are attempting to develop a set of multiple choice questions to measure pediatric nurses' knowledge of growth and development theory and that you wish to identify the items that best measure mastery of the subject matter. Let us suppose that you have 100 questions on the test and that you wish to identify the best 50 questions for a future test. The issue is to select the items that best discriminate between high and low performance on the test. Let us suppose that we have given the preliminary test to 200 nurses working in pediatric settings.

We could proceed by grading the test and computing the total correct responses for each nurse. If the "marking" were done

with a computer program, we would use a matrix that has nurses and questions on the dimensions. Each cell would identify a correct or an incorrect response to each question for a particular nurse. Now we could order the nurses by the number of correct responses and then choose the top and bottom quartiles. Table 13.8 shows the percent from each quartile getting each question correct.

The next step is to select those items in which the performance of top and bottom nurses differs most. We assume here that, overall, the questions measure knowledge of the subject matter and that we are simply choosing those items that discriminate best.

The first two questions discriminate well—the high scorers do considerably better on those items than the low scorers. The third question would be rejected; although 55 percent of the nurses in the top quartile gave the right answer, so did 60 percent of the bottom group. Similarly, question 4 would be dropped because a similar proportion of top and bottom nurses answered correctly.

Similar procedures may be used to select high discrimination items for indexes. Suppose, for example, that we had 15 items for an index measuring nurses' job satisfaction and we wished to deter-

Table 13.8 Discrimination Ability of 100 Items: Percent Correct for Each Item by Quartile

Question#	Percent Correct Each Item	
	Bottom 25%	Top 25%
1	40.0	80.0
2	5.0	95.0
3	60.0	55.0
4	80.0	80.0
5	10.0	40.0
6	20.0	60.0
—	—	—
100	30.0	20.0

mine which items to include in the index. We want items that do two things: (1) validly reflect the dimension of the concept they are supposed to and (2) discriminate between high and low scorers. We might want to do the following:

- Include the items that have face validity.
- Add them together, coming up with a total score for each individual.
- Split the sample into the top and bottom quartiles in job satisfaction scores.
- Test each item's ability to discriminate between high and low job satisfaction.
- Select that items that best differentiate high scorers from low scorers.

b. Selecting Index Items

Indexes are constructed by combining several individual questions and represent an attempt to summarize, in one score, a measure of a variable. Indexes are constructed in situations in which we have a single-dimension variable but where one question might not adequately measure the variable. Indexes can be constructed by combining a number of similarly formatted questions or combinations of questions with different formats. In all cases, the indicators are combined and possibly weighted to sum to a single index score. The steps involved in developing an index are identified below.

Step 1. Review conceptual definition. As in developing other measures, the first step is to review the conceptual definition of the variable. Some sense of the "range" or the dimensions involved in the variable should be developed. The chances are that several questions can then be designed to measure the variable, reflecting each of the dimensions in the conceptual definition.

Step 2. Develop measures for each dimension. Here the same principles apply as for the development of individual measures. For example, in measuring attitudes toward the use of nurse prac-

titioners, one might identify which, if any, events would lead a respondent to favor use of nurse practitioners. Items may initially be selected on the basis of face validity—that is, if the item appears, on the face of it, to represent a part of the theoretical continuum being measured, then an effort should be made to get a measure of that item. Items usually consist of a *stem statement* relating to the phenomenon being measured, a *set of scale values,* and *anchors* at each end of the scale values. These aspects are illustrated in the following example:

Stem statement: I support the use of nurse practitioners for treatment of common health problems.

Anchors: Strongly disagree   Strongly agree

Scale values: 1 2 3 4 5 6 7 8 9

The following three items on the use of nurse practitioners may form part of an index:

I support the use of nurse practitioners in underserviced areas of the healthcare system.

Strongly disagree 1 2 3 4 5 6 7 8 9 Strongly agree

I support the use of nurse practitioners in all sectors of the health-care system.

Strongly disagree 1 2 3 4 5 6 7 8 9 Strongly agree

I support the use of nurse practitioners in family practice centers.

Strongly disagree 1 2 3 4 5 6 7 8 9 Strongly agree

Step 3: Pretest index. Index items should always be pretested. A pretest is simple; all you have to do is complete the index yourself and then sit beside individuals who are within the population being studied and have several complete the index items.

Encourage these pretest respondents to ask questions, telling them in advance that you are trying to find out if all the questions are clear. Reword questions to achieve clarity. Pretests almost always lead to revisions in the wording of index items.

Step 4. Pilot test index. If time permits, indexes should be pilot tested. A **pilot study** involves having a number of respondents complete a questionnaire containing the proposed index items. In a pilot study, you take what you consider to be the final version of the index to a sample of respondents similar to those in the proposed study. The results are analyzed to see if the index items discriminate and if they are internally consistent. Items may be dropped or altered on the basis of a pilot study.

If time is not available to do a pilot test, at least ensure that a full range of possible variability is represented by the index items. When the data are being analyzed, the various items can be evaluated using the SPSS procedure of RELIABILITY. This procedure provides a method of checking the internal consistency of index items. Items may be dropped if they do not prove to be internally consistent.

Gillis (1990) developed and pilot tested the Knowledge of Growth and Development Test (KGDT), a 35-item, multiple choice test designed to measure a nurse's knowledge of child development on three conceptual dimensions: (1) knowledge of play, (2) teaching and procedure preparation, and (3) the stages of psychosocial development across the five stages of childhood. The KGDT was pilot tested on a sample of senior baccalaureate nursing students. The effectiveness of each item was determined by an item analysis. Item analysis provided information about the percentage of the group that answered the item correctly and the discrimination index or ability of the item to differentiate between nurses of high and low ability. All items with a D value (discrimination index value) of 0.65 were maintained. Three items were reworded because of their initial negative D values. The KGDT had good internal consistency (Cronbach alpha = 0.80).

c. The Rationale for Using Several Items in an Index

Suppose we are interested in measuring nurses' attitudes toward abortion. Would it be better to use one question or several questions in our measure? The general consensus among most researchers is that measures with multiple items have an advantage over single-item measures in attaining precise measurement. Jackson (1999) has summarized the arguments in favor of using multiple items in measurement:

- An attitude toward abortion would almost certainly be complex, and one would want to reflect this complexity in any measurement (e.g., would nurses have the same attitude toward abortion if the pregnancy threatened the life of the mother, was the result of a rape, or was economically inconvenient?).
- A single item may lack precision, may lack a sufficient range in values (a question such as, "Are you in favor of abortion?" with yes or no response categories would be inadequate. Even with more response categories, it would still be weak because the question does not identify conditions in which a person might favor or not favor abortion).
- Single items are also less reliable and more prone to random measurement error. If a question like the one above were repeated in a questionnaire, the respondent, having indicated opposition to abortion the first time, might well change her answer the second time because she thinks: "Well, it depends on the situation. If the female was raped and is 14 years old, I would be in favor of her right to have an abortion."
- With multiple items, it is possible to evaluate the reliability and validity of the index; with single indicators, it is more difficult to gauge the amount of measurement error.

2. Likert-Based Indexes

Rensis Likert (1931) proposed that indexes or scales could be constructed by summing respondents' answers to a number of related items. This type of question is widely used in nursing research. In the original format, the respondent is asked to (1) strongly disagree, (2) disagree, (3) be undecided or neutral, (4) agree, or (5) strongly agree with a statement. Such items were, and continue to be, popular in measuring attitudes and perceptions. Box 13.4 illustrates some of these questions.

Readers should note that the items in Box 13.4 deviate somewhat from the original format. Given a preference for increasing the variability in such items, the number of response categories has been increased from five to nine. This increase does not take more space on the questionnaire or more space when entered into a computer. Using more response categories (9 point rather than 5 point) should lead to slightly higher correlations between index items and prove to be somewhat better at reflecting true underlying values. (See the earlier discussion on the effects of reduced levels of measurement.) When there are only a few items in an index, increasing the number of scale values usually increases the reliability of the scale. When there are many items, fewer values are needed to achieve high levels of reliability.

a. Tips for Constructing a Likert-Based Index

The following tips may be helpful in constructing such items for use in a **Likert-based index.**

Tip 1. Avoid the word "and" in Likert items if such usage makes the item multidimensional. In such indexes, we are attempting to measure a single variable, so it is important for us not to add a second dimension inadvertently. Suppose we asked a respondent to assess how well he or she gets along at home by making the following statement:

I get along well with my mother and father.
Strongly disagree 1 2 3 4 5 6 7 8 9 **Strongly agree**

What number is the respondent to circle if he or she gets along well with mother but fights continuously with father? The question has to be subdivided into two questions, one asking about relations with mother and one asking about relations with father. Watch out for the word "and" in a Likert item. Most of the time, you will have to change the item.

Tip 2. Place the "Strongly Agree" on the

BOX 13.4 *Likert Index Example: Job Satisfaction of Nurses*

In the following items, *circle a number* to indicate the extent to which you agree or disagree with each statement.

16. I enjoy working with the types of patients I am presently working with.
    Strongly disagree 1 2 3 4 5 6 7 8 9 Strongly agree
29. I would be satisfied if my child followed the same type of career I have.
    Strongly disagree 1 2 3 4 5 6 7 8 9 Strongly agree

30. I would quit my present job if I won $1,000,000 through a lottery.
    Strongly disagree 1 2 3 4 5 6 7 8 9 Strongly agree
31. This is the best job that I have had.
    Strongly disagree 1 2 3 4 5 6 7 8 9 Strongly agree
32. I would like to continue the kind of work I am doing until I retire.
    Strongly disagree 1 2 3 4 5 6 7 8 9 Strongly agree

SOURCE: McCabe, C. (1991). Job Satisfaction: A Study of St. Martha Regional Nurses. St. Francis Xavier University, Sociology 300 Project. Cited with permission.

right-hand side of the scale, with 9 indicating strong agreement. Some researchers prefer to vary the response categories, by, for example, reversing the side on which the agree and disagree labels are placed. This is done to prevent **response set,** a situation in which the respondent tends to answer all items similarly. Although switching the side on which the agree and disagree categories are placed may reduce the tendency to respond in a set manner, it may also introduce additional errors in response. (Respondents may not notice that you have switched the agree and disagree categories.) This author's preference is to maintain a uniform presentation. Response sets are best avoided by wording some questions positively and others negatively.

Tip 3. Avoid multiple negatives that may confuse respondent (e.g., statements such as, "I *don't* think the university administration is doing a *bad* job" will almost certainly confuse and slow down respondents). If the respondent thinks the university administration is doing a good job, should the respondent circle the 9 for Strongly Agree, or the 1 for Strongly Disagree? A direct simple statement is better: "The university administration is incompetent" or "The university administration is excellent."

Tip 4. Vary the "strength of wording" of questions to produce variation in response. Most items should be stated as moderately positive or negative. Statements that reflect extremes or are neutral produce less variance in response and consequently are not effective in discriminating participants on the construct being measured. Similarly, if there is uncertainty as to where responses will fall, use more than one item with different intensities in the wordings.

Tip 5. Before the first Likert-type item is presented, provide a brief explanation of how respondents are to indicate their answers. Likert items result in an ordinal level of measurement. Typically, such items are combined to form indexes by adding together the values on individual items (after having reversed the scores on the negative measures). For example, when scoring a scale measuring the construct "satisfaction" with a distance education nursing course, the scale values for the negatively stated items would be reversed so that the highest value reflects satisfaction rather than dissatisfaction. The values for the negative items would then be summed and added to the values for the positive items. Likert indexes are frequently referred to as **summated rating indexes.** In such indexes, the scores for each item are summed or summed and averaged to yield each individual's score. Typically, the resulting scores are considered to have been transformed into ratio level data that permits the use of more sophisticated data analysis procedures.

b. Evaluation of Likert-Based Indexes

We have assumed that the summation score reflects the true underlying variable. If an item does not correlate with this score, we assume that the item is not appropriate. It is, however, possible that the other items are in error. If index items are not well thought out, the chances are that the correlations between the items will generally be low and that this information may then be used to reject items.

To perform this analysis using SPSS, see the RELIABILITY procedure in Appendix A.

Likert-based indexes are widely used in nursing research. Their popularity is because of these factors:

- They are easy to construct.
- There are well-developed techniques for rigorously assessing the validity of potential items.
- They are relatively easy for respondents to complete.

- They require fewer items than other indexes to achieve the same level of reliability when 9-point scales are used.
- They can be used for group and individual comparisons.
- They can be administered in oral or written formats.

The disadvantages of Likert-based indexes include susceptibility to: (1) *social desirability response set bias,* the tendency to give an answer that is consistent with current social values; (2) *extreme response set bias,* the tendency to select an attitude at the extreme; and (3) *acquiescence response set bias,* or the tendency to always agree with statements regardless of their content (Massey, 1995).

3. Semantic Differential Procedures

Osgood (1957) is most associated with the development of the **semantic differential** measurement technique. There are numerous index applications for this type of measurement technique in nursing. Originally, these measurement techniques were used to study subjective feelings toward objects or persons. For example, stereotyping behavior, measuring how respondents view various out-groups, has been investigated using this approach. More recently, the semantic differential index has been used in nursing to measure attitudes toward such constructs as caregiving roles, menopause, smoking, risk-taking behavior, computer-assisted learning, self-concept, and maternal–child bonding. The format of semantic differential questions is shown in Box 13.5. These questions consist of a series of bipolar adjectives, indicating two extremes, placed at the margins of the page; the respondent is asked to indicate where, between the two extremes, he or she would place the group, individual, or object being evaluated by selecting a value on a 9-point scale. For example, respondents might be asked to indicate

---

BOX 13.5 *Semantic Differential*

62. Circle a number to indicate where you think *you* fit on a continuum between the two opposites.

621 Shy 1 2 3 4 5 6 7 8 9 Outgoing
622 Passive 1 2 3 4 5 6 7 8 9 Dominant
623 Cautious 1 2 3 4 5 6 7 8 9 Daring
624 Bookworm 1 2 3 4 5 6 7 8 9 Social butterfly
625 Quiet 1 2 3 4 5 6 7 8 9 Loud
626 Serious 1 2 3 4 5 6 7 8 9 Humorous
627 Conformist 1 2 3 4 5 6 7 8 9 Leader
628 Cooperative 1 2 3 4 5 6 7 8 9 Stubborn

---

where a group would be placed on an honest/dishonest continuum or on a hot/cold dimension. Respondents are encouraged to answer the questions quickly, letting their guards down, and thus revealing how they "see" various categories of individuals or objects.

Factor analytic studies (see Chapter 18) of semantic differential indexes suggest that such scales assess three factors of meaning. These include (1) evaluation, (2) potency, and (3) activity. Table 13.9 presents the pairs of adjectives frequently used to define these factors. There are a variety of traditional and nontraditional uses for such items. Researchers can compare participants' scores for rating various constructs or compare various groups of respondents' scores. Questions can be used to measure individual variables or be combined to create indexes. The items are scored similarly to items on a Likert index. Remember to take into account the direction of the positive–negative bipolar adjective pairs.

4. Magnitude Estimation Procedures

Magnitude estimation procedures are useful when *comparative judgments* are re-

Table 13.9   Anchors for Semantic Differential Factors

	Factor		
	Evaluation	Potency	Activity
Bipolar adjectives	Good/bad	Strong/weak	Active/passive
	Fair/unfair	Tense/relaxed	Quick/slow
	Positive/negative	Large/small	Severe/lenient
	Honest/dishonest	Hard/soft	Sharp/dull
	Successful/unsuccessful	Rigid/flexible	Stimulating/boring
	Valuable/worthless		
	Useful/useless		

Source: Adapted from Waltz, C., Strickland, O., and Lenz, E. (1991). *Measurement in Nursing Research* (2nd ed). Philadelphia: F.A. Davis.

quired. When these procedures are used, a respondent compares the magnitudes of a series of stimuli. These techniques emerged out of work done by S.S. Stevens (1966a, 1966b, 1951), who attempted to examine the relationship between physical stimuli (e.g., the physically measured roughness of different sandpapers) and respondents' perception of their roughness. This powerful technique is useful when comparative judgments are required. The technique results in ratio level measurement and should be in the repertoire of the nurse researcher. This technique is used best in interview or in group-administered questionnaires. The instructions need to be reviewed carefully with the respondents, so it is necessary to have a researcher present when the instrument is administered.

Typically, one of two methods is used to do magnitude estimations. The first is to have respondents provide numerical estimates. If one were estimating the relative popularity of different students in a residence, for example, one might begin by having respondents compare the popularity of each student with that of a student the researcher has identified as being about average in popularity. The researcher would then assign this average student 100 units of popularity. The respondent would be asked to proceed

through a list of students, indicating in each case the amount of popularity each has relative to that of the "average student." If the respondent thinks that Joan is two and a quarter times as popular as the average, a value of 225 would be assigned. Alternatively, if the respondent thinks that Joan has three quarters the popularity of the "average student," then a value of 75 would be assigned.

A second approach is to have respondents draw different length lines to indicate their perceptions of the differences between stimulus objects. In this case, a standard line is given, and the respondent is asked to draw lines relative to the standard line. (Sample instructions for using the "line method" are presented in Box 13.6.)

a. Tips for Using Magnitude Estimation Procedures

Some tips for the utilization of magnitude estimations are:

Tip 1. Only use magnitude estimations when a researcher is present to explain the method. The mailed questionnaire is not a suitable vehicle for using this technique.

Tip 2. Use magnitude estimations when comparative judgments are required.

BOX 13.6 *Sample Magnitude Estimation Instructions: Perceptions of Hospitals*

Now we would like to have you rate the various local hospitals on a number of dimensions. The way you will do it will be to draw different lengths of line to indicate how each of the hospitals compares with one another. If you draw a line twice as long as the "standard" line, it means you think that particular hospital is twice as good as average for the particular dimension being rated. For example, suppose you were asked to indicate how far each hospital is from your home. You would then draw lines indicating the relative distances from your home. You might draw the following lines:

IF THE AVERAGE HOSPITAL IS _____
THIS FAR, HOW FAR IS: (suppose you then drew the following lines)
Breckenridge _____
Dallas General _____
Mount Royal Hospital _____
Mount St. Vincent _____
St. Francis Xavier ____
St. Mary's _____

We would interpret your lines to mean that you think that Breckenridge Hospital is about 1.5 times further than the average local hospi-

tal from your home; Dallas General, Mount Saint Vincent Hospital, and St. Mary's are about average; and St. Francis Xavier Hospital is about one third as far as the average hospital.

Now we would like you to give us estimates on the following 25 aspects, using the technique that was described above.

How good are the family room facilities for family members of hospitalized clients?
Standard = _____
Breckenridge
Dallas General
Mount Royal Hospital
Mount St. Vincent Hospital
St. Francis Xavier Hospital
St. Mary's Hospital

How good a professional reputation do you think the nursing staff at each hospital has?
Standard = _____
Breckenridge
Dallas General
Mount Royal Hospital
Mount St. Vincent Hospital
St. Francis Xavier Hospital
Saint Mary's Hospital

Tip 3. Use a stimulus category somewhere near the middle of the range you intend to use as a standard. Avoid choosing a standard that is near the extreme high or low.

Tip 4. After the standard has been assigned, leave the respondent free to assign all other values.

Tip 5. Randomize the order of presentation and avoid starting with the extremes of the continuum.

Tip 6. Before the session begins, tell the respondent how to indicate a "zero" response or a "nonapplicable" one.

Tip 7. Data derived from magnitude estimations generally require three columns of space for each variable entered. When lines or numbers are

used, the value "999" is used to indicate an item that has not been answered; "001" generally is used to indicate a zero response. Lines are generally measured in millimeters, and numerical estimates are entered directly without change.

b. Evaluation of Magnitude Estimations

The exciting part of this technique is its ability to provide ratio level measurement for perceptions about social and psychological phenomena of interest to nurses. It is possible, for example, to measure the status of occupations and people with different incomes and education levels

(Hamblin, 1971); the perceptions of those who have migrated (Jackson, 1999); the relative attractiveness of universities to high school students (Jackson, 1973); the difficulty of adopting selected activities in meeting a goal (Sennott-Miller and Miller, 1986); dyspnea in clients with obstructive lung disease (Janson-Bjerklie et al., 1986); and the difficulty of caregiving tasks (Waltz et al., 1991).

In collecting data, respondents sometimes use numbers incorrectly, rank ordering the stimuli rather than maintaining the proportionality between the stimulus items. One has to be careful to make certain that respondents understand the procedure. A further limitation is that a researcher must be present to train the respondents in the use of the technique and, hence, it is not applicable to mailed questionnaires or phone interviews.

5. Visual Analogue Scales

Visual analogue scales (VAS) were developed more than 60 years ago to measure various subjective phenomena. Today they are gaining increasing popularity in nursing research as an easily administered tool appropriate for most clinical populations. VAS measure the intensity of participants' sensations and feelings about the strength of their attitudes, beliefs, and opinions about specific stimuli such as pain, fatigue, nausea, quality of life, health status, appetite, and self-care ability. VAS requires participants to place an "x" or mark on a line or linear scale that reflects the intensity of their feelings, beliefs, or opinions. Usually a 100-mm line is used with two anchor words or phrases at each end of the line to describe the endpoints of the scale. The line can be drawn vertically or horizontally. A mechanical format visual analogue scale is now available. It is similar to a slide rule plastic device that shows a 100-mm horizontal line on the front and a movable tab that provides im-

mediate feedback of numerical measures on the back side (Frank-Stromberg and Olsen, 1997).

a. Steps for Constructing and Using a Visual Analogue Index

Step 1: A VAS measures only one dimension of a phenomenon at a time; therefore, in constructing a scale, the researcher must first decide which dimension is to be measured with the scale. For example, you may be interested in measuring the intensity of pain experienced by participants. If other dimensions of pain are to be measured by the researcher, additional visual analogue scales will be required for each dimension.

Step 2: Identify the bipolar anchors that will appear at each end of the scale. They are placed beyond each end of the scale, not above or below the line. The anchors should reflect the entire continuum of responses possibly related to the phenomenon of interest. For example, if you are measuring intensity of pain, one anchor may be "no pain" and the other anchor may be "the worst possible pain."

Step 3: Draw the scale. The scale is a line of 100 mm in length with right angle stops at each end.
For example:
No pain |————————| **Worst possible pain**

Step 4: Some researchers prefer a vertical format for the scale because it eliminates problems with left–right discrimination and is more analogous to the "more" (high, top) and "less" (low, bottom) ends of the continuum measure by a visual analogue scale. The participant in the sitting position should mark the scale. It is not known what the impact of reclining in the supine position may be on the perception of scale length for bedridden clients.

Step 5: For children, pictures may be

used at each end of the scale as anchors. The pictures should represent

the two extremes of the dimension being measured. For example:

Step 6. Printing is preferred to photocopying visual analogue scales because photocopying the instrument may cause small alterations in the length of the line, which may produce invalid data if not corrected.

Step 7: Instructions should be clear and include a written example of how to mark the scale. "Place a mark on the line that indicates the degree of pain you are having at this moment," is the type of instruction you would provide to participants.

Step 8: To score the visual analogue scale, measure the distance of the mark from the end of the scale in millimeters. Usually the low end of the scale is used as the zero point. If more than one scorer is measuring the points marked, it is important to have identical rulers so that systematic bias is avoided.

b. Evaluation of Visual Analogue Indexes

A major advantage of the VAS is its ease of administration and its sensitivity to changes in levels of the stimulus. They are readily understood by participants and can be completed quickly and easily. They do not limit participants to a defined number of responses but rather enable them to make fine distinctions in responses. In this manner, they are more sensitive than categorical scales. Reliability and validity are similar to more time-consuming measures. Validity is determined by using the contrasted groups' approach or by correlating the VAS scores with other measures of the phenomenon. Reliability is assessed using test–retest procedures.

6. Delphi Technique

The Rand Corporation (a think tank in California) originally developed the Delphi technique in the 1950s as a means to structure group opinion and discussion (Waltz et al., 1991). It has been used in nursing research to assess priorities such as national research directions, determine goals and plans for curriculum revision in nursing education programs, and obtain the opinions of experts on a variety of topics without the necessity of meeting face to face. It is especially useful in exploring planning options; identifying the pros and cons of expert nurses related to health reform policies; and developing national agendas around issues such as nursing education, research, or professional practice roles.

a. Steps in Using the Delphi Technique

Step 1: The first step is to identify and select a panel of experts on the topic of interest to the investigator. The panel should be as representative of various demographics and expertise as possible so that bias is avoided in the membership. For example, if you applied the Delphi technique to determine national nursing research priorities, you should have a panel composed of nurse researchers from across the country, including large urban centers as well as rural areas, nurses from various sectors of health care and academia, and nurses with expertise in various research methods and interests.

Step 2: Next a questionnaire that focuses on the phenomenon of interest is developed and circulated to the expert participants. Usually the questionnaire is administered by mail, interview, or an interactive computer conference line. The respondents do not discuss issues face to face at any time. The questionnaire is developed according to the guidelines presented in Chapter 14 and contains a set of instructions for participants. Most Delphi questionnaires contain close-ended questions, but the opportunity can easily be provided for open-ended statements as well as scales. For example, in generating research priorities, you may begin by asking respondents to list research questions they consider to be of major importance. In subsequent rounds of the questionnaire, you may present lists and have respondents prioritize the items.

Step 3: Returned questionnaires are analyzed and results tabulated and returned to participants. Anonymity of participants' responses is protected, although the researcher may list names as part of the study. Descriptive statistics, frequencies and measures of central tendency, and dispersion for each item are usually circulated to participants. Occasionally participants with extreme responses may be asked to explain their choices.

Step 4: After the primary round of questionnaires, the experts again respond to a second questionnaire developed by the researcher. Participants respond to the new information in the questionnaire that has resulted from the statistical analysis of the primary questionnaire and return it to the researcher for subsequent analysis. The experts can adjust their opinions based on feedback received after each questionnaire. This procedure is repeated until the data reflect a consensus of opinions or beliefs among the panel. The questionnaire-analysis cycle may take three to five times to reach consensus. It is not advisable to go beyond five cycles because of the risk of panelists' attrition because of disinterest.

The Delphi technique is flexible, can accommodate a variety of research topics, and obtains the opinion of experts without the financial cost or the time inconvenience of bringing experts together. The opinions of a variety of experts can be concisely condensed into a precise statement. Honest opinions are likely because anonymity is protected. It is unlikely that verbally aggressive experts will unduly influence the group. The disadvantage is that the procedure is costly in terms of multiple data analysis and processing and mailing and printing costs. Also, the time requirement for collection of data depends on busy experts' returning questionnaires so that subsequent rounds of data collection and analysis can proceed. Panel members may become bored and withdraw before completion of the study if data collection does not proceed at a reasonable pace. This creates problem with sample size.

Box 13.7 illustrates the use of the Delphi technique to predict changes in nursing education. The phases in the questionnaire analysis cycle are described. For a complete discussion of the procedure and findings, consult the original source.

7. Physiological Measures

Nurses use physiologic measures on a regular basis to assess the health status and physiological functioning of their clients. Data such as blood pressure values, temperature, pulse rate, respiratory rate, height, weight, percent of body fat, muscle strength, electrocardiogram and electroencephalogram readings, pulmonary artery pressure, cardiac output, salivary enzyme levels, urinary or serum glucose and ketone levels, and oxygen saturation levels are a few of the many physiologic

BOX 13.7 Nurse Researchers at Work

THE DELPHI TECHNIQUE: A POSSIBLE TOOL FOR PREDICTING FUTURE EVENTS IN NURSING EDUCATION

The purpose of this study was to explore the potential of the Delphi technique in predicting events of the next 50 years in nursing education. Experts were selected on the basis of educational level, rank in educational institution, or position in agency. The selected panel consisted of 16 members representing education, practice, the professional association, and government. The Delphi technique included four rounds, each involving a questionnaire and questionnaire analysis, conducted in the following manner.

Round I: Panelists were requested to make a maximum of 10 predictions regarding the future of nursing education in the next 50 years. A grouping and collation was done to reduce the number of predictions to a manageable size.

Round II: The predictions were presented and the panelists were asked to predict in which time interval they would occur. Results were tabulated and reported for each statement in terms of number and predictions in each time interval.

Round III: Panelists received feedback from their Round II predictions plus the corresponding response from the total group for each statement. If a panelist's prediction differed from the group response, he or she was requested to revise his or her prediction or to support his or her position. The results were again tabulated and reported for each statement. Statements achieving consensus were announced. Reasons for dissenting opinions were incorporated into the next questionnaire.

Round IV: Panelists were asked to reconsider their predictions in view of the dissenting opinions and to revise them if they so desired. The additional predictions that achieved consensus were identified. A description of the events that would occur in the future, as predicted by the consensus of the panel of experts, was composed and sent to the panelists.

For a discussion of the results, interested readers are referred to the original source.

SOURCE: Summarized from Bramwell, L., and Hykawy, E. (1999). The Delphi technique: A possible tool for predicting future events in nursing education. *The Canadian Journal of Nursing Research, 30*(4), 47–59.

measures that clinical nurses quantify on a regular basis to assess the level of functioning of their clients.

These measures are of value to nurse researchers as well. Physiologic measurement is particularly appropriate in studies designed to assess the impact of nursing interventions on bodily functions. Traditionally, nursing research has tended to use psychosocial measures because of problems inherent in physiological measurement strategies. Often nurses do not have control over or access to the equipment or resources available to monitor changes in physiological functioning. The situation is changing, however, and many nurse researchers are now engaged in studies that use physiological measures and scientific equipment to yield biological data.

For example, Kang and associates (1998) studied the relationship of social support to stress responses and immune function in healthy and asthmatic adolescents. They drew blood samples and measured the natural killer (NK) cell function in the immune response. Monitoring the numbers and types of NK cells in the circulation is important for evaluating changes in immune responses. Results indicated that high social support appeared to attenuate the magnitude of examination-induced reduction in NK cell function activity, suggesting that social support plays a protective role against immune decrements during times of stress.

Well-designed and appropriately implemented physiological measurement devices are among the most precise methods of measurement one can use in nursing research. They provide objective and sensitive measurements that are difficult for the participant to distort. They usually yield ratio level data that can accommodate a range of statistical procedures. The disadvantages include the expense, storage requirements, additional training requirements, and the intrusiveness created by some devices. Error is also a potential concern because of environmental factors such as temperature or barometric pressure changes that may affect readings; different users and procedures that lead to inconsistency in measurements; changes in calibrations of equipment that affect precision of measurement; or carelessness on the part of those recording the measurement values.

8. Observational Measurement

Observational measurement is frequently conducted in nursing research to determine how participants respond in specific situations. It is a data collection method that is particularly well suited to phenomena that are best viewed from a holistic rather than a reductionistic perspective. For example, if one is interested in studying the impact of caring behaviors by nurses on separation anxiety in hospitalized children, a researcher could elect to interview the child or administer a questionnaire, but direct observation of the child's behavior would most likely yield the best data to comprehensively answer the research question. A distinction must be made between the general types of observations that nurses engage in as part of the nurse–client interaction and the *scientific observation* that is associated with research measurement. To be scientific, observations must meet four conditions as outlined by LoBionda-Wood and Haber (1998, p. 313). These include:

1. The observations undertaken must be consistent with the study's objectives and aims.
2. There is a systematic and standardized plan for the observation and the recording of data.
3. All of the observations are checked and controlled.
4. The observations are related to scientific concepts or theories.

Observations may be structured, semistructured, or unstructured. They may occur in natural settings or in controlled laboratory settings. In structured observations, the researcher carefully defines what observations are to be made and how they are to be recorded and coded (see Fig. 7.1). Usually a category system is devised for organizing and sorting the data. Tally sheets, checklists, and rating scales are also used. Consistency of observations and recording is very important. Usually interrater reliability is established and monitored periodically throughout the study if observation is the primary means of data collection. This is important in terms of determining the degree of confidence to place in the data.

In qualitative investigations, unstructured observations are conducted. These involve spontaneously observing what occurs in natural settings with little preplanning. Participant observation is a special type of unstructured observation used in qualitative investigations. It enables the researcher to collect information that otherwise may go unrecorded. Detailed field notes, logs, and narratives are used to record such data.

Observation is difficult at the best of times because the very presence of the observer may change the situation so that one is not certain of what they are observing. Participants may behave in atypical ways that may distort the study findings. If one proceeds to observe participants without informing them about the study, ethical dilemmas may result. Although observations tend to be more subjective than other measurement techniques, studies using these techniques remain as some of the best available means to capture the complexity of both the subjective and the objective complexity of human behavior. The advantages include the flexibility they provide to the researcher in reconceptualizing the problem based on emerging data. They provide a direct, first-hand measurement of events. For a complete discussion of observational measurement, see Chapter 7, which considers both overt and naturalistic observational field studies.

9. Interviews

The interview is the data collection method used most frequently by nurses to obtain information from clients and their families. An **interview** is defined as a face-to-face verbal interaction in which the researcher attempts to elicit information from the respondent, usually through direct questioning. Because nurses use the interview technique so frequently in their practice, the dynamics of interviewing are well known to them. Similar to scientific observation, however, care and precision are required in conducting interviews for purposes of research. The interpersonal skills of the researcher are an important asset in collecting interview data. The response rate from interview studies is usually higher than from questionnaires. A skilled interviewer can elicit rich and accurate descriptions from respondents that would not be possible by other means. Because interviews are self-reports, the researcher must assume that the data reported are an accurate account of the phenomenon under investigation.

The interview is classified according to the degree of standardization implicit in the interview questions. The interview may be (1) structured with the researcher exercising a maximum amount of control by predetermining questions and the range of response categories that can be recorded; (2) semistructured with specific topics focusing the discussion; or (3) nonstructured, in which questions are not predetermined but are left to the discretion of the researcher, who frequently takes his or her lead from the respondents' cues. Usually a broad research question such as, "Tell me what your experience was like with . . . " is used to initiate the discussion.

Interviews have the advantage of soliciting more in-depth data than would be available through questionnaires; they provide the opportunity for probing of responses; and they can be used with participants who are not able to read or write. They are limited by time and cost factors that make it difficult to use large sample sizes unless adequate financial and human resources are available. When more than one interviewer is used to collect data, it is important that sufficient time be spent training the interviewer in data collection procedures. Inconsistencies in data collection procedures and subject selection bias are always potential threats to the validity of findings.

If you are planning on using an interview to collect data for your research project, you are advised to refer to Chapter 7 for a discussion of in-depth and focus group interviews.

10. Questionnaires

The **questionnaire** is a self-administered form designed to elicit data from the respondent through written or verbal responses. Questionnaires have many important uses in nursing research. Chapter 14 provides a comprehensive discussion of questionnaire development and administration.

G. DEVELOPMENT OF AN INSTRUMENT

Because nursing research is still evolving, nurses frequently encounter the problem of not being able to locate a measurement tool for a construct of interest. When this occurs, the nurse researcher is faced with the challenge of developing an instrument or modifying the study. The process of instrument construction is a complex one. It involves the following steps:

1. Define the construct to be measured.
2. Create the instrument items.
3. Assess the content validity of the items.
4. Pretest and pilot test the items.
5. Assess the validity and reliability of the instrument.
6. Publish results so that others can avail themselves of the measurement tool.

Let us consider the development of the Adolescent Lifestyle Questionnaire (ALQ) as an example of each of these steps. Gillis (1997) sought to develop a valid and reliable instrument to measure healthy lifestyles in adolescents. Before this, no instrument was available to measure healthy lifestyles in adolescents.

Step 1: Define the construct. Gillis defined healthy lifestyle as a multidimensional pattern of discretionary activities and perceptions that are part of an adolescent's daily approach to living and that significantly affect health status in a positive manner.

Step 2: Create the items. Items for the ALQ were developed from qualitative research interviews with 30 adolescents. Two broad interview questions were posed: (1) "What does it mean to you as a teen to live a healthy lifestyle?" and (2) "What kinds of things do teens your age do on a regular basis to keep healthy?" Item development was guided by a review of the adolescent and adult health promotion literature and by analysis of the qualitative interviews. Factors were selected that *a priori* were congruent with the definition of lifestyle and were sufficiently general enough to apply to large numbers of adolescents. The pilot

form of the ALQ comprised 66 items in seven categories: physical participation, nutrition, safety, social support, health awareness, stress management, and identity awareness. The seven categories were considered dimensions of a healthy lifestyle in adolescents. The instrument used a five-point response format of 1 = never; 2 = rarely, 3 = sometimes, 4 = often, and 5 = almost always to obtain an ordinal level of measurement.

Step 3: Assess the items for content validity. Content validity was assessed by eight nurses with expertise in adolescent health promotion. Four were asked to rate each item using four criteria: readability, cultural relevance, age appropriateness of items, and conceptual congruence with the construct of a healthy lifestyle. The remaining four nurses were asked to place the items in the seven categories according to definitions provided by the researcher. Items were added, modified, and deleted based on input from the panel of nurse experts. The resulting instrument contained 56 items.

Step 4: Pretest and pilot test the instrument. The pilot version of the instrument was tested on a sample of 73 school-based adolescents over a 3-week period for reliability, item clarity, and response variance. Results of reliability testing using the test–retest procedure yielded a coefficient of 0.76 for the total instrument, indicating stability. Cronbach's alpha was calculated as a measure of internal consistency. The alpha coefficient for the total instrument was 0.93 and ranged from 0.60 to 0.87 for the subscales.

Examination of frequency distributions indicated that the full range of responses was used for the majority of items. Some items were deleted or reworded because of confusion over meaning and terminology. As a whole, the instrument appeared to have sufficient reliability to warrant further development.

Step 5: Estimate reliability and validity. Empirical validation of the ALQ followed the process suggested by Nunnally (1978). This included item analysis of the pool of 56 items to determine which contributed most to the internal consistency of the measure; factor analysis to define the factorial composition of the item pool and establish validity; and reliability measures to estimate the internal consistency of the final version of the ALQ. Box 13.8 provides detailed results of the reliability and validity testing of the final version of the ALQ.

Step 6: Publish the results. Nursing's ability to study phenomena of concern to the discipline and thereby advance the science of nursing is limited by our ability to measure such phenomena. Hence, it is important that researchers who invest considerable time and resources in instrument development studies share their results with others. (This study is published in the following source: Gillis, A. (1997). The adolescent lifestyle questionnaire: Development and psychometric testing.

BOX 13.8 *Nurse Researchers at Work*

RELIABILITY AND VALIDITY TESTING OF THE FINAL VERSION OF THE ADOLESCENT LIFESTYLE QUESTIONNAIRE: RESULTS

Item Analysis

Five items were eliminated from the 56-item instrument on the basis of evaluation of the results of the item analysis. Corrected item-total correlations were calculated both for the total scale and for each of the seven subscales in a series of analyses. At each step, items that depressed the reliability as measured by coefficient alpha of either the total scale or the subscale to which they were assigned were deleted from the item pool for that scale and the item-total correlations of the revised set were recalculated. Of the remaining 51 items, 47 had item-total correlations of 0.25 or higher, levels considered acceptable by Nunnally (1978). The interitem correlation matrix was examined to identify redundancy among items. No correlations above 0.70 were found; hence the **51 items** were retained.

Factor Analysis

The 51 items were subjected to factor analysis. This was the initial assessment of the construct validity of the Adolescent Lifestyle Questionnaire (ALQ). It was guided by the hypothesis that seven subscales did exist. A stepwise solution with the principal axis factoring (PAF) extraction method and oblique rotation was used . . . Ten factors were extracted and rotated. Intuitively, it appeared the 10 factors could be combined into seven conceptually valid subscales, as hypothesized. Eight items that did not load strongly on a single factor were eliminated. The remaining **43 items** were entered into a factor analysis. All 43 items loaded on the expected factors at a level of .45 or higher. The seven-factor solution explained 56 percent of the variance of the revised **43-item** ALQ . . . Correlations among the seven factors were low to moderate, suggesting that each factor represents a distinct dimension related to other dimensions of healthy lifestyle, without being redundant.

Reliability

The final structure of the **43-item** ALQ was tested for internal consistency using Cronbach's alpha (see Table 13.4). Test–retest reliability was again examined by administering the ALQ to 65 adolescents at an interval of two weeks. Pearson r was 0.88 for the total score and ranged from 0.80 to 0.88 for the subscales.

SOURCE: Gillis, A.J. (1997). The adolescent lifestyle questionnaire: Development and psychometric testing. *The Canadian Journal of Nursing Research, 29*(1), 29–46. Cited with permission.

Canadian Journal of Nursing Research, 29(1), 29–46.)

Data collection and measurement strategies constitute critical aspects of the research process. They mark the transition from the theoretical to the empirical phase of the research study. Much of the success of a research project depends on the care and attention that the researcher pays to appropriate data collection and measurement issues. Determining what measurement tool to use and confirming that the tool validly and reliably reflects the construct of interest is central to doing good science and to advancing nursing.

E X E R C I S E S

1. Would it be possible to have a valid measure that is not reliable? Could you have a reliable measure that is not valid?

2. Discuss sources of random and non-random measurement error in reactive research designs. To what extent are such errors caused by different perceptions of the question being posed or differences in image management? Is image management more likely to lead to random or nonrandom errors?

3. "In our culture, teenage males will overestimate their weights; teenage females, however, slightly underestimate their weights but show less variability in their estimates of their true weight."

   Discuss this quotation, making clear the differences between true value, random error, and systematic error in measurement.

4. Develop and pilot test one of the following types of indexes or scales: Likert, semantic differential, visual analogue, or magnitude estimation. Report fully on the methods you used to develop the scale or index.

RECOMMENDED READINGS

Carmines, E.G., and Zeller, R.A. (1979). *Reliability and Validity Assessment.* Beverly Hills: Sage. This is an excellent introduction to the assessment of reliability and validity.

Frank-Stromberg, M., and Olson, S. (1997). *Measurement in Nursing Research* (2nd ed.). Boston: Jones and Bartlett Publishers. An excellent resource for both the development and use of instruments in nursing research and clinical practice.

Montgomery, K. (2000). Getting organized: Qualitative data collection. *Applied Nursing Research, 13*(2), 103–104. This article describes an organizational schema researchers can use to prepare for qualitative data collection.

Lodge, M. (1981). *Magnitude Scaling: Quantitative Measurement of Opinions.* Beverly Hills: Sage. Another in the Sage series; this introduction to magnitude estimation procedures neatly summarizes the alternative procedures and reviews the findings that have resulted.

Sandelowski, M. (2000). Combing qualitative and quantitative sampling, data collection, and analysis techniques in mixed method studies. *Research in Nursing and Health, 23,* 246–255. This article provides examples of data collection combinations, including the use of instruments for fuller qualitative descriptions, for validation, and as elicitation device interviews.

Strauss, A., and Corbin, J. (1997). *Grounded Theory in Practice*. Thousand Oaks: CA: Sage. This book provides an updating on the development of grounded theory along with recent illustrations of the work done using this tradition.

Waltz, C., Strickland, O., and Lenz, E. (1991). *Measurement in Nursing Research* (2nd ed). Philadelphia, PA: F.A. Davis. This comprehensive text describes the process involved in selecting, testing, and designing instruments for use in nursing investigations.

Chapter 14

Questionnaire Development

CHAPTER OUTLINE

KEY TERMS

Closed-ended questions

Likert-type questions

Open-ended question

Pilot study

Precoded single-choice questions

Presence–absence questions

Questionnaires

Rank-ordering questions

Response set

As discussed in Chapter 5, a **questionnaire** consists of an organized set of written questions that are presented to respondents for their reply. Questionnaires have many applications; they are used to do interviews, conduct research, and compare outcomes of different programs among other applications. A review of the literature suggests that nursing research has relied heavily on questionnaires as a primary means of collecting data for the past 40 years. This trend is likely to continue in the new millennium.

A well-designed questionnaire does not impose on the patience of the respondent. It should be possible to move through the questionnaire rapidly, without becoming bored and without having to reread questions because of ambiguity. An easy-to-complete questionnaire is more likely to be filled out successfully. For those doing a survey, Chapter 5 contains a discussion of how to administer different types of surveys. Although Chapter 13 discusses issues related to validity and reliability of questionnaires, this chapter focuses on the development of questionnaires. All questionnaires contain the following components: (1) a cover letter, (2) a set of directions to respondents, (3) a set of questions, (4) a set of response categories, and (5) a demographic section. Each of these elements is addressed in this chapter. We begin our consideration with some general issues, then pay attention to the phrasing of specific questions, and conclude with issues of layout and format.

A. GENERAL GUIDELINES FOR QUESTIONNAIRE DEVELOPMENT

The following section presents a set of general guidelines for developing a questionnaire. In some situations, the guidelines should not be followed in detail; simply use them with intelligence and a good dose of common sense.

Guideline 1. Consult the participant. All questionnaires are an imposition on those who are asked to complete them. It is important, if you wish to have a high completion rate, not to impose on your respondents. Above all, respondents must be made to feel that they are being consulted and can freely express opinions. The cover letter, questionnaire, and interview schedule should be designed to be inclusive—that is, designed to make all participants feel that their opinions are both valued and acceptable.

Guideline 2. Keep it short. Frequently projects involve a group of researchers and there may be considerable difficulty in keeping the questionnaire from becoming too long. Asking too many questions not only is an infringement on the respondent's time but also creates additional work in data entry and error detection. To overcome this problem, it takes a careful negotiator to persuade a colleague that some of the proposed questions be left for a later study. One test when such difficulties arise is to request individuals to indicate precisely how the variable will be used to meet the objectives (hypothesis) of the study. Such discussions force some careful thinking about the survey, the objectives, and the analysis. All too often a number of variables remain unanalyzed, either because they are considered to be poorly measured or because their relationship to the study is unclear.

There cannot be any strict rules for the length of a questionnaire. It may be useful to develop a guide that identifies:

- The variables that need to be measured
- The content that is interesting but not essential to the study
- The approximate number of questions needed to cover the study variables
- The maximum number of questions

that are practical to ask in the study, given who your respondents are and taking into account their needs and attention spans

- An estimate of the time it will take to complete the instrument

From this guide, researchers can decide to increase or reduce the number of questions to truly reflect the study variables.

If the questions are easy to answer and the respondents have a particular interest in the survey, it is possible to extend the length of the questionnaire. However, it is always wise to use as few questions as possible and never ask questions merely for interest's sake. Table 14.1 suggests guidelines for maximum lengths for typical questionnaires.

The table can only be a guide because enormous variations may exist in the complexity of the questions, in the sophistication of the respondents, and in the respondents' interest in the survey.

Phone surveys have to be particularly easy to respond to. Each question must have simple response options because the respondent will have difficulty trying to remember all the response categories if many are presented. Keep phone questionnaires simple and short.

Other questionnaires can involve more questions and greater complexity. Mailed questionnaires need to be kept somewhat shorter than the others are because the researcher is not present to provide encouragement. Interviews using a questionnaire can safely be extended to about 60 questions and take as much as an hour to complete. It should be remembered

that interviews, whether using structured or semistructured questionnaires, take much more time because of the tendency of respondents to stray from the topic. Questionnaires administered to an assembled collection of individuals can involve 70 or more questions. Here, as long as the questions are well designed, respondents can move through the instrument rapidly. But no matter how the data are to be gathered, the researcher should strive for brevity and simplicity. There is no point in gathering data that you do not have the theoretical or analytical skills to process.

Guideline 3. Achieve precise measurement. Generally, researchers should try to obtain the most precise measurement possible. Collect data in the rawest form, such as income to the dollar, precise occupation rather than a general category, and age to the nearest year rather than an age category that spans 10 years. This recommendation has to be moderated where other factors argue against precise measurement. You might avoid precision when it would entail asking for information that is too personal, require respondents to make distinctions beyond those they normally use, or when the methods needed to ensure such precision would be too cumbersome. Arguments in favor of precise measurement are presented in Chapter 13.

When asking about income, for example, the question should be clearly stated to determine if the income is individual income or household income. Also, the researcher may consider ask-

Table 14.1 Maximum Number of Questions on a Questionnaire

Type of Questionnaire	Maximum Length	Maximum Time
Phone questionnaire	20 questions	10 to 20 minutes
Mailed questionnaire	50 questions	15 to 20 minutes
Group administered	70 questions	20 to 30 minutes
Interview	60 questions	60 to 90 minutes

ing the source (e.g., base pay from the primary employer or from extra jobs or overtime). Some people consider income and age as personal information. Researchers need to determine the importance of the measurement scale (ordinal versus ratio data) because the measurement scale determines the statistical analysis. Researchers take a chance of not getting any response or a nonresponse on those items if the information asked appears too personal.

B. TYPES OF QUESTIONS ILLUSTRATED

This section illustrates a variety of formats for typical questionnaire items. Although it is not possible to anticipate all types of questions, the same principles can be applied to many questions. (A compendium of questionnaires designed by students in our research methods course is available for review on the Internet at the following address: *http// www.stfx.ca/people/wjackson*).

I. Precoded, Single-Choice Questions

In **precoded, single-choice questions,** the respondent is asked to indicate with a checkmark which category applies to him or her. Box 14.1 provides illustrations of such questions. Note that only the question is numbered; it would look too cluttered if the categories are also numbered. After the category label, a dashed line is used so that the respondent's eye moves laterally to the check-off category; the number beside the square box is the value that will be used when the data are entered into the computer. To avoid a cluttered look, there should be no space between the number and the square box.

The next items in Box 14.1 illustrate slightly more complex forms of the check-off question. Question 5 illustrates how to accommodate two columns of check-off categories; in this case, the questionnaire provides one for the mother's and one for the father's educational level. Once again, the computer codes are placed next to the categories because it facilitates data en-

---

BOX 14.1 *The Simple Precoded Question*

4. What year of school are you in?
   Freshman ------------------1☐
   Sophomore --------------2☐
   Junior ----------------------3☐
   Senior ----------------------4☐

5.1/5.2 What is the highest education completed by your mother and father?

	Mother	Father
Grades 0–6	------------1☐	------------1☐
Grades 7–9	------------2☐	------------2☐
Grades 10–12	------------3☐	------------3☐
Some post-secondary	------------4☐	------------4☐
University graduate	------------5☐	------------5☐

11. What was the approximate population of your home area before you began college?

Rural area	---------------01☐
Small town under 999	---------------02☐
Between 1000–4999	---------------03☐
Between 5000–9,999	---------------04☐
Between 10,000–19,999	---------------05☐
Between 20,000–29,999	---------------06☐
Between 30,000–49,999	---------------07☐
Between 50,000–74,999	---------------08☐
Between 75,000–99,999	---------------09☐
Between 100,000–249,999	---------------10☐
Between 250,000–999,999	---------------11☐
More than 1,000,000	---------------12☐

try. Similar space saving can be achieved by splitting long category lists into two and placing them side by side.

The question on population size simply illustrates that when there are more than nine categories, it is important to place the leading zero in the computer codes. If the leading zero is omitted, data entry errors will almost certainly occur. The particular population categories would, of course, have to be altered, depending on the target population.

Two points also need to be mentioned that are not illustrated in Box 14.1. Frequently, it is not possible to name all the possible responses that would be appropriate (e.g., religious affiliation) and the researcher will have a final category that says:

Other —— 12☐
Please specify _____.

The most obvious reason for using a "please specify" category is that there would not be sufficient room to list all possible religions. However, even more importantly, you do not wish to insult your respondent by not having included his or her religion. In actual fact, if the major religious groupings have been included, the person who specifies a category not included in the questionnaire will simply be coded as an "Other."

Finally, please note that the response categories provided should cover the full spectrum of possible responses and it should not be possible for a respondent to check off two of the categories. Note in Box 14.1 that the population categories are *mutually exclusive*—no category overlaps another one. A common error is illustrated in Example 1, Box 14.2.

Example 1 illustrates a situation in which the researcher has failed to provide mutually exclusive categories; Example 2 corrects the error.

Precoded, single-choice questions are also referred to as **closed-ended questions.** The major advantage of such ques-

---

BOX 14.2 *Two Versions of Population of My Home Town*

Flawed Version: Categories Are Not Mutually Exclusive

Example 1. The population of the place I considered my hometown when growing up was:

Rural area	---------------------1☐
Town up to 5000	--------------------2☐
5000 to 20,000	--------------------3☐
20,000 to 100,000	--------------------4☐
100,000 to 1,000,000	--------------------5☐
1,000,000 or over	--------------------6☐

Better Version: Categories Are Mutually Exclusive

Example 2. The population of the place I considered my hometown when growing up was:

Rural area	---------------------1☐
Town under 5000	--------------------2☐
5000 to 19,999	--------------------3☐
20,000 to 99,999	--------------------4☐
100,000 to 999,999	--------------------5☐
1,000,000 or over	--------------------6☐

---

tions is they ensure comparability of responses and facilitate analysis of responses. They are particularly easy to administer, but this advantage must be balanced with the time-consuming challenge of questionnaire construction.

2. Open-Ended Questions

An **open-ended question** asks the respondent to answer some question or to offer a suggestion or opinion, but to do so without any preset categories being provided for the answer. There are at least six reasons for including some open-ended questions in a questionnaire: open-ended questions are preferred if:

- The responses are too numerous (e.g., year of birth).

- The researcher does not wish to impose response categories on the respondent.
- The researcher wishes to create the sense that the respondent is really being consulted, by being asked to offer his or her opinions.
- The researcher wishes to provide a qualitative dimension to the study—open-ended responses are often used as a source of quotations for the final report.
- The study is being done as a pilot and the appropriate response categories have not been determined.
- You wish to change the pace or format for the reader.

Although open-ended data are not always analyzed when writing the final report on a project, they can provide insights to the researcher that might be missed if such questions were not asked.

Box 14.3 illustrates some variations in typical formats. Questions 20 and 22 are questions where the space for the response indicates that two numbers are expected. By providing two blanks, the respondent is being prompted to enter two numbers. The percent symbol in question 20 also helps to indicate exactly what is expected. This helps to prevent frivolous replies, such as writing in "average" in the case of question 20, which asks about the respondent's average in the final year of high school, or writing in "a long time ago" in the case of question 22, which asks about year of birth.

Question 21 illustrates a method of asking about occupation. The additional line (Brief Job Description) is included to ensure that the respondent provides sufficient detail to enable the researcher to attach an occupational rating code to the response. If such specification is not requested, some respondents will simply indicate the employer (e.g., writing in "Microsoft") and the researcher will not be able to attach an occupational rating to that kind of response. When detail is re-

BOX 14.3 Sample Open-Ended Questions

20. Approximately, what was your average in your final year of high school? _ _ %
21. What is (or was) your father's occupation? (e.g., foreman, railway machine shop . . . supervises work of about 25 people)?
    Job _____
    Brief job description _____
    _____
    _____
    _____
22. In what year were you born? 19 _ _ .
23. What is the one thing that you would like to see changed at the university health and counseling center?
    _____
    _____
    _____
24. In your opinion, what is the single best thing about the health and counseling center?
    _____
    _____
    _____

quired, the researcher must be careful to request it.

Questions 23 and 24 simply seek the opinion of the respondent on two issues. Typically, the responses that are given would either be listed (simply typed) or coded. If they are coded, the categories would be determined after the data have been collected and the responses examined.

A good rule to follow is to minimize the number of open-ended questions. Many researchers minimize the number of opinion-seeking, open-ended questions because they are time consuming to code; tend to generate responses that are inconsistent; and are more likely to be left blank. Indeed, respondents frequently fail to complete a questionnaire that has too many such questions. Many respondents appear to believe that asking them to write a sentence or two is too much of an imposition.

When a pilot study is conducted and the research team is uncertain about the appropriate response categories, it is a good idea to pose the question in an open-ended form. After you analyze the results, you can then base the categories to be used in the final study on those suggested in the pilot study.

Placing an open-ended question at about the two-thirds mark of a long questionnaire may well provide the relief needed to sustain the respondent's interest and ensure completion of the questionnaire. If both open-ended and fixed-choice questions are asked, it is advisable to place the open-ended version first so that the respondent is not influenced by the fixed-choice options.

Michael D. Smith (n.d) has explored the effectiveness of open versus precoded questions in revealing the incidence of physical abuse. Both formats were equally effective in detecting abuse; however, it was noted that if questions about abuse were asked a second time, some 21 percent of the victims revealed their victimization on the second question. The findings suggest that, with questions of a personal nature, it is a good idea to repeat a question a second time, using a variant. Some may object that such persistent questioning may create an expectation (demand characteristic) that the respondent should make a positive response. However, if the question is properly worded this should not be a problem.

Use opinion-seeking, open-ended questions sparingly, but keep in mind that they are an excellent vehicle for providing a change in pace for the respondent or for exploring new issues in detail.

3. Presence–Absence Questions

Presence–absence questions request respondents to check off which items in a

list do or do not apply to them. Box 14.4 provides examples of such questions. Of the two versions presented, the second one is preferable. In it, either a "yes" or a "no" is expected for each item. Although this is a little more work for the respondent, the researcher can then be more confident that each item has been considered. In question 24, if an item is left blank, does that mean that the respondent is opposed to eating that item? Or did the respondent simply fail to consider that item?

In contrast to the questions presented in Box 14.1, in which the respondent was asked to check one of a set number of answers, square boxes are not used for the

---

BOX 14.4 *Presence/Absence Check-Off Questions*

Flawed Version: Possible Ambiguity of Items Left Blank

24. On a day you consider routine, which of the following food choices would you include in your diet for a 24-hour period? (Check as many as appropriate.)

Dairy products	_____	
Meat products	_____	
Whole grain products	_____	
Fruit products	_____	
Vegetable products	_____	

Better Format: Less Ambiguity About Items Left Blank

23. Have you ever had contact with handicapped people in any of these groups? (Circle to indicate "yes" or "no" for each group.)

	Yes	No
Community	1	0
Family	1	0
Relatives	1	0
Elementary school class	1	0
Junior high school class	1	0
Senior high school class	1	0
University class	1	0
As coworker	1	0

answer in Box 14.4. Instead, respondents are asked to circle a 1 (for yes) or a 0 (for no). Readers should also note that the computer codes used involve "1" for presence and "0" for absence. During analysis, a "total experience" variable may be created by simply adding the score on each item together. A total score of 5, for example, would mean that the individual has had experience with disabled people in five of the settings identified in the question.

4. Rank-ordering Questions

Rank-ordering questions are those in which a respondent is asked to indicate an ordering of response items, usually from most preferred to least preferred. Asking respondents to rank order a list has to be done with great care. In this case, detailed instructions should be provided for the respondent. Box 14.5 includes an example of such a question.

First, note that respondents are only asked to pick out the three most important items; in most cases, respondents will not be able to accurately pick more that the top three (Jackson, 1999). These are difficult types of questions for re-

---

BOX 14.5 Rank-ordering Questions

31. **RANK ORDER** the three most important things you want in your nursing job. (Place a 1 beside the most important one; a 2 beside the next important one; and a 3 beside the next most important one.)

High salary _____
Satisfaction _____
Continued interest _____
Power _____
Prestige _____
Excitement _____

---

spondents, and they should be kept as simple as possible.

Second, it should be noted that the instructions are embarrassingly explicit. Although "rank ordering" may be an obvious and simple idea for many people, the detailed instructions will minimize the number of respondents who will simply place a checkmark beside three items or check just one of the items. It is suggested that you use bold type for "rank order" with a larger size font.

Note that the respondents are given a short line on which they are to write their answers. Again, it is important to provide a different look for the item in order to cue the respondents that this is not a "check-one" question. Be assured that if you use a "check-one" format, a good number of questionnaires will be returned with one of the items checked.

One suggestion for coding these responses into the computer is to use the values provided by the respondents (i.e., 1 = 1, 2 = 2, and 3 = 3) and code all items left blank as a 4. In this way, means can be computed during analysis. (This is a situation in which it seems to make sense to compute a mean using ordinal data.) In the few cases in which respondents simply tick off three items, each one ticked can be given a 2. Of course, if the whole item is left blank, the researcher is forced to assign the missing value code to each of the items.

Avoid overusing rank-ordering items in questionnaires. They slow down respondents and increase the risk of losing the respondents' cooperation.

5. Likert-type Questions

Chapter 13 presented Likert-type questions under the discussion on index construction. Readers are referred to that chapter for a more extensive discussion of these items. But because they are used as stand-alone items, a brief comment will be made on them here. **Likert-type questions** are those that ask respondents to indicate the strength of their agreement or disagreement with a statement. This type of question is widely used in social science research. In the original format (Likert, 1931), respondents are asked to react to a statement by indicating whether they (1) strongly disagree, (2) disagree, (3) are undecided or neutral, (4) agree, or (5) strongly agree. Such items were, and continue to be, popular in measuring both matters of fact and attitudinal issues. Box 14.6 provides some examples of these questions.

Readers should note that the items in Box 14.6 deviate somewhat from the origi-

nal format. Given a preference to increase the variability in such items, the number of response categories has been increased from five to nine (see Chapter 13 and Jackson, 1999). This increase does not take more space on the questionnaire or more space when coded into the computer.

The following tips may be helpful in constructing such items:

Tip 1. Avoid the word "and" in such items if its usage makes the item multidimensional.

Tip 2. Place the "Strongly agree" answer on the right-hand side of the scale, with 9 indicating strong agreement. Some researchers prefer to vary the response categories, such as reversing the side on which the agree or disagree labels are placed. This is done to prevent **response set**—that is, a situation in which the respondent tends to answer similarly to all items. Although switching the side on which the agree and disagree categories are placed may reduce the tendency to respond in a set manner, it may also introduce additional errors in response. (Respondents may not notice that you have switched the agree and disagree categories.) Our preference is to maintain a uniform presentation. Response set is best avoided by wording some questions positively and wording others negatively.

Tip 3. Avoid negatives that may confuse respondents. For example, statements such as: "I don't think the hospital administration is doing a bad job" will almost certainly confuse and slow down respondents. Use direct statements such as: "The administration at my hospital is terrible:" or "The administration at my hospital is outstanding."

Tip 4. Select a "strength of wording" to produce variation in response. For example, if you were asking patients about the quality of care given by nurses in a hospital, you might ask several questions, varying the strength of the word-

---

BOX 14.6 *Likert-type Items*

In the following items, *circle a number* to indicate the extent to which you agree or disagree with each statement.

52. I believe self-confidence represents the most effective determinant of healthy lifestyle.
Strongly disagree 1 2 3 4 5 6 7 8 9 **Strongly agree**

53. I believe alcoholics can be rehabilitated to lead healthy lifestyles.
Strongly disagree 1 2 3 4 5 6 7 8 9 **Strongly agree**

54. I believe daily exercise is one of the most effective ways of lowering blood pressure.
Strongly disagree 1 2 3 4 5 6 7 8 9 **Strongly agree**

55. I believe a positive attitude is important in shaping a healthy lifestyle.
Strongly disagree 1 2 3 4 5 6 7 8 9 **Strongly agree**

56. I believe a mother's lifestyle is a powerful determinant of lifestyle choices in children.
Strongly disagree 1 2 3 4 5 6 7 8 9 **Strongly agree**

57. I believe a father's lifestyle is a powerful determinant of lifestyle choices in children.
Strongly disagree 1 2 3 4 5 6 7 8 9 **Strongly agree**

ing in each item. You might well suspect that nursing care will be rated high, so you might wish to strengthen the wording from:

Version 1: The nursing care I received at St. Martha's was good.

Strongly disagree 1 2 3 4 5 6 7 8 9 Strongly agree

To

Version 2: The nursing care I received at St. Martha's was perfect in every instance.

Strongly disagree 1 2 3 4 5 6 7 8 9 Strongly agree

The *strengthening* of the wording in version 2 will almost certainly produce more variation in response. Version 1 would be expected to produce 8s and 9s almost exclusively. (A further illustration is provided in Rule 7 below.)

Tip 5. If there is uncertainty about where responses will fall, use more than one item with different intensities in the wordings.

Tip 6. Before the first Likert-type item, provide a brief explanation of how respondents are to indicate their answers.

Tip 7. When respondents fail to answer a question, use the 0 value as a missing value code. (The 9, which is usually used for missing values, reflects a real value in the case of a 9-point Likert item.)

Likert items result in an ordinal level of measurement. Such items are frequently combined to form indexes by adding together the values on individual items (after having reversed the scores on the negative measures) and researchers conventionally treat such scores as ratio level data (see Chapter 13).

6. Index Development

Indexes are constructed by combining several individual questions. They represent an attempt to summarize, in one score, a measure of a variable. Indexes are constructed when we are dealing with a single-dimension variable, but in contexts in which one question may not measure the variable adequately. Indexes can be constructed by combining a number of similarly formatted questions or combinations of questions with different formats. In all cases, the indicators are combined and possibly weighted, so that they add up to one index score. (See Chapter 13 for details on different methods of constructing indexes. Appendix A contains illustrations for index construction using the Statistical Package for the Social Sciences [SPSS].)

C. STEPS IN DEVELOPING A QUESTIONNAIRE

This section reviews the steps that need to be taken in developing your questionnaire.

Step 1. Make a list of variables. A comprehensive questionnaire designed to reflect the variables of a study can be thought of as consisting of four major groupings:

- The background characteristics or demographics
- The dependent variable or variables
- The independent variables
- The other types of variables; that is, intervening, antecedent, and sources of spuriousness variables

Questions to measure variables in each of these groups have to be developed. Some researchers prefer to use four or more separate questionnaires for each separate grouping rather than combine items into one major instrument.

The first task is to create a list of variables; during this stage it is not necessary to worry about how the variables will be measured; a list is all that is required. The list may be derived by:

- Applying relevant theoretical models and identifying variables that should apply.
- Reviewing the literature, paying particular attention to which variables were measured by other researchers.
- Examining other questionnaires for ideas as to which variables should be included.
- Reviewing the causal models that have been developed for the current project.
- Thinking about which variables "make sense," given the topic of the research.

Step 2. Anticipate how data will be analyzed. After the list of variables is developed, it is important to discuss what statistical procedures will be used to analyze the data when they are collected. Indeed, it is possible to set up proposed analysis tables showing the relationships that are to be analyzed and indicating the procedures that will be used to examine each of them. It is critical to have some understanding of how the analysis is to proceed because the methods used to ex-

amine relationships are constrained by the level of measurement attained in operationalizing each of the variables. This discussion may also include how the analysis will proceed, given different outcomes of preliminary runs on the data. Important new variables frequently emerge as a result of this process. Table 14.2 indicates the types of procedures that would be appropriate given different levels of measurement of the variables involved in the study. The procedures outlined in the table are explored in greater detail in Chapter 16.

Suppose that you wished to do regression analyses on the data. In such cases, you would prefer to have ratio level measurement of all the variables. You might want to figure out how to use magnitude estimation procedures or how to construct indexes that would meet—or be close to meeting—the standard for ratio measurement. On the other hand, if the nature of the dependent variable (nominal measurement) dictates a reliance on cross-tabular analysis, then you would be content to get ordinal and nominal level measure-

Table 14.2 Appropriate Analysis Procedures by Levels of Measurement

DEPENDENT	INDEPENDENT VARIABLE		
	Nominal	Ordinal	Ratio
Nominal	CROSSTABS	CROSSTABS	CROSSTABS MEANS*
			DISCRIMINANT
Ordinal	CROSSTABS	CROSSTABS	CROSSTABS
		SPEARMAN R	SPEARMAN R
			DISCRIMINANT
Ratio/Interval	MEANS	MEANS	CORRELATION
	ANOVA	ANOVA	GRAPH
	T TEST	T TEST	PARTIAL CORRELATION
			MANOVA
			REGRESSION

*In SPSS for this case, run the independent variable as though it were the dependent variable; the interpretation of the test of significance would be standard.

ments of your variables. The majority of questionnaire items tend to be measured at the nominal or ordinal level.

Questionnaire items often address a wide variety of topics. Because of this, researchers frequently analyze individual items, rather than summing items and getting a total score. Likert scales and summated rating scales are exceptions to this.

Step 3. Write the proposed questions on index cards. During the development of a questionnaire, it is a good idea to write proposed questions on index cards (usually 3 × 5 inch cards are large enough). Using cards facilitates both the quick editing of items and rearranging their location in the questionnaire. The researcher should develop a checklist of positive and negative attributes of questionnaire items and check each question against the list. The placement of items on the index cards facilitates this checking. Box 14.7 illustrates the positive and negative characteristics of questionnaire items.

Step 4. Double-check to make certain you have all the variables. It is essential to ensure that all the variables that play a part in the hypotheses and models related to the project have been included. The list of variables must be checked and double checked. It is not unusual for a researcher to discover that a key variable has become lost in the shuffle. With checking completed, it is now time to begin drafting the questions themselves. Once again, there are some rules to keep in mind as this process begins.

Step 5. Review conceptual definitions. When developing the wording for a particular question, it is important to review the conceptual definition of the construct that is being measured. Knowing the conceptual definition provides an important guide as to what the question is to measure. To illustrate, suppose one

---

BOX 14.7 *Positive and Negative Characteristics of Questionnaire Items*

Positive Characteristics

- **Clarity:** Questionnaire item has only one meaning.
- **Brevity:** Question is as brief as possible yet it retains its clear meaning.
- **Simplicity:** Vocabulary in questionnaire items is no higher than a grade seven level.
- **Applicability:** Respondents have the ability to answer the questions appropriately.
- **Relevance:** Items are congruent with and reflective of the variable to be measured.

Negative Characteristics

- **Double-barreled questions:** Does the question ask two questions in one and have a hidden premise?
- **Double negatives:** Avoid use of words such as "don't" and "not."

- **Sensitive questions:** Do not phrase the question in a manner that angers or emotionally upsets the respondent or family members.
- **Jargon-filled items:** Does the question use jargon, technical terms, professional literature, or slang with which respondents are not familiar.
- **Complex questions:** Does the question use long phrases or complex clauses that are not understood by the general public?
- **Biased questions:** Does the question lead the respondent in one direction to answer the item? Does the item contain emotionally charged words such as "abortion?"
- **Inappropriate questions:** The respondent does not have sufficient information to respond to the item.

SOURCE: Adapted from Seaman, C.H. (1987). *Research Methods: Principles, Practice, and Theory for Nursing.* Los Altos, CA: Appleton Lange.

is attempting to measure socioeconomic status. And suppose that, in the conceptual definition of socioeconomic status, reference is made to a hierarchical continuum of respect and prestige. Given this conceptual definition, the researcher might be led to adopt a measure particularly designed to reflect the relative amount of prestige an individual has. In this case, one might opt to use an occupational prestige scale such as the one developed by Featherman and Stevens in the United States (1982) or Pineo and Porter in Canada (1967). Although this procedure might yield a valid measure of the concept in general, experienced researchers would realize that the measure may be weak on the "respect" aspect of the definition. It would also run into some serious difficulties if there were a number of housewives or single stay-at-home parents in the sample (such individuals are not assigned scores in occupational prestige scales). Therefore, one might choose to measure the "respect and prestige" an individual has by getting a number of individuals to rate each individual compared with others. Perhaps the latter approach would yield the most valid measure of the concept even though it would be rare for a research design (probably a study of a particular group) to allow for the practical use of this method.

Suppose, alternatively, that the proposed conceptual definition of socioeconomic status stressed variations in access to scarce resources. In this case, one might attempt to reflect the variable by obtaining an indication of the individual's total income. Here the assumption is that an individual's total income would be a good reflection of that individual's ability to buy access to scarce items in the society.

The more general point is that researchers must pay careful attention to conceptual definitions because they provide invaluable and crucial guides to valid measurement.

Step 6. Develop wording for questions.

There are a few tips to keep in mind as you commence writing drafts of the questions to be included in your questionnaire.

Tip 1. Words must be understood. All respondents must understand the words used in questionnaires. Err on the side of simplicity. If a survey is being done on high school students, play it safe and use words that a student in grade 7 can handle. Most word processing programs can assess the reading level of your questionnaire. Furthermore, the words selected should be those that have but one unambiguous meaning. Showing off an impressive vocabulary has no place in a questionnaire that is intended to produce valid and reliable data. At the same time, using slang or jargon that is unfamiliar to respondents may be offending and lead to a refusal to answer the question. For example, if you are interested in determining the amount of drug use by respondents, it is better to ask, "Approximately how often do you take sedatives or tranquilizers per week?" rather than, "Approximately how often do you get high on drugs per week?"

Tip 2. Pay attention to the "and" alert. Individual questions should be unidimensional. Avoid the trap involved in a question such as:

My lifestyle choices are similar to those of my mother and father.
Strongly disagree 1 2 3 4 5 6 7 8 9 Strongly agree

The problem with the question, as worded, is that some respondents will not make choices that are similar to both their mother's and father's choices. As a result, some respondents may indicate a 1 or a 2 if they do not make choices similar to both; others might indicate a 6 or 7 as a kind of average of the relationship between their choices and those lifestyle choices of their mother and father. The point is that two dimensions have been introduced—the lifestyle choices of the mother *and* the lifestyle choices of the father. Such questions should be divided into two separate questions. It is always useful to scan one's questions to eliminate such unwanted confusion; double check any question that has the word "and" in it.

Similar to the "and" alert, avoid **double-barreled questions** that ask two questions in one statement. They are recognized by words such as "either/or," "and/both," and "therefore."

Tip 3. Vary wording to produce variability. It is important that the items in a questionnaire produce variability in response. If most respondents provide similar responses to a question, then the question will have little use during analysis. Try to ensure that the respondents will scatter themselves across the response continuum. A simple example will illustrate the point:

Women play an important role
    in shaping the health of family
    members.

Strongly disagree 1 2 3 4 5 6 7 8 9 Strongly agree

Using common sense alone, one could anticipate that most respondents will be in strong agreement with this statement and will circle 8 or 9. If, indeed, respondents do not vary their responses much, the question will not prove useful in discriminating between respondents' views about the role of women. In this case, what one does to produce more variability in response, is to "strengthen" the wording of the item, so that more respondents will move toward the "disagree" end of the continuum. For example, the researcher could use a statement such as, "Women play a more important role in shaping family health than men," or "Women play the single most important role in shaping the health of family members." In both examples, we have made it less likely that all respondents will remain at the "Strongly agree" end of the continuum.

In dealing with a variable such as job satisfaction in nursing, a review of the literature will reveal that most respondents will report themselves to be relatively satisfied with their jobs. Knowing this, researchers strive to identify items that will induce some participants to report that they are less than fully satisfied—perhaps the researcher will ask if the respondent would like her or his child to have a job similar to their own or ask if they think they are paid the "right amount" for the responsibilities that they have.

Similarly, a question about the satisfaction of clients with services in an acute care facility will need to ensure that the questions ferret out the slightest dissatisfaction. Otherwise it is likely that virtually everyone will rate the service as "good" or "excellent."

When one is phrasing questions so as to ensure that respondents vary in their scores, one is not attempting to distort reality—to show dissatisfaction when none is present; rather, one is attempting to develop measures that are highly sensitive. And if one is attempting to understand what leads clients to be relatively more, or relatively less, satisfied with their treatment in a health care facility, one would need highly sensitive measures, given the fact that participants generally tend to respond positively. If all participants simply reported that they were "satisfied," we would not be able to identify what factors influence levels of client satisfaction.

Tip 4. Avoid complexity. Try to keep questions simple; avoid asking participants to do difficult tasks. When it is necessary, for example, to have participants rank order a list, it is usually best to ask them to rank order the three most important items rather than asking them to go through the whole list. In most cases, the slight reduction in discriminatory power will be offset by a higher response rate to the question.

Tip 5. Use existing wordings for comparative analysis. When a researcher wishes to compare data that he or she is generating to data reported by other researchers, it is important that the wording of questions be identical. Here one has to weigh the advantages of improving the wording of a question against the advantage of maintaining identical wordings to facilitate comparative analyses.

Tip 6. Take the edge off sensitive questions. Using a combination of experience and common sense, the survey researcher soon learns that there are some issues that respondents may be reluctant to report. Illegal activities, evaluating friends or neighbors, and indicating age or income can all be sensitive issues. By asking for the respondent's year of birth rather than age, the researcher makes the question sound scientific and more likely to be answered; if age is asked, the respondent may feel some invasion of privacy is occurring; the same with income. Here many researchers will ask respondents to indicate into which broad category of income they fall. Alternatively, if income is a key question and if the question is located among those dealing with conditions of work, respondents will generally provide the information. However, if the income question is being used as a measure of socioeconomic status, then other indicators, such as years of education or occupational prestige, might be considered preferable to income itself—simply to avoid prying unnecessarily into what may be perceived to be a highly personal matter.

Show acceptance of socially undesirable behavior and attitudes by using strategic leads such as "Many adolescents have suicidal tendencies. Have you ever thought about suicide?" This is more likely to get an honest response than if you bluntly ask how many times the respondent has thought about suicide.

Tip 7. Avoid asking participants to speculate on why they act the way they do. Generally we are not interested in polling participants' opinions on whether certain relationships exist. For example, if you were studying the relationship between participation in regular physical activity and levels of self-esteem, you would normally not ask participants if they think there is a relationship between these two variables. Instead, the researcher would get separate measures of the two variables (among others) and would then analyze the data to determine if there is any relationship.

Tip 8. Be precise and highly specific when choosing wording. If you wish to measure, for example, how much people smoke, ask questions that pinpoint the number of cigarettes smoked in a given period and the occasions when they "light up." Here the time period will have to be reasonable. It is silly to ask how many cigarettes someone has had in the past 2 years; few people could make a reasonable estimate without considerable thought. Box 14.8 illustrates some possibilities in asking about smoking patterns.

Question 1 suffers because of variations in what respondents consider light, moderate, or heavy smoking behavior. Question 2 is better be-

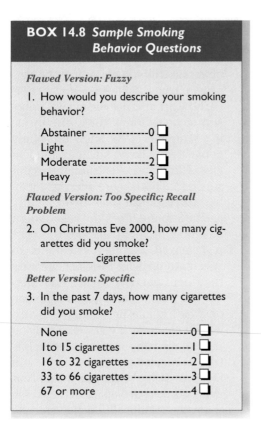

BOX 14.8 *Sample Smoking Behavior Questions*

Flawed Version: Fuzzy

1. How would you describe your smoking behavior?

    Abstainer ----------------0 ☐
    Light   ----------------1 ☐
    Moderate ----------------2 ☐
    Heavy   ----------------3 ☐

Flawed Version: Too Specific; Recall Problem

2. On Christmas Eve 2000, how many cigarettes did you smoke?
    _____ cigarettes

Better Version: Specific

3. In the past 7 days, how many cigarettes did you smoke?

    None   ----------------0 ☐
    1 to 15 cigarettes   ----------------1 ☐
    16 to 32 cigarettes ----------------2 ☐
    33 to 66 cigarettes ----------------3 ☐
    67 or more   ----------------4 ☐

cause it pins down a specific time period, but perhaps it goes overboard; it is possible to become too specific. Question 3 offers a reasonable compromise because it is specific and refers to a reasonable and recent time period.

Tip 9. Pretest the questionnaire. It is important to have a few individuals complete the questionnaire or the interview before settling on the final wordings of the questions. Start by filling it out yourself. Make any necessary corrections and then administer it to a few other people. Generally it is best to sit with the individuals completing the questionnaire. Before they begin, tell them exactly what you are doing (try to remove any ambiguity in the questionnaire) and encourage them to ask for any clarifications. Perhaps, as they complete the

questionnaire, they may inquire, "When you ask about the size of my family, do you mean the family I was born into or the one I have with my husband? Also in that question, do you want me to include the parents in the count?" If so, clearly you will need to change your wording of the question. With experience, you will learn to be highly specific in your wording of questions. The goal is to minimize variations in participants' understanding of each question. It is always a good idea to review your questionnaire and search for possible ambiguities. The goal, although actually impossible to achieve, is to have all participants understand each and every question in an identical manner.

Tip 10. If resources allow, do a pilot study. It is recommendable that researchers use pilot studies in a number of situations. A **pilot study** involves having a small sample of respondents complete the questionnaire or undergo the interview. Pilot studies are used to determine items to be included in indexes and to determine, from open-ended questions, which categories should be used in a fixed-choice format. Further refinements in questionnaires may be achieved through the use of a pilot study.

D. ORDERING QUESTIONS, FORMATTING, AND PRESENTATION

1. Ordering Questions

Rule 1. Introduce the questionnaire to respondents. Normally, questionnaires contain a brief statement introducing the study to the respondent. It should be short (usually three or four lines is sufficient) and should inform the respondent about who is doing the study, who is sponsoring it, and what the study is about. These few lines should attempt to establish the legitimacy of the project. By identifying who is doing the study and who is sponsoring it, the idea is conveyed that the survey is important. Such identification also provides the respondent with some additional information that he or she can use to decide whether to fill out the questionnaire. The researcher should not identify the specific hypotheses of the study; to do so might well bias the responses. Finally, if the survey is anonymous, respondents should be assured that their anonymity will be protected. A good way to achieve the latter goal is simply to ask respondents not to write their names on the forms (see Box 14.9 for a sample wording).

In a mailed questionnaire, a letter describing the project and requesting the cooperation of the recipient is generally included. Ideally, this letter should be written on letterhead stationery and be signed by the head of the organization. One attempts to communicate the importance of the project by identifying its sponsors and by the professional appearance of the mailing. Normally, a stamped, return envelope is included for the respondent's convenience.

Figure 14.1 illustrates a sample letter that might accompany a mailed questionnaire. It is important that the intro-ductory statement on a questionnaire and the letter of introduction do not replace an informed consent form. The researcher must provide evidence that respondents have given free and informed consent to participate in the study. This evidence is ordinarily obtained in writing. Figure 14.1 includes an informed consent form that should be signed by respondents as evidence of their consent. (For a review of protecting subjects' rights, see Chapter 10.)

Rule 2. Ease them into it. In deciding the order of questions, consideration should be given to starting with questions that are easy to answer. It is important not to start by asking questions that may be regarded as "too personal." Background information questions are usually placed at the end of questionnaires (Dillman, 1999; Erdos, 1983; Jackson, 1999). However, when students are being surveyed or in situations in which there is little problem with refusals, it is possible to begin with items that reflect the respondent's place of birth, gender, and the size of the community in which the respondent lives. Perhaps then it will be possible to move to issues such as the respondent's year of birth.

Whether one begins with background information or other questions, it is important that the respondent be able to move quickly through these first items, creating the impression that it will take

---

BOX 14.9 *Sample Introductory Questionnaire Statement*

We hope that you will be willing to complete this important survey of health behavior being conducted by a group of nursing students as part of their course requirements. We hope you will find the questions interesting. Please complete the questions in the order in which they are presented. You have the right to skip any question you do not wish to answer, and you may stop completing the questionnaire at any time you wish without penalty. We hope, however, that you will complete it in its entirety. There are no right or wrong answers. Please be as truthful as possible. Your answers are completely confidential. You do not need to put your name on the questionnaire, and no one will know how you answered the items.

comes to formatting each page of the questionnaire for optimal appearance. When choosing font size, consider the age of the expected respondent; older respondents, in particular, will appreciate a somewhat larger print.

Rule 10. Do not squeeze too much onto one page. Avoid trying to squeeze too much onto a single page; questionnaires should permit the respondent to move through each page rapidly. Squeezing material looks bad and discourages your respondent. Moreover, if it is squeezed too tightly, it will be harder to code.

E. EVALUATION OF QUESTIONNAIRES

1. Advantages

The questionnaire is one of the most popular tools for data collection in nursing research. It enables the researcher to collect self-report data from respondents either through written or verbal responses. Questionnaires are especially useful when one wishes to collect a broad range of descriptive information from respondents about phenomenon such as attitudes, knowledge, behaviors, opinions, or facts about events or people. Questionnaires are economical in that they can be distributed to large samples through the mail or directly; they can be administered with ease; and they can be completed and analyzed in a limited time period. They present items in a consistent manner; minimize bias that is often present in interviews and other forms of data collection, and offer the possibility of anonymity.

2. Limitations

Although questionnaires provide many advantages, they are not without limitations. Questionnaires require considerable thought, planning, and testing to create a valid and reliable data collection instrument. Because individual items often address a variety of different topics within one questionnaire, it is difficult to determine the reliability of all items (see Chapter 13). Table 14.3 outlines some questions that may be asked in helping beginning researchers to assess various questionnaire items.

Table 14.3   Queries to Help Judge Questionnaire Items*

Item	Query
Format	In fixed choice questions, are the question response categories mutually exclusive? Does the formatting make data entry easy? Is the length of the questionnaire likely to discourage completion of the instrument?
Language	Will the wording be easily and consistently understood by the respondents? Are the questions culturally appropriate, not offending some respondents? Does the language invite the respondents to express their opinions? Does the strength of the wording provide for sufficient variation in response?
Indexes	If the index was developed by other researchers, has its reliability been tested? Has the index been used on respondents drawn from similar populations? Does the content of the items cover the essential variables of the study?
Validity	Are the proposed measures congruent with the definitions implied by the constructs? Have other researchers established the validity of the measures?

*If you answer "yes" to all these queries, then you can be confident that the questionnaire is appropriate to use in your study. If you answer "no" to one or more of these queries, then you should revise the questionable items. If you are considering the use of an existing instrument designed by another researcher and you answer "no" to some of the queries, you should consider developing a new instrument.

Clear written instructions must accompany the instrument so that the respondent responds appropriately to the items provided. Data collected by questionnaires tend to be less in depth and more superficial than those collected by interviews. Even open-ended questions that allow respondents to express their perspectives do not probe for deeper meanings.

3. Challenges

Questionnaires require researchers to provide, in addition to clear, coherent questions, a sense of motivation that inspires respondents to complete the instrument. It is often a challenge to get respondents to complete and return questionnaires. This is particularly true with mailed questionnaires. The response rate for mailed questionnaires is often low (25 to 30 percent). To be respectable, a mailed questionnaire should hope to elicit a 50 percent response rate (Seaman, 1987; Jackson, 1999). Others indicate that a 60 percent rate is good and a 70 percent rate is very good (Babbie, 1992). Hand delivery and pick up of completed questionnaires may be a feasible way to increase response rates. An alternate method may be to mail the questionnaires and then visit with respondents on prearranged dates to pick up the completed questionnaires.

To increase response rate, the researcher may use inducements. A variety of approaches have been used with varying success. Items such as a small payment to compensate for time consumed by the questionnaire completion, the placement of a pencil in the envelope to ease completion, the promise of a summary of the study results, and an appeal to the altruistic nature of the respondent to contribute to knowledge development or increase understanding of some phenomenon important to society may yield respectable return rates. In addition, a nonresponse questionnaire procedure can be used; in 2 weeks, the researcher may send a postcard to remind the participants to return the questionnaires; 4 weeks after the initial mailing, the researcher may send another questionnaire.

E X E R C I S E S

1. Develop a series of background information questions that would be appropriate for a study you would like to do. Be careful to obey as many of the rules for questionnaire construction as you can.

2. Using the questions developed in question 1:
   a. Complete the questionnaire yourself. Decide which changes you would make, based on problems that emerged when you completed the questionnaire. Revise the questionnaire.
   b. Sit down with a fellow student and have him or her complete the revised questionnaire. What changes resulted from having another person complete the questions? Revise the questionnaire to remove any ambiguities.

3. Develop a series of items for an index that is of interest to you. Define the conceptual aspects of the index and suggest indicators.

Nurse researchers are interested in studying elements of the nursing world. One way to do this is to take measures on the relevant variables for all people in the population of interest. Although this solution is possible if one is studying a small population (e.g., clients who received nursing care in the emergency department of the local hospital), when the concern is to understand how people from larger aggregations such as a community, region, or country feel about certain health issues, then it is necessary to figure out ways to get a sense of their beliefs and attitudes without having everyone complete a questionnaire or agree to be interviewed. In such cases, a sample that can reflect or represent the views of the larger population may be drawn. A **sample** represents a microcosm of the population you are interested in studying. It is a way of representing the variability within a large population through the study of a smaller number selected from that population. If the sample is representative of the population from which it is drawn, the researcher can have confidence in concluding that the results are generalizable to the entire population and setting studied. This chapter discusses sampling techniques, procedures for selecting samples, and methods for estimating sample size.

Sampling is done to save time and money. If you can estimate who is going to benefit from a health promotion program with a sample of 250, why poll 1000 people? And although common sense suggests that larger samples would be more accurate than smaller ones, this is not necessarily the case. The key issue is that a sample must be representative—it must reflect the population accurately. Box 15.1 reports a classic case of an inaccurate sample. In this famous case, a huge sample (more than two million people) failed to predict the winner of the 1936 American presidential election (Simon and Burstein, 1985, p. 108).

The *Literary Digest* poll described in Box 15.1 was deficient in that:

- It lacked a representative sample of the general population.
- Circumstances altered substantially between the time of data collection and the time of the election.

The lesson to be learned from the *Literary Digest* debacle is that, for reasons of both economy and accuracy, a well-selected small sample is to be preferred to a large, poorly selected sample.

Sampling may involve the selection of people, events, organizations, periods of time, records, and many other phenomena of concern to the field of nursing. It is used in a great variety of nursing research projects, such as choosing which client records will be subjected to a content analysis, choosing and then assigning nurse volunteers to different conditions in experimental designs, or deciding which members of an HMO are to be included in a telephone survey.

A. THE TERMINOLOGY OF SAMPLING

To begin our discussion, some terms need to be distinguished:

- **Population.** The population is the entire group that you wish to describe. In Box 15.1, the population would be the American electors of 1936. If you were studying clients with asthma, the population might be defined as "all people with asthma residing in the United States." Other examples of research populations of interest to nurses include successful code blue procedures at hospital X in 1999; preschool children with hearing disorders in Ontario, Canada; nurses with clinical specialist registration in the state of California; 5-year survivors of breast cancer in North America; state-funded baccalaureate

BOX 15.1 *Predicting the 1936 American Election*

In 1920, 1924, 1928, and 1932, the New York–based *Literary Digest* conducted polls in an effort to predict the winner and the winning margin in the American presidential elections. The polls were accurate (within 1 percent in 1932), so it was with considerable confidence that the *Literary Digest* conducted its 1936 poll. On October 31, 1936, the magazine published its results based on mailings to some 10 million Americans. The results indicated:

Literary Digest Prediction of 1936 American Presidential Elections*		
Candidate	**Number of Votes**	**Percentage of Votes**
Landon	1,293,669	57.1
Roosevelt	972,897	42.9
TOTAL	2,266,566	100.0

*Responses from more than 10,000,000 ballots mailed out (under 23 percent response rate).

The poll suggested that Landon would easily win the presidential election, but it turned out that Roosevelt won by a substantial margin. So why, with a sample of more than 2 million, did the *Literary Digest* miss the mark so badly?

The founder of the American Institute, George Gallop, predicted in July of 1936, some months before the *Literary Digest* began mailing out its ballots, that it would not be accurate. Gallop pointed to the flaw of using mailing lists based on telephone listings and listings of automobile owners. Gallop pointed out that such lists largely favored the more economically prosperous; during the years of the Depression, the new voters came largely from poorer groups (few of whom owned cars or telephones). Gallop also noted that those most likely to return their ballots would overrepresent the better educated and the higher socioeconomic categories.

Gallop thus challenged the *sampling frame* used by the *Literary Digest.* The sampling frame is the target population from which the researcher draws a sample. The sampling frame did not accurately reflect American electors; rather, it favored the more prosperous elements in society, and Roosevelt's strength was among the poorer elements of American society.

Source: Summarized from Simon J.L., and Burstein P. (1985). *Basic Research Methods in Social Science* (3rd ed). New York: Random House, pp. 107–110.

nursing programs; or health records of all women diagnosed with depression at hospital X in the year 2000. As the examples suggest, a population may be defined broadly and potentially include millions of people, phenomena, or events, or it may be defined narrowly and include only a few hundred people or events. The terms "population" and "universe" are used interchangeably.

- **Accessible population.** This is the population that is feasible for the researcher to access. For example, you may be interested in studying perceptions of caring in clients who receive care in emergency departments. The research population is all clients who receive care in emergency departments. It is impossible to get a complete list and contact all such clients. Therefore, you should choose your sample from the *accessible population;* that is, those clients to whom the researcher has feasible access. You may have access to clients in emergency departments of the four general hospitals in your county, the regional trauma center, and the local hospital emergency department. Any of the clients at these six centers would constitute the accessible population for the study.

- **Sampling frame.** This is the list (or lists) from which you draw a sample. In Box 15.1, the sample frame included all those people listed as automobile owners plus all those who had a phone. Ideally, the sampling frame and the population are identical; in practice, however, it is often not possible to get a complete list of the population, so the sampling frame may not perfectly reflect the population. Almost any list will not be exactly up to date; some people will be left off and other people may be listed twice. The goal is to get as accurate a sampling frame list as possible. In evaluating the accuracy and completeness of the sampling frame, you should consider the following:

1. What systematic omissions from the list have resulted from the enumeration method? For example, are seriously ill clients, socially disadvantaged, or illiterate clients omitted?
2. Will omissions bias the study findings and generalizability of results? For example, if seriously ill clients are omitted from a list of clients receiving care in emergency departments, will this bias results of a study of perceptions of caring by emergency clients?
3. Is there any systematic bias inherent in the ordering of the sampling frame? For example, if the sampling frame systematically alternates all names by gender, a sample may be selected that is all male or all female. This is certain to happen in systematic sampling if every second name is selected from the list.
4. Does the list of potential participants represent the population of

interest to the research study? For example, if you are interested in studying smoking behaviors in disadvantaged women and you select your sampling frame from a list of women attending a private clinic, you most likely will miss many disadvantaged women who cannot afford to attend a private smoking cessation clinic.

If the above four factors are considered, it is likely you will increase the probability of getting a representative sample of the population you wish to study.

- **Sample.** The sample refers to those individuals (or units) selected for a study.
- **Response rate.** The response rate refers to the percentage of delivered questionnaires that are completed and returned.
- **Biased sample.** The sample is not representative of the population it is intended to reflect.
- **Sampling error.** This represents the difference between the values emerging from the sample and those emerging from the population on some phenomenon.

B. FUNDAMENTAL SAMPLING TECHNIQUES

There are two categories of sampling procedures used in quantitative studies: probability sampling techniques and nonprobability sampling techniques. Table 15.1 summarizes the major quantitative sampling procedures. You may wish to refer to this table as you read about each sampling method. Qualitative studies for the most part use nonprobability sampling techniques. These are discussed in Chapters 6 and 7. Table 15.2 presents a typology of common sampling strategies used in qualitative research.

Table 15.1   Summary of Quantitative Sampling Procedures

Type	Description of Procedure	Strengths and Limitations
Probability		
Simple random	All members of a population are enumerated and then the sample is selected from the sampling frame using random procedures	Risk of bias is low Representativeness is enhanced Time consuming to draw sample
Stratified random	Selection of participants from two or more strata	Tedious to draw sample Requires knowledge of underlying structure of population Representativeness is high Bias is low
Systematic	Selection of every kth person in the sampling frame	Requires a list of the sampling frame Observe for systematic bias in the ordering of the sampling frame Representativeness limited if bias is present in the sampling frame
Cluster	Multistage sampling in which large clusters are sampled first, followed by successive sampling of smaller and smaller units	Efficient way to draw a large sample if elements in a population are not available Higher sampling error than simple random
Convenience	Participants selected because they are in the right place at the right time	Easily accessible High risk of bias Questionable representativeness
Quota	Inclusion of participants based on predetermined characteristics; a type of convenience sampling	Uses knowledge of population to enhance representativeness of sample Bias is present
Snowball	Participants are referred by earlier participants	Facilitates access to difficult-to-find subjects Representativeness is suspect Bias is high
Purposive	Selects subjects on the basis of personal judgment about representativeness	Bias may be high Limited ability to generalize results Easy to draw sample
Expert	Subjects selected on the basis of their expertise	Representativeness is questionable Achieves consensus efficiently and effectively

1. Probability Sampling Techniques

Probability sampling techniques are used in selecting sampling units so that each unit has a known chance of being included. It is important to appreciate that tests of statistical significance assume that sampling has been done using some form of probability sampling (see Chapter 12). If your study involves the use of such tests, be certain to meet the sampling assumption. The sampling units usually are individuals, but may also be other levels of analysis, such as communities or countries. Probability sampling usually yields samples that are representative of the population from which they were drawn and

Table 15.2   Typology of Sampling Strategies In Qualitative Inquiry

Type of Sampling	Goal
Maximum variation	Deliberate selection of participants who are outliers from the norm to see if the commonalities exist with the larger group
Homogenous	Deliberate selection of participants with a range of similar experiences; this facilitates cohesion during the interview process
Critical case	Important case that permits generalization of findings to other cases
Theory based	Selection of the sample is determined by the goal of finding examples of a theoretical construct; participants are selected on the basis of whether or not they present an instance of the theoretical construct
Confirming and disconfirming cases	Sample is selected to maximize both deviant and typical cases
Snowball or chain	Sample selected by participants referring the researcher to other people who share common experiences
Deviant case	Selection of outlier cases that show great variation in the phenomenon from the majority of the sample
Typical case	Represents what is normal or average in the sample
Politically important case	Participants selected for their "value-added" potential to anticipated issues in the analysis
Random purposeful	When a potential purposive sample is too large, a random purposeful sample is used to select a sample of appropriate size
Stratified purposeful	Uses subgroups to select participants that represent dimensions on which variability is sought
Criterion selection	All cases meet some criterion
Reputational case	Selection of participants on the basis of reputable key informants
Convenience	Selection of participants on the basis of ease and convenience but at the expense of information and credibility

Source: Summarized from Miles, M.B., and Huberman, A.M. (1994). *Qualitative Data Analysis* (2nd ed). London: Sage.

avoid bias. Representativeness of the sample is necessary if the researcher is to make generalizations about study results to the larger unmeasured population.

Probability sampling involves the techniques of simple random sampling, systematic sampling, stratified sampling, and multistage or cluster sampling. The procedures for selecting each of the major types are listed below.

a. Simple Random Sample

A **simple random sample** provides each unit (usually a person) in the population an equal chance of being selected for participation in a study. This procedure is the best-known probability approach. It requires that a list of the potential respondents is available to the researcher. Such lists might include student lists, lists of clients from a health-care facility, lists of employees, lists of nursing programs, and so forth. The following steps are necessary when selecting a *simple random sample:*

Step 1. Number the units on the list.

Step 2. Computers are typically used to generate the random numbers used in sample selection. Alternatively one may use a table of random numbers such as the one provided in Table 4.1

(Chapter 4) to select the required number of units. (Sample size determination is discussed later in this chapter.) To use a table of random numbers, shut your eyes and place a pencil mark on the table. The number closest to where the mark is made is used as the starting point. From this point, one reads the numbers systematically (perhaps reading down the column, continuing at the top of the next column, and so forth), placing a checkmark beside the cases whose number shows up on the random number table. This process continues until a sufficient number of cases for the study has been selected.

Step 3. Additional replacement units should be selected and kept on a separate list, so that when a sampling unit cannot be contacted or an individual or program does not participate, then that unit will be replaced by the first replacement unit. Replacements should be identified and numbered because they will be used in the order in which they have been selected. Numbering them as R1, R2, and so on is a convenient way of noting them.

b. Systematic Sample

A **systematic sample** provides each unit (usually a person) in the population an equal chance of being selected for participation in a study by choosing every *n*th unit, starting randomly. The systematic sample provides a somewhat easier way of selecting cases from a list of potential respondents. In this case, names listed in birth announcements, phone books, health maintenance organization directories, street maps, dormitory diagrams, nurse registration lists, student lists, or surgical lists all might be sources from which one might draw a systematic sample. In the case of systematic samples, it is even possible to proceed with sampling when no list exists before sampling.

For instance, one could choose students living in every fourth residence room and, as long as one numbers the rooms systematically, one could proceed without a list of the students.

The critical issue is that every person must have a known (usually equal) chance of being selected. The steps in selecting a systematic sample are as follows:

Step 1. Get a list, map, or diagram as appropriate.

Step 2. Having determined the sample size required plus the additional number for replacements (for the refusals or for those with whom contact cannot be made), these two figures should be added together and be regarded as the total sample requirement.

Step 3. Divide the total sample requirement into the total number of units in the population being surveyed. This number should then be rounded to the nearest, but lower, round number. (e.g., if the number you get is 8.73, round it to the nearest, lower, whole number; in this case, 8). This number represents what is known as the **skip interval** or the **sample interval.**

One caution that must be mentioned in the use of systematic samples is that if the list is ordered in some fashion, there may be a problem. Suppose you have a listing of couples with the name of the man always listed first. In such a case, if the skip interval were an even number, then all those selected would be women. If the list is patterned, as in the example discussed, a different sampling procedure will have to be used.

Step 4. Using a table of random numbers, select a number between 1 and the value of the sample interval. The number selected becomes the starting case, the first one selected to participate in the survey. Suppose we were doing a survey of nursing students living in campus dormitories and we have determined the skip interval to be 8 and the starting case to be 3. In this case, we would develop a systematic procedure for numbering the dormitory rooms and for moving from floor to floor, dormitory to dormitory. We would begin with the third door, then go to the eleventh, nineteenth, and twenty-seventh. In rooms with two nursing student residents, we would ask both to participate; otherwise, students in double rooms would have less chance of being selected for the study. However, caution has to be exercised because, in some universities, nursing students may select their roommates and, if this is the case, there would be a lack of independence in some of the units sampled. If this is a problem, the researcher would be well advised to obtain a list of all nursing students in residence and then use a random sampling procedure.

When systematic samples are being selected from lists, it is a rather straightforward matter to go through the list, placing checkmarks beside cases that have been selected, perhaps marking every fifth one. Additional units should be selected for use as replacements and marked with R1, R2, and so on to indicate the order in which they should be used.

c. Stratified Sample

There are times when a simple random or systematic sample would not provide an appropriate solution to sample selection. This is true if you are interested in studying a *stratum* or subpopulation such as juveniles with diabetes, people with congenital heart defects, or individuals in a particular age group. Suppose, for example, that you are doing a survey of lifestyle patterns among the adolescent age group (early, mid, and late adolescent *strata*) attending public schools. Although it would be possible to do a random sample of ado-

lescents in the public school system, such a procedure might be somewhat wasteful because some schools will be made up predominantly of young adolescents, others will be made up of middle adolescents, and others will be made up of older adolescents. As a result, a very large sample would be required to provide a sufficient number of respondents to allow generalizations about lifestyle patterns across the adolescent age span. In situations such as this one, it is useful to draw a **stratified sample.** A stratified sample gives respondents within each of the three adolescent age groups an equal chance of selection, but at the same time, ensures that an equal number will be selected from each of the three age groups or strata.

Step 1. Determine the sample size required from each of the categories.

Step 2. Develop a list for each of the age strata from which you wish to draw your sample.

Step 3. Using either a systematic or random sampling procedure, choose the cases for the sample along with the required number of replacements.

Samples may be stratified by more than one variable. In order to achieve more precise estimates, we might also have stratified the previous sample by gender and by grade level. The procedures are identical; simply identify the stratification dimensions an then select respondents using an equal probability procedure. The number of adolescents in each stratum should be the same as the proportion of the group in the total population. For example, if the population is the total adolescent age span and the strata are early adolescents (33.3 percent of the population), mid adolescents (40.7 percent of the population), and late adolescents (26.0 percent of the population), the sample selected should reflect similar proportions. Figure 15.1 illustrates the use of proportional stratified random sampling to select a sample of adolescents.

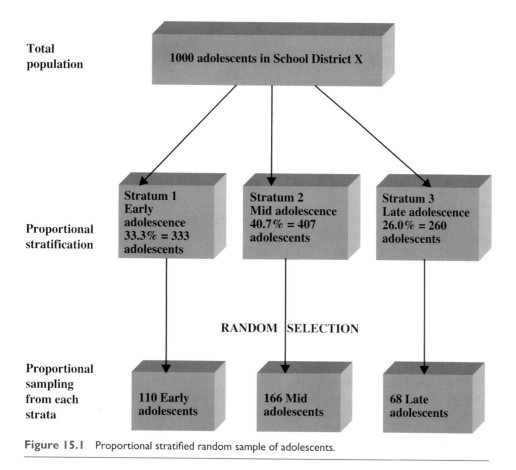

Figure 15.1 Proportional stratified random sample of adolescents.

d. Multistage Area Sample

When the task involves developing a sample to reflect a large unit such as a state, province, or country and no list of the population is available, then one develops a **multistage area sample** or **cluster sample.** The key point is that at each successive stage of the sampling process, every individual (or unit) must have a known chance of being selected. The difference between a simple random sample and a cluster sample is that a simple random sample is a one-stage process: a population is listed and items are selected from it at random. In a cluster sample, the population is divided into groups or *clusters;* the first units or clusters to be sampled are the largest, followed by smaller and smaller units selected at random. You

eventually get down to the level of the individual who is randomly selected from the smallest cluster. In a simplified form, the procedures for large-scale surveys such as a national surveys may be summarized as follows:

Step 1. Identify **primary sampling units** (these may be census tract areas or other similar units, normally several hundred of them); these units are numbered, and a selection of units is made from them, using an equal probability technique.

Step 2. Within the selected areas, identify the city blocks (in urban areas) or square miles (rural areas). From these, choose an appropriate number of units, making sure to use an equal probability technique

Step 3. Within the selected areas, number the housing units and select the units that will be used randomly from among these.

Step 4. For each household, list the people who fall within the desired sampling parameters (e.g., adults, older than age 18 years who have lived in the community for 1 month or more). Table 5.2 (Chapter 5) gives an example of a sample form.

Step 5. An equal probability procedure such as simple random or stratified methods is then used to select respondents from a list of those who are eligible.

Cluster or multistage sampling has many applications in nursing research. For example, it may be used by a school health nurse who is interested in studying lifestyle patterns in school-aged children. The school nurse may work with a nurse researcher to select a random sample of schools from the school district; within the schools, she may randomly select classrooms and within classrooms, she may randomly select children. This may yield a representative sample more efficiently than randomly selecting children from all schools in the district. Cluster sampling may also be used by community health nurses to study family health practices. In this case, the researcher would randomly select census tracts within his or her district, then blocks of households within the census tracks, and then families within the household blocks.

When it is impossible to obtain a list of all the elements in a population, cluster sampling is a practical approach to ensure the representativeness of the sample. For example, if you are interested in studying student nurses' attitudes toward mandatory registration in your state, you may not have the ability to get a list of the names of all nursing students. You could, however, get a list of nursing programs in your state and randomly select schools from that list, then randomly select nursing students from the schools.

It should be noted, however, that *no sampling choices should be made by data collection personnel*. All choices should be made by probability procedures. When a selected participant is not available (e.g., he or she has moved away, not home after three callbacks, or refuses to cooperate), then replacements are used, *in the order selected*. It is critical that interviewers not simply replace the unavailable respondent with the nearest, most convenient replacement. This would bias the sample toward those who are at home or are more cooperative. Whatever rules are established, these should be communicated clearly to those doing the data collection and should also be made clear in any technical reports on the research project (see Table 5.2 for a sample form that may be used).

Box 15.2 presents the telephone introduction instructions for the 1993 Alberta Survey (Kinzel, 1992). Although the telephone numbers selected for dialing were randomly determined, the procedures favored interviewing men, particularly those who happen to have answered the phone call from the interviewer. In their procedures, any time a man answered the phone, he was invited to participate in the interview. This procedure was an attempt to compensate for the overrepresentation of teenagers and women, who typically were found to be more likely to answer the phone. These procedures were followed to create a greater equality in the participation rates of male and female respondents.

2. Nonprobability Sampling Techniques

Nonprobability sampling techniques are commonly used by nurse researchers. These procedures do not provide potential respondents with a known chance of being asked to participate in a study. They are, nonetheless, important to know about

BOX 15.2 *The Alberta Survey*

Telephone Introduction Sheet 1993

1. Hello, I'm calling (*long distance*) on behalf of the Population Research Lab at the University of Alberta. My name is . . . (full name or Mrs. XXXXX)
2. I have dialed XXX-XXXX. Is this correct?
3. Your telephone number was selected at random by computer.
4. Just a moment of your time to explain why I'm calling.
5. The lab at the university is currently conducting an important study on current issues (e.g., the family, health and well-being, AIDS, credit cards, crime, work, and social issues).
6. In order to determine who is eligible for the study, please tell me how many women and men aged 18 years or older live on a regular basis at this number?
NUMBER OF WOMEN _____ and NUMBER OF MEN _____ This total includes yourself as a member of this household over the age of 18.

Requesting an Interview with Person who Answers the Phone

7. I would like to interview you. I'm hoping that now is a good time for you. Your opinions are very important for the research that is being done at the University of Alberta.
8. Before we start, I'd like to assure you that your participation is voluntary and that any information you provide will be kept confidential and anonymous. As I mentioned, there is a wide variety of questions. If you do not wish to answer any of them, please feel free to point these out to me and we'll go on to the next question. Of course, you have the right to terminate the interview at any time.

(Optional Read)

We do not need your name, so no one will know your answers to these questions. If you have any questions about the survey, you can call the study supervisor in Edmonton at XXX-XXXX for further information.

Refusal

9. It is extremely important for the university study to have the highest number of people who have been selected take part.
10. I can't replace your household with another one without destroying the randomness of the survey.
11. Do you think anyone else in the household could take part (*either now or later*)? (do not pause) Could someone assist us with the study?

Requesting to Speak to Someone Else in the Home

12. We don't always interview the person who answers the telephone. In your household, it is one of the (*male/female*) members we need to talk to.
13. May I please speak to (*him/her*) (one of them who is free at the moment)?
14. Hello, I'm calling from the Population Research Lab at the University of Alberta. My name is . . . (full name or Mrs. XXXXX)
15. The lab at the university is currently conducting an important study on current issues (e.g., the family, health and well-being, AIDS, credit cards, crime, work and social issues).
16. Your telephone number was selected at random by computer. I'm hoping that now is a good time for you. Your opinions are very important for the work that is being done at the University of Alberta.
17. Before we start, I'd like to assure you that your participation is voluntary and that any information you provide will be kept confidential and anonymous. As I mentioned, there is a wide variety of questions. If you do not wish to answer any of them, please feel free to point these out to me and we'll go on to the next question. Of course, you have the right to terminate the interview at any time.

(Optional Read)

We do not need your name, so no one will know your answers to these questions. If you have any questions about the survey, you can call the study supervisor in Edmonton at XXX-XXXX for further information.

because much nursing research involves nonprobability sampling techniques.

a. Quota Sample

In a **quota sample,** respondents are selected on the basis of meeting certain criteria. Quota sampling requires some underlying knowledge of the population structure so that the researcher proportionately represents the strata in the sample. However, no list of potential respondents is required; the first respondent to meet the requirements is asked to participate and sampling continues until all the categories have been filled—until the quota for each has been reached. Suppose one were asked to compare food preferences of young adults with those of elderly individuals. One might do a survey of nutrition clinic clients, selecting the first 75 who meet the "young adult" criteria and the first 75 who meet the criteria for inclusion in the comparison group. Note that this sampling procedure is the nonprobability twin of stratified sampling. It is useful in providing adequate representation of different groups in a population such as various age groups, ethnic groups, gender, or socioeconomic levels. The major distinction between quota sampling and stratified sampling is that the elements are not randomly selected in each strata of a quota sample.

The steps in selecting a quota sample are as follows:

Step 1. Define precisely the criteria for inclusion into each of the categories.

Step 2. Select participants on a first-come, first-included basis until the quota for each category has been met.

Quota sampling may also employ **matched pairs.** To do so, the researcher predetermines significant characteristics in the sample that might influence the dependent variable and matches the sample according to those characteristics. For example, if a researcher is interested in measuring the impact of a health promotion program on participants, the researcher would try to "match" each program participant with another person with similar predetermined characteristics at the outset of the program. Subjects may be matched for current health status, similar patterns of health-related lifestyle, age, occupation, and so on. Matching pairs is a time-consuming and demanding challenge, but it enables control for bias in the interpretation of findings and reduces sampling error (see Chapters 4 and 9).

b. Convenience Sample

Convenience samples involve selection on the basis of ease or convenience. If you were to "poll" people entering a shopping mall on their attitudes toward current health reform initiatives, you would be selecting a convenience sample. Such samples may, however, involve particular categories of individuals. For example, by asking a couple of classes of tenth grade students to complete questionnaires on health behaviors, you would obtain a convenience sample of the students present. Convenience samples may be atypical of the population with regard to the phenomenon of interest; therefore, caution must be used in interpreting the findings. Moreover, generalizability of results from studies using this sampling technique is not possible. The researcher has no control over sampling biases or the representativeness of the sample. For this reason, convenience sampling is not encouraged unless no other alternatives exist or the phenomenon of interest is homogenous with respect to the characteristics studied.

c. Snowball Sampling

Snowball sampling is a name for a referral sampling procedure. As you complete one interview, you ask if there is anyone else known to the respondent who might be appropriate for the study. This technique is frequently used in situations in which one cannot get a list of the individuals who share some characteristic. Some examples in which you may choose to use this sampling procedure are:

- A study of the marital adjustment of couples whose first child was born before the couple married. In this case, you would not easily find a list of this population. But through referrals, you could identify individuals who would be appropriate for your study.
- A study of prostitutes who are under age 16 years
- A study of people convicted of white-collar crimes
- A study of "closet" homosexuals

d. Purposive Sampling

Purposive sampling, also referred to as *judgmental sampling,* uses the researcher's expertise and knowledge of the population to hand pick the cases to be included in the sample. The researcher usually selects participants who are considered typical of the population of interest. This subjective sampling technique is common in qualitative studies. For example, in a qualitative study, Baker (1996) used purposive sampling to select 15 participants with schizophrenia to collect narratives about their inner experiences with schizophrenia. In addition, participants were purposively selected so that the sample would include individuals of both genders, various age groups, varying abilities to recognize signs of relapse, and different lengths of time since diagnosis.

This approach is useful when a researcher is interested in understanding the experiences of certain segments of a population. Some examples include the use of extreme cases. These are sought when one wishes to better understand a rare or unusual phenomenon such as a group of participants with a rare diagnosis

such as sickle cell anemia. It is also useful when one wishes to examine different ends of a continuum on some variable. For example, to explore the concept of independence, one may sample a group of early adolescents and a group of senior citizens and compare the findings. Purposive sampling is frequently used in instrument development studies in which the researcher is interested in testing the validity of an instrument using the known-group technique (see Chapter 13) or pretesting the instrument with a purposive sample of divergent types of people. A limitation of purposive sampling is the inability to assess the representativeness of the participants in relation to the population. The researcher often assumes that errors of judgment in overrepresenting or underrepresenting elements of the population in the sample tend to balance out, but there is no way to test this assumption.

e. Expert Sampling

Expert sampling is actually a type of purposive sampling used with the Delphi technique (see Chapter 13). The researcher handpicks a sample of participants because of their expertise in the study phenomenon. A series of questionnaires are distributed to the expert sample and responses analyzed. After the analysis of the questionnaires, questions are reformulated and redistributed to the expert sample for completion and subsequent analyses. This is a means to achieve experts' consensus on an issue.

f. Advantages and Disadvantages of Nonprobability Techniques

Note that none of these nonprobability techniques leads to independent, randomly selected units. But for some research problems, this type of sampling is the only feasible one.

Convenience, quota, and snowball samples are reasonable approaches to

sampling when one is investigating relationships among variables (e.g., the relationship between exercise participation
and self-esteem) and one is interested in
trying to understand the conditions under
which there is (or is not) a relationship between the major variables rather than generalizing to the entire population. Purposive sampling is especially useful when
one is interested in understanding the experiences of special segments of the population rather than the typical experience
of the entire population. Explanatory studies, in fact, frequently use nonprobability sampling procedures. However, when
tests of significance are an important tool
in one's research, it should be noted that
such tests assume that probability sampling procedures have been used. Therefore, tests of significance are not appropriately used when quota, convenience,
snowball, purposive, or expert samples
have been used.

3. Qualitative Sampling Techniques

Although there is considerable overlap
between the sampling techniques used by
quantitative and qualitative researchers,
most of those used by qualitative researchers are variants of nonprobability
procedures. Table 15.2 presents a typology of the more commonly used sampling
procedures used in qualitative studies.
An examination of the table indicates that
although some focus on showing differences, others focus on showing the typical, the extreme, or ones that identify politically important cases. Given that these
are nonprobability sampling procedures,
it is inappropriate to conduct tests of significance on the data or to attempt extrapolations to larger populations.

In most situations, qualitative researchers are interested in samples of participants who have experienced the phenomenon being studied and who are able
and willing to share their interpretation

of the experience with the researcher.
Because the goal is understanding the
meaning of the participant's experience,
qualitative researchers are typically not
interested in attempting to generalize
their results to larger populations. Therefore, they typically do not use probability
sampling procedures.

C. SAMPLE SIZE DETERMINATION

A variety of factors influence the size of
the sample that is appropriate for any
study; thus, no simple rule can be applied
in determining an appropriate sample
size. If someone tells you that samples
should be 10 percent of the population,
the advice is not sound. Sample size determination involves a series of trade-offs
between precision, cost, and the numbers necessary to do the appropriate
analyses. At the same time, it is necessary
to take into account the amount of variability in the factors studied and, sometimes, even the size of the population.

A general guideline is the larger the
sample, the more accurate the findings.
This is because a larger sample is more
likely to be representative of the population. A second guideline is the more heterogeneous the population, the larger the
sample required. This is because there
will be much variability among variables
in a heterogeneous population so many
participants are required to ensure you
get subjects that are typical of the population from which they are drawn.

Research design also influences sample
size. Designs such as experimental or evaluation studies that involve a number of different groups or cells require the investigator to estimate the number of subjects
required for each cell as well as the total
study. To compare an experimental group
with a control group on the dependent
measure, it is necessary to figure out how

many participants are required for each cell. If the number in each cell is too small (< 10), atypical values will change the treatment mean dramatically. Guidelines for the number of participants per cell range from 10 to 30 (Woods and Catanzaro, 1988; Wilson, 1993). Using cell sizes of 20 or more enables more options during statistical analysis. Other designs such as surveys require more participants than experimental designs and challenge researchers to compensate for the problem of low response rate; in contrast, qualitative designs using observation and in-depth interviews require fewer participants than experimental designs. Therefore, one sees that the answer to the straightforward question, "How many should the sample include?" is never straightforward.

This section outlines steps that are useful to beginning researchers in determining sample size (1) when the variable you are making your estimates about is measured at the ratio level; (2) when the variable is measured at the nominal level; and (3) when doing a *power analysis* as a means of estimating sample size. In addition to the methods presented here, interested readers may wish to consult statistical texts for guidance on sample size (Fleiss, 1973; Kraemer and Theimann, 1987; Polit, 1996; Ritchey, 2000). Cohen (1977) has generated a collection of tables for estimating sample size for a variety of statistical tests. The tables are based on anticipated effect size of the study variables, significance level, and the power associated with the test.

1. Steps in Determining Sample Size and Estimating a Ratio Variable

Sample size determination involves eight basic steps, some of which are statistical and some of which are pragmatic. For this illustration, we will focus on a situation in which we are making estimates about a ratio level variable. It is usually best to begin with the statistical ones, estimating the required sample size, and then modify this number to take practical considerations into account.

Step 1. Decide on the confidence level to be used. If you would like to be confident that your result will fall within a given range of precision 95 percent of the time, use the value 1.96. (Recall that in a normal distribution, 95 percent of the cases fall ± 1.96 standard deviation units from the mean.) If you wish to be 99 percent confident, a larger sample will be required. (Here

---

BOX 15.3 *Estimating the Standard Deviation*

Suppose you wished to estimate the standard deviation of a variable such as the weight of male undergraduates. Try doing the following steps:

Step 1. Estimate the average weight of male undergraduates. **Estimate: 160 lb.**

Step 2. Within what weight range would you expect to find about two-thirds of the male students? **Preliminary estimate: 145 to 175 lb.**

Step 3. Because two-thirds of the cases represents 1 standard deviation on either side of the mean weight, this indicates that our preliminary estimate of the standard deviation is 15 lb.

Step 4. Double the estimate in Step 3 (30 lb). Does it make sense that about 95% of all cases will fall within the range defined by the mean ± twice the estimate at Step 3 (i.e., 160 ± 30; range, = 130 to 190 lb)? If the band is not wide enough, how much wider should it be? If it is too wide, how much narrower should it be? Suppose you decide that it should be slightly wider, arguing that about 95% of the cases will fall between 125 and 195 lb. Divide this range by 4 to get the estimated standard deviation (70 ÷ 4 = 17.5). **Standard deviation estimate: 17.5 lb.**

the appropriate value will be 2.58.) Most nurse researchers use the 95 percent level in determining sample sizes. With this level, you can be confident that your sample mean will be within a given precision 19 out of 20 times.

Step 2. Select a major variable to determine sample size. Normally you focus on the main dependent variable of the study in computing the required sample size. And if the dependent variable is measured at the ratio level, it will be easier to determine sample size requirements. Such a variable may include the percentage of surgical clients readmitted with complications after early discharge or an attitude score. You will need to estimate the population standard deviation (sd pop) for this variable. This estimate can be made by examining results from other surveys or, failing that, simply by using common sense, noting the mean and the range within which one expects to find two thirds of the cases (Box 15.3). Another suggestion for estimating an unknown population standard deviation is to approximate it by taking the range of values (excluding extreme cases) and dividing this value by two. This method generally provides a reasonable estimate. Finally, it must be acknowledged that in studies with a large number of variables involved, it is impossible to make claims, with any certainty, about the precision of all the variables. Most of them have unknown sampling distributions.

Step 3. Determine the minimum precision that would be acceptable. Do you want to be within 3 lb of the true mean when estimating weight, within two percentage points in predicting number of clients with complications, or within three points on a scale with a maximum score of 75? The measure of precision should be expressed in the same units as the standard deviation.

For example, if the mean is measured in pounds, the standard deviation also has to be measured in pounds.

Step 4. Compute the sample size. Compute the required sample using the following formula:

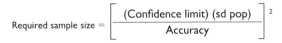

$$\text{Required sample size} = \left[\frac{\text{(Confidence limit) (sd pop)}}{\text{Accuracy}} \right]^2$$

Suppose, for example, that you wished to determine the sample size required to estimate the average weight of male university graduates. You wish to be 95 percent confident (Z = 1.96) and be within 2 lb of estimating the true weight. The estimated standard deviation of the population is 14.0 lb. The values would be plugged into the equation, as in:

$$\text{Required sample size} = \left[\frac{1.96 \ (14.0)}{2.0} \right]^2 = 188$$

The indicated sample size is 188 and should result in an estimate of the population's average weight within 2 lb, being confident that the estimate will be within this margin 95 percent of the time.

Step 5. Compute the sampling fraction. The **sampling fraction** is the sample size in relation to the population (see Monette et al., 1990, p. 149). Thus, if you have a population of 800,000 and a sample of 188, the sampling fraction would be:

$$\text{Sampling fraction} = \text{Sample size/Population}$$
$$= 188/800,000$$
$$= 0.0002 \ (0.02\%; \text{ go to Step 7})$$

If the sampling fraction is less than 5 percent, go to Step 7. Alternatively, if the population was 1200 residence students, the sampling fraction would be:

Sampling fraction = 188/1200
= 0.157 (15.7%; go to Step 6)

If the computed sampling fraction is more than 5 percent of the population, an adjustment may be made in your sample size. To compute the adjustment, go to Step 6.

Step 6. Make the small population adjustment. When the sampling fraction is greater than 5 percent, the required sample size may be reduced according to the following formula:

Adjusted sample size = $n \div [1 + (n \div N)]$

$$= 188 \div [1 + (188 \div 1200)]$$

$$= 188 \div 1.157$$

$$= 162$$

where n = sample size estimated in Step 4;
N = estimated size of universe.
See Monette, Sullivan, and Dejong, 1990.

Step 7. Are there sufficient cases for the analysis? The required sample size must now be scrutinized to ensure that it will provide a sufficient number of cases for the most complex analysis that is to be done. For example, if one intends to do a series of cross-tabulation tables with three categories in each of the independent and dependent variables, with a maximum of one control variable with two categories, then one is proposing a number of 18 cell tables ($3 \times 3 \times 2$). With 188 cases, the maximum expected frequencies would be just over 10 cases per cell ($188 \div 18 = 10.44$). This would hardly prove adequate and, therefore, one would want to increase the sample size or rethink the proposed types of analyses that are to be performed. Correlational techniques place less stringent demands on one's sample so that, to the extent model testing can be done using those techniques, fewer cases are required.

Step 8. Adjust the sample size for cost and time factors. A final step is to adjust the sample to take time and cost into account. If one requires a sample of 3000 but has only the resources to deal with 1000, then one will have to do some rethinking on the precision that will be possible. If, on the other hand, one has sufficient resources to increase the sample size, then one usually does so because some additional precision is likely to result.

2. Steps in Determining Sample Size and Estimating a Nominal Variable

A common situation for a researcher is to be trying to estimate a population proportion for a nominal level variable. Pollsters attempting to predict the vote for a particular candidate in an upcoming election may want to know the required sample size to provide an estimate of the likely vote and to be within perhaps 5 percent of the percent likely to support the candidate. Once again, the researcher may want to be 95 percent certain that the estimate will be within this margin of error. Suppose you believe the support for the given candidate is probably somewhere between 35 and 55 percent. How might you determine how many must be called in a phone survey to more precisely pin down the level of support?

For nominal or ordinal variables, the estimate may be calculated using the following formula:

n = (Success) × (failure)
× (confidence limit Z value)^2/(Accuracy)^2

where n = required sample size;
success is the estimated proportion voting for the candidate;
failure is the estimated proportion not voting for the candidate;
95% confidence limit (Z score: use the value

1.96 for the test; 2.58 for the 99% confidence limit);
and accuracy is the range within which you want the estimate to be.

Thus, if we thought a reasonable estimate of our candidate's vote would be 40 percent and we wish to be 95 percent confident (i.e., our population estimate will be within the accuracy parameter 19 out of 20 times), we wish to be within 5 percent of the vote for the candidate. These values are plugged into the equation, and we note that we will need to complete 369 phone surveys to provide our answer.

n = (Success) × (failure)
  × (confidence limit Z value)^2/(Accuracy)^2

$$n = \frac{(0.40 \times 0.60) \times (1.96)^2}{0.05^2}$$

$$n = \frac{0.24 \times 3.84}{0.0025}$$

$$n = 369$$

Thus, to be within 5 percentage points, it will be necessary to interview 369 persons. If you wish to change the parameters, simply adjust the values in the formula accordingly. You will note that gaining accuracy requires substantial increases in sample size.

3. Power Analysis and Sample Size

Power is the ability of a study to identify relationships or detect real differences among variables. **Power analysis** is a procedure used to determine the power of a statistical test; in other words, to determine the probability that an inferential statistical test will detect a significant difference that is real or correctly reject a null hypothesis. The minimum acceptable power for a study is 0.80. If one does not have sufficient power to detect a real difference that is present in a population,

then one must question the ethics of conducting the study as presently designed. Power analysis is used to estimate the sample size needed to obtain a significant result and allow the researcher to conclude that the research hypothesis is supported. Let us use a research example to demonstrate how power analysis is used to determine sample size.

Suppose you are interested in measuring the impact of a health promotion program on health attitudes. You recruit participants into the intervention group and the comparison group through the same process and randomly assign persons to the two groups from the same pool of eligible participants. You wish to test your null hypothesis that states that *there is no difference in health attitudes between those exposed to the program and those not exposed to the program.* To test the null hypothesis, you must determine how many participants you need in the intervention and comparison group to detect differences in health attitudes. You conduct a power analysis to determine how many participants you need for each group.

Power consists of four elements: significance level or alpha, sample size, effect size (ES), and power. If any three are known, the fourth can be calculated using the power analysis formulas. Let us briefly describe each element. **Alpha** refers to the probability of making a type I error (Chapter 12). This is a situation in which you detect a difference in health attitudes between the two groups even though no difference exists. In this case, the null hypothesis is rejected when it should have been accepted. The conventionally accepted level for a type I error rate is 0.05. This means you are willing to accept the risk of committing an error five times out of 100. A stricter alpha level such as 0.01 or 0.001 would decrease the power.

A type II error could result if you concluded that there is no difference in health attitudes between the two groups and a difference actually exists. As a result, you erroneously accept the null hypothesis. **Beta** refers to the probability of making a type II error. A rule of thumb for selecting beta is that it be no more than four times the value of alpha. Hence, if you are willing to take a chance of finding a difference in health attitudes 5 percent of the time when there really is no difference, then you would be willing to risk missing a true difference about 20 percent of the time (beta = 0.20). The *power* of a statistical test is determined by the following formula: 1 − beta = power (1 − 0.20 = 0.80). The conventional standard accepted for power is 0.80.

Effect size is concerned with the strength of the relationship among study variables. It is a measure of how false the null hypothesis is, or in other words how strong the effect of the independent variable is on the dependent variable. Most nursing interventions have small effects; therefore, small samples are not likely to detect small differences or relationships between variables. Four strategies exist for determining effect size (Polit and Sherman, 1990):

- A review of the literature that has examined similar phenomena enables the researcher to estimate the strength of the effect size based on prior studies. If a substantial number of studies have been conducted on the phenomena of interest, a *meta-analysis* (a process for statistically combining the results from multiple studies on a research topic)

may be conducted to estimate the effect size of the relationships of interest.

- A pilot study may be conducted to determine the effect size. The results of the pilot test can then be used to estimate the effect size for the main study.
- A "dummy table" analysis can be created to estimate effect size when no prior information is available. In the dummy table, the researcher calculates the smallest effect size that would still be considered sufficiently large to have practical or theoretical value. For example, if an exercise program resulted in a 10 percent weight loss for participants, it would be considered worthwhile and cost effective. An effect size estimate could be determined based on this information.
- Estimate on the basis of clinical experience or prior research whether you consider the effects small, medium, or large. The qualitative labels can then be attached to quantitative effect size values to conduct a power analysis. Effect sizes are usually small in new areas of research. A medium effect size should only be estimated when you can see the effect with the naked eye. In estimating effect size, it is prudent to be conservative because most nursing interventions have modest effects.

The effect size is estimated differently depending on the type of statistical test that is performed. Table 15.3 presents Cohen's (1977) estimation of small, medium,

Table 15.3 Definitions of Levels of Effect Size for Common Statistical Tests

Test	Effect Size Values		
	Small	Medium	Large
T test for two-group means	0.20	0.50	0.80
F test for k independent means	0.10	0.25	0.40
r $(r \neq 0)$	0.10	0.30	0.50
F $(R^2 \neq 0)$	0.02	0.15	0.35

Source: Adapted from Polit and Sherman (1990) and Cohen (1977).

and large effect sizes for four frequently used statistical tests.

After decisions have been made about alpha or significance level (α), population effect size (γ), and power ($1 - \beta$), it is possible to determine the sample size. Let us return to our example and determine the sample size needed to test the null hypothesis that there is no difference in health attitudes for those exposed to a health promotion program and those in the comparison group. The following steps are required:

Step 1. Estimate the population effect size (γ). In a two-group situation in which the difference of means is of interest, the formula for the effect size is

$$\gamma = \frac{\mu^1 - \mu^2}{\sigma}$$

where γ is the difference between the population means divided by the population standard deviation. But we do not know this information beforehand; therefore, we must estimate the population means and standard deviation based on whatever information is available to us.

Step 2. To estimate the population effect size, review the literature to see if earlier studies examined the effect of a health promotion program on health attitudes. One study is found that reported mean scores on a health attitude survey for seniors engaged in a 6-month health promotion program and a comparison group of seniors. The results of this study were:

X_1 (health promotion program) = 5.70
X_2 (no health promotion program) = 5.30
σ (pooled standard deviation) = 0.50
Calculation = 5.70 − 5.30 = 0.40

$$\gamma = \frac{5.70 - 5.30}{0.50} = 0.80$$

Thus, the value of τ would be 0.040.

Step 3. Consult a table of sample size requirements available in statistical texts. Table 15.4 represents such a table and provides approximate sample size requirements for various effect sizes and powers, and two values of α (for two-tailed tests), in a two-group mean difference situation. The table demonstrates that for α of 0.05, the estimated sample size needed for an effect size of 0.40 and a power of 0.80 is 99 participants per group—that is, 99 participants assigned to the health promotion group and 99 participants assigned to the comparison group for a total sample size of 198 participants. A sample smaller than 198 has an unacceptable probability of resulting in a type II error.

Step 4. If no previous research is available to calculate the effect size, the next step would be to estimate the expected effect size based on experience, intuitive knowledge, and literature. By convention, the value of γ in a two-group test of mean differences is estimated at 0.20 for small effects, 0.50 for medium effects, and 0.80 for large effects (Cohen, 1977). Again, consult the table of

Table 15.4 Approximate Sample Sizes* to Achieve Selected Levels of Power as a Function of Estimated Effect Size for Test of Difference of Two Means

Power	Estimated Effect†			
	0.20	0.40	0.60	0.80
$\alpha = 0.05$				
0.60	246	62	28	217
0.70	310	78	35	20
0.80	393	99	44	25
0.90	526	132	59	34
0.95	650	163	73	41
0.99	919	230	103	58

*Sample size requirements for each group; total sample size would be twice the number shown.
†Estimated effect (γ) is the estimated population mean group difference divided by the estimated population standard deviation.

sample sizes to determine that with an α of 0.05 and power of 0.80; the total sample size (number of subjects in both groups) for studies with expected small, medium, and large effect sizes would be 784, 126, and 50, respectively. Most nursing studies cannot expect effect sizes in excess of 0.50. The 0.20 to 0.40 effect size is a realistic expectation for nursing studies. Polit and Sherman (1990) conducted a power analysis on 62 articles published in nursing research journals and reported that the average power for small effects was under 0.30. The average effect size for t-test situations was 0.35.

Power analysis is an advanced statistical technique that is often required when applying for external funding. Several computer software packages are now available for performing power analysis on personal computers. These include programs such as POWER (Borenstein and Cohen, 1988), EX-SAMPLE (Brent et al., 1988), and SPSS for Windows. Beginning researchers should consult a statistician for advice in determining appropriate sample sizes.

To perform this analysis using SPSS, see the WEIGHT command in an SPSS manual.

D. OTHER SAMPLING ISSUES

Besides simply estimating the number of cases that will be needed in order to meet the needs of the research project, there are a few other issues related to sampling. These are explored here.

1. Sample Size and Accuracy

The relationship between sample size and precision of estimations is a simple one. To double accuracy, sample size must be quadrupled. In the illustration concerning the weights of graduating male college students, if we wished to be

within 1 lb of estimating the true value of the population, we would need a sample four times as large as the one proposed for a sample that would get us within 2 lb. For example:

$$\text{Required sample size} = \left[\frac{1.96 \ (14.0)}{1.0} \right]^2 = 753$$

The original sample size required was 188 or one quarter of 753. Note that "accuracy" is referred to in statistics texts as the confidence interval. In the previous example with a sample size of 753, we can be 95 percent confident that the true population mean weight is within 1 lb of the sample mean.

2. Sample Size and Confidence Limits

The relationship between precision and confidence limits means that to move from the 95 percent confidence limit to the 99 percent level, one may simply multiply the sample size by 1.73. Thus, in the illustration on graduating male college students, to be within 2 lb of the average weight but to be 99 percent confident, one would need to multiply the original sample size of 188 by a factor of 1.73 (188 $\times$ 1.73 = 325). A sample of 325 will be required to be 99 percent confident that the estimate will be within 2 lb of the true population mean. Conversely, to move from the 99 percent confidence limit to the 95 percent limit, the sample size determined for the 99 percent level may be multiplied by 0.58.

3. The Impact of Refusals

Although the evidence from studies examining different response rates under controlled conditions shows little variation in the descriptive accuracy independent of response rate, tests of significance assume probability sampling techniques and assume that there is no systematic bias in who chooses to complete the form. Such tests also assume that any measurement error is random. Because we cannot know what impact refusals and measurement error have on our data, researchers make every effort to get completed questionnaires from all respondents. It is not clear what conclusions one could legitimately arrive at if one had a response rate of 20 percent.

4. Confirming Representativeness

Steps, however, may be taken to confirm that one's sample is indeed representative of the population about which one is attempting to make generalizations. For example, one might compare the age, gender, and marital status distributions of one's sample with known distributions for the population from census data. If one's sample is not wholly representative, there are techniques for weighting results to get a better reflection of the population whose characteristics one is trying to estimate. However, when there has been a high nonparticipation rate, there is no guarantee that the sample will be representative for other variables, even if it is representative for the age or gender distributions that have been checked.

An alternative procedure that can be used to confirm representativeness of a sample when the population characteristics are not known is to take a random sample of the nonrespondents, interview them by telephone on key descriptive items, and then compare the respondents' with nonrespondents on these items. If there is little difference between the two, you can be confident that your sample is representative of the population from which it was drawn (Martof, 2000).

E X E R C I S E S

1. Suppose that you have census information indicating that the mean income of a population is $37,000 with a standard deviation of $21,000. You wish to draw a sample that will be within $2000 of the true population mean 95 percent of the time. How large a sample would be required?

2. Assuming the same population values as in the above question, determine the sample size required to produce 99 percent confidence that you will be within $2000 of the true mean.

3. If the most complex cross-tabulation table you wish to run in an analysis is a $2 \times 2 \times 2$ table, what sample size would produce 20 expected cases in each cell (assuming breaks at the midpoint)?

4. Suppose you wish to sample staff nurses' opinions of a hospital that has 400 staff nurses. You wish to be 95 percent confident that you will be within 5 percent of estimating the true attitude of the nurses. How large a sample size would you recommend? Show your computations for determining the sample size.

5. You wish to estimate the popular support of a local candidate for political office who is running ahead of the competition. You are asked to do an estimate that will be within 4 percentage points 19 out of 20 times. How large should your sample be?

RECOMMENDED READINGS

Kish, L. (1965). *Survey Sampling.* New York: Wiley.

Konrad, T.R., and De Friese, G.H. (1990). On the subject of sampling. *American Journal of Health Promotion, 5*(2), 147–153.

O'Connell, A. (2000). Sampling for evaluation. *Evaluation and the Health Professions, 23*(2), 212–234.

Polit, D. (1996). *Data Analysis and Statistics.* Stamford, CT: Appleton & Lange.

Polit, D., and Sherman, R.E. (1990). Statistical power in nursing research. *Nursing Research, 39*(6), 365–369.

Having collected the data, it is now time to analyze them. We will approach this task in two ways. We begin with a method of hand tabulating the results and then move on to a discussion of how computers may be used to analyze data.

A. ANALYZING DATA WITHOUT USING A COMPUTER

Some analyses that we do with a computer could also be done easily by hand. And sometimes it is even faster to analyze results manually if one does not have easy access to a computer. Chapters 11 and 12 present a number of statistics that can readily be hand computed if the data set is small. This section provides a method of collecting and processing information from field studies.

1. Manual Analysis of Field Study Data

We will work through a manual analysis of behavior in a hospital emergency waiting room. The student researchers who conducted this naturalistic field study were interested in whether family members in an emergency situation would communicate (signal) the nervousness they felt while waiting for their family member to receive care. "Signaling" was defined as any "nervous and/or unnecessary actions per-

formed by people who feel out of control of the situation at hand." Signaling included such common behaviors as frequent staring or fidgeting with their wrist watches, demanding that the charge nurse have their family member seen immediately by the attending physician, pacing the corridor, or commenting on nervous feelings and concerns to other waiting room clients. Three hypotheses were proposed for the study:

- Females would be more likely to signal than males.
- The more people present in the waiting room, the higher the amount of signaling.
- The closer the family member's relationship to the client, the higher the amount of signaling.

The data were collected on **tally sheets** such as those described in Chapter 7. The student observers indicated on the tally sheet whether or not family members in the waiting room signaled. Also entered on the tally sheet were the gender of each family member, the person's relationship to the family member (i.e., spouse, parent, child, other) and the number of people in the waiting room.

Figure 16.1 illustrates how the tally sheet was set up. Note that each line on the tally sheets records the information for one subject. Column 1 records whether the family member signaled in some way; column 2 records the gender of the family member, column 3 records the number of people present during the observation;

ID #	Signaling		Gender		Relationship				Number in Waiting Room	
	Yes	No	Male	Female	Spouse	Parent	Child	Other	8 or <	9 or >
1		√	√		√				√	
2	√			√	√				√	
3	√			√			√			√
4	√			√						
5 etc.	√		√				√			√

Figure 16.1   Tally sheet for emergency waiting room study.

and column 4 records the relationship of the family member to the client.

Having recorded the information on the sheets for 150 family members, the task now is to analyze the results. One way to do this is to set up a **master table** for the results, enter the observations into the master table, and then derive the results tables from the master table. By using a master table, you will only need to make one pass through the raw data. From the master table you can create any other required tables showing the relationship between the independent variables and the dependent variable. Here are some steps for hand analyzing this type of data.

Step 1. Set up a master table. A master table is generally set up on 8½″ by 14″ paper. Using the paper so that the long side is across the top, arrange the categories of the dependent variable on the left side of the sheet. In this case, the categories "Signal Given" and "No Signal Given" are labels. Categories of the independent variables are arranged across the top of the master table. In this case, we have three independent variables: gender, relationship to client, and number in the emergency waiting room. Each observation ends up in one—and only one—cell of the master table. Thus a mother, who is one of five people in the waiting room, and nervously paces up and down the corridors, would end up in one cell only.

Step 2. Transfer data to the master table. After observations have been completed, the tally sheet data are transferred to the master table. Normally each observation is entered into the applicable cell with a short stroke; these are grouped together so that the fifth line entered into a cell is a line across the other four. Each group then reflects five observations falling into the cell (Fig. 16.2 shows a master table; see Fig. 7.2 for another one). Later these can be counted and a total for each cell entered and circled at the bottom of the cell.

Step 3. Create the individual tables. To test the three hypotheses, three tables would be created, each showing the relationship between signaling or nonsignaling and gender (Table 16.1), rela-

Number	MALE								FEMALE							
Present	8 or less				9 or more				8 or less				9 or more			
Relationship Status	S	P	C	O	S	P	C	O	S	P	C	O	S	P	C	O
Signal Given (tally)	丗丗‖	丗丗丗‖	‖	‖‖‖	‖‖‖‖	‖‖‖‖		‖	丗丗丗‖	丗丗丗‖	‖	‖‖‖	‖‖‖‖	丗‖	‖	‖
Signal Given (total)	12	17	2	3	4	4	0	2	17	16	2	3	4	6	1	2
No signal Given (tally)	‖	‖	‖‖	‖‖‖	‖	‖	‖	‖‖‖‖	丗‖	丗	‖‖‖‖	丗‖	‖‖‖‖	丗‖‖‖‖	‖‖‖	‖‖‖‖
No signal Given (total)	1	1	2	3	1	1	1	4	6	5	4	6	4	9	3	4

Relationship categories: S = Spouse
P = Parent
C = Child
O = Other

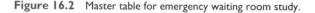

Figure 16.2 Master table for emergency waiting room study.

Table 16.1   Signaling Behavior by Gender

	Gender					
	Male		Female		Total	
Signaling Behavior	N	%	N	%	N	%
Signaling	44	75.9	51	55.4	95	63.3
Nonsignaling	14	24.1	41	44.6	55	36.7
Totals	58	100.0	92	100.0	150	100.0

Chi-square = 6.449; degrees of freedom = 1; probability = < 0.05 (reject null hypothesis).

tionship status, and number of people in the waiting room (Table 16.2). To determine the number of cases for each cell of the new table, you simply add up the count in the appropriate cells of the master table. For example, to find out how many males versus females were seen signaling, one simply adds together the count in all the cells for males (the first eight cells) and then the cells for females (next eight cells). These two numbers would then be incorporated into the number of observations of males and females who signaled. Similar procedures are then followed to get the count on the number of males and females not signaling.

Step 4. Format the tables. Tables 16.1 and 16.2 show the format for two of the tables. Various features of these tables are to be noted:

- **Table title:** The title reports the name of the dependent variable (signaling behavior) followed by the independent variable (group size). Any control variables would follow. Sometimes it is a good idea to report where

and when the observations were made (see Table 16.2).
- **Lines to separate sections of the table:** After the table title, draw two closely spaced lines to separate the table title from the body of the table. Single lines will be used to separate other sections of the table.
- **Independent variable across the top of the page:** Arrange categories of the independent variable (group size) across the top of the table, using easily understood category labels.
- **Dependent variable arranged on the vertical axis:** Notice that the dependent variable (signaling behavior) is arranged along the side of the page. Once again, use labels that are easy to understand and that will communicate clearly to your reader what would be included in each category.
- **Calculate column percentages:** Note also that the percentages are calculated on each of the columns. The rule is to calculate percentages toward the independent variable (adding up to 100 percent on each category of

Table 16.2   Signaling Behavior by Number of People in Hospital Waiting Room

	Number of People					
	Eight or Fewer		Nine or More		Total	
Signaling Behavior	N	%	N	%	N	%
Signaling	72	72.0	23	46.0	95	63.3
Nonsignaling	28	28.0	27	54.0	55	36.7
Totals	100	100.0	50	100.0	150	100.0

the independent variable). For example, if we wished to calculate the appropriate percentages for looking at the relationship between gender (independent variable) and signaling (dependent variable), we would calculate what percentage of males signal or do not signal. We would then do a similar calculation for the females. In this way, we can compare the percentage of males signaling with the percentage of females doing likewise. The reason you would not calculate the percentage toward the dependent variable is that we are not so much interested in the distribution of signaling by gender (we might have a different proportion of males and females in our sample and therefore more males might signal simply because there were more male family members present in the waiting room).

Occasionally tables are created when the percentages are run across the page; this is usually done to accommodate situations in which there are a number of categories of the independent variable and, in order to have enough space, the table is turned sideways.

To calculate the percentage, divide the cell value by the marginal total (this is the column total if the dependent variable is arranged on the vertical axis) and multiply by 100. In Table 16.1, the first cell percentage would be calculated by $(44 \div 58) \times 100 = 75.9$ percent. These percentages should be reported to an accuracy of one decimal point. The total should report the actual total—either 99.9, 100.0, or 100.1.

- **More complex tables:** More complex tables containing control variables may also be created from the master table. However, before constructing such tables, the materials in Chapter 17 should be consulted in order to establish what model is being tested

and how the results should be interpreted. For ease of interpretation, arrange the dependent variable along the vertical axis, with categories of the independent variables on the horizontal axis.

Step 5. Calculate tests of significance and measures of association. Tests of significance and measures of association may be calculated manually. Chapter 12 provides examples of how such computations may be done. The results of these computations may be entered below the table, as shown in Table 16.1.

Step 6. Interpret the results. In interpreting the results of the analysis, we typically focus on just one of the categories of the dependent variable; in the case of the emergency waiting room study, we would simply compare the percentage of males who are seen to signal in the waiting room with the percentage of females who are seen to do likewise. In the case of Table 16.1, we would note that "although 75.9 percent of the males signal, 55.4 percent of the females signal." It is unnecessary to report the "Not Signal" categories because these are simply the remaining cases adding up to 100.0 percent. The writer of a report should also note whether the differences between the gender categories are statistically significant, whether the differences observed were in the direction predicted in the hypotheses, and report on any measures of the strength of the association. A chi-square test of significance could have been performed on this data using the procedures outlined in Chapter 12 (see Box 12.4).

2. Manual Analysis of Experimental and Survey Data

Using the manual analysis procedures outlined in Chapters 11 and 12, it should be possible for the researcher to analyze experimental and survey data without using a computer. Suppose you do a between-subjects experiment; you could compute the dependent variable *means* and *standard deviations* for your treatment group and for your control group (see Chapter 11 for information on calculating means and standard deviations).

Box 12.5 may be used as a model to calculate a between-subjects t test. If you have a within-subject design, refer to Box 12.6. If you require a one-way analysis of variance, use Box 12.7 as a model. If you require an ANOVA, you will probably find that it will save time to enter the values into a computer and have the machine, equipped with appropriate software such as Statistical Package for the Social Sciences (**SPSS**), do the calculations.

Although survey type data could be analyzed by recording the information on a master table, generally the number of variables measured is substantial and it would usually be advisable to learn how to use a computer to process the information. However, if there are just a few variables measured, even with a large number of cases, it is possible to transfer the information to a master table and then derive cross-tabular tables from it. But if you wanted to calculate means, standard deviations, or correlations among the variables, the chore of hand computing the results would be onerous unless there were few cases in the study. In most situations, use of computer technology is advised.

B. ANALYZING DATA USING A COMPUTER

The remaining sections of this chapter apply if a computer is to be used to assist in the analysis. Although this process is relatively straightforward, there are a number of points to keep in mind so that data entry and error checking will proceed efficiently.

In most cases, the contemporary researcher will be working either on a personal computer (PC) or Macintosh (MAC) or on a terminal that is connected to a computer network. Students need not understand much about computers in order to use them—just as you do not need to know much about engines in order to drive a car.

A simple analogy that has been found useful by past students with minimal computer experience introduce readers to computers. ("Cyber space cadets" may skip the next paragraph.)

Think of entering a large, strange house. It is a little frightening at first, but after a while you will find that it is fun exploring it. The first thing you will have to do is get inside. You will need a key, such as a secret password, in order to enter. Let us imagine that you have been provided with a password so you can get into the house. Looking down the hall, you realize that there are many rooms in this house. The hall represents the computer's operating system; there are many procedures and utilities available to the user in the various rooms. Having entered the house, you now have to decide which room to explore. The first room is marked *Editor;* here you can make and modify files. The second room is marked *Storage;* you can save files here and get them later. A third door is marked *SPSS;* nursing research data are analyzed here. A fourth door is marked *Word Processing;* here reports are written and modified. A fifth door is marked *Printing;* here files get copied onto paper so that they will be available to the user. There are many other doors in the house, but these need not be explored immediately by beginning research students.

Before suggestions are given for the entry of data into a computer, we need to introduce the idea of *files.* When data, or the text of a report, are entered into a computer, they are stored in a file. Computer files are just like those found in a filing cabinet, they contain information on some topic and are arranged so that they can be retrieved easily. Many computers use a two-word naming convention for files. The first part consists of the file name and type, and the second part consists of the file extension. The two parts are separated by a ".". Typically, one is allowed eight character spaces for the file name and type with the last three characters before the "." representing the file type and the three characters after the "." the file extension. For the data collected in a study, one might use the name JOAN-DAT.SPS. If Joan were involved in a number of studies, she would need to use unique names for each of them. However, she would always use the same file type label for data—perhaps "SPS". Later, we will need to know about other kinds of files, so additional file types will be introduced then.

Contemporary nursing students usually use computers that are using Microsoft Windows operating systems. Typically students control the computer by using keystrokes and by manipulating the mouse to point and click on desired options. For purposes of this book, we will assume that the computer used is also equipped with a Windows version of SPSS.

The Statistical Package for the Social Sciences is undoubtedly the most popular, and widely available, statistical package used by social scientists. It was developed in the 1960s, has gone through a series of embellishments over the years, and now contains a great number of statistical and data manipulation procedures. There are versions for mainframe computers (SPSS^x), personal computers (SPSS/PC+), and versions that take advantage of the capabilities of Microsoft Windows. The version featured in this Appendix is the one designed for Windows and it is known as SPSS for Windows (Version 10.0).

A number of manuals are available from SPSS that detail the many additional features and options that are available for the various commands. Some of these manuals are listed at the end of Appendix A; you

may wish to consult them as you develop your facility in working with SPSS.

I. Using SPSS for Windows (Version 10.0)

You will probably be using the point-and-click method of issuing the various SPSS commands. A few general tips for this method include:

- After each procedure is run, the results are sent to the SPSS Viewer, which will be displayed on your monitor. You can save, edit, and print your results from the SPSS Viewer.
- To select one variable. simply click on it when it is highlighted.
- To select multiple variables from a list, hold down the Ctrl button and click on the variables.
- To start using SPSS, turn on a computer that is using a Windows operating system and is equipped with SPSS for Windows. After you are logged on, you are ready to start.

a. To Begin an SPSS Session

- Click on **Start.**
- Point to **Programs.**
- Point and click on **SPSS.**

A screen similar to the one shown in Figure 16.3 should now appear on your monitor. Note that there are a number of blank cells displayed on the screen. You could start a new SPSS file by entering data at this point or you could access an existing SPSS file. We will begin by accessing an SPSS file that has the data entered.

b. To Access an Existing SPSS File

- Click on **File.**
- Click on **Open.**

A screen will now appear (Fig. 16.4) and you identify the location of the file

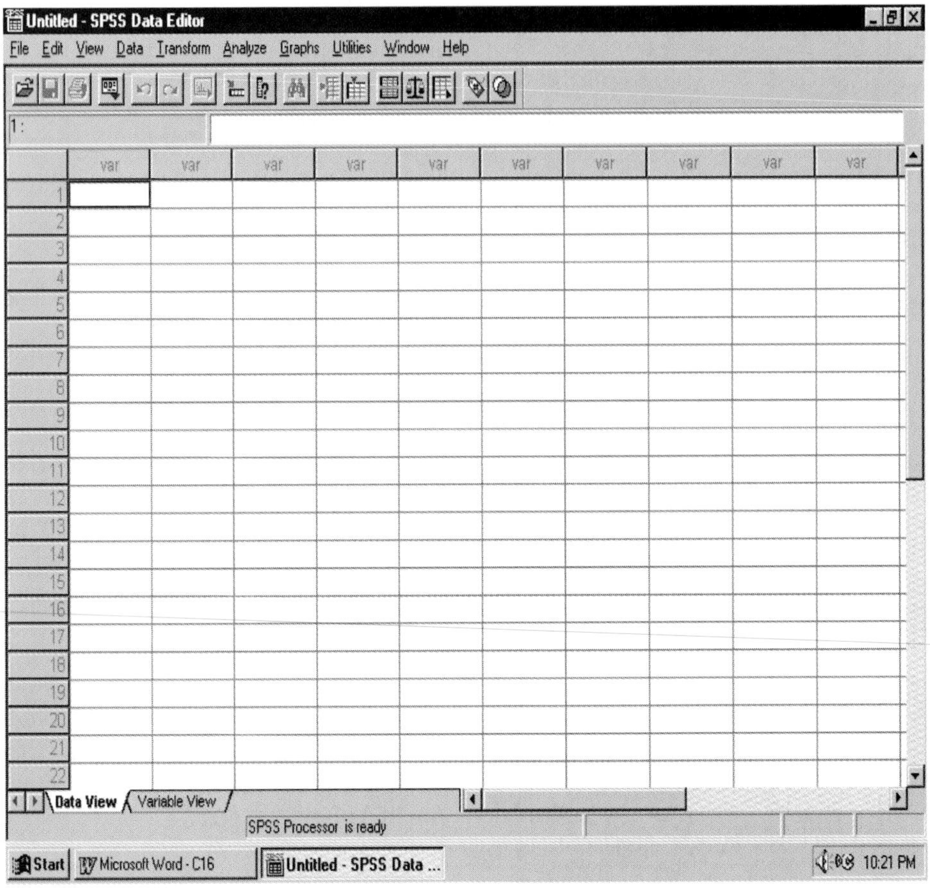

Figure 16.3 SPSS opening image.

and its name. You may need to specify where the file is located as well as its name. For our practice sessions, we will assume the file is called **C:\internl.sav.** After you enter the name of the required file (**C:\internl.sav**), click on **OK.**

The blank boxes on the screen grid will now be filled with numbers and you are now ready to begin analyzing the data set. This is a data set collected from social research methods students in Canada, New Zealand, and Australia. The questionnaire used to collect the information is included in Appendix B of the text. Figure 16.5 displays the screen after the **C:\internl.sav** has been accessed.

There are two methods of using SPSS:

- The **point-and-click** method, which simply involves choosing options from among those provided on a screen menu and clicking on them
- The **syntax** method, which involves typing in SPSS commands

c. Using the Point-and-Click Menu Method

Assuming you now have the SPSS file loaded (see Fig. 16.5), you now must decide what procedures you wish to run on the data. Here are some of the basic things you might want to do (click on that standard toolbar item and then click on each item in the order listed).

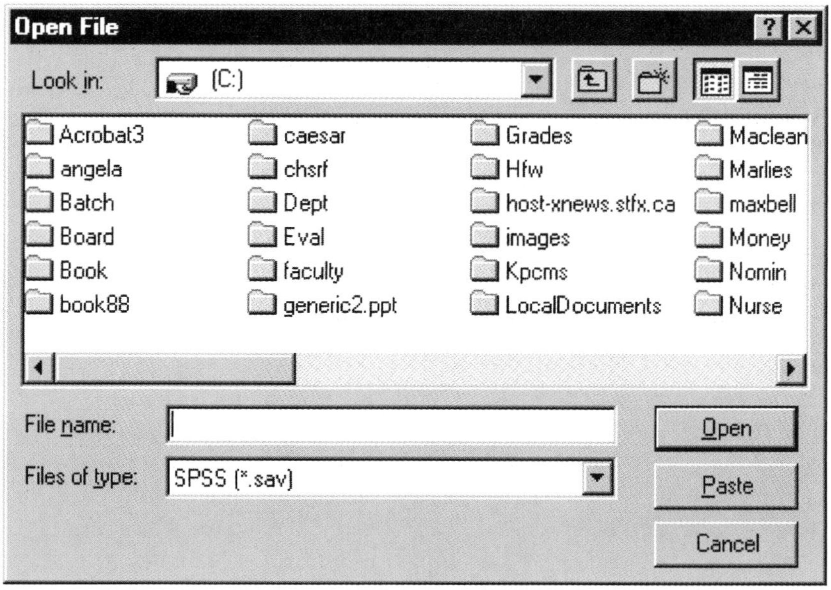

Figure 16.4 SPSS: getting the file.

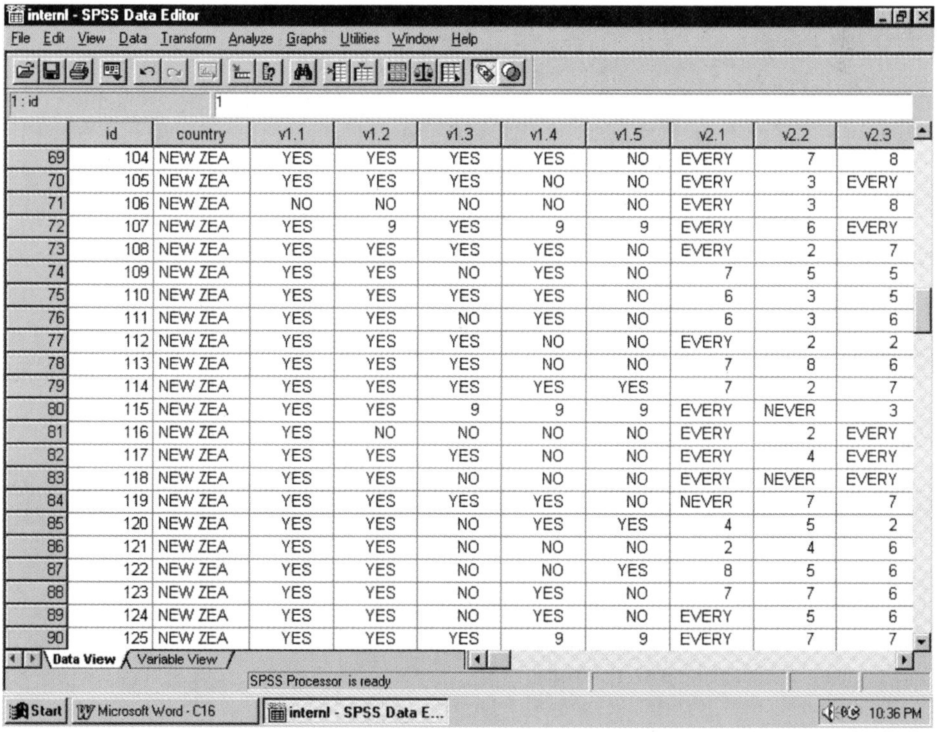

	id	country	v1.1	v1.2	v1.3	v1.4	v1.5	v2.1	v2.2	v2.3
69	104	NEW ZEA	YES	YES	YES	YES	NO	EVERY	7	8
70	105	NEW ZEA	YES	YES	YES	NO	NO	EVERY	3	EVERY
71	106	NEW ZEA	NO	NO	NO	NO	NO	EVERY	3	8
72	107	NEW ZEA	YES	9	YES	9	9	EVERY	6	EVERY
73	108	NEW ZEA	YES	YES	YES	YES	NO	EVERY	2	7
74	109	NEW ZEA	YES	YES	NO	YES	NO	7	5	5
75	110	NEW ZEA	YES	YES	YES	YES	NO	6	3	5
76	111	NEW ZEA	YES	YES	NO	YES	NO	6	3	6
77	112	NEW ZEA	YES	YES	YES	NO	NO	EVERY	2	2
78	113	NEW ZEA	YES	YES	YES	NO	NO	7	8	6
79	114	NEW ZEA	YES	YES	YES	YES	YES	7	2	7
80	115	NEW ZEA	YES	YES	9	9	9	EVERY	NEVER	3
81	116	NEW ZEA	YES	NO	NO	NO	NO	EVERY	2	EVERY
82	117	NEW ZEA	YES	YES	YES	NO	NO	EVERY	4	EVERY
83	118	NEW ZEA	YES	YES	NO	NO	NO	EVERY	NEVER	EVERY
84	119	NEW ZEA	YES	YES	YES	YES	NO	NEVER	7	7
85	120	NEW ZEA	YES	YES	NO	YES	YES	4	5	2
86	121	NEW ZEA	YES	YES	NO	NO	NO	2	4	6
87	122	NEW ZEA	YES	YES	NO	NO	YES	8	5	6
88	123	NEW ZEA	YES	YES	NO	YES	NO	7	7	6
89	124	NEW ZEA	YES	YES	NO	YES	NO	EVERY	5	6
90	125	NEW ZEA	YES	YES	YES	9	9	EVERY	7	7

Figure 16.5 SPSS: filled screen.

ANOVA: Analyze/General Linear Model/Univariate
CORRELATE: Analyze/Correlate/Bivariate
CROSS-TABS: Analyze/Descriptive Statistics/Cross-tabs
DESCRIPTIVES: Analyze/Descriptive Statistics/Descriptives
DISCRIMINANT: Analyze/Classify/Discriminant
FACTOR: Data Reduction/Factor
FREQUENCIES: Analyze/Descriptive Statistics/Frequencies
GRAPHS: Graphs/Scatter/Define
MANOVA: Analyze/General Linear Model/Multivariate
MEANS: Analyze/Compare Means/Means
SPEARMAN CORRELATION: Analyze/Correlation/ Spearman
REGRESSION: Analyze/Regression/Linear (Method = Backward)
RELIABILITY: Analyze/Scale/Reliability (Model=Alpha)
t TEST PAIRS: Analyze/Compare Means/Paired-Samples t Test
t TEST GROUPS: Analyze/Compare Means/Independent Samples t Test

Some other basic procedures that you will need to know are:

COMPUTE: Transform/Compute
IF: Transform/Compute
LIST: Use Syntax Editor to issue command
RECODE: Transform/Recode/Into Different Variables
SORT CASES: Data/Sort Cases
SELECT CASES: Data/Select Cases

Appendix A discusses each of the above procedures and provides guidelines for interpreting the output that results from each analysis. Note that the SPSS Windows version uses the following file types:

- .sav an SPSS windows **system file** (when you access a .sav file, the data will show on the SPSS Data Editor screen). A system file contains all of your data and all of the labels describing the variables in your file.
- .sps an SPSS Windows **syntax file** (when you access an .sps file, you are automatically in the Syntax Editor). Syntax files are used to contain instruction commands that are then sent to SPSS for processing.
- .spo an SPSS Windows **output file** (when you access an .spo file, you are automatically in the SPSS Viewer Editor). An output file contains the results of your analyses. You can modify, print, or copy these files to a word processor.

d. Using the Syntax Method

In the syntax method, the user types in the desired commands. This method appeals to experienced SPSS users who know SPSS commands and the command structure. New users will probably find it easier to use the "point-and-click" approach. To use the Syntax method, follow these steps:

- Click on **File**
- Click on **New**
- Click on **Syntax**

Now a blank screen should appear and you simply type the commands onto the screen. Remember that after each command is completed, you must end the line with a period (.) Having entered the commands, you can then position the cursor (the flashing vertical line) where you wish SPSS to begin processing. To have SPSS process the commands, do this:

- Click on **Run**
- Click to choose from among options shown

It is a good idea to maintain a copy of the syntax files used. If data errors are found or if additional data are added to the file later, then the syntax files can simply be resubmitted to SPSS without having to go through the whole process a second time. When you leave the program, you will be asked if you wish to save a copy of the syntax file; if you respond "yes," you will also be given an opportunity to name the file.

2. Data Entry

Data entry is simply the process of transferring the information collected in a study to a computing device. In survey research projects, which include a large number of variables, it is usually best to enter the data into a word processor such as Word or WordPerfect. Later you can highlight the text, and using the Edit/Copy command, paste it into an SPSS syntax file. Alternatively, data may be entered directly into the Syntax Editor that is part of SPSS for Windows. Using the Syntax Editor has the advantage of being able to enter all the data on one line for each case as opposed to having to use two or more lines if you have quite a few variables. The Syntax Editor approach is the preferable one, especially if you have a large survey to process.

We will assume that you have figured out how to use one of the above approaches and you are now ready to begin data entry. The following rules provide guidelines for data entry if you are creating a separate raw data file.

a. Creating a Separate Raw Data File

Guideline 1. Number the questionnaires, forms, and data sources. Questionnaires or data collection forms are numbered, normally beginning with 001 (or 0001 if there are more than 1000 cases). This *ID number* is written on the front page of the instrument (usually the top right-hand corner). This number will be entered into the computer and provides the only link between the particular form and the data that are entered into the computer file. If an error is found in the data, the original form can be located by using the ID number, the information can be checked, and the error can be corrected. Keep the questionnaires or forms sorted by their ID number.

Guideline 2. Code any uncoded questions. If there are questions that have not been precoded (e.g., occupational codes or open-ended opinion questions), they should now be coded and the values written on the questionnaire (or form) in the margin next to the question. In the case of occupational prestige codes, they would be looked up and a value entered onto the questionnaire.

Guideline 3. Do a column count. Using a blank copy of the questionnaire (or form), go through it, and, opposite each question, indicate where it will be entered onto the terminal screen. Typically, screen widths are 80 columns wide. This means that you can enter 80 digits across the screen before you run out of space. Thus, if you were entering your data into a Word file, you would need to start a second line of data for the questionnaire if it exceeds 80 characters. If you are using SPSS for Windows, you need not worry about the screen width; the Syntax Editor will allow you to use as many columns as is necessary for your data set.

The first three columns will be used for the ID number of the questionnaire, and the fourth column will be used to identify the record number for the respondent. (This is required only for questionnaires that require more than 80 columns to enter the data. Record #1 refers to the first line of data, record #2 the next set of data for the respondent, and so forth. The ID number is repeated on each line of data followed by the record number.) If a question can have values between zero and nine, then one column will be required to record the data; if the values range up to 99, then two columns will be required; if the values range up to 999, three columns will be required. On the right-hand margin of the questionnaire (or form), these values are recorded. The right-hand margin might look something like this:

Variable	Columns
ID	1–3
Record #	4
Blank	5
Gender	6
Yr of Birth	7–8
Income	9–14
Occupation	15–16

In a short questionnaire, the informa-tion for each variable will fit onto one 80-column line; each questionnaire will occupy one line of data. If more than one record (or line) is required, then a second record is used, with the first three columns being saved for a repeat of the ID number. The fourth column will contain a "2," meaning that it is the second record for the questionnaire. In the case of a questionnaire requiring two records, the data might be set in a way similar to the example below:

```
0011476989232333 2322211112221111 222456345644556666663339
0012453437676722112222111 1122299122876321453213345222
0021456338992212 212221132221112 22334110033445565443221 1
0022234343445857463748 4985050595211222333423334444
```

Note the first four columns. The first three contain the ID number (which has also been written on the questionnaire), and the fourth column refers to the record number. What we have here is respondent 001 first record; then the same respondent 001, second record; this is followed by respondent 002, first record, followed by respondent 002, second record. It is not critical that the ID numbers be in sequence, but the case must be together—record 1 must be followed by record 2 for each case The reason we enter the ID number and then the record number is that most computers' sorting routines will be able to sort your file with one simple command. The blanks in the data set are discussed below.

Guideline 4. Enter data with the help of a partner. Inexperienced computer users will find that data entry will be much easier and will be done with fewer errors if two people work together on entering the data. One person can read the numbers off the questionnaire, and the partner can enter the values into the computer.

Guideline 5. Leave internal blanks to mark a new page. Errors can be identified more quickly if, after the end of each page in the questionnaire, a blank is left in the data. The column of blanks must always line up when the data are printed out; if the blanks do not line up, then an error has been made and must be corrected. The first six lines of a data set are listed in the following example, showing how the blanks line up:

page 1	page 2	page 3	page 4

```
00112435445523 211212333448976999 123232111123212 23411112
0021123123I234 3222132221222322I2 43223533321I232 34532432
0031432I234443 2334453244333212I2 332122341122233 23323222
00413444688822 12222211223212332I9 234433221222321 34521211
00513335543221 2233322211141242I1 3321114221I1212 32121223
00614322345432 2311433211221221 21 11221I222111231 22132454
```

Note that the fourth line of data contains an error; by examining the listing, it becomes apparent that the error is somewhere in the data entered from page two of the questionnaire (there are too many digits in the space reserved for page two). The introduction of blanks to mark the end of pages is enormously helpful in error detection, so researchers should be sure to use them.

Guideline 6. Simplify missing value codes. If respondents do not answer a question or if a question is not applicable, a **missing value code** is used. These should be kept as simple and as consistent as possible. When possible, use the values 9, 99, or 999 for variables that require one, two, or three columns, respectively. Suppose a respondent is asked to indicate gender as either male or female and leaves the question blank. Instead of leaving the column blank, a 9 would be inserted into the appropriate column. See Appendix A for additional details on missing values.

Although it is possible to use alternate codes (when a question is not answered or a question is not applicable), such as "8" for not answered and "9" for not applicable, such discrimination should only be made where it is known that the information will be used later; if it is not going to be used, keep matters simple by using the single code "9" to cover both cases. In occupational codes, it may be necessary to provide special codes for "housewife" if values are not provided in the occupational code system being used. For the nine-point Likert attitudinal scales, 0 is used for the missing value code.

A code must be entered for every question, even if it is not answered. The reason for this is that when instructions are given to the computer, each question is identified with particular columns in the data; each question, therefore, must be in the identical position in all lines of data. (Actually, most programs allow the use of a space or a comma to separate questions but because error detection is easiest when questions occupy the identical columns in each question, we will use the same-column method.)

Guideline 7. Document research decisions. When data are being entered into a computer, a number of decisions are required. A questionnaire may have a lot of missing data, and the person entering the data might decide that it would be better to discard the questionnaire. When this happens, the questionnaire or form should be set aside and fellow researchers should be consulted to determine whether that data should be used. Cases may arise in which a respondent has checked two items on a question when only one was expected. Generally, these discrepancies are rare enough for it to be appropriate to "flip a coin" to decide which of the two will be taken. (One would not systematically take the highest placed item on the list because that would systematically bias the results toward those items listed first.) When such a decision has been made, the decision should be marked clearly on the questionnaire and initialed by the person making the decision. With such documentation, it is then possible for others to check through the data and understand what coding decisions were made and by whom.

Guideline 8. Code for information not on the questionnaire. Frequently, there will be information that is not coded on the questionnaire that should be appended to the data. It is always recommended that provision be made to include a code to identify who collected the original information, who did the coding on the questionnaire, who did the data entry, and any other information that may be useful in the later data analysis or in error checking. The reason why it is helpful to code who did the coding is that if there are systematic differences between coders in dealing with different questions, then the cases dealt with by each coder can quickly be identified and compared. Appropriate corrections can then be made without too much trouble.

Guideline 9. Use double data entry. When resources allow, it is recommended that different individuals enter data twice. A computer program can then be used to compare the two files, flagging any differences between the files. This technique is extremely helpful in reducing data entry errors.

Guideline 10. Save the data. When data entry is complete, save the file as an ASCII or DOS file (if using WordPerfect, use Ctrl F5 and Save; if using Microsoft Word, use the Save As command; on the Save As window, click on Text Only). Alternatively, you can highlight the data and do an Edit/Copy on it and then do an Edit/Paste of the data into a syntax file. If you have entered the data into a syntax file in SPSS, save it as an .SPS file, which will allow for easy entry into the Syntax Editor. (Saving the file is easy; when you exit from the program, SPSS will ask you if you wish to save the file. Simply respond "yes" and provide a name for the file. The machine will automatically append .SPS to the file name, indicating that this is an SPSS syntax file.)

Guideline 11. Error checking. This is a process used to locate and correct errors in the data before data analysis. Programs are available for identifying out-of-range entries and for locating non-numerics, such as O for 0, or a l (lowercase letter "l") instead of a 1 (one). If you have access to such a utility program, use it.

b. Point-and-Click Raw Data Entry

If the data are being entered directly into SPSS, click on File/New/Data, move the cursor to the cell you wish to start with (the cell will be highlighted), and enter the data for each variable moving across the row. The value will show on the screen just above the matrix. To move from variable to variable after the value has been entered, either hit the Tab key or the right arrow key to move from case to case and use the down arrow key after the value has been entered.

(i) Inserting a New Case

If you wish to add a new case, position the cursor on the case below where you want to insert the new case. On the toolbar, click on Data and then Insert Case. Enter the data for the new case.

(ii) Inserting a New Variable

If you wish to add a new variable, position the cursor on the variable after the spot where you want to insert the new variable. On the toolbar, click on Data and then Insert Variable. Enter the data for the new variable for all the cases. Note that if you do not enter any value for a case, the system will add a "."indicating that this case has a MISSING VALUE.

3. Creating and Saving an SPSS.sav File

If you have a modest to large survey to process, it is probably worth learning how to use the Syntax Editor to enter the commands to define the variables, attach labels, and indicate the missing value codes. Variable lists may be used to give many variables the same labels (e.g., yes or no questions). Lists may also be used to identify variables with the same missing values. This approach to data entry is described below under the section called "The Syntax Method." If the data being analyzed involve just a few variables (< 10 or 15), the direct entry method may be used comfortably. This approach will be described under the "Point-and-Click Method" section.

a. Point-and-Click Method for Creating and Saving an SPSS System File

Hit File, then New, then Data. A screen with blank cells will now appear. Click on Variable View tab at the bottom of the data screen. Your first task will be to name each variable. Usually we start with an ID as the first variable name and it will give us a place to enter the number for the questionnaire (or observation form); these should correspond to the number written in the top left-hand corner of the questionnaire. Figure 16.6 shows the appropriate window.

(i) Defining and Labeling Variables

At the bottom of the Data Editor screen, there are tabs for Variable View and for Data View. Click on the Variable View tab, and the screen will display the variables along the vertical axis of the screen. The definable characteristics are arranged along the top of the screen. By clicking on one of the characteristics, Labels for example, you can then attach the labels for that particular variable. On the gender variable, you would attach the labels "Male" and " Female."

Hint: In studies with a lot of variables (as in most surveys), it is a good idea to use the question numbers for variable names. Because the names must begin with an alphabetical character, it makes sense to call them v1, v2, v3, and so on. For multipart questions, use v4.1, v4.2, v4.3, and so on. When analyzing data, you can quickly find the variable names by just looking at the questionnaire.

(ii) Missing Values

See Guideline 6 for suggestions on the treatment of missing values. It is best to use 9, 99, 99.9, and so on to indicate values to indicate a refusal to answer a question or to indicate a question that does not apply to a respondent. If it is going to be relevant to distinguish the reason for the missing value, other code numbers may be applied. If you are using the syntax approach to defining the missing values, a variable list is made up for each missing value. If the point-and-click approach is used, declare the missing value when the variable labels are attached.

Hint: In large surveys, if the point-and-click approach is used to define the variable, it speeds up the process to put on value labels and missing values after the .sav file has been created. Simply put on the variable names and labels, save the file, enter the Syntax Editor, and enter the VALUE LABELS and MISSING VALUES,

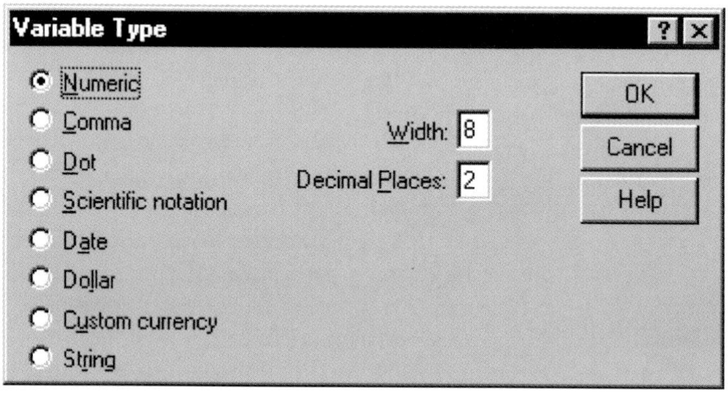

Figure 16.6   SPSS: defining variables.

and then save the output. Because variable lists may be used for VALUE LABELS and MISSING VALUES, it is much quicker to do these in the Syntax Editor.

Hint: You can change the default settings for variables (type of variable, size of field) by clicking on the Variable View (bottom of screen), select the case you would like to have similar settings, do an Edit/Copy, then highlight the variables you want it applied to and do an Edit/Paste and those definitions will be applied to the cases that that have been highlighted. For example, if you are dealing with survey data and most variables are one character wide, you would reset the defaults to show Numeric 1, MISSING VALUES as 9. Only when you encounter 2 column variables would you have to redefine the settings for these variables.

(iii) Saving or Updating the SPSS System File: The .sav File

Whenever you wish to save or update your SPSS system file, click on the toolbar File and click on Save. You will be able then to specify where you want it saved and change the name of the file if you wish. Anytime you compute new variables or transform old ones, you may want to save the changes, so remember to update the file with the Save procedure. Be certain to maintain backup copies of your .sav file on disks as well as on the hard drive of your computer.

b. *The Syntax Method of Creating and Saving an SPSS System File*

In order to use the syntax procedure to create a system file, access the Syntax Editor:

- Click on **File**
- Click on **New**
- Click on **Syntax**

Now a blank screen should appear. Simply type the commands onto the screen. For researchers who are familiar with the SPSS command structure, the main difference between what you are familiar with and the Windows versions is that you have to remember that after each command is completed, you must end the line with a period. After entering the commands, you can then position the cursor (the flashing vertical line) where you wish SPSS to begin processing. To have SPSS process the commands do this:

- Click on **Run**
- Click to choose from among options shown

It is a good idea to maintain a copy of the various syntax files used. If data errors are found or if additional data are added to the file later, then the syntax files can simply be resubmitted without having to think through the whole process a second time.

Box 16.1 shows the command structure that will identify, name, and label all the variables in a study. A key shortcut to remember is that data lists may be used when several variables have the same labels. This saves the researcher from entering labels more than once. Examples of the various commands necessary to define an SPSS system file are shown in Box 16.1. This method is probably the quickest one for data sets involving many variables and many cases. Smaller data sets can be entered directly using the point-and-click method discussed in the preceding section.

(i) Saving or Updating the SPSS System File: The .sav File

Whenever you wish to save or update your SPSS system file, click on the toolbar File and then on Save. Then you will be able to specify where you want it saved and change the name of the file if you wish. Anytime you compute new variables or transform old ones, you may want to save the changes, so remember to update the file with the Save procedure. Be certain to maintain backup

---

BOX 16.1 *Sample Syntax Commands to Create an SPSS System File*

Title system file creation, Nursing Faculty Review, Winston
Data list file = 'C:\oia\nursing\nursedat.sps' Records = 1
/id 1–5 v1 8 v2 9 v3 10 v4 12 v4.1 to v4.7 13–19 v5 20 v6 22 v8 23 v9.1 to v9.6 24–29 v10 to v12
30–32 v13 34 v16 35 v17 36 v18.1 to v18.5 37–41.
Variable labels id "identification number"
/v1 "Year of Graduation"
/v2 "Program"
/v3 "Honors Thesis"
/v4 "Further Education"
/v5 "Current Employment"
/v6 "Employed in Field of Choice"
/v8 "Different Field of Study"
/v9.1 "Quality of Content for Nursing"/ v9.2 "Quality of Instruction for Nursing"
/v18.4 "Audio-Visual Aids"
/v18.5 "Quiet Study Space"
value labels /v1 0 "1995 or earlier" 1 "1996" 2 "1997"
3"1998" 4 "1999" 5 "2000" 6 "2001" 7 "2002" 8 "2003"
/v2 1 "Major" 2 "Advanced Major" 3 "Honors"
/v4 0 "Yes" 1 "No"
/v4.1 to v4.5 0 "No" 1 "Yes"
missing values v1, v2, v3, v4, v4.1 to v4.5, v5, v6, v8, v13 (9)
/v4.5, v4.6, v9.1 to v9.6, v10 to v12, v16, v17, v18.1 to v18.5 (0).
Frequencies var= v1.

---

copies of your .sav file on disks as well as on the hard drive of your computer.

4. Data Cleaning Using SPSS

After the data have been entered into the computer and saved in a file, it is time to begin the systematic search for errors so they can be corrected before analysis of the data begins. This process is referred to as **cleaning the data.** If you have specialized software, then you would proceed by using this program. (The instructor's manual contains a program for detecting non-numerics, and out-of-range entries.) If you do not have access to such data cleaning programs, the following steps will help you detect errors in the data.

Step 1. Assuming you have entered the data into a file, the first job is to list

that file on a printer. The printout should be examined and any irregularities circled. Check the following:
- All lines must end in the same column. If there are too few or too many columns in a line, it means that questions were either missed or entered twice. Mark discrepant lines so that they can be checked against the original questionnaire and the errors located. The file must be "rectangular" with no ragged edges.
- Any internal blanks must line up vertically. If end-of-page blanks have been used, one can quickly identify situations in which there have been too many or too few entries made from a particular page on the questionnaire. Once again, mark any discrepancies.
- When there are two or more files to

be checked, ensure that the file lengths are equal. For example, if 165 questionnaires have been completed, there must be 165 lines in each of the files.

- Proofread ID numbers (columns one through three) to ensure that there are no repeated or missing ID numbers. Again, mark any errors. (Some cases may have been withdrawn, so those ID values will be missing.)
- Finally, there must be no blank lines or partial lines left in the data set. (SPSS reads a blank line as a case and assigns a missing value to all variables. If you find that you always have one or two missing cases even though you know there should be none on certain variables, your problem may be that you have blank lines somewhere in your data file.)

Step 2. When the file that includes the variable labels and other file definition commands is run, SPSS will alert you to any inappropriate non-numerics in your raw data file. The output will indicate which case has the problem. Note the case numbers, examine your data, and make corrections to the data. Sometimes you will have included non-numeric data intentionally but may have forgotten to indicate this on your DATA LIST commands. Remember, you can use non-numerics, but when identified on the DATA LIST command you must put an "(A)" after the column numbers for the variable, as in "v27 17–18, **v28 19–40 (A),** v29 to v31 41–43."

Step 3. On all nominal and ordinal data, run the frequencies procedure. Examine the output (you need not print it out at this point because you are simply scanning it for errors), looking for any categories that are not labeled or any out-of-range values for that variable. For example, on the gender variable, there should be only two categories, one for male respondents and one for females. If there are any other

values included, the case must be identified and the data corrected before you proceed with further analysis. To locate the problem case (or cases), go to the SPSS grid with your data listed and click on the column (top of grid) where the variable name is identified; the whole column should then be highlighted. If you want to find a 3 in your gender variable, click on the icon for find (binoculars) and tell the machine to find 3. The machine will now highlight the problem case. Note the case number listed under ID, go to your sorted pile of questionnaires, and find the questionnaire with the same ID number and note the value that should be included for gender. Correct the value by highlighting the gender cell for the case in error by entering a 2 or a 1 as appropriate. While doing this check, make certain that the missing values are properly flagged as missing. In the case of the gender variable, 9s probably were used as the missing value code, make certain any 9s are flagged as missing on the frequency distribution. But note that if there are no missing cases for a variable, the frequencies will not list the category for missing values.

Continue checking the frequency distributions looking for out-of-range entries, correcting them as you go along. It is a good idea to keep a record of these changes and then go back to your raw data file and correct that file as well.

Step 4. The ratio variables should be listed on the descriptives' window (Analyze/Descriptive Statistics/Descriptives). Check the lowest and highest values for each variable. Are they within range? Note especially that the MISSING value is not listed as the highest value. If it is, you have made an error in your missing values. Problem cases may be identified by bringing up the SPSS data grid, highlight the variable that has an error, and use the binoculars icon to find the value you wish to find. Corrections may be made directly on the SPSS grid, but should also be made in the raw data file.

Hint: If you make the corrections in the raw data file, you can resubmit the MAKER file (i.e., the one containing the data list, variable labels, and so on) and this will update your SPSS System file.

Step 5. After correcting the errors, you are now ready to proceed with your analysis.

5. Steps in Analyzing Data for a Project

When doing your analysis, it is a good idea to use the Paste command to save the procedures you have run in a Syntax file. The reason for this is that if you have errors in your data and it becomes necessary to re-run a job after corrections have been made, you can then quickly re-submit your jobs without having to re-think your whole analysis.

Step 1. Be certain to have the questionnaire or the recording form on which you have recorded the column numbers for each variable, printouts of your FREQUENCIES (nominal and ordinal variables) and DESCRIPTIVES (ratio variables) with you. If you have not run these analyses, run them.

Step 2. If you need to construct any indexes, it should be done at this point. Review the procedures for creating indexes (see Chapter 13); if you are using RELIABILITY, click on the appropriate icons to do the job, and determine the items that are to go into the index. Do a COMPUTE to create the index. Add VARIABLE LABELS (and VALUE LABELS, if appropriate). Save the SPSS (.sav) file so that the next time you sign on, the new variable (or variables) will be available.

Step 3. Examine your causal models. Select the appropriate procedures for testing the models. Do the procedures to test the various relationships indicated by the model. Note that you may need to RECODE some variables. If most of the relationships are examined using one method (say MEANS), you should probably do all of them using that procedure, even though a few could be examined using correlations. Enter the commands to do the basic runs and, if recoding of variables has been done, retain the recodes for future use by updating your system file by clicking on **File/Save.**

Hint: When doing RECODES, create a new variable to contain the information and add an "r" to the name of the original variable. For example, if you recode v9, call the new variable v9r; using this method will remind you that any variable name with an "r" appended to it is a recoded version of the original variable.

Step 4. If you have any intervening or sources of spuriousness models, these should be processed. Review Chapter 17 for suggestions on interpreting results.

Step 5. After you have assembled the computer output, you should consider how you will present the results. (See various summary tables in Chapter 19 for possible ways of setting up your tables for presentation.) Note that it is helpful, particularly in small sample studies, to indicate whether the trends in various relationships go in the directions predicted.

Step 6. Write your report in sections, following the outline suggested in Chapter 19.

6. The 3M Approach to Selecting Analysis Procedure

As a way to remember how to decide which procedure to use to analyze any relationship, use the three steps in the **3M approach.**

Step 1. Model. The first step is to decide which variable is to be treated as the dependent variable and which one as the independent variable. Because the researcher typically is trying to understand what causes variations in a dependent variable, common sense alone can generally determine which variable should be designated as the dependent variable. However, there are other cases where it is not obvious. In such cases, try to decide which variable occurs last in a temporal sequence. It is entirely possible that the two variables mutually influence one another. If this is the case, one will nonetheless have to be designated as the "dependent" variable. It is a good idea to diagram the relationship using greater than (>) and less than (<) symbols as well as a line with an arrow pointing toward the dependent variable.

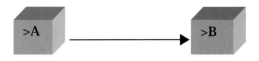

Step 2. Measurement. The second step is to identify the level of measurement attained in the dependent and in the independent variable. Recall that there

are three levels of measurement: nominal, ordinal, and ratio.

Step 3. Method. Having identified the measurement levels, the third step is to examine Table 16.3 to determine which method should be used to examine the relationship. The methods listed are the names of SPSS procedures.

Having identified the appropriate procedure to use, you are now ready to proceed with the analysis. The reader may wish to review Table 16.3, which indicates the appropriate analysis procedure for given levels of measurement in the independent and dependent variables. Appendix A presents the basic procedures along with the most commonly used options and statistics. For full details of SPSS procedures, consult the appropriate SPSS manual listed in the suggested readings section at the end of the Appendix A.

7. When You Get Errors and Warnings

If you are using the Syntax method of entering SPSS commands, expect to get error and warning messages when you run SPSS jobs. Some of these errors lead to the termination of the job; other less serious ones (warnings) simply lead SPSS to ignore an instruction. SPSS has error

Table 16.3   SPSS Procedures for Multivariate Analysis

Dependent	Independent Variable		
	Nominal	Ordinal	Ratio
Nominal	CROSSTABS	CROSSTABS	CROSSTABS
			DISCRIMINANT
Ordinal	CROSSTABS	CROSSTABS	CROSSTABS
		SPEARMAN	SPEARMAN
			DISCRIMINANT
Ratio	MEANS	MEANS	CORRELATION GRAPH
	ANOVA	ANOVA	PARTIAL CORRELATION
	T TEST	T TEST	MANOVA
			REGRESSION FACTOR

checking routines that identify the error immediately after the line on which the error occurs.

Later in this section, Table 16.4 presents a listing of some of the more common errors and warnings and what procedures might be taken to solve them. But before you examine this table, we will review some basic strategies in error detection.

Tip 1. Expect errors. The first thing to realize is that you will make errors. Even after many years of using SPSS, you will continue to make errors. SPSS errors are just part of your life as a data analyst.

Tip 2. Examine error and warning messages carefully. The errors and warnings are listed on the output immediately after the problem has been encountered. To assist the researcher, the characters or symbols creating the problem are quoted. A key point is to carefully examine the description SPSS provides of the error that will assist you in identifying your mistake.

Tip 3. Make certain SPSS is accessing the necessary files. A common error a new users often encounter is that SPSS is not able to access the file (or files) required. This means that you may have an error on your Get File command line. In SPSS, the computer will do an error search and identify all the problems it has with the instructions. Of course, if the machine has not been able to find your system file (*.sav), every variable you mention will produce an error because the computer has not found a file containing the named variables. The first thing to do when you get an error at the beginning of a job is to check to see that the machine was able to access the necessary files for the task.

Tip 4. Fix first errors first. When correcting errors in a syntax command set, begin with the first errors identified. Often when you fix an error at the be-

ginning many of the subsequent errors will be fixed. For example, you do a COMPUTE to create a new variable known as TOTALS, but on all your subsequent commands you refer to the variable as TOTAL. Each time the machine encounters TOTAL, it will give you an error. If you change the name of the variable on the COMPUTE statement to TOTAL and resubmit the job, all the subsequent references to TOTAL will be correct. Sometimes it is a good idea to resubmit a job after you have fixed the first few errors to see how many have been eliminated. Proceed then by again fixing the first errors that show up and then resubmit the job until you get an error-free run.

Tip 5. Stuck? Reenter the command line. Sometimes you can stare at an error line and cannot see what is wrong with it. Perhaps you used a letter "O" rather than a number "0," as in v1O when you meant v10. SPSS does not have a variable called v1O, but it is hard to see the difference on some monitors. Do not waste a lot of time; just reenter the command line.

Tip 6. Examine results on screen before sending to a printer. Sometimes you may inadvertently do something very silly and produce an enormous, meaningless output file. Suppose, for example, that you are running CROSSTABS and you are examining the relationship between two variables with a control for occupational prestige of the respondent. In error, you failed to use the recoded version of the occupational prestige variable and you accidentally produced a monster output file because for each occupational code (there may be 70 or 80 distinct numbers), the computer generated a table showing the relationship between your main variables. If you look at the results on the screen before you print them, you will avoid wasting paper on foolish output.

Tip 7. Double check variable list. When the output reflects an inappropriate analysis, check the list of variables submitted. A common mistake is to RECODE a variable for use in an analysis but then use the original form of the variable rather than the recoded one when the variable is mentioned on the command line. This mistake will not generate an error or a warning, but it will generate a lot of useless output!

Tip 8. Check for a premature FINISH command. If part of your job is run but is terminated before all the expected

output is completed, check to make sure that you have not left a FINISH command in the middle of your job. Often when previously used .sps jobs are modified and resubmitted, we forget to take out the old FINISH command. SPSS will ignore any commands after the FINISH command.

The left side of Table 16.4 lists a few common errors and warnings, and the right side of the table suggests possible corrections.

Table 16.4   Common SPSS Syntax Errors and Warnings and How to Fix Them

SPSS Error or Warning	Double Check This
Error: Unexpected end of file encountered	Check *data file* (.DAT file) eliminate blank lines (watch end and beginning of file particularly
Error: Variable name not recognized	1. If this happens on the first and subsequent variables mentioned, make certain system file was accessed (check for correct file names). 2. Check the spelling of the variable name.
Error: Unrecognized commands due to incorrectly spelled words	A common error is a misspelled command such as STTSTICS for STATISTICS
Warning: The (ADD) VALUE LABELS command. Be certain to include the values for each category	Correct: VALUE LABELS rv43 1 "No" 2 "Yes".
Warning: Incorrectly enclosed literal	Incorrect: VALUE LABELS rv43 "No" 2 "Yes".
Error: Text: Dependent. In regression analysis, this warning occurs if you fail to include the slash before the dependent variable is identified. The machine will try to read DEPENDENT as a variable if the / is omitted. If the / is missed, other consequent errors may result, such as the machine's attempting to do a BACKWARD solution but with no dependent variable identified.	Correct: VARIABLE LABEL v43 "Place of Birth". Incorrect: VARIABLE LABEL v43 "Place of Birth'. Correct: REGRESSION VARIABLES=v34 v12 V56 /DEPENDENT=v34 /BACKWARD. Incorrect: REGRESSION VARIABLES=v34 v12 V56 DEPENDENT=v34/ BACKWARD.

E X E R C I S E S

1. Using the information presented in Figure 16.2, set up a properly formatted table to test the null hypothesis for the relationship between signaling and whether the person is a parent or spouse (grouped together) compared with child or other (grouped together). Hand compute a test of significance for the relationship. What do you conclude about the null hypothesis?

2. The following figure shows a portion of the data for a study. Reviewing the section of the chapter dealing with error detection methods may help you locate some of the *eight* errors that can be found in scanning the data file. Two of the errors are hard to see, so it is understandable if you only find six. The computer could find the others in a flash. *Hint: check for non-numerical entries.* Good luck.

Display 16.3 Partial Printout for Data

```
00112435445523 211212333448976999 123232111123212 23411112
00211231231234 322213222122232212 432235333211232 34530432
00314321234443 233445324433321212 332122341122233 23323222
00413444688822 122222112232123219 234433221222321 34521211
00513335543221 223332221114124211 332111422111212 321212
00513335543221 223332221114124211 332111422111212 32121223
00614322345432 231143321122122121 112211222111231 22132454
00812234342334 6545645646-0988777 793787987987423 98798777
00917879879877 878777778723442343 789987987777987 79879879
01018977772221 987798798778778987 798798777A97777 77788777
```

RECOMMENDED READINGS

George, D., and Mallery, P. (2000). *SPSS for Windows Step by Step: A Simple Guide and Reference 9.0 Update* (2nd ed). Boston: Allyn & Bacon.

Kinnear, P., and Gray, C. (1999). *SPSS for Windows Made Simple* (3rd ed). East Sussex, UK: Psychology Press.

SPSS. (1999). *SPSS Base 10.0 Applications Guide.* Chicago: SPSS Inc. This basic manual contains the basic procedures covered in *Doing Nursing Research.*

SPSS. (1999). *SPSS Advanced Models 10.0.* Chicago: SPSS Inc. This advanced techniques manual will be of interest to those doing GLM repeated measures, loglinear, and other advanced techniques.

SPSS. (1999). *SPSS 10.0 Syntax Reference Guide.* Chicago: SPSS Inc. For those who prefer to use syntax commands, this is the complete reference guide—some 1412 pages are included!

Chapter 17

Testing Simple Causal Models

KEY TERMS

Four-variable causal models

Intervening variable model

Jackson's rule of thirds

Source of spuriousness model

In *nonexperimental research* (correlational and comparative surveys, case studies, and so on), how do we test whether a proposed explanation for some relationship has any merit? Suppose, for example, that you want to see if your data support the idea that expectations among parents who value health explains the observed link between health value and adolescents' engagement in healthful lifestyles. This chapter describes procedures for evaluating causal models such as the one suggested above. First, the type of model being dealt with must be determined—that is, is it a source of spuriousness, an intervening variable, or a candidate variable model? (See Chapter 3 for a description of these models.) Second, the appropriate statistical procedures for the analysis must be determined. This determination is based on the level of measurement of the variables involved in each proposed analysis.

To establish a causal relationship, three conditions must be met:

1. The variables must be *associated.*
2. They must be in a plausible *causal sequence.*
3. They *must not be spuriously connected.*

To show that two variables are *associated,* one has to demonstrate that they vary together: To argue that one variable is producing changes in another, one has to demonstrate that as one changes, so does the other. Empirical association is reflected through cross-tabulation table analysis (CROSSTABS), differences in means across categories (MEANS, *t* TEST, ANOVA, MANOVA), and various correlational techniques (CORRELATION, REGRESSION).

To demonstrate a plausible *causal sequence* is largely a matter of theory or of common sense. What is meant here is not only that the independent variable precedes the dependent variable in time but that the ordering is believable. Usually, giving a little thought to the causal order

will provide an answer. For example, it would be foolish to argue that the "size of your present community" influences the size of the "community in which you were born." The causal sequencing is wrong; the present cannot influence the past. On the other hand, the size of community one has chosen to live in as an adult may, of course, be influenced by the size of community in which one grew up. To demonstrate that a relationship is not *spurious* is always a challenge, one that can never fully be met. (Recall that a spurious relationship is one in which a third factor is influencing both the independent and the dependent variables; thus, their covariation may be the result of the common connection to the source of spuriousness.) A critic may always point to some potential *source of spuriousness* for the relationship between the variables. The best the first-time researcher can hope to achieve is to deal with the more obvious potential sources of spuriousness.

We begin this chapter with some techniques for testing three-variable causal models. Later in the chapter, we examine causal models with four variables.

A. TESTING THREE-VARIABLE CAUSAL MODELS

In nonexperimental research, identical analyses may be used to test different **three-variable causal models.** Such models generally attempt to explain or elaborate on a relationship that is known to exist or that a research project expects to demonstrate. These models introduce a third variable to explain the relationship between two other variables. We will use some sample data to illustrate. Suppose we have done a survey on 395 senior high school students concerning factors that influence healthful lifestyle choices. Table 17.1 presents the results.

Table 17.1 is a standard cross-tabulation table whose computations could be

Table 17.1   Percent of Senior High School Students Who Make Healthful Lifestyle Choices by Health Value Background*

Type of Lifestyle Choices	Low Health Value Background N	Low Health Value Background %	High Health Value Background N	High Health Value Background %	Total N	Total %
Healthful choices	144	73.1	176	88.9	320	81.0
Unhealthful choices	53	26.9	22	11.1	75	19.0
Total	197	100.0	198	100.0	395	100.0

$^{*}X^2 = 16.021$; df = 1; significant at the 0.001 level.

done with the CROSSTABS procedure. A shorter version of the table is also possible and will be used to illustrate the model testing to be presented later. The shorter version is illustrated in Table 17.2.

With the information provided, it is possible to reconstruct the original table. Because 73.1 percent of 197 students with low health value backgrounds report healthful lifestyle choices, it is possible to determine the number of students who fall into the category ($0.731 \times 197 = 144$). Similar calculations could be done to reconstruct Table 17.1.

The much simplified Table 17.2 is easy to read and focuses attention on the two percentage figures that are to be compared. Although some 88.9 percent of the students with high health value backgrounds report healthful lifestyle choices,

73.1 percent of those with low health value backgrounds make similar choices. Note that there is a 15.8 percentage point difference by health value categories in those making healthful lifestyle choices. We will use this table in discussing the first causal model, the intervening variable model.

1. Testing for Intervening Variables

In an **intervening variable model**, the interest is in understanding the relationship between X and Y—understanding the mechanism by which X is connected to Y. Frequently, a researcher will be testing a number of alternative explanations of how X influences Y. In the case of one intervening variable, the relationship could be diagrammed as follows:

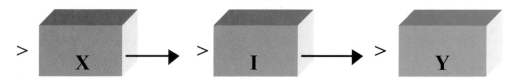

Table 17.2   Percent of Senior High School Students Who Make Healthful Lifestyle Choices by Health Value Background*

	Low Health Value Background	High Health Value Background
Healthful lifestyle choices, %	73.1	88.9
Cases, n	197	198

$^{*}X^2 = 16.021$; df = 1; significant at the 0.001 level.

In this diagram, *I* is the *intervening variable,* or the linking variable between *X* and *Y.* The hypothesis is that variations in *X* cause variations in *I,* which, in turn, influences *Y.* Typically, one would propose a number of possible intervening variables, so the following diagram would be more appropriate:

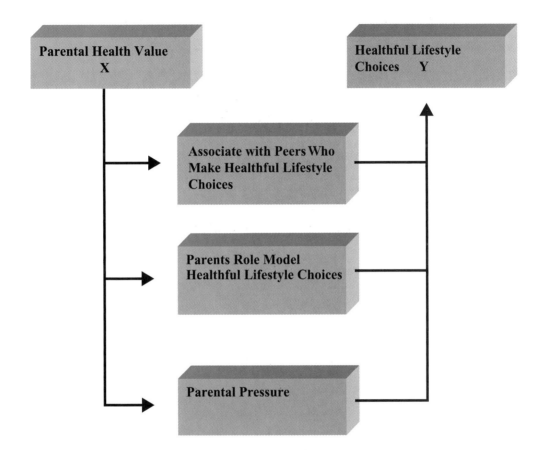

In this diagram, three alternative explanations are suggested for the connection between *X* and *Y.* The researcher would collect data that measure each of the variables involved and conduct the appropriate statistical tests to determine, which, if any, of the proposed alternative explanations, or intervening variables, explains the connection between *X* and *Y.*

Let us suppose, for example, that three alternative explanations are proposed for the relationship between parental health value and likelihood of making healthful lifestyle choices:

1. Students with high health value backgrounds associate with peers who make healthful lifestyle choices.
2. Students with high health value backgrounds have parents who role model healthful lifestyle choices.
3. High health valuing parents are more likely to put pressure on their children to make healthful lifestyle choices.

a. The Rationale Behind the Tests

The thinking behind the test is as follows: if we have a *causal relationship* between *X* and Y (health value and healthful lifestyle choices) and propose a link to explain how X influences Y, then X (health value) should not be able to influence Y (lifestyle choices) if we hold the linking variable constant. The argument is that X influences Y through I. A plumbing analogy may be helpful. Water can only flow from X to Y through a pipe. If you turn off a valve located between X and Y, then increasing the volume of water flowing into the pipe at point X will have no influence on Y because the valve has been turned off. However, if we open the valve, then changes in the pressure at X will influence the flow at Y. Keeping the analogy in mind, let us now see if we can "control" for the intervening variable.

Our first explanation for the relationship between parental health value and likelihood of making healthful lifestyle choices is that students with parents who have high health values tend to associate more with peers who make healthful lifestyle choices. How can we analyze the data to see if the results are consistent with this model? Using a cross-tabulation table analysis (CROSSTABS), we run the relationship between health value and lifestyle choices, controlling for the intervening variable, association with peers who make healthful lifestyle choices. We wish to see what happens when the control is applied. In this case, we wish to see

whether the original 15.8 percent difference in the relationship between health value and healthful life-style choices (1) increases, (2) stays the same, (3) decreases or disappears, or (4) is mixed.

b. Jackson's Rule of Thirds

According to **Jackson's rule of thirds,** if the original difference between the categories increases by one third or more, we will interpret this as an *increase,* or a strengthening, of the original relationship; if the difference remains within one third of the original, we will interpret this as an indication that the relationship has *remained the same;* if the difference decreases by more than one third, we will interpret this as a *decrease or disappearance* of the relationship; finally, if the relationship is markedly different when different control categories are compared with one another (e.g., it disappears in one category, but stays the same in the other), the result is *mixed* (Jackson, 1999).

To apply the rule of thirds to the case under examination, we must first decide where the cutpoints are between the thirds. To do this, we take the original difference of 15.8 and divide by 3; this yields a value of 5.3. Table 17.3 presents these values and shows how the differences would be interpreted.

Table 17.3 Applying Jackson's Rule of Thirds

Sample Data Results	Interpretation
Original difference: $88.9 - 73.1 = 15.8$	
Determining thirds: $15.8 \div 3 = 5.3$	
Outcomes	
1. If new difference is greater than 21.1 ($15.8 + 5.3 = 21.1$)	Increased
2. If new difference is between 10.5 and 21.1 (15.8 ± 5.3)	Stayed the same
3. If new difference is less than 10.5	Decreased or disappeared
4. If new differences vary markedly across categories of the control variable	Mixed

c. Using CROSSTABS to Test for an Intervening Variable

But what are our expectations? If the model being tested is correct, we would expect the relationship between health value and healthful lifestyle choices to decrease or disappear when the relationship is run, controlling for the intervening variable. If health value influences healthful lifestyle choices through the linking variable (peers' lifestyle choices), then if we hold the linking variable constant, there should be no relationship between health value and lifestyle choices. Differences in healthful lifestyle choices by health value category should decrease or disappear when the control is applied. All other outcomes are interpreted as not supportive of the model. Table 17.4 presents summary data for five possible outcomes.

To interpret the outcomes, it is necessary to determine whether the original relationship has *increased, stayed the same, decreased or disappeared,* or is *mixed.* The beginning researcher should keep the interpretation of the data as simple as possible. Only when the difference *decreases or disappears* do we have possible support for an intervening variable model. Let us look at the five outcomes and suggest an interpretation for each one.

Outcome 1. According to the rule of thirds, the relationship has *decreased or disappeared* (i.e., the new difference is less than 10.5, so it has decreased by more than one third of the original). The original difference has been reduced to one percentage point in the case of those whose best friends engage in healthful lifestyle choices and to

Table 17.4 Percent of Senior High School Students Who Make Healthful Lifestyle Choices by Health Value Background, Controlling for Healthful Lifestyle Choices of Best Friend, with Five Possible Outcomes

Outcomes	Best Friend with Healthful Choices		Best Friend with Unhealthful Choices*	
	Low Health Value Background	High Health Value Background	Low Health Value Background	High Health Value Background
First outcome	92.0	93.0	71.0	69.0
Difference		1.0		−2.0
Second outcome	74.0	92.0	71.0	86.0
Difference		18.0		15.0
Third outcome	85.0	92.0	68.0	76.0
Difference		7.0		8.0
Fourth outcome	74.0	96.0	61.0	82.0
Difference		22.0		21.0
Fifth outcome	90.0	92.0	60.0	82.0
Difference		2.0		22.0

*The original difference, with no control for healthful lifestyle choices of best friend, is shown below:

	Low Health Value Background	High Health Value Background
Percent who make healthful lifestyle choices	73.1	88.9
Difference		15.8

two percentage points for those whose best friends do not engage in healthful lifestyle choices. This is the only outcome—one in which the original relationship decreases or disappears—that we consider to be consistent with the intervening variable causal model.

Outcome 2. The relationship *stays the same* (the new difference is between 10.5 and 21.1), so the intervening variable model is to be rejected.

Outcome 3. This outcome supports the intervening variable model. The difference *decreases or disappears* (i.e., the new difference is less than 10.5, so it has decreased by more than one third of the original); the interpretation is that the independent variable influences the dependent variable through the tested intervening variable.

Outcome 4. This outcome would lead us to reject the intervening variable model; the relationship is *strengthened* (i.e., the new difference is greater than 21.1), so this suggests that the proposed alternative explanation is having an independent influence on the dependent variable.

Outcome 5. This outcome would also lead us to reject the intervening variable model. The difference *decreases or disappears* in one of the control categories but *increases* in the other, suggesting a conditional effect—the intervening variable is probably having an independent influence but only at certain levels of the intervening variable. This is an example of a *mixed* result.

To perform this analysis using SPSS, see the CROSSTABS procedure in Appendix A.

d. Using MEANS to test for an Intervening Variable

The second explanation proposed for the connection between health value and healthful lifestyle choices is that the students with high health value backgrounds make healthful lifestyle choices because their parents role model healthful behaviors. We will assume for this example that healthful lifestyle choices are measured in terms of the number of healthful behaviors selected on the adolescent lifestyle questionnaire (ratio level measurement, Gillis, 1997), permitting the use of the MEANS procedure.

The logic is identical to that used in the previous procedure. We will examine the difference in the number of healthful choices between health value categories. We will then re-run that relationship, controlling for parents' role modeling of healthful lifestyle choices. Once again, we will apply the rule of thirds to provide a guideline for the interpretation of the data. Table 17.5 indicates that there is a 14.0 difference in the number of healthful lifestyle behaviors selected by health value categories. The question is will this difference increase, stay the same, decrease, disappear, or be mixed when the control for parental role modeling of healthful life style choices is applied?

Table 17.5 shows different outcomes. Once again, we look at the control table, examine the difference between the levels of parental role modeling of healthful lifestyle choices, and contrast this difference with the original difference of 14.0 healthful behaviors.

Outcome 1. For students whose parents do not role model healthful lifestyle choices, the data indicate a 19.1 healthful behavior difference between health value categories in total number of healthful lifestyle choices. Among those who perceive their parents to role model healthful lifestyle choices, the difference between the categories is 19.6 healthful behaviors. By applying the rule of thirds, we see that the difference in both health value categories has increased by more than one third (i.e., the new difference is greater than 18.66 [$14.0 \div 3 = 4.66$]; $14.0–4.66 = 18.66$).

Table 17.5   Mean Number of Healthful Lifestyle Choices by Health Value Background, Controlling for Parents' Role Modeling of Healthful Lifestyle Choices, with Five Possible Outcomes

Outcomes	No Parental Role Modeling		Parental Role Modeling*	
	Low Health Value Background	High Health Value Background	Low Health Value Background	High Health Value Background
First outcome	14.9	34.0	33.0	52.6
Difference		19.1		19.6
Second outcome	22.3	36.6	25.5	39.8
Difference		14.3		14.3
Third outcome	15.6	22.7	34.2	41.0
Difference		7.1		6.8
Fourth outcome	23.5	24.8	37.7	39.2
Difference		1.3		1.5
Fifth outcome	16.4	31.3	38.9	40.1
Difference		14.9		1.2

*The original difference, with no control for parental role modeling, is shown below:

Healthful Lifestyle Choices	Low Health Value Background	High Health Value Background
Mean number of healthful lifestyle choices	24.7	38.7
Difference	14.0	

Therefore, we argue that the relationship has been intensified; we must reject the intervening variable model.

Outcome 2. In the second outcome, in both the "No Healthful Role Modeling" and "Healthful Role Modeling" categories, the difference between the students with low and high health value backgrounds remains almost the same as the original difference of 14.0 (i.e., the new difference is between 9.34 and 18.66; 14.0 ± 4.66). Therefore, we reject the intervening variable model.

Outcome 3. In the third outcome, the difference has been reduced by more than one third (the new difference is less than 9.34); therefore, we conclude that there is some evidence to support the intervening variable model.

Outcome 4. In both the "No Healthful Role Modeling" and "Healthful Role Modeling" categories, the differences in number of healthful lifestyle choices have decreased or disappeared (dropped by more than two thirds); this outcome supports the intervening variable model.

Outcome 5. The final outcome suggests a mixed result. The difference decreases or disappears within the "Healthful Role Modeling" category but remains the same within the "No Healthful Role Modeling" category. We reject the intervening variable model. The data here suggest that parental role modeling of healthful choices has a conditional impact on the number of healthful lifestyle choices made by students.

To perform this analysis using SPSS, see the MEANS procedure in Appendix A.

e. Using PARTIAL CORR to Test for an Intervening Variable

Partial correlations are measures of the strength of an association that take into account one or more additional variables. (Refer to Chapter 11 for a more detailed discussion.) Partial correlations measure how closely two variables are associated when the influence of other variables is adjusted for; a first-order partial is one that takes into account one additional variable and a second-order partial takes into account two additional variables. Partial correlations are presented as $r_{12.3}$. This indicates that you are measuring the correlations between variables 1 and 2 with the effect of variable 3 removed from both the variables being correlated. By combining CORRELATIONS and PARTIAL CORR, we can test for an intervening variable.

In this case, we wish to test whether parental influence intervenes between health value and healthful lifestyle choices by adolescents. Using correlational techniques, we would first establish that there is an association between health value and adolescents' healthful lifestyle choices. If there is an association, we would then proceed with the analysis to test whether the data are consistent with an intervening variable model.

If the intervening variable model is correct, we should at least expect the following:

- That the correlation between adjacent variables will be greater than between non-adjacent categories ($r_{XY} < r_{XI}$ or r_{IY})
- That if I is controlled, the relationship between X and Y should be reduced or disappear; this could be tested with a partial correlation coefficient.

The model will be tested using two correlational techniques, CORRELATIONS and PARTIAL CORR. Table 17.6 presents the correlations between three variables: parental pressure index (I), health value score (X), and number of healthful lifestyle choices (Y).

The first test is to see if the magnitude of the correlations is consistent with the model being tested. The prediction was that adjacent correlations would be higher than nonadjacent ones. The adjacent correlations are I-X and I-Y and the correlations are 0.31 and 0.46, respectively. The nonadjacent correlation is X-Y and the correlation is 0.22. So far, the data are consistent with the intervening variable model.

The next question is whether the partial correlation will increase, will stay the same, or will decrease/disappear when I is controlled. For this analysis, a partial correlation would be computed. When this calculation is done (see Chapter 11 for the formula), we find that the partial ($r_{XY.I}$) is 0.10. By applying the rule of thirds, we see that the original relationship between X and Y is 0.22 and because the partial is about one half of the original value, we note that the association has *decreased or disappeared*. Therefore, we find support for the model.

To perform this analysis using SPSS, see the PARTIAL CORR procedure in Appendix A.

2. Testing for Sources of Spuriousness

The next major type of causal model is the **source of spuriousness model**. Here the

Table 17.6   Correlations Between Variables in Model

Parental Pressure	Health Value	Number of Healthful Lifestyle Choices	
	(I)	(X)	(Y)
Parental pressure (I)	1.00		
Health value (X)	0.31	1.00	
Healthful lifestyle choices (Y)	0.46	0.22	1.00

researcher proposes that although there is a statistically significant relationship between the variables X and Y, this relationship may be a noncausal one, only existing because some third variable is influencing both X and Y. The argument is that the only reason X is related to Y is that a third factor is influencing both of them. Having observed a statistically significant relationship, the researcher will want to ensure that the relationship is not spurious and, therefore, will run a number of spuriousness checks. The source of spuriousness model may be diagrammed as follows:

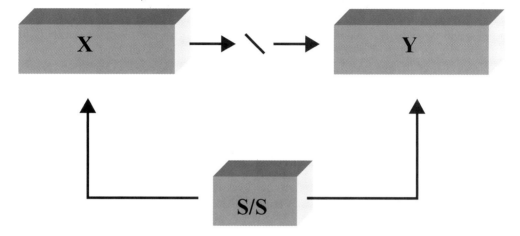

a. The Rationale Behind the Tests

How do we go about testing a source of spuriousness model? The idea is that if X and Y are spuriously associated, the reason they vary together is that a third variable (a source of spuriousness) is influencing both X and Y. Therefore, if we control for the source of spuriousness (S/S), there should no longer be any association between X and Y. This suggests that we need the same kind of analysis that we used for testing intervening variables. To test for a potential source of spuriousness, the steps are:

● Test the original relationship between X and Y; if this demonstrates a robust relationship (probably statistically significant); then,
● Controlling for the source of spuriousness, re-run the relationship between X and Y. As in the intervening variable model, we can then apply Jackson's rule of thirds to determine if the relationship has increased, stayed the same, decreased/disappeared, or become mixed. In order to conclude that the original relationship is spurious, the difference between the categories must decrease/disappear.

b. The Dilemma: The Models Are Not Empirically Distinguishable

The difficulty is that it is possible for two researchers working with the same data and with the same three variables to establish two different causal models, one proposing that the variables are connected in an intervening variable model and the other proposing that the variables may be associated spuriously. They might then do the identical analysis but come to totally different conclusions. Let us suppose that when the control is applied, the original difference decreases/disappears. In this case, one researcher would conclude that the intervening variable model has found support in the data and the other would conclude that the relationship is spurious. Both would be correct.

Because the two models are not empirically distinguishable, the importance of precisely specifying models in advance becomes clear. If we develop the models after analyzing the data, the interpretation of the data is little more than a flight of fancy; if the difference disappeared, we could argue either for an intervening variable explanation or for a source of spuriousness explanation. Because the test results equally support both models, we must specify in advance which model we are, if fact, testing.

c. Using MEANS to Test for Spuriousness

To illustrate a test for spuriousness, we will use the same variables as in the previous example. Table 17.7 presents sample data showing how the analysis turned out for the relationship between health value and healthful lifestyle choices.

Readers should note that there is a 14.0 difference between the students with low and high health value backgrounds in the number of healthful lifestyle choices made. Now suppose that we wanted to make certain that this relationship was not caused spuriously by the rural or urban backgrounds of these students. The type of home community (rural versus urban) may be influencing the health value level achieved by the families and may also be influencing the lifestyle choices of the students. It would, therefore, be the urban or rural location that is influencing both variables rather than the

health value level that is influencing the students' lifestyle choices.

Table 17.8 reports five different outcomes for this analysis. These should be examined carefully, the rule of thirds should be applied, and a decision should be made as to which outcome lends support to the spuriousness model of the relationship between the variables. To apply this rule, simply divide the original difference by 3 (14.0 ÷ 3 = 4.66). Next, compare the difference in healthful lifestyle choices by health value categories for each of the rural and urban categories.

Outcome 1. Here the differences (21.1 and 19.3) have both grown by more than a third; therefore, we reject the source of spuriousness model.

Outcome 2. The original difference between the number of healthful lifestyle choices by students with low versus high health value backgrounds was 14.0 choices. When the control for rural versus urban background is applied, the difference remains much the same; therefore, we reject rural versus urban background as a source of spuriousness.

Outcome 3. The original difference in this result has been reduced to 6.1 for both categories. Because the difference has decreased/disappeared, we find support for the source of spuriousness model.

Outcome 4. In this case, the original difference has been reduced to less than one third of its original value, so we can-

Table 17.7   Number of Healthful Lifestyle Choices by Senior High School Students, by Health Value Background

Healthful Lifestyle Choices	Low Health Value Background	High Health Value Background
Mean number of healthful lifestyle choices	24.7	38.7
Difference	14.0	
Cases, *n*	197	198

Table 17.8   Mean Number of Healthful Lifestyle Choices by Health Value Background, Controlling for Rural and Urban Backgrounds, with Five Possible Outcomes

Outcomes	Rural Background		Urban Background	
	Low Health Value Background	High Health Value Background	Low Health Value Background	Health Value High Background
First outcome	8.7	29.8	33.3	52.6
Difference		21.1		19.3
Second outcome	22.7	36.7	25.8	39.6
Difference		14.0		13.8
Third outcome	23.0	29.1	37.1	43.2
Difference		6.1		6.1
Fourth outcome	17.3	19.1	37.4	39.7
Difference		1.8		2.3
Fifth outcome	21.6	22.7	27.4	40.4
Difference		1.1		13.0

not reject the source of spuriousness model. Outcomes 3 and 4 both lend support to the spuriousness model.

Outcome 5. Here the result is mixed. The difference disappears among the rural students but is only slightly reduced among the urban students. We reject the source of spuriousness model.

In order to do the analysis, we need a table showing the difference in healthful lifestyle choices by health value categories. Second, we will need to re-run this relationship, controlling for rural and urban backgrounds.

To perform this analysis using SPSS, see the MEANS procedure in Appendix A.

d. Using CROSSTABS to Test for a Source of Spuriousness

To use CROSSTABS in a test for a source of spuriousness, one runs the original relationship and then re-runs the relationship, controlling for the source of spuriousness. The rule of thirds would then be applied and we only consider the original relationship to be spurious if the difference *decreases/disappears.*

To perform this analysis using SPSS, see the CROSSTABS procedure in Appendix A.

e. Using PARTIAL CORR to Test for Spuriousness

This test requires ratio level variables. It simply involves running the zero-order correlation followed by a partial correlation controlling for the potential source of spuriousness. The analysis should be run and the data interpreted according to the rule of thirds. We only consider the original relationship to be spurious if the relationship decreases/disappears.

When procedures are being selected for evaluating causal models and the researcher believes that the vast majority will only require one type of procedure, it is sometimes best, in the interest of simplicity, to use the same procedure throughout rather than shift back and forth between techniques in a way that may confuse readers. This usually means some underutilization of the data because the procedure selected must meet the measurement requirements of the variable with the lowest level of measurement. For example, if you have only one test that could be done using the MEANS procedure but all the rest require CROSSTABS, then you would probably use CROSSTABS throughout even though you could use the MEANS procedure on one of the tests. Your decision would be based on keeping the analysis as simple as possible for your readers.

To perform this analysis using SPSS, see the PARTIAL CORR procedure in Appendix A.

B. TESTING FOUR-VARIABLE CAUSAL MODELS

In the classic work entitled *Causal Inferences in Nonexperimental Research* (1964), Hubert M. Blalock, Jr., presented a number of ideas on testing causal models. The procedures for testing four-variable causal models parallel the ideas presented in the earlier section of the chapter and should be seen as an extension of them. In the case of **four-variable causal models,** there may be two intervening variables (plus an independent and dependent variable). Figure 17.1 illustrates a four-variable model.

Suppose the model that you wish to examine is the one presented in Figure 17.1. This model suggests a specific causal ordering of the variables. Or $A \rightarrow B \rightarrow C \rightarrow D$. What could one do to test this model? A number of properties that should hold true if the model is accurate are:

- Correlations between adjacent variables should be higher than between nonadjacent variables; if the model is correct, the following should hold:

$$r_{AB} > r_{AC}, r_{AD}$$
$$r_{BC} > r_{BD}$$
$$r_{CD} > r_{AC}$$

- The weakest correlation in a causal chain should be between the variables

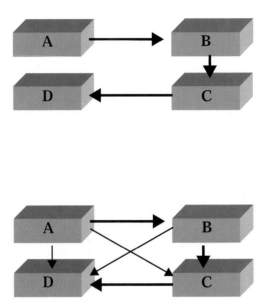

Figure 17.1   Four-variable causal model.

furthest apart causally. If the model is correct, the following should hold:

$$r_{AD} < r_{AB}, r_{AC}$$
$$r_{AC} < r_{AB}$$
$$r_{BD} < r_{AB}, r_{BC}$$

- The strength of relationships should diminish if intervening variables are controlled for; if the model is correct, the following partial correlation results should hold:

$$r_{AC.B} = 0$$
$$r_{BD.C} = 0$$
$$r_{AD.BC} = 0$$

Let's look at the steps necessary to test the simplest model. First, we will examine the magnitude of the various correlations. Are they consistent with the four-variable model? Namely:

- Are the correlations between causally adjacent variables higher than between nonadjacent variables?

- Do correlations drop when intervening variables are controlled?

Suppose that we have the following correlation matrix between the variables *A, B, C,* and *D*.

Correlation Matrix

Variables	A	B	C
B	0.56		
C	0.21	0.61	
D	0.10	0.18	0.63

Step 1. Does the causal order make sense? The first step in assessing a causal model is to ensure that the causal ordering is plausible. The model should pass a commonsensical test, indicating that the variables are in a temporal sequence that is possible. For example, the first variable in the model should occur before other variables and should represent a possible cause of variation in variables that occur later in the model.

Step 2. Compare the correlations. Inspect the correlations to see if correlations between adjacent variables are higher than those between nonadjacent variables. In this case, we note the following:

Model Predicts	Observed Correlations	Conclusions
$r_{AB} > r_{AC}, r_{AD}$	0.56 0.21 0.10	Supports model
$r_{BC} > r_{BD}$	0.61 0.18	Supports model
$r_{CD} > r_{AC}$	0.63 0.21	Supports model

Step 3. Eliminate causal links not implied by the model. There are three causal links that are not implied by the model. These include the *AC* link, the *BD* link, and the *AD* link. (These are marked with thinner lines in Figure 17.1.) The first two are tested using first-order (one control) partial correlations, and the last one is tested by means of a second-order partial correlation. The tests reveal the following:

Model Predicts	Observed Partial Correlation	Conclusion
1. Testing *AC* link: $r_{AC.B} = 0$*	0.10	Reduced by more than one third: Supports model[†]
2. Testing *BD* link: $r_{BD.C} = 0$	−0.33	Reduced by more than one third: Supports model
3. Testing *AD* link: $r_{AD.BC} = 0$	0.01	Reduced by more than one third: Supports model

*The formulas used to hand compute the partials are as follows:

$$\text{First order: } r_{AC.B} = \frac{r_{AC} - (r_{AC})(r_{BC})}{\sqrt{1 - r_{AC}^2}\sqrt{1 - r_{BC}^2}}$$

$$\text{Second-order: } r_{AD.BC} = \frac{r_{AD.B} - (r_{AC.B})(r_{CD.B})}{\sqrt{1 - r_{AC.B}^2}\sqrt{1 - r_{CD.B}^2}}$$

[†]The causal inference uses the *rule of thirds* used in this text. Hubert Blalock bears no responsibility on this point!

The evidence in this case is consistent with the proposed model. If any of the results had failed the test, then the interpretation would be that the evidence is not consistent with the proposed model.

Although it is possible to test complex causal models using cross-tabulation tables, the procedure requires a large number of cases when additional control variables are added. Once again, however, the principle remains the same: observe what happens to the original relationship when the control variables are applied simultaneously. Does the original difference increase, stay the same, decrease/disappear, or is it mixed?

To perform this analysis using SPSS, see the CORRELATION and PARTIAL CORR procedures in Appendix A.

Chapter 18 introduces some other basic techniques that are used when attempts are made to deal with multiple variables simultaneously. The chapter includes regression, discriminant, analysis of variance, and factor analyses.

E X E R C I S E S

1. Working with a two-variable relationship that you think would be relatively strong, diagram four models (two intervening variables and two possible sources of spuriousness) that may explain the original two-variable relationship. Describe in detail how you would go about testing the four proposed models. What outcomes would lend support to each of your models, and what kinds of evidence would lead you to reject them?

2. Compare the procedures used by a researcher using an experimental design to arrive at causal inferences with those used by a nonexperimental researcher. Using the same three variables, illustrate an experimental and a nonexperimental approach by outlining a possible design each might use in exploring the relationship between the same three variables. For the particular relationship you have explored, discuss the reasons why you prefer one of the designs.

RECOMMENDED READINGS

Blalock, H.M., Jr. (1964). *Causal Inferences in Nonexperimental Research.* Durham: The University of North Carolina Press. Undergraduates will find this book challenging but nonetheless rewarding to work through the methods for testing models with four or more variables.

Brink, P., and Wood, M. (1998). *Advanced Design in Survey Research.* Thousand Oaks, CA: Sage. This book contains a comprehensive chapter on structural equation modeling, a means of testing hypothesized relationships between concepts.

Hyman, H. (1955). *Survey Design and Analysis.* New York: The Free Press. Paul Lazarsfeld's foreword to Hyman's book contains the classic statement on interpreting three-variable causal models. Because most undergraduates find the terminology difficult to sort out, the authors of this text do not follow the Lazarsfeld approach.

Munroe, B., and Page, E. (1993). *Statistical Methods for Health Care Research* (2nd ed). Philadelphia: J.B. Lippincott. Several helpful chapters present theory testing approaches using path models and structural equation models.

Musial, C.M., Jones, S.L., and Warner, C.D. (1998). Structural equation modeling and its relationship to multiple regression and factor analysis. *Research in Nursing and Health, 21,* 271–281.

Chapter 18

Four Multivariate Techniques

CHAPTER OUTLINE

KEY TERMS

b Coefficient

BACKWARD (stepwise) solution

Beta weight

Confirmatory factor analysis

Correlation matrix

Covariates

Data reductioin

Discriminant function analysis

Dummy coding

Dummy variable

Eigenvalue

Exploratory factor analysis

Factorable

Factor analysis

Factor extraction

Factor loadings

Hierarchical regression

Instrument development

Instrument validation

Linear regression equation

Marker variable

Multicollinearity

Multivariate analysis of variance (ANOVA or MANOVA)

Multiple regression analysis

Principal components method

Principal factors method

R^2

Stepwise entry solution

Theory development

This chapter extends some of the techniques for analysis introduced in the previous chapters. The four sections of this chapter cover regression analysis (an extension of the correlation discussion in Chapter 11); discriminant function analysis, which is a multivariate extension used in the analysis of nominal dependent variables (see Chapter 11); multivariate analysis of variance (an extension of analysis of variance in Chapter 12); and factor analysis, which is used primarily in index construction (an extension of the discussion in Chapter 13). In all likelihood, you have already encountered these four techniques in reading the nursing literature and, therefore, you need to have an understanding of each of them. Fundamentally, they all rely on the basic ideas surrounding the concept of correlation.

As discussed throughout this text, phenomena nursing researchers wish to understand are complex and multivariate in nature. This means that the analytical techniques we use must allow us to take into account many variables simultaneously. With the exception of factor analysis, these techniques provide for the analysis of multiple independent variables. Factor analysis allows one to determine the similarities and differences among sets of separate measures; therefore, it is an important technique used in the development of indexes. Although bivariate (two-variable) analyses have their place, nurse researchers ultimately need to use basic multivariate techniques if they are to tackle the complexity inherent in their subject matter.

The selection of the appropriate technique should be guided by a consideration of (1) the level of measurement attained in measuring the variables and (2) what the analysis is attempting to reveal. We will begin our consideration of multivariate analysis by exploring multiple regression analysis. An understanding of regression is helpful when examining the other approaches featured in this chapter: discriminant analysis, multivariate analysis of variance, and factor analysis. An examination of these basic multivariate techniques reveals that they have much in common.

A. MULTIPLE REGRESSION

Multiple regression analysis attempts to predict variations in a dependent variable from two or more independent variables. And just as we did with correlation, there are two basic elements—a measure of the strength of the association and an equation that describes the relationship. Multiple regression involves two or more independent variables in contrast to the simple linear regression that involved one independent variable.

I. The Rationale

Regression is a powerful tool in the hands of nurse researchers because of its ability to provide:

- An estimate of the *relative importance* of independent variables in influencing a dependent variable
- A *mathematical equation* that describes the relationship between the independent variables and the dependent variable
- A measure of how much *variance is explained* by the combination of independent variables

For example, if you are trying to estimate the relative contribution of three variables when predicting cigarette smoking behavior, a regression analysis might indicate that exposure to cigarette advertising accounts for 22 percent of the variation, that friends' smoking status accounts for 37 percent of the variation, and that annual income contributes another 14 percent of the variation in smoking behavior. Taken together, the three variables account for 73 percent of the variation in cigarette smoking.

Alternatively, the relationship between smoking behavior and exposure to cigarette advertising could be analyzed simply by comparing the average number of cigarettes smoked across categories of advertisement exposure (MEANS analysis). This would permit the researcher to show a significant relationship between cigarette smoking and advertisement exposure but would not enable the researcher to say that exposure to cigarette advertising is about one half as important as friends' smoking status. Because regression analysis provides this additional information, it is a powerful tool. Besides allowing the researcher to examine the relative importance of the various factors producing variation in a dependent variable, it also allows the researcher to express the relationship in the form of an equation, giving the researcher the ability to predict values for a dependent variable, given values for the independent variables.

As in correlational analysis (see Chapter 11), we are interested in both the equation that describes the relationship as well as a measure of the strength of the association. We will only consider the simplest version of regression—that of an additive or linear relationship among the variables. Regression analysis assumes that the variables are normally distributed and that measurement is at the ratio level. Special procedures, however, do permit the inclusion of variables not achieving ratio measurement.

Although regression analysis assumes ratio level measurement and normally distributed variables, researchers sometimes include ordinal and even nominal variables. However, the price one pays for reduced levels of measurement is almost certainly a weakened ability to predict variation in the dependent variable, as well as a greater instability in the coefficients associated with the independent variables

(see Box 13.1 for an example of the impact of reduced levels of measurement).

2. The Linear Regression Equation

In Chapter 11, we examined the relationship between two variables using a correlation approach. The equation describing the relationship between X (independent variable) and Y (dependent variable) consisted of an a value and a b coefficient as in:

$$Y = a + bX$$

To take into account two or more independent variables, this basic equation is extended as follows:

$$Y = a + b_1X_1 + b_2X_2 + \ldots b_kX_k$$

In the equation, the a is a constant and, if the values for each case were calculated and plotted, would represent the point where the regression line crosses the Y axis. The **b coefficients** refer to the slopes of the regression lines. If small increases in the X variable lead to large increases in the Y variable, the b value will be higher (see the relationship between cigarette smoking and number of cigarette advertisements shown in Fig. 18.1); on the other hand, if it takes large increases in X to produce an increase in Y, the b value will be smaller (see the relationship between cigarette smoking and annual income shown in Fig. 18.2). In the two-variable case (Figs. 18.1 and 18.2), the b value in the case of number of cigarette advertisements is higher than the b value for the case of income predicting cigarette smoking behavior. The reason is that the values for number of cigarette advertisements have a smaller range, perhaps from 0 to 50 per year approximately, but the range in the values for income is considerable, perhaps from \$18,000 to \$80,000. Thus, the b values tend to be much lower. Even though the correlation between cigarette smoking and number of cigarette advertisements

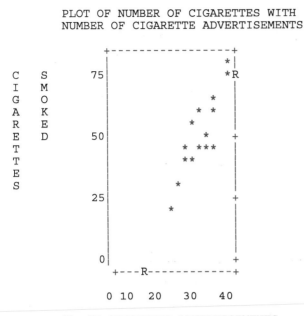

PLOT OF NUMBER OF CIGARETTES WITH
NUMBER OF CIGARETTE ADVERTISEMENTS

No. OF CIGARETTE ADVERTISEMENTS

15 cases plotted

Regression statistics of CIGARETTES SMOKED on NUMBER OF
ADVERTISEMENTS
        Correlation   .89
        R Squared   .79
        S.E. of Est   7.68
        Significance   .0000

Intercept (*a* value) -21.64   Standard Error   10.64
Slope (*b* value)   5.97   Standard Error   .86

**Equation: No. of cigarettes smoked = -21.64 + 5.97(No. of
advertisements)**

Figure 18.1   Prestige and years of education. (*continued on next page*)

and between cigarette smoking and income may be similar (e.g., 0.90 in both cases), the *b* value for income will be much lower than the *b* value for number of cigarette advertisements.

If standardized slopes are of interest, these will be referred to as β weights or **beta weights.** In this case, think of all the variables in the equation as being standardized—think of them as *Z scores*—so that it does not matter if the independent variables have different ranges (as in the case of income and number of cigarette advertisements). Each independent variable is standardized (reassigned values so that each has a mean of 0 and a standard deviation of 1), which then allows us to compare the beta values directly. The β's represent the amount of change in *Y* (the dependent variable) that can be associated with a given change in one of the *X*s, when the influences of the other independent variables are held constant. Regression programs provide the researcher with both the *b* and the β (beta) coefficients (see Fig. 18.2).

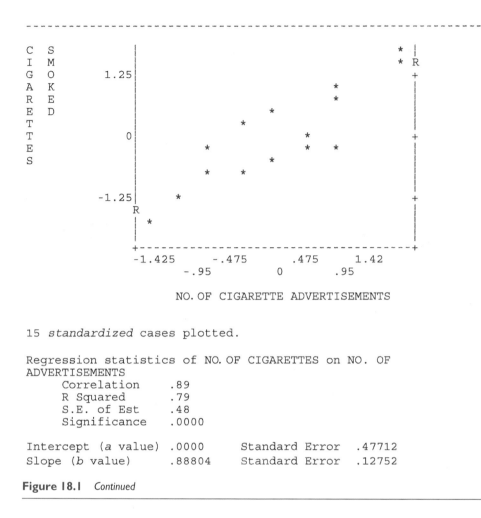

```
C  S                                                    *  |
I  M                                                    * R
G  O        1.25                                           +
A  K                                              *        |
R  E                                              *        |
E  D                                      *                |
T                                    *                     |
T           0|                                 *           +
E                               *         *  *             |
S                                     *                    |
                           *     *                         |
                                                           |
           -1.25|          *                               +
              R                                            |
                |   *                                      |
                |                                          |
              +--------------------------------------------+
             -1.425      -.475       .475      1.42
                    -.95          0         .95

            NO. OF CIGARETTE ADVERTISEMENTS
```

15 *standardized* cases plotted.

Regression statistics of NO. OF CIGARETTES on NO. OF
ADVERTISEMENTS
        Correlation   .89
        R Squared   .79
        S.E. of Est   .48
        Significance   .0000

Intercept (*a* value) .0000   Standard Error .47712
Slope (*b* value)   .88804   Standard Error .12752

Figure 18.1 *Continued*

The strategy of multiple regression involves determining the slopes for each of the independent variables while simultaneously holding constant, or adjusting for, the other independent variables. The slopes (*b* coefficients) are determined to maximize our ability to predict variations in the dependent variable. Thus, we may define a **linear regression equation** as one that describes a relationship between a number of independent variables and a dependent variable and that provides for the best linear (additive) weightings of the independent variables and a constant calculated so as to maximize the prediction of the dependent variable.

3. The Strength of the Association, R^2

The R^2 is a measure of the amount of variation in the dependent variable that is explained by the combination of independent variables. Recall that when two variables are involved, the measure is r^2 (see Chapter 11). The two statistics are directly comparable and would yield identical results if, in a case in which there are multiple independent variables, one simply took the values for each variable, plugged them into the equation, and then computed the "predicted value" for the dependent variable. If one then correlated

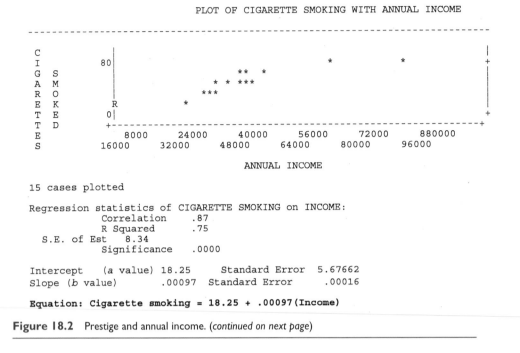

Figure 18.2   Prestige and annual income. *(continued on next page)*

the predicted and the observed values of the dependent variable, the problem is reduced to a simple two-variable correlation, and the r^2 would equal R^2. Both of these statistics vary from 0 to 1. The higher the value, the higher the explained variance; the higher the value, the higher the predictability of the dependent variable by the independent variables.

Regression analysis is an important technique for both applied and pure research. Applied researchers are particularly interested in identifying the independent variables that are:

- Important in influencing the dependent variable
- Modifiable through policy changes

Applied researchers are most concerned with the *b* coefficients because they indicate how much change in the independent variable will be required for a unit change in the dependent variable.

Pure researchers, on the other hand, usually focus on the βs because, generally, theorists are more concerned with the relative impact of each independent variable on the dependent variable.

4. Using Variables Not Meeting the Measurement Assumption

Researchers frequently wish to include, along with ratio level variables, variables measured at either the ordinal or nominal levels. It is possible to do this, but one must exercise greater caution in interpreting the results.

a. Using Ordinal Variables

The price one pays in using ordinal variables is generally a weakened ability to predict variations in a dependent variable. In general, the fewer the categories in an ordi-

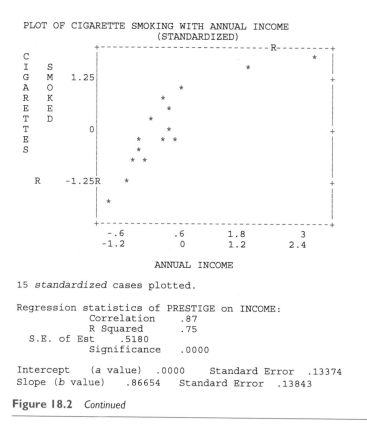

```
PLOT OF CIGARETTE SMOKING WITH ANNUAL INCOME
                (STANDARDIZED)
      +----------------------------R--------+
C                                         *  |
I   S                              *          |
G   M   1.25                                  +
A   O                      *                   |
R   K                   *                      |
E   E                     *                    |
T   D                  *                       |
T       0                 *                    +
E                    *   *  *                   |
S                     *                         |
                  *   *                         |
     R    -1.25R     *                          +
                                                |
               *                                |
                                                |
      +----------------------------------------+
          -.6        .6        1.8         3
          -1.2        0        1.2        2.4

                  ANNUAL INCOME
```

15 *standardized* cases plotted.

Regression statistics of PRESTIGE on INCOME:
          Correlation   .87
          R Squared   .75
    S.E. of Est   .5180
          Significance   .0000

Intercept   (a value) .0000   Standard Error .13374
Slope (b value)   .86654   Standard Error .13843

Figure 18.2 *Continued*

---

nal variable, the lower its correlation with other variables. Thus, more categories in the ordinal variable are preferable. If regression analysis is anticipated, using nine-point Likert items rather than five- or seven-point categories is recommended. When ordinal variables are placed into competition with ratio level variables for explaining variance, the resulting equation will tend to underestimate the relative importance of the ordinal variables (see Box 13.1 for more details on the effects of using fewer categories).

b. Using Presence–Absence Questions

In the case of presence–absence questions, one really has an ordinal variable with two values. Such questions are normally coded so that "0" refers to the absence and "1" refers to the presence of the

characteristic. Again, these variables are at a disadvantage in explaining variation in the dependent variable. Indeed, with only two categories, these variables are at a particular disadvantage (e.g., when compared with another ordinal variable with nine values or a ratio variable). Again, the coefficients are likely to underestimate the importance of such variables when they are in competition with variables measured at the ordinal or ratio levels.

c. Using Dummy Variables for Nominal Variables

Nominal level variables may be included in a regression analysis, but they must first have special coding methods applied to them so that they can be properly interpreted in the regression analysis. Suppose you have a religious affiliation vari-

Table 18.1   Recoding the Religion Variable into Three Dummy Variables

Case #	Original Coding, Religion Variable	Coding for Three New Dummy Variables		
		Catholic	Protestant	Jewish
1	1 (Catholic)	1	0	0
2	2 (Protestant)	0	1	0
3	3 (Jewish)	0	0	1
4	3 (Jewish)	0	0	1
5	2 (Protestant)	0	1	0
6	1 (Catholic)	1	0	0
7	4 (atheist)	0	0	0
8	9 (no answer)	0	0	0
9	4 (Mormon)	0	0	0
10	2 (Protestant)	0	1	0
178	4 (agnostic)	0	0	0

able (nominal) and wish to include it in a regression analysis. For purposes of illustration, suppose religion is arbitrarily coded into four categories: Protestant = 1; Catholic = 2; Jewish = 3; and other = 4. It would not be advisable to enter this variable into the regression equation in this manner because it would be treated as if the numbers really meant that 2 was twice as big as 1, 4 was twice as big as 2, and so on. Rather, the researcher should apply a special coding method referred to as **dummy coding.** In dummy coding, new variables are created out of the original variable in such a way that there will be one fewer new variables than the number of categories in the original variable. In this example, we would create three new variables (there were four categories in our nominal religious affiliation variable). The new variables are coded as either presence or absence of the characteristic by assigning the value of "1" to the cases with the characteristic and "0" to those without the characteristic. The reason we can fully describe the religious affiliation variable with three rather than four new variables is because the fourth (in this case) is "other," and "other" will

be accounted for by the combined values in the "absence" category. It should be noted that you always need an "other" in this type of situation. In other words, even if your variable has 20 categories in it, you would still need a final category called "other." Note that if you use gender as a **dummy variable,** either the males or the females will be assigned to the "other" category.

The dummy-variable coding procedure uses 1s and 0s. Thus, we will have a "Protestant" variable, and it will be coded into presence (1) or absence (0); a "Catholic" variable using 1s for Catholics and 0s for non-Catholics; and a "Jewish" variable similarly coded 1 and 0 (Table 18.1). There is no distinction among members of a category—that is, all 1s are considered equally Catholic and all 0s are considered equally non-Catholic. These three new variables would then be entered into the regression analysis as independent variables along with the other relevant independent variables.

Another example of a dummy variable is the inclusion of a gender variable into a regression analysis. In this case, either the males or the females would be assigned a value of 1, and those not assigned would be given a 0. Thus, if females were assigned the value of 1, then the males would be given the value 0. In this case, only one new variable is needed to represent the two categories of gender (recall that we use one fewer dummy variable than categories of the original variable).

5. Some Tips for Using Regression Analysis

Tip 1. Ensure that variables are theoretically independent of one another. What this means is that you cannot use aspects of the dependent variable as independent variables. Ensure that you are including only meaningful potential causes of the dependent variable, *not alternate measures of it.*

Tip 2. Watch out for highly correlated independent variables. The weighting that is attached to the variables will be unstable if the independent variables are highly correlated with one another. The program will print out a warning if there is a problem in this area. The term **multicollinearity** is used to refer to the extent of the correlation among the independent variables. To achieve high predictability of a dependent variable, it is preferable to have the independent variables correlated with the dependent variable but not with one another. If you have a number of highly intercorrelated independent variables, it is usually advisable either to develop an index out of them (if it makes sense to do so) or to select one of the measures and use it to represent the others.

Tip 3. Try to achieve ratio level measurement. If you intend to use regression analysis, attempt to collect data in as raw a form as possible, at the ratio level if possible; if ordinal data are collected, use more categories, rather than fewer.

Tip 4. Use raw data. Do not use recoded variables (dummy variables are an exception) in regression analysis. For ex-

ample, if you have a variable such as age coded as age at last birthday, then use the raw age variable data (e.g., 24, 19, 37, 54, and so on) rather than recoded age categories that may have used three categories to represent those under age 30 years, those age 30 to 49 years, and those age 50 years of age or older.

Tip 5. Use the BACKWARD solution in the REGRESSION procedure. In nursing research, a great deal of intercorrelation exists among variables. In regression, one wishes to find the smallest group of variables that best predicts the dependent variable or accounts for the largest proportion of variance in the dependent variable. By using the **BACKWARD (stepwise) solution,** all the variables are included in the regression equation; then the least important variable is dropped and the equation is recalculated. This procedure is repeated until only significant variables remain. The advantage of this format is that variables that are important when in combination with other variables will remain in the equation; in other formats, they might never be included. This is the method used in the computer analysis example presented in this chapter (see Table 18.2).

Other commonly used formats for entering variables include hierarchical and stepwise with the forward solution. In **hierarchical regression,** the researcher determines the order of entry, or hierarchy, of the variables into the regression equation. This technique is used in creating path models (see Chapters 2 and 3). There is usually a theoretical rationale for the order in which the variables are entered. Hierarchical entry is often used when you have a set of given variables that are beyond the control of the researcher (e.g., such as age, gender, or socioeconomic status [SES]) and you are interested in determining if a specific nursing intervention will impact a nursing outcome, above and beyond the factors that you cannot change. For example, if you wanted to know if a relaxation class reduces the number of cigarettes smoked by participants, you would enter the given variables (age, gender, SES) first followed by your intervention last.

With the **stepwise entry solution,** the independent variable that has the greatest correlation with the dependent variable is entered first. The next variable entered is the one that will increase the R^2 the most above the first variable's contribution. Because there are inter-correlations among the independent variables, we cannot simply select the independent variable with the next highest correlation with the dependent variable; rather, we must first calculate partial correlations between the remaining independent variables and the dependent variable. The partial correlation removes the effect of the first variable from the correlation. The variable that has the highest partial correlation with the dependent variable enters the regression next and so on until no remaining independent variables contribute significantly to the R^2 value. At this point, the analysis is ended.

At times, the stepwise forward solution is combined with the backward solution to overcome the weakness of each approach. When this happens, the variables are entered into the regression according to the forward solution method but they are assessed at each step using the backward method to determine whether their contribution remains significant given the influence of the other variables in the equation.

Tip 6. Interpret weightings with care. Understand that the weightings are designed for the particular combination of independent variables in a particular sample and that they may not be reliable if applied to other samples. One has to be particularly cautious in situations in which the independent variables are substantially correlated with one another. (In such situations, with another sample, it is quite likely that different variables will be selected as significant predictors of the dependent variable.)

Tip 7. Monitor number of cases carefully. By default (i.e., if you do not provide a specific instruction to the contrary), SPSS deletes a case if it has a missing value in any of the variables in the equation. Thus, if there are a lot of variables in an analysis, there is a danger of losing many cases. And as the number of cases drops close to the number of variables, the R^2 increases dramatically. *To determine the number of cases used in the analysis, add one to the total degrees of freedom reported in the table.*

If a large number of cases have been dropped, one should attempt to detect if there is a pattern to the missing cases. If one subcategory of respondents is more likely to respond to a question, one might wish to analyze the data these respondents provide separately from those subcategories of respondents whose responses are less complete. However, if it appears that the missing values are random, consider using one or more of the following techniques:

- **Repeat analysis:** After an initial regression analysis (using the BACKWARD option) has identified the significant variables, rerun the analysis, naming only the significant variables, plus perhaps two or three that were dropped in the last few steps. This will preserve the cases that were dropped because of missing values in variables that are not in the final equation. Frequently, many fewer cases will be dropped if this procedure is followed.
- **Pairwise solution:** Try running the analysis using PAIRWISE treatment of missing cases. In this solution, the

correlations are determined for all the pairs of variables for which data are available. (On the linear regression screen, click on the Options button to choose the PAIRWISE treatment).

- **Means solution:** A third approach is to try the MEANS treatment of missing values, which will substitute the mean of the variable for any missing cases. (On the linear regression screen, click on the Options button to choose the MEANS solution).

Tip 8. Deal with interactions among independent variables. If you have reason to suspect that the joint effect of two independent variables is important but that, individually, they may not be significant predictors of the dependent variable, there are two relatively easy approaches to this problem:

- Create a new variable by multiplying the values of the two variables suspected of interaction and include the new variable in the regression analysis along with the variables from which it was constructed. If the new variable is a significant predictor, it will remain in the equation when the analysis is done; if it is not, it will be dropped.
- Convert all the variables to log function variables (this converts the equation to a *multiplicative power function*). By doing so, any interactions will be taken into account in the weightings of the independent variables. In effect, what this procedure does is to raise the weightings to a power. This is accomplished by transforming the elements to log functions, as in:

$$\log Y = \log a + \log X_1 + \log X_2 + \log X_k$$

The consequence of using log transformations is that each independent variable is raised to a power rather than multiplied by the value of the independent variable, as in the linear regression equation.

6. Presenting and Interpreting Regression Results

Table 18.2 presents a sample of a regression results table. Note that both the b coefficients and the beta weights are reported. It is possible to hand compute an estimate of the impact of each independent variables by using the following formula (Hamblin, 1966):

$$\frac{\% \text{ Variance explained}}{\text{by each variable}} = \frac{\beta_1 \times R^2}{\Sigma \beta s} \times 100$$

This estimate represents the impact of each variable in the equation. However, if other variables were included, the percentages would change.

The regression equation is included in Table 18.2. This equation will help you identify where each of its elements are found in a printout; note that the b coefficients (not betas) are used along with the constant term.

Pure researchers have particular interest in the beta weights because they provide a basis for directly comparing the impact of the different independent variables on the dependent one. Applied researchers are usually more concerned with b coefficients, especially those that can be changed through policy alterations. They provide the basis for understanding how much change in the dependent variable may be produced for each change in the independent variable. Variables can be grouped for presentation to illuminate the degree to which different variable types influence the dependent variable (e.g., how much of the variation in the dependent variable is caused by socioeconomic variables in comparison to the variety of experience variables?).

A second method for estimating the relative importance of variables is to calculate a *part correlation coefficient*. This coef-

Table 18.2   Multiple Regression Analysis for Registered Nurses' Salaries

Variable	b Coefficient	Beta Coefficient	Percent Explained
Qualifications	794.0	0.038	3.1
Contract status	1326.0	0.065	5.3
Age in current year	94.0	0.092	7.5
Years in position	263.0	0.153	12.5
Professional age	210.0	0.172	14.0
Years at hospital	264.0	0.250	20.4
Professional rank	-4570.0	-0.372	30.3
Constant	38504.0	% Explained	93.1
Multiple R	0.964		
R^2	0.930		

The variables are:
Qualifications: Baccalaureate degree = 1; no degree = 0
Contract status: Permanent contract = 1; nonpermanent contract = 0
Age = Age in 2001
Years in position: Years in position in 2001
Professional age: Years since RN license earned
Years at hospital: Years working as RN at institution
Rank: General practice nurse = 1; specialty practice nurse = 2; advanced practice nurse = 3; clinical nurse practitioner = 4
Salary = 38504 + 794 (qual) + 1326 (contract status) + 94 (age) + 263 (rank) + 210 (proage) + 264 (years) − 4570 (rank)

ficient is calculated for each independent variable and represents the difference in the R^2 when the variable is included versus when it is not included. The variables may then be ordered in terms of the unique contribution of each independent variable. To get part correlations in SPSS, click on Statistics and click on the Part and Partial Correlations window.

B. DISCRIMINANT FUNCTION ANALYSIS

Discriminant function analysis attempts to predict the category of the dependent variable into which each case falls by using the combined information from the independent variables. For example, suppose you wished to predict which children would initiate a smoking habit in adolescence. The independent variables included tobacco use by parents, siblings, friends, and teachers; students'

leisure time activities; and psychosocial variables of self-esteem and coping mechanisms. Based on a study of school-aged youths, discriminant analysis would then be used to predict whether each case would fall into the "smoking" or "no smoking" categories of cigarette smoking behavior.

1. The Rationale

Discriminant function analysis has some similarity to regression analysis. This alternative is used in situations in which:

- The measurement of the dependent variable is at the nominal level.
- Regression analysis is inappropriate because the assumption that the dependent variable is normally distributed is not met.

Discriminant analysis is a valuable tool for nurse researchers and has applications in many situations. To illustrate some of these situations, let us consider applications that might be made of the technique in various areas of nursing research:

- **Epidemiology:** Studies of the distribution of residence patterns of families who have tested positive and those that have tested negative for tuberculosis
- **Community health:** Studies of rates of participation and nonparticipation in pre- and postnatal education, of participation in a parenting class, or of the rates at which adolescents drop out of school or stay in school
- **Health promotion:** Attempts to determine whether individuals are exercisers or nonexercisers or smokers or nonsmokers and the distribution of clients who favor the use of nurses, nurse practitioners, or physicians for annual health assessments
- **Psychiatric nursing:** Classifying clients as mentally ill or mentally healthy or to differentiate between leaders and nonleaders in group therapy sessions
- **School health:** Attempts to distinguish between healthful and nonhealthful behavior in school-aged children

2. Comparison with Multiple Regression Analysis

Similar to multiple regression analysis, discriminant analysis has the ability to simultaneously deal with multiple independent variables. So, if your dependent variable has two, three, or four categories; your independent variables are ratio variables; and you wish to assess the extent to which you can correctly classify category membership on the dependent measure, consider using discriminant function analysis. And as with regression analysis, if you wish to use nominal or ordinal independent variables, it is possible to do so (using dummy-coded variables), as long as caution is exercised in interpreting the results.

The coefficients computed are based on a regression-like linear equation:

$$D = B_0 + B_1 X_1 + B_2 X_2 + \ldots + B_k X_k$$

The X values are the values of the independent variables, and the B values are the coefficients associated with each independent variable, weighted to maximize the prediction of D, the categories of the dependent variable. The B values are weighted to maximize the ratio of the between-groups sum of squares to the within-groups sum of squares. The output for the analysis will display the discriminant function score for each case. Plugging in the observed values for each variable and multiplying it by the coefficient derives the score for each case. Suppose the discriminant equation was as follows:

$$D = 0.013 + 0.003(X_1) + 0.004(X_2) + 0.078(X_3) + 0.056(X_4)$$

Table 18.3 displays the values for each variable, the coefficients, and the resulting discriminant score for the first case in the file.

Discriminant scores are calculated for each case, and each case is then classified into one of the groups (in this example, participating or not participating in prenatal education). The printed output indicates the actual group each case belongs to, and asterisks are used to indicate the cases that were misclassified.

3. Presenting and Interpreting Results

A basic statistic provided by discriminant analysis is the percentage of cases that can be classified correctly using information from the combination of independent variables. The statistic calculated is similar to that of *Lambda*, which was described in the section dealing with cross-tabular table analysis (see Chapter 11). You may recall that Lambda computes the

Table 18.3   Calculating the Discriminant Score, Case 1

Variable	Observed Value	Coefficient	Discriminant Score
D dependent variable*	1		
Constant		0.013	0.013
X_1 maternal identity score	72.6	0.003	0.218
X_2 family socioeconomic score	47.0	0.004	0.188
X_3 family size	3	0.078	0.234
X_4 number of previous pregnancies	0	0.056	0.000
Sum of values, case #1		0.653	

*Dependent variable is "Participating" or "Not Participating" in prenatal education.

error reduction in estimating a dependent variable, given knowledge of an independent variable. In our example, using the computed discriminant function equation, we determine that 85.2 percent of the cases were correctly grouped according to the discriminant function analysis.

As with regression analysis, the computed coefficients are available in standardized and unstandardized forms. The unstandardized coefficients are used when calculating the discriminant scores for each case. When the researcher wishes to compare the relative impact of each variable, standardized coefficients are used (this is to take into account the different ranges of the variables). Indeed, if there were two categories in the dependent variable, we would have achieved similar results if we had used regression analysis. The b coefficients in regression analysis have a similar ratio to the B discriminant coefficients. However, when there are three or more categories in the dependent

variable, the results are different. Table 18.4 provides a sample of the way in which discriminant analyses may be presented.

Bertrand and Abernathy (1993) used discriminant function analyses to predict three categories of smoking behavior among school-aged children. Data were collected over a 3-year period and included the predictor variables of peer influence, self-esteem, mental health, leisure time activities, and parent–child relationships. The investigators hoped to identify groups of children at risk of initiating smoking so that they could be targeted early and offered effective smoking prevention programs. Children were classified into the categories of "never smoked," "tried but quit," and "current smoker." Results indicate that the highest rates of correct classification were with students who fell into the categories of "never smoked" and "current smoker." The group "tried but quit" was less likely to be correctly classified. Table 18.5 presents the "hit" rate for clas-

Table 18.4   Discriminant Analysis, Sample Presentation

Actual Group	Cases, n	Predicted Group Membership 1	2
Participate (1)	261	221	40*
Not participate (2)	83	11*	72
Total	344	232	112

Percent of "grouped" cases correctly classified: 293 out of 344 cases = 85.2%. (221 + 72 = 293)
*Cases misclassified

Table 18.5   Discriminant Analysis, Number of Children Correctly Classified into Smoking Categories

	Predicting from Sixth Grade					
	Never Smoked,		Tried and Quit,		Current Smoker,	
	N	%	N	%	N	%
Grade 7	1074	64.5	72	20.9	33	52.4
Grade 8	792	59.7	70	15.4	126	49.6
Grade 9	613	53.4	152	30.4	148	40.9

These percentages reflect the number of students correctly classified out of the total number actually falling within that smoking category ("hit" rate).

sification among the three smoking categories produced from the analyses. When the accuracy of prediction is examined for each category, we see that approximately 53 percent of students who reported they had never smoked in ninth grade were correctly classified on the basis of their sixth grade responses. The percentages rise to 65 and 58 percent for seventh and eighth grades, respectively.

C. MULTIVARIATE ANALYSIS OF VARIANCE

Multivariate analysis of variance (MANOVA) is a method used in examining the relationship between ratio level dependent variable (or variables) and two or more nominal, ordinal, or ratio level independent variables, treatments, or covariates.

1. The Rationale

Although regression analysis is appropriate in many situations, there are several situations in which multivariate analysis of variance (ANOVA or MANOVA) would be more appropriate than regression analysis. For example, as Kachigan (1986) points out, if you had predictor variables that have qualitative differences (e.g., three different countries) or if, rather than having a ratio variable measuring the amount of time spent watching TV, you had a variable that indicates whether

someone watched TV or went to the movies, you again would probably opt for analysis of variance. In short, if an independent variable is made up of values that differ in *kind* rather than in *quantity,* you would opt for analysis of variance.

A second situation that is better handled with analysis of variance is one in which the relationship between the independent and the dependent variable changes over the continuum. Perhaps the relationship is nonlinear and, once again, analysis of variance should be considered as an alternative to regression. For example, suppose you were examining the relationship between job satisfaction and size of the institution in which respondents work. Perhaps satisfaction increases as one moves up the size scale, levels off, and then declines in work places above 500 employees—a nonlinear relationship. In this case—and particularly if other covariates such as worker's age and size of home community are included in the analysis—one would perhaps choose a multivariate analysis of variance technique.

It should be noted that multivariate analysis of variance is appropriate under the following conditions:

- When the dependent variable is measured at the ratio level
- When one or more of the treatment variables is measured at the ratio level and others are measured at the nominal or ordinal levels
- If you have multiple dependent measures that you wish to examine simul-

taneously; this is often the case in nursing and health-related research in which one is interested in the impact of an intervention on more than one outcome variable
- In nonexperimental designs in which you wish to examine whether there are

significant interactions among independent variables

In these cases, you would consider using MANOVA. The ratio level treatment variables are called **covariates.** Box 18.1 presents sample results. Note how

---

BOX 18.1 MANOVA Analysis, Sample Presentation: Analyzing Egalitarianism

Source of Variation	Analysis of Variance				
	Sums of Squares	Mean Square	df	F	Significance of F
Within cells [error]	11539.00	69.10	167		
Regression	127.71	63.85	2	0.92	50.399
Country [A]	932.68	466.34	2	6.75	0.002
Gender [B]	2.18	2.18	1	0.03	0.859
Country by gender[A × B]	87.92	43.96	2	0.64	0.531

Regression analysis for within cells error term:
Dependent variable: Egalitarianism

Covariate	Beta	T Value	Significance of T
Socioeconomic status	−0.024	−0.311	−0.756
Family size	0.100	1.290	0.199

The variables are as follows:
Dependent variable: Egalitarianism
Independent variables: Country (Canada, United States, Australia); gender (males, females)
Covariates: Socioeconomic status (occupational prestige rating); family size (number of children in family)

Understanding the Values in the Summary Table
a. The **degrees of freedom** are calculated as follows:
- Regression: df = number of covariates in analysis (in this case: 2)
- Main effect (A): df = 1 less than number of levels in that factor (in this case: 3 − 1 = 2)
- Main effect (B): df = 1 less than number of levels in that factor (in this case: 2 − 1 = 1)
- Interaction effect (A × B): df = product of the dfs making up the interaction (in this case: 2 × 1 = 2)
- Error term: df = total number of cases minus the product of number of levels of A and B (in this case, 173 − [3 × 2] = 167)
b. To compute the **mean square for an effect,** divide the sum of squares for the effect by its df (for the effect of Country: 932.68 ÷ 2 = 466.34)
c. To compute the **F value for each effect,** divide the mean square by the mean square error term (the F for Country: 466.34 ÷ 69.10 = 6.75)

continued on next page

BOX 18.1 *MANOVA Analysis, Sample Presentation: Analyzing Egalitarianism (Continued)*

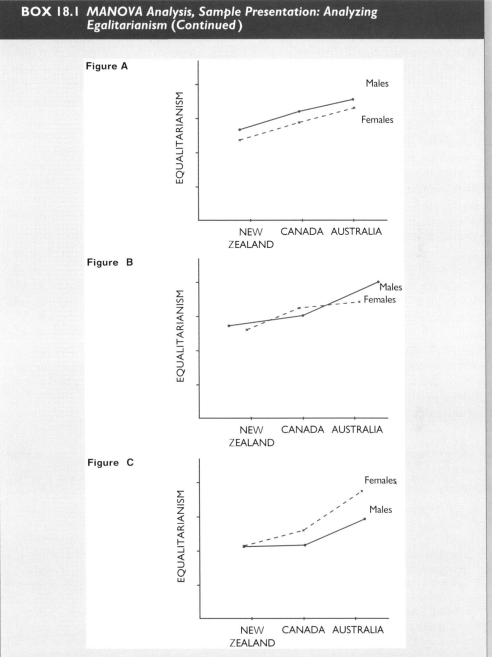

Figure A

Figure B

Figure C

A No interaction. This chart illustrates a situation in which there is a significant main effect of Country on Egalitarianism, but the plot of the means of egalitarianism by Gender categories indicates that because the males in each country remain about the same distance above the mean scores for the females, there is no interaction between gender and country. **B** Nonsignificant interaction. Similar to the previous chart, this one features a significant main effect (Country) and shows a weak but not significant interaction of Gender by Country. (This is the data from those reported in Figure 18.1.) **C** Significant interaction. This chart indicates a significant Gender by Country interaction, as well as a significant main effect (Country). In this case, there appears to be no difference between the genders in terms of egalitarian scores in the United States, but the gap between the genders in egalitarianism increases as one moves from the Canadian data to the Australian data.

MANOVA results combine standard analysis of variance results along with regression analysis. (See the discussion of analysis of variance in Chapter 12.)

2. Comparison with Multiple Regression Analysis

Although the strength of regression analysis lies in its ability to take many variables into account simultaneously and determine the mathematical equation that best describes the relationship between independent variables and the dependent variable, the strength of analysis of variance lies in its ability to assess interactions among variables and estimate the extent to which the results of a study might be caused by random sampling fluctuations. Hence, analysis of variance is most associated with tests of significance (see Chapter 12), and regression analysis focuses on predictive equations. Regression analysis uses analysis of variance as a test of significance for the influence of the independent variables in the equation.

It is possible to analyze a data set using both analysis of variance and regression techniques. The regression analysis would simply use dummy-coded variables to match the categorization used in the analysis of variance. The key difference between the two techniques is shown in Box 18.2.

Although the residuals in regression analysis are measured in terms of deviations from the regression line (see Chapter 11), the residuals in analysis of variance are measured as deviations from group means. As Iversen and Norpoth point out:

> *If the regression line passes through all group means, the residual sum of squares will turn out the same for the regression analysis as for analysis of variance. But if the relationship between X and Y is not linear, then the regression line will not pass through all group means, and as a result, the regression residual sum of squares will exceed the analysis of variance residual sum of squares. (1976, p. 91)*

BOX 18.2 *Comparing the Correlation Coefficient and Analysis of Variance*

A. Correlation coefficient. In the case of the correlation coefficient, the sum of the squared deviations in the numerator refer to deviations from predicted values; the denominator uses sum of squared deviations from the mean of Y. The denominator measures within category variation. Note that the correlation coefficient refers to the ratio of the two types of variation measured subtracted from 1.

$$r^2 = 1 - \frac{\text{Variations around regression}}{\text{Variations around mean of } Y}$$

B. Analysis of variance (f score).

$$F = \frac{\text{Variation within category} + \text{Variation between categories}}{\text{Variation within category}}$$

In the case of analysis of variance, treatment effects are reflected by the sum of squared deviations between treatment categories; random error refers to the sum of squared deviations within the treatment categories. The F represents the ratio between the two types of deviations.

Note that in both cases, we use the sum of squared deviations from relevant means. For both statistics, the denominator reflects variations within a category. The numerators are different. For the correlation coefficient, the value reflects deviations from predicted values; in the case of analysis of variance, the numerator reflects variations between categories.

Thus, if there is a substantial difference in the residual sums of squares between analysis of variance and regression analysis, it would indicate a nonlinear relationship between the variables. If there is not much difference in the residual sums of squares, it would lead us to conclude that the relationship is, indeed, linear.

Although generally seen as the technique associated with experimental and quasi-experimental designs, analysis of variance can also be used in a variety of nonexperimental situations, particularly those in which there are a limited number of independent variables. In all cases, however, the dependent variable should be measured at the ratio level.

3. Presenting and Interpreting Results

In inspecting your results shown in Box 18.1, you should examine two issues as you begin to interpret your results. First, you will want to know if your treatment (or independent) variables had a significant effect; if there are covariates, is the regression effect significant? If there are significant treatment effects, you should see if there is any interaction between the treatments.

a. **Main effects.** To decide if a treatment or covariate was statistically significant, you will need to examine the "significance of F" column to see if the value is less than 0.05. (If this value is not shown, you will need to compare the F value with the values found in Table 12.4 using the appropriate degrees of freedom. If the value you obtained is larger than the one reported in Table 12.4, you have a statistically significant effect. To use Table 12.4, you will need values for the required degrees of freedom. Use the smaller value across the top of the table and the larger one on the vertical axis.)

b. **Interaction effects.** If you have a sig-nificant main effect, you should then inspect your results for any interactions between the effects. Your job is simple if there is no significant interaction effect: you simply report that none was present. It is more complicated with an interaction; in this case, the effect of a treatment is not independent of the other treatment. Rather, it may be that under the high condition of treatment A, we find that treatment B does not enhance the impact on the dependent variable. Here you need to indicate the conditions in which the interaction occurs. You might, for example, create a plot of the relationship between the variables, such as one of the ones shown in Box 18.1 figures A, B, C.

Some aspects of analysis of variance were also discussed in Chapters 11 and 12.

D. FACTOR ANALYSIS

Variables that are correlated can be grouped together into a *factor*. A factor is a hypothetical entity that represents related concrete measures taken on research participants. For example, in a study of the effectiveness of a variety of nursing interventions in reducing postchemotherapy pain in patients with breast cancer, the reported excellence of the experience with meditation, guided imagery, and chanting may be grouped together into a factor called "spirit-centered interventions." **Factor analysis,** then, is a multivariate empirical procedure used to determine the underlying structure of a *set* of variables— that is, to show how variables cluster together to form a *unidimensional* construct. It determines the structure of a set of variables by analyzing the intercorrelations among them. It sorts the variables into categories according to how closely related they are to other variables. Within a given data set, a varying number of factors may emerge. For example, in this example, we may have spirit-centered interventions, body-centered interventions, family and social interventions, and so on.

I. The Rationale

Factor analysis provides a measure of the amount of variance in the data set explained by a particular factor as well as the amount of variance in the factor explained by a particular variable. It is a somewhat controversial procedure because it involves a greater degree of subjectivity than is associated with most statistical analyses. After a factor is identified mathematically, the researcher provides a name for it (this is the subjective part) by examining the variables included in the factor and deciding what the underlying factor is all about. He or she then labels it accordingly. Another researcher may, of course, apply a somewhat different label to the identified factor.

The major applications of factor analysis include:

- **Data reduction.** A researcher may collect a large amount of data, particularly in survey research, and then reduce the data through factor analysis. A single composite variable or several variables measuring different dimensions of a concept may be created out of a conglomerate of variables through factor analysis. It may be used to sort out meaning from a large number of survey items on a questionnaire and reduce a large number of variables into a smaller, more manageable set of measures. For example, a survey may collect data on 50 indicators of an individual's perceived health status. Through factor analysis, the data may be reduced to three dimensions or factors, namely a physical dimension, a psychological dimension, and a social dimension. The reduced data can then be analyzed fur-

ther using procedures such as regression or analysis of variance.

- **Instrument development.** The development of new instruments is a major use of factor analysis. Instrument development usually proceeds with a large number of items used to represent the research phenomenon. The item pool can be factor analyzed to determine which items cluster together and should be retained and which items should be discarded. Gillis (1997) used factor analysis to reduce 66 items into a 43-item measure that isolated seven dimensions to a healthy lifestyle.
- **Instrument validation.** Factor analysis is an important tool for validating new research instruments (see Chapter 13). In nursing research, it is used most frequently for this reason. Factor analysis offers an empirical method of identifying the underlying factors that compose a construct. Although the researcher may *a priori* identify various dimensions to the research construct, only factor analysis can offer empirical support for the researcher's conclusions.
- **Theory development.** Factor analysis is used to identify structures of variables or constructs that can be interpreted meaningfully by the researcher. The researcher explains why variables that have been defined mathematically are clustered together the way that they have emerged. It can also lead to the conceptualization of research phenomena and their underlying dimensions and show important intercorrelations and relationships among constructs. These are important steps in theory development.

There are two types of factor analysis, exploratory and confirmatory analysis. **Exploratory factor analysis** is used when a researcher does not *a priori* identify the factor structure of the variables in the data set. It is similar to stepwise regression analysis in that the variance of the first factor identified is partialed out before analysis of the second factor proceeds. **Confirmatory factor analysis** is usually conducted after an exploratory analysis has occurred or when a researcher has a hypothesis about the existing factor structure that is to be tested. It is usually based on theory.

Computer programs provide many options when doing a factor analysis. Typically, a researcher can specify the variables to be included; the basis on which variables are selected for inclusion; and how the second and additional factors should be identified to be independent of the first (orthogonal rotation) or simply the second-best factor (oblique rotation).

Factor analysis is a complex, widely used technique in nursing research. A full discussion of the method is beyond the scope of this chapter. Interested readers are referred to statistical texts referenced at the end of this chapter and to the work of Ferketich and Muller (1990), who provide a comprehensive decision tree that describes the key decision points and options available to researchers who wish to conduct factor analyses.

2. Basic Terminology of Factor Analysis

Factor analysis begins by computing a **correlation matrix** (a table showing the correlation coefficients between all designated variables). As such, the analysis is assuming ratio level measurement of variables and normal distributions of variables. Ordinarily correlations between variables need to average 0.25 or higher in order for the data set to be considered *factorable*.

Factor loadings are the *b* weights (similar to the *b*s in regression analysis) in the factor analysis equation. Factor loadings may be combined to yield a *factor score,* which measures the extent that factor scores are similar thus reflecting the underlying common factor(s). A factor is defined mathematically as a linear combination of variables in a data matrix and is represented by the following equation:

$$F = b_1 X_1 + b_2 X_2 + b_3 X_3 + \ldots b_k X_k$$

where F = a factor score (each factor is computed separately); X_1 to X_k = values on the k original variables; and b_1 to b_k = weights (these are the factor loadings).

An **eigenvalue** is the sum of the squared factor loadings for any one factor. Thus, the eigenvalue is a measure of how much of the total variance is explained by a given factor. The higher the eigenvalue relative to other ones, the greater the variance explained by that factor.

A correlation matrix is said to be **factorable** if there are reasonably robust correlations among the items. Ordinarily, one would expect the interitem correlations to average above 0.25 to consider the variables to be worthy of factor analysis. Any lower than that and you may not find that any factors would be extracted.

In **factor extraction,** the analyst seeks to determine the number of factors that need to be extracted in order to capture or explain the variation in the data set. To proceed, the analyst will then select a method for how additional factors will be identified through a process of factor rotation.

A **marker variable** is one that produces the highest correlation with the underlying factor that is identified in the analysis. The marker variable is useful to researchers in attempting to label the underlying factor.

In determining the second factor, a rotation is required, either (1) an orthogonal (varimax is the most common version of orthogonal rotations) forces a 90 degree rotation, producing an entirely independent solution or (2) an oblique rotation that selects the second best solution but does not insist on the 90 degree rotation.

There are two main ways in which factors are extracted: (1) the **principal components method,** which includes an analysis of all the variance in the observed variables, not just the shared variance among the variables; and (2) the **principal factors method** (known in SPSS as the Principal Axis Factoring method). This approach relies on the shared variances of the variables included in the analysis and appears to be the most commonly used approach.

3. Presenting and Interpreting Results

Tables 18.6 to 18.8 report results from a factor analysis of variables designed to measure "liberalism." There were seven variables included, and these were based on nine-point Likert-type questions (Strongly Disagree to Strongly Agree) posed to students in three countries. The items were as follows:

1. My government should increase its provision for foreign aid.
2. Quotas in job hiring should be used to increase the numbers of visible minorities in good jobs.
3. Visible minorities in this country are not given an equal chance in education compared with those in the majority.
4. The immigration policies of this government are too strict.
5. Abortion should be entirely the personal choice of the woman involved.
6. There is nothing wrong with being homosexual.
7. The government does not pay enough to welfare recipients.

Using the *principal factors method,* the analysis extracted two factors, which account for a total of 55.4 percent of the variance (see Total Variance Explained in Tables 18.6 to 18.8). The *marker variable* (i.e., the one with the highest correlation to the underlying dimension measured) for the first factor, with a factor loading of 0.636, is item 7, "The government does not pay enough to welfare recipients." As indicated by the factor loadings, five items loaded predominantly on this first

factor (1, 2, 3, 4, 7). The second identified factor included items 5 and 6. In this case, the marker variable is item 5, with a factor loading of 0.610, "Abortion should be entirely the personal choice of the woman involved." The other variable that loads on this factor is item 6, "There is nothing wrong with being homosexual."

At this point, the researcher's task is to identify and label the factor that seems to underlie the two identified liberalism dimensions. Examining the marker variables and the other variables that loaded on the two factors, the researcher might label the first one as a *public policy liberalism* factor because all of the variables have to do with government programs and spending that might be used to increase the equality of participation of minority groups. The second factor made up of two variables appears to have more to do with *individual rights liberalism.*

If the researcher wishes to compute *factor scores* for individual cases, one could proceed in one of two ways:

1. Simply add together the individual raw scores on the 5 variables in factor 1 (public policy liberalism).
2. Multiply the raw scores by the factor loading for each variable and add these together.

Suppose the first two individuals in the file had the following raw values on the seven questions:

Question #	1	2	3	4	5	6	7
Respondent 1:	7	8	7	6	3	4	9
Respondent 2:	3	4	3	5	8	9	5

1. **Simple Addition Method for Determining the Factor Score:** Here we simply added together the raw scores for the appropriate variables. To get the result on the public policy liberalism factor, we would add the following numbers together to get the result for the two respondents:

Table 18.6   Factor Analysis of Liberalism Measures

	Initial Eigenvalues			Extraction Sums of Squared Loadings			Rotation Sums of Squared Loadings		
Factor	Total	% of Variance	Cumulative %	Total	% of Variance	Cumulative %	Total	% of Variance	Cumulative %
1	2.471	35.295	35.295	1.842	26.320	26.320	1.622	23.165	23.165
2	1.405	20.075	55.370	0.839	11.993	38.313	1.060	15.148	38.313
3	0.801	11.449	66.810						
4	0.650	9.283	76.102						
5	0.642	9.167	85.269						
6	0.549	7.841	93.109						
7	0.482	6.891	100.00						

Table 18.7   Factor Matrix*: Factor 1: Public Policy Liberalism

	Factor 1	Factor 2
Government increase foreign aid	0.546	−0.360
Increase number of visible minorities in jobs	0.535	−0.179
Visible minorities are not given equal education	0.550	−4.76E-02
Immigrant policies too strict	0.513	−0.243
Abortion is a woman's personal choice	0.310	0.610
Homosexuality is okay	0.438	0.490
More money should be given to welfare	0.636	6.161E-02

Extraction method: principal axis factoring.
*Two factors extracted; 16 iterations required.

Table 18.8   Rotated Factor Matrix*: Factor 2: Individualism Rights Liberalism

	Factor 1	Factor 2
Government increase foreign aid	0.651	−6.20E-02
Increase number of visible minorities in jobs	0.556	9.243E-02
Visible minorities are not given equal education	0.508	0.216
Immigrant policies too strict	0.567	2.612E-02
Abortion is a woman's personal choice	−1.20E-02	0.684
Homosexuality is okay	0.157	0.639
More money should be given to welfare	0.533	3.53

Extraction method: principal axis factoring; rotation method: varimax with Kaiser normalization.
*Rotation converged in three iterations.

a. **Public Policy Liberalism Factor Score**
Respondent 1: 7 + 8 + 7 + 6 + 9 = **37**
Respondent 2: 3 + 4 + 3 + 5 + 5 = **20**

b. **Individual Rights Liberalism Factor Score**
Respondent 1: 3 + 4 = **7**
Respondent 2: 8 + 9 = **17**

2. **Multiply Factor Loadings by Raw Scores to Determine Factor Scores.** This is the preferred method because it weights the individual scores according to their relationship to the underlying factor. In this case, we use the factor scores to weight the raw scores. Some analysts use all of the factor weightings to determine these scores, but others simply use the ones related to the underlying factor. We will use the latter method because it more clearly represents the factor alone. Using the information in Factor Loadings in Tables 18.6 to 18.8, the following calculations are made to demonstrate how these factor scores can be computed. (If you were using SPSS, these could be done quickly with a COMPUTE procedure.)

    a. **Public Policy Liberalism Factor Score (Weighted by Factor 1 Loading)**
    Respondent 1: $(7 \times 0.546) + (8 \times 0.535) + (7 \times 0.550) + (6 \times 0.513) + (9 \times 0.636) =$ **20.754**
    Respondent 2: $(3 \times 0.546) + (4 \times 0.535) + (3 \times 0.550) + (5 \times 0.513) + (5 \times 0.636) =$ **11.173**

    b. **Individual Rights Liberalism Factor Score (Weighted by Factor 2 Loading)**
    Respondent 1: $(3 \times 0.684) + (4 \times 0.639) =$ **4.608**
    Respondent 2: $(8 \times 0.684) + (9 \times 0.639) =$ **11.223**

4. Comparison with Cronbach's Alpha Procedure

The seven variables that were designed to measure liberalism were also run using the RELIABILITY procedure in SPSS. This analysis indicated that the abortion and homosexuality items should be dropped from the index in order to maximize Cronbach's alpha score. In short, both factor analysis and reliability analysis led to similar conclusions regarding the appropriate items for the "first factor" in measuring liberalism.

5. Comparison with Regression Analysis

Factor analysis is similar to regression analysis in that it involves the formation of linear combinations of variables. In regression analysis, the researcher develops equations that test hypotheses composed of independent and dependent variables. In factor analysis, equations are developed that test the interrelationships among a large number of variables and produce clusters of variables (factors) that are closely related to each other. Factor analysis requires larger sample sizes than regression analysis. Nunnally (1978) suggests a minimum of 10 participants for each variable. Thus, if there are 50 variables being factor analyzed, the sample should be approximately 500 cases.

The equation for computing the factor loadings is similar to the one used for linear regression analysis. Indeed, the b coefficients are used as the factor loadings for factor analysis. If you prefer, the regression equation is the same as the equation for the first factor in factor analysis. One should also note that both regression analysis and factor analysis use the correlation matrix as a starting point and both share common assumptions about ratio measurement of variables and normally distributed variables. The major difference between the two methods is that in the case of regression analysis, we are computing weightings on independent variables to maximize the prediction of a dependent variable for which we have values. In the case of factor analysis, we do not have a measured dependent variable; instead, in the computation of the first factor, we have a calculated value that produces the maximum association between all the variables. The second and succeeding factors produce the next best fit and depends on whether the researcher specifies an orthogonal or an oblique rotation.

E. THE FOUR TECHNIQUES COMPARED

Table 18.9 summarizes some of the characteristics of each of the techniques considered in this chapter.

Table 18.10 identifies the SPSS techniques and their associated levels of measurement. This table should be consulted when deciding which form of analysis

would be most appropriate for your project.

The advanced techniques presented in this chapter represent the main ones likely to be required by beginning researchers. Particular research questions and the levels of measurement achieved in the variables determine the appropriate technique that should be used. Note that most of these techniques rely primarily on variables measured at the ratio level. The major exception is that in discriminant function analysis, the dependent variable is assumed to be a nominal variable.

Each technique has its unique strengths, limitations, and appropriate usages. When in doubt consult an experienced researcher or a statistician.

Table 18.9   Characteristics of the Four Multivariate Techniques

Technique or SPSS Procedure	Measurement or Distribution Assumptions	Major Strength	Major Weakness
Multiple Regression REGRESSION	Ratio level on all variables; use dummy variables for nominal independent variables; assumes normal distribution of all variables	Dealing with multiple variables simultaneously, predictive equations	Instability of weightings from study to study if independent variables share much common variance
Discriminant Function Analysis DISCRIMINANT	Nominal dependent; ratio independent variables; similar to regression, can use dummy independent variables; normal distribution of independent variables; population covariance matrices must be equal	Does regression-type analysis using a nominal dependent variable; provides a measure of predictive accuracy of model	Similar to regression, an instability of weightings assigned if the independent variables share much common variance
Multivariate Analysis of Variance MANOVA	Ratio level dependent variable; handles treatment and control variables measured at all measurement levels	Deals well with interactions among variables	Deals well with interactions among variables
Factor Analysis FACTOR	Ratio level variables; however, Likert measures commonly used	Identifying factors with a common variability	Labeling of factors is subjective

Table 18.10   SPSS Procedures for Multivariate Analysis

DEPENDENT	INDEPENDENT VARIABLE		
	Nominal	Ordinal	Ratio
Nominal	CROSSTABS	CROSSTABS	CROSSTABS
			DISCRIMINANT
Ordinal	CROSSTABS	CROSSTABS	CROSSTABS
		SPEARMAN	SPEARMAN
			DISCRIMINANT
Ratio	MEANS	MEANS	CORRELATION GRAPH
	ANOVA	ANOVA	PARTIAL CORR
	t TEST	t TEST	MANOVA
			REGRESSION FACTOR

E X E R C I S E S

1. Suppose you wish to predict exercise behavior in a group of sedentary adult women. You have nonexperimental data on a number of psychosocial and biometric variables such as age, motivation levels, attitude toward exercise, belief in ability to successfully adhere to an exercise regimen, body weight, and percent of body fat. Of the methods outlined in this chapter, which one would seem to be most appropriate for this problem? Provide the rationale for your choice.

2. Suppose you are examining variations in serum cholesterol levels using socioeconomic status and region of country as independent variables. Also suppose that you suspect that there is an interaction between region of country and socioeconomic status. What factors would you need to take into account in deciding which method of analysis you would use? How might you deal with the suspected interaction between the two independent variables?

RECOMMENDED READINGS

Ferketich, S., and Muller, M. (1990). Factor analysis revisited. *Nursing Research, 39*(1), 59–62.

Iverson, G.R., and Norpoth, H. (1976). *Analysis of Variance*. Beverly Hills: Sage. This is a fine introduction to analysis of variance emphasizing the link between regression and analysis of variance techniques.

Kachigan, S.K. (1986). *Statistical Analysis: An Interdisciplinary Introduction to Univariate and Multivariate Methods*. New York: Radius Press. This text includes a detailed discussion of the techniques included in this chapter.

Munro, B., and Page, E. (2000). *Statistical Methods for Health Care Research* (2nd ed). Philadelphia: J.B. Lippincott. This is a good review of the statistical techniques most commonly used in health research. It contains clear explanations of computer printouts of various statistical procedures.

Neter, J., Wasserman, W., and Kutner, M. (1985). *Applied Linear Statistical Models*. Homewood, IL: Irwin. This is a more advanced presentation that is, however, excellent in explaining the principles of regression and analysis of variance techniques.

Polit, D. (1996). *Data Analysis and Statistics for Nursing Research.* Stamford, CT: Appleton & Lange. This practical statistics textbook for nursing students focuses on how to understand and interpret statistics rather than how to calculate them.

SPSS Inc. (1999). *SPSS Base 10.0 Advanced Models.* Chicago: SPSS Inc. This manual includes details on using MANOVA as well advanced regression techniques.

SPSS Inc. (1999). *SPSS Base 10.0 Applications Guide.* Chicago: SPSS Inc. This manual covers all the basic procedures plus discriminant function analysis, factor analysis, reliability, regression and analysis of variance.

SPSS Inc. (1999). *SPSS Base 10.0 Syntax Reference Guide.* Chicago: SPSS Inc. This manual provides the syntax for all SPSS 10.0 procedures.

SPSS Inc. (1999). *SPSS Base 10.0 User's Guide.* Chicago: SPSS Inc. This manual provides the basic instructions for using SPSS 10.0 and includes many of the same procedures presented in the *SPSS Base 10.0 Application Guide.*

Chapter 19

The Research Report

CHAPTER OUTLINE

KEY TERMS

Audience

Clinical significance

External validity

Generalizability

Implications

Nonparallel construction

Plagiarism

Pronoun problem

Review of literature

Research report

Sexist language

Summary tables

However well designed, well executed, and brilliant a research project is, its impact depends, above all, on the quality of the written report. Unless the researcher communicates clearly and disseminates results widely, the research effort will yield little in terms of knowledge development or improved practice. This chapter presents some general guidelines for communicating results to the research community and users of nursing knowledge. Suggestions for the organization and presentation of both quantitative and qualitative research reports are provided.

A. GENERAL ORIENTATION

Writing the research report is the final stage in the research process. No project is complete until the research report is submitted. The **research report** is usually a comprehensive description of key aspects of the project and includes a minimum of four major sections: the introduction, methods, results, and discussion. Some sections may contain subsections depending on the nature of the project and source of the publication. The most popular types of reports include dissertations or theses, reports on class-assigned research projects, reports to funding agencies, evaluation research reports, papers presented at scientific or professional conferences, and articles in research or professional journals. Reports may range in length from 15 pages for a journal publication to 300 pages for a doctoral dissertation. In preparing a report, consider the specific audience that will receive the report, the intended effects you hope the reader will get from the report, and the differentiated uses that will be made of the report. Although there is considerable consistency in report structure, variations reflect intended audience, style of writing, type of research project, and mode of publication or dissemination. Let us consider how these factors influence report writing.

I. Audience

Reports are written for a variety of audiences, and the particular characteristics of your audience should be taken into account when you are preparing one. Audiences may include staff nurses, other researchers, policy makers, legislators, professors, colleagues in an academic field, health-care administrators, allied health professionals, or the general public. Your **audience** will help to determine what content to include, the level and complexity of ideas to present, and the areas to be emphasized.

If a report is intended for a professional journal, then it should be organized in a manner similar to material found in the journal to which the report is to be submitted. Often journals provide guidelines for the submission of manuscripts. In cases in which they are not included, you can contact the journal editor to obtain guidelines and inquire about their interest in the manuscript topic. Use a model article from the journal as a helpful guide for preparing your report. If the journal is a "popular" one, then the report should avoid the use of technical terminology. For example, if you were writing an article on parenting styles for a professional journal, it would be appropriate to use such terms as "authoritative" and "laissez-faire"; however, in a popular magazine article, such terms would have to be explained.

There are different kinds of journals—some are thematic, others are specialty journals, and still others are broad in scope and publish a wide range of papers. It is important to recognize publishing opportunities that each may present for the manuscript you are preparing. For example, thematic journals, such as *Advances in Nursing Science,* often indicate in advance a schedule of topics that will be presented in forthcoming issues of the journal. Specialty journals, such as *JOGNN* and *Health Care for Women International,* publish manuscripts that relate to women's health. Research journals such as *Nursing Research* publish on a broad range of topics. Finally, some journals are more eclectic, such as the *Journal of Professional Nursing,* and regularly publish sections on research, policy, and educational issues related to nursing.

Most often, it is best to write for the general audience, to assume the audience has no prior knowledge of the project, and to convey ideas clearly and simply. Students who are submitting a paper for a course requirement are well advised to write not for the professor, but rather in a manner that any intelligent person would be able to follow. One hint is to write for your "Aunt Martha" or your "Uncle John," not for your professor. Your aunt and uncle have no knowledge of your research project, are not nurse scientists, and have only a high school education, but they are very smart. If you explain things clearly, they will understand your project. A side benefit of this is that your professor will also be able to figure it out!

Why would writing for an aunt or uncle be helpful? There is a tendency when preparing a report to use too many computer terms, to use technical jargon, and to fail to explain either the logic behind your research design or the logic behind the inferences you have made from your data. If you write for Aunt Martha, you will be less likely to fall into some of these traps. And, in the process, you will probably write a better report, whether it is intended for a journal, a term paper, an international research conference, or for the president and CEO of your health agency.

If you know your audience, you will also know what questions will come to their minds and you will be able to address issues of concern to them. Above all, explain your points clearly and fully.

Do not assume specialized knowledge on the part of your reader.

2. Style

Edit your material carefully. Read it slowly, perhaps out loud, and eliminate redundant words, sentences, and paragraphs. Editing should shorten the document considerably. Do not sacrifice readability and brevity for the sake of saving a nice turn of phrase. Keep it short.

It is a good idea to provide headings and subheadings to help guide your readers through the material. When technical details that would detract from the flow of the main text are nonetheless required, footnotes should be used. For purposes of editing, it is easier to place footnotes at the end of the paper.

Tables should be numbered and titled for easy reference. They should include sufficient information to permit the reader to read tables rather than text. Text should compliment important aspects of the table and not present redundant information. Generally, it is preferable to locate tables and figures on separate sheets and place them on the page after the first reference to them in the text. In manuscript preparation, tables are also placed on separate sheets so that the editor may move the material to the nearest convenient spot in the text. Because tables take extensive resources to typeset, it is best to limit them to a maximum of four or five tables per manuscript, if considering a journal publication.

Style is always influenced by the publication source. Most editors impose a specific style that has been adopted by their journal. For example, the American Psychological Association Manual (1998) is widely adopted by nursing journals such as *Nursing Research, Applied Nursing Research, Research in Nursing and Health,* and the *Canadian Journal of Nursing Research.* Authors need to consult the editor or the journal's "guidelines for authors" to determine what specific style a journal prefers.

3. Type of Report

The classic criteria of clarity, conciseness, simplicity, and ease apply to all writing, whether it is qualitative or quantitative research one is reporting. Differences exist in style depending on the type of research. Quantitative reports traditionally use objective stances rather than subjective or emotionally laden statements, and impersonal pronouns rather than personal pronouns such as "I," "me," or "we." Colloquialisms are avoided. Quantitative researchers attempt to convey a dispassionate accounting of exactly what was studied and what was discovered.

Qualitative researchers, in contrast, use a variety of narrative forms and techniques to engage the reader. The researcher is present in the writing of qualitative reports and uses specific strategies to disclose his or her own biases, values, and the context that have shaped the narrative. This may include an epilogue, reflective footnotes, interpretive commentaries, or a section on the role of the researcher (Creswell, 1998). The researcher attempts to give the flavor of the "lived experiences" being studied and to provide enlightening examples that illuminate the phenomena explored. Quotations are frequently used to bring in the voice of participants and convey complex meanings and understandings. Such devices result in a lively and interesting report. The writing style is usually personal, familiar, "up-close," highly readable, friendly, and applied for a broad audience (Creswell, 1998). If the writing style is effective, it should transport the reader into the world of the study. A careful description of the settings, people, events, and the interactions among them is one of the main contributions of qualitative research (Streubert and Carpenter, 1999).

The type of research report influences the structure. Quantitative reports conform to the following classic format or some rendition of it:

- Problem statement
- Theoretical framework
- Research question or hypotheses
- Methodology
- Results
- Discussion

Qualitative reports use a format that varies depending on the specific research tradition. That is, the structure for reporting an ethnographic study varies from a grounded theory report or a phenomenological study. Each qualitative researcher must craft a structure that is appropriate to the particular study. The literature is increasingly producing more and more diverse ways of reporting such studies. A variety of choices are available to the researcher. Box 19.1 illustrates some alternatives available for the organization of a qualitative study.

4. Avoiding Plagiarism

In writing papers, you must scrupulously avoid plagiarism. **Plagiarism** is the unacknowledged borrowing of other authors' ideas or words. Most academic disciplines have now adopted the method of referencing used by the American Psychological Association. This method requires you to identify the source from which the material has been taken in the body of the text and to include the complete bibliographic information in the list of references at the end of the paper. This is the referencing method used throughout this text.

a. Short Quotations

When fewer than 40 words are being directly quoted, the material should be enclosed in quotation marks. After the quotation, reference should be made to the name of the author, year of publication, and the page number. For example: "The

BOX 19.1 *Alternative Structures for Qualitative Reports*

Emami, Torres, Lipson and Ekman (2000): A four-part ethnographic report consisting of an "Introduction," "Methodology" (including "Data Collection," "Sample," and "Analysis"), "Findings," and "Discussion."

Orne, Fishman, Manka, and Pagnozzi (2000): A four-part phenomenological report composed of an "Introduction," "Method" (including "Study Participants," "Procedures," and "Thematic Analysis"), Findings" (including four separate theme clusters), and "Discussion"

Gray and Smith (1999): A five-part grounded theory report starting with the - "Introduction"; followed by "The Study," which is subdivided into a heading called "Materials and Methods" (containing "Design," "Sample and Data Collection," "Ethical Issues," and "Data Analysis"); a "Findings" section that describes the five phases that emerged from the core category of professional socialization; a "Discussion" section (in-

cluding a subheading of "Limitations"); and, finally, the "Conclusion" section

Gates (2000): A seven-part phenomenological report composed of an "Introduction/Context," "Researcher's Perspective," "Methodology" (including "Participants," "Data Gathering," and "Data Analysis"), "Findings," "Discussion," "Research and Practice Implications," and "Conclusion."

Dickson (2000): A participatory action research report composed of seven sections beginning with an introduction that is untitled; followed by a section entitled "Grandmothers" that describes the context in which the study occurred; a section called "The Grandmothers' Project"; followed by the "Methodology" section ("Data Collection," "Data Analysis," and "Trustworthiness"), the "Findings and Discussion of Effects of Participation" section, a "Study Strengths and Limitations" section, and concluding with an "Implications" section

difference between mores and folkways lies in the nature of the reaction the violation of the norm produces, and not in the content of the rule" (Jackson, 1999, p. 19).

b. Long Quotations

When more than 40 words are directly quoted, the material is indented an additional five spaces on the right side of the page and the material is single-spaced, with a reference to the author's name, date, and page at the end of the quotation (unless the author has been introduced earlier in the paragraph). For example, if the quote is introduced, Gillis and Jackson (2002) noted . . . then only the page number is needed at the end of the quotation.

c. Paraphrased Material

When using paraphrased material by borrowing ideas that you are not quoting di-

rectly, you are nonetheless required to cite your source. Once again, you should include the author's name and the year of publication but not the page number.

d. Citing Secondary Sources

Occasionally you find a study that is discussed in a journal article or book (a secondary source) but you are unable to locate the original (primary source) in which the study was first published. When a secondary source is used, cite the original author first, followed by a reference to the secondary source. For example, "Gillis, cited in Jackson (1999)." In this case, Gillis is the primary source and Jackson is the secondary one.

e. Multiple Authors' References

When there are three, four, or five authors, the first reference includes all the names, and subsequent references to their work use only the first author's name, followed by "et al." When there are six or more authors, use only the first author's name followed by "et al." and the year for the first and subsequent citations.

f. Reference List

At the end of the paper, provide a reference list that includes all references cited in alphabetical order. Notice how books and articles are cited in this text. Additional examples may be noted in the bibliography that is included at the end of this text.

Sample article reference: Parsons, K. (1997). The male experience of care giving for a family member with Alzheimer's disease. *Qualitative Health Research, 7*(3), 391–408. (The italicized material may be underlined if you do not have an italic font on your printer.)

Sample book reference: Norwood, S. L. (2000). *Research Strategies for Advanced Practice Nurses.* Uppersaddle River, NJ: Prentice Hall Health.

Sample chapter from an edited book reference: Israel, B.A., and Schurman, S. (1990). Social support, control and the stress process. In Glanz, R., Lewis, F., and Rimer, B. (Eds.): *Health Behavior and Health Education.* San Francisco: Jossey-Bass.

5. Avoiding Sexist Language

In the past few years, there has been an increasing awareness of **sexist language.** We will briefly look at some of the major pitfalls in gender references.

a. The Pronoun Problem

The **pronoun problem** encourages stereotypic thinking by referring to such people as doctors, managers, and patients as he

and nurses, secretaries, and parents as she. There are a number of solutions to the pronoun problem. To illustrate, suppose we have the following sentence: "A doctor has to be especially careful; otherwise, he can be sued for malpractice." (The problem is characterizing the doctor as a he.) This sentence can be changed in any one of the following ways:

- "A doctor has to be especially careful; otherwise, he or she can be sued for malpractice." (This is a somewhat awkward solution but is acceptable if not used too frequently.)
- "Doctors have to be especially careful; otherwise, they can be sued for malpractice." (This is a common solution, converting to the plural form avoids the use of *he or she.*)
- "If not especially careful, doctors can be sued for malpractice." (This sentence avoids the pronoun all together by reconstructing the sentence.)

b. The "Man" Problem

Traditionally, many words and expressions in the English language used *man* or *men* to refer to persons of either gender. In a manner similar to the pronoun problem, such usage may unintentionally suggest, for example, that a *foreman* should be a man. Table 19.1 includes a few examples and some alternative forms that could be considered.

c. The Nonparallel Construction Problem

Language may frequently put one gender at a disadvantage. For example, a man may be referred to more formally than a woman, suggesting a power or importance differential. More generally, **nonparallel constructions** can result in confusion or misrepresentation by violating the principle that parts of a sentence that are parallel in meaning should be parallel

Table 19.1   Neutralizing Gender Terms

Traditional Usage	Alternative Forms
Chairman	Chair, chairperson, coordinator, head, leader, moderator, presiding officer
Clergyman	Cleric, member of the clergy, minister
Fisherman	Fisher
Foreman	Boss, supervisor
Mailman	Letter carrier, postal worker
Mankind	Human beings, humanity, people
Manmade	Artificial, manufactured, synthetic
Manpower	Personnel, workers
Salesman	Sales agent, salesperson
To man	Operate, to staff
Workman	Employee, laborer, worker

Table 19.2   Nonparallel and Parallel Gender References

Inappropriate Usage (Nonparallel)	Alternative Forms (Parallel)
Man and wife	Husband and wife
Men and ladies	Men and women
Men's and ladies' teams	Men's and women's teams
Males and women	Males and females

in structure. Table 19.2 provides some illustrations of nonparallel gender references and more appropriate, parallel forms.

B. ORGANIZATION OF QUANTITATIVE REPORTS

A paper should be organized into sections. As previously noted, there are a variety of reporting formats for qualitative reports associated with each perspective and method (see Box 19.1). This section relates primarily to quantitative reports. The final section of the chapter presents some minimum guidelines for qualitative reports with an example of the structure of a qualitative research report. An effort should be made to cover the material discussed under each of the following headings, but it should be noted that there are somewhat different traditions for the reporting of experimental studies versus surveys and other descriptive designs.

1. Introduction

The introduction should inform your reader what the project is about, indicate the general approach that has been used to solve the problem it tackles, and suggest the critical problems the project raises. Also mention interesting questions and unresolved issues that you propose to answer in your research.

2. Review of the Literature

The **review of the literature** tries to provide an overview of the "state of scientific knowledge" in your area of study. Consider reviewing the theoretical models that are appropriate and the empirical findings that bear on the particular relationships you will be examining or, if such material is not available, give the reader some sense of the variables that have been related to the major dependent variable in your study. The review should highlight the areas in which there are inconsistencies in the conclusions of other studies and indicate which of these inconsistencies you intend to address.

Generally, it is best not to present summaries of articles; instead, it is good to focus on what the consensus is on the relationship between particular variables and the dependent variable. For example, suppose that you were examining factors related to nurses' job satisfaction. It would be useful for your reader to know whether there is any agreement in the scientific literature on whether "satisfaction" is related to such variables as age, type of educational program, nursing practice settings, level of decision making, and years of work experience. When there are inconsistencies, do you have any observations as to why they emerged? Different regions, different measurement or analytic procedures, or systematic variations in the compositions of the populations studied might all account for the variations between studies. If inconsistencies are present, they can be noted and you can heighten your reader's interest in your project by proposing to answer some of the questions that have been raised.

The review of the literature varies in length and style depending on whether it is being prepared for a thesis or dissertation, a conference presentation, a scholarly paper, or a journal publication. Journal editors often limit the length of the review because of cost and space limitations. Chapter 3 contains a discussion of how a review of literature can be developed and presented. Readers are referred to that chapter for additional suggestions.

3. Hypotheses and Research Questions

The review of literature section should lead into a section defining the hypotheses, questions, or relationships that are to be examined. These should be precisely stated and connected to the literature of the discipline. It is almost always best to diagram the research models that are being evaluated in the research: not only does this permit the presentation of hypotheses clearly but additional precision is achieved by drawing in causal arrows and "greater than" and "less than"

symbols. Figure 19.1 presents the diagram used by Murray (1999) in a study of unwanted intimacy.

4. Methods

The methods section details the research plan that was used to answer the research question or test the hypotheses. It includes a description of what was done in sufficient detail so that another researcher could replicate the study. It is usually divided into subsections including descriptions of the sample, data collection procedures, and indexes and measurement procedures used. The rationale given for the design selected should state the advantages the chosen design has over alternative designs. What designs have typically been used by other investigators looking at similar relationships?

a. Description of the Sample

Readers should be introduced to the results by reporting some of the background characteristics of the individuals involved in the study. Gender distribution, rural or urban location, and average age all may be reported if judged to be relevant by the researcher. If efforts are to be made to ensure the representativeness of the sample, this is the stage in the report that such material would be introduced appropriately. If you know from census material, for example, that 54 percent of the region's population above age 15 years is female and your sample is 59 percent female, this fact should be noted. In experimental studies, a detailed description of the method of randomization used should be included.

b. Data Collection Procedures

After determining the questions and the design, the next step in the methods sec-

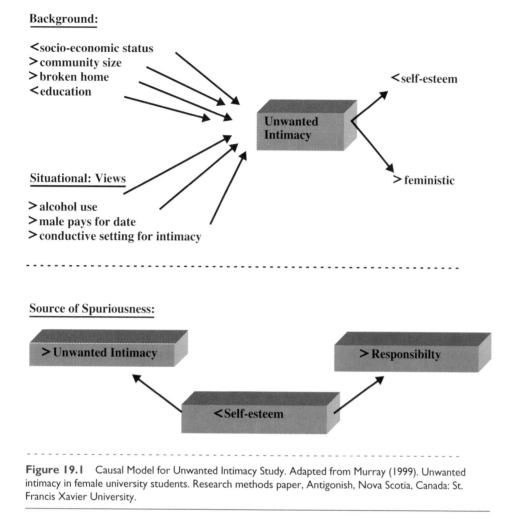

Figure 19.1   Causal Model for Unwanted Intimacy Study. Adapted from Murray (1999). Unwanted intimacy in female university students. Research methods paper, Antigonish, Nova Scotia, Canada: St. Francis Xavier University.

tion is to describe the measurement, sample design, and data collection procedures. A description of the methods used to collect the data is critical to evaluating the study. A description of the instruments and procedures and the rationale for their selection is usually included. In describing a questionnaire, it is not necessary to discuss every question; however, sufficient detail should be provided so that it is evident how the variables were operationalized. It is helpful to focus attention on nonstandard items and, if possible, include a copy of the questionnaire in an appendix to the report. If the instrument was developed for use in the study, the procedure for development and testing of the quality of the instrument should be described. Also indicate what revisions were made and what scoring procedures were followed. Any comments on problems in data collection should be mentioned at this point in the report.

c. Description of Indexes and Measurement Procedures

A description and evaluation of indexes or scales constructed and a preliminary report on the mean results should be made at this point. If you have used an index that was administered in a previously published study, comparisons may be made between the mean results of your study and those of other researchers. Details for the measurement of other key variables should also be included. If the study involves repeated measures, what steps were taken to ensure that the measurement process itself was not contaminating the results?

5. Presenting Results

The results section is usually a combination of narrative description and statistical reports. If descriptive and inferential statistics have been used, the descriptive statistics are reported first. When reporting statistical findings, three pieces of information are required: the test value, the level of significance, and the degrees of freedom. For example, it may be reported that depression was experienced at 1 month postpartum in new mothers and significantly lower levels of depression were reported in 3-month follow-up measures. The following statement reflects the three pieces of statistical information to communicate this: "The ANOVA for repeated measures indicated a statistically significant reduction in depression by time ($F = 12.12$; df $= 2$; $P = < 0.001$)."

The narrative presentation of results should be written in the *past tense*. This is because research studies do not prove or confirm that hypotheses are correct; rather, hypotheses are supported or not supported by the findings. It is inappropriate to write: " Adolescents who take peer pressure resistance classes engage in healthier lifestyles than those who do not." The use of the present tense implies the results apply to all adolescents rather than just the sample whose behavior was observed in the past (Thomas, 2000). The verbs "take" and "engage" should be changed to "took" and "engaged." The results should read as follows: "Adoles-

cents who *took* peer pressure resistance classes *engaged* in healthier lifestyles than those who *did* not."

Clinical significance of findings should also be discussed. Findings may or may not have statistical significance (findings are unlikely to be caused by chance) and yet still have importance for nursing practice. If the difference is great enough to make an impact on client care or on a phenomenon of concern to nursing, then it is clinically significant, even if analysis procedures do not produce *statistically significant* results. For example, the use of a certain sedative in combination with an analgesic consistently reduces the perception of pain in a variety of postoperative conditions in comparison with pain perception levels for those only receiving the analgesic. Although the differences between the two groups may not be statistically significant, the trend consistently favors the use of the sedative in combination with the analgesic; therefore, the results have clinical significance because the treatment leads to reduced pain levels. In small sample studies (those with fewer than 200 subjects), it is particularly important to report on whether the data trend is in the direction predicted by the various research hypotheses.

Generally, the Statistical Package for the Social Sciences (SPSS) output is not in an appropriate form for presentation. Tables placed in a final report need to be reformatted. Their format should conform to those shown throughout this book or be modeled on those presented in journal articles or books. Although it is possible to control the SPSS output format, beginning researchers will probably find it easier to retype the tables.

In qualitative reports, the results section often contains a summary of themes and narrative descriptions of phenomena. Extensive quotations may be used to substantiate the major themes identified. Models, figures, and diagrams are useful in concisely illustrating complex ideas, theories, and relationships that emerge from qualitative investigations.

a. Organizing Summary Tables

The variations in the dependent variable should be explored at this point. Any basic analyses that explore the formal hypotheses of the study should be presented. A challenge for the researcher is to compress this information into as few tables as possible. Well-designed **summary tables** can add a lot to your report without sacrificing anything. When possible, use summary tables to compress the results of many analyses into one table. Remember to focus on the relationships being ex-

plored when reporting findings. If you are using tests of significance, report whether the findings are statistically significant. If a particular relationship is not statistically significant, is there a trend in the data? It is misleading simply to report "significant" findings. As noted earlier, relationships that are not statistically significant may well have substantive significance.

Let us look at some formats for reporting single-variable information, cross-tabulation tables, differences of means, and correlations into summary tables.

(i) Summarizing Univariate Statistics

Table 19.3 presents one way of compressing the information on a number of vari-

Table 19.3 Summarizing the Sample Characteristics

A. Nominal or Ordinal Variables	Number	Percentage
Gender		
Male	82	48.0
Female	89	52.0
Status		
Student	26	15.2
Retired	2	1.2
Unemployed, looking for work	13	7.6
Unemployed, not looking for work	4	2.3
Employed part time	19	11.1
Employed full time	107	62.6
Population of home community		
Under 5000	17	9.0
5000 to 19,999	24	12.7
20,000 to 99,999	16	8.5
100,000 to 999,999	108	57.1
1,000,000 or more	24	12.7

B. Ratio Variables	Mean	Standard Deviation	Cases, n
Age, years	29.6	14.7	183
Income, dollars	43,257	16,419	77
Seniority	8.87	3.76	104
Children, n	1.37	1.06	78

ables into a single table. Note that nominal variables can simply have the frequencies listed for each category. These kinds of listings are useful in summarizing descriptive characteristics of the cohort studied. The mean values and the standard deviations can be used to summarize the ratio variables.

(ii) Summarizing Cross-tabulation Tables

Table 19.4 shows one method for reporting a series of cross-tabulation table results (CROSSTABS procedure in SPSS). Note that only the percentage of smokers is reported, along with the number of cases in the column, the chi-square probability, and whether the results have a trend in the predicted direction (+) or in the opposite direction (−).

(iii) Summarizing Mean Values for a Dependent Variable

Table 19.5 provides an illustration of how you can compress a number of analyses of ratio variables into one table. The analysis by Annette Fougere compares the academic performance of grade 12 students who did or did not regularly eat breakfast. Note that Table 19.5 includes the mean grade performance, standard deviations, number of cases, probability level, and an indication of whether the data have a trend in the predicted direction (+) or in the opposite one (−).

(iv) Summarizing Correlations

Table 19.6 shows a correlation matrix for variables related to first-year university performance. Note that a report on many relationships can be compressed into such a table. By using asterisks, it is also possible to indicate which of the correlations are statistically significant.

(v) Tables and Figures in Qualitative Reports

Table 19.7 and Figure 19.2 show examples of the type of "word" items that are frequently presented in qualitative research reports to portray results. Tables in qualitative studies are often conceptual or thematic. Table 19.7 presents five thematic areas that represent changes found in a group of native grandmothers who participated in a health promotion project. Figure 19.2 visually presents some findings from a grounded theory study designed to build a theory about individuals' perception of being psychiatric patients. The figure highlights the patients' experiences before hospitalization that were shaping their responses, including medication noncompliance, lack of social capitol, and substance abuse.

b. Using Graphs and Charts

When feasible, it is a good idea to present data using graphs and charts to make a greater visual impact on readers. Figures 19.3 and 19.4 show some alternative forms of reporting information. Figure 19.3 uses a bar graph to show the relationship between country of origin and having suicidal thoughts. Respondents' countries of origin are grouped into three categories: Canada, New Zealand, and Australia.

Figure 19.4 uses a plot to show the relationship between prestige and income. The visual information conveys much about the strength of the association between the two variables. To seasoned researchers, the correlation of 0.83 between the two variables reveals much, but for most readers, the plot of the information reveals additional information. Notice, for example, that the prestige ratings tend not to increase much as incomes rise above the $90,000 mark.

c. Evaluating Hypotheses and Models

The reader should now be well prepared, and anticipating the results of the hypothesis and model testing. If diagrams described the original relationships, they should be used again when the findings are reported. If you are testing a theory

Table 19.4 Summarizing Cross-tabulation Tables: Respondents' Smoking Behavior by Selected Independent Variables*

Independent Variables	Smokers, %	Cases, n Column Total	Probability (Chi-Square)	Trend
Residence				
On campus	19.8	101	0.93283	?
Off campus	20.4	54		
SES of father				
Low SES	22.2	54	0.61304	+
Mid to high SES	18.8	101		
Respondents' age, y				
19 or younger	19.7	76	0.93597	+
20 or older	20.3	79		
Level of self-esteem				
Low	19.5	77	0.87237	−
High	20.5	78		
Level of stress				
Low	19.4	67	0.90052	−
High	18.6	86		
Home community, population				
Under 30,000	17.8	118	0.22068	−
30,000 or more	27.0	37		
Gender				
Male	17.6	68	0.51734	+
Female	21.8	87		
Type of program				
Arts	23.3	60	0.48859	+
Science	18.7	91		
Exercise/week				
Less than three times	29.6	71	0.00613	+
Three or more times	11.9	84		
Father smokes				
Yes	29.3	41	0.8363	+
No	16.7	114		
Mother smokes				
Yes	45.5	33	0.00004	+
No	13.1	122		

Source: Adapted from Michelle Lee (1992). Smoking Behaviors. Antigonish: St. Francis Xavier University, Research Methods Paper.

Table 19.5   Summarizing Means: Grade Performance of Grade 12 Students

Independent Variables	Mean	Standard Deviation	Cases, n	Test of Significance	Trend
Eats breakfast					
No	68.9	12.7	46	0.0003	+
Yes	76.3	10.0	95		
Breakfast eaten in past 7 days					
No	69.5	9.9	39	0.0049	+
Yes	75.4	11.5	106		
Breakfast maker					
Others	72.7	14.4	42	0.2731	−
Self	75.1	10.0	85		
Lunch maker					
Others	73.8	11.7	105	0.8412	*
Self	74.3	11.6	29		
Supper maker					
Others	74.1	11.6	117	0.6416	*
Self	72.9	10.6	27		
Gender					
Male	71.4	11.7	85	0.0026	+
Female	77.2	10.0	58		
Community population					
≤ 5000	73.7	11.9	103	0.8024	−
> 5000	74.2	10.2	42		
Career plans					
University	78.2	9.0	92	0.0000	+
Nonuniversity	66.2	11.1	53		
Extracurricular activities					
No	70.9	12.0	70	0.0015	−
Yes	76.8	9.9	74		
After-school job					
No	73.4	11.8	88	0.5825	−
Yes	74.5	10.8	57		

+ Trend predicted correctly; − trend predicted incorrectly; * trend not predicted.
Source: Adapted from Annette Fougere (1992). Effects of Eating Breakfast on Grade Performance. Antigonish: St. Francis Xavier University, Research Methods Paper.

and have derived a hypothesis, then you should report the finding of the test, even if the relationship is not statistically significant.

In cases in which you are investigating alternative explanations for a relationship you have initially assumed to be statistically significant, you would only con-

Table 19.6   Correlations Between First Year University Average, Average High School Grade, and English High School Grade (*n* = 3617)

Correlations	First Year University Average	Average High School Grade	English High School Grade
First year average	1.000		
Average high school grade	0.573*	1.000	
English high school grade	0.464*	0.662*	1.000

*$P < 0.001$

tinue to test the alternative explanations if the relationship turned out to be statistically significant. You would, of course, include the intervening variable model in your report; however, if no relationship has emerged, you would not proceed with an evaluation of the alternative explanations—you have no relationship to explain. All you would do is note in your report that the alternative explanations will not be explored because the original relationship was not sufficiently strong.

If it turns out that the primary relationship is not statistically significant, it is then appropriate to explore the relationship of independent variables to the dependent variable. If you are forced to this "fall back" position and have not established the various hypotheses in advance, then you should indicate that your

Table 19.7   Categories and Components: Effects on Grandmothers of Participation in a Health Promotion Project

Category	Component
Cleansing and healing	Self-healing
	Self-care
Connecting with self	Self-understanding
	Well-being, self-esteem, and self-respect
	Identification of strengths and needs
	Cultural and spiritual identity
Acquiring information and skills	Health education
	Assertiveness
	Learning about and securing resources
Connecting with the group	Group identification
	Mutual understanding and respect
	Mutual learning and inspiration
External exposure and engagement	Willingness to influence the system
	Speaking up
	Community honoring

Source: Dickson, G. (2000). Aboriginal grandmothers' experience with health promotion and participatory action research. *Qualitative Health Research, 10*(2), 188–213.

Substance abuse, lack of social capital, medication noncompliance

↓

NORM VIOLATIONS

↓

Voluntary nature, familiarity, inevitability, utility

↓

HOSPITALIZATION

Figure 19.2   Basic conditions, intervening factors, and individual responses to psychiatric hospital admission.

explorations are being conducted without the guidance of hypotheses. The reader is then alerted to the fact that you are on a hunting expedition. Hunting is fine as long as the reader is alerted.

6. Discussion

At this point, an effort should be made to tie together the whole project. The discussion section accomplishes this by focusing on the interpretation of the results; the limitations of the study; and the implications of the findings for practice, education, theory, and future research. Again, references should be made to the review of literature section, showing how the results of your research fit into the general picture. Such references also help tie the paper together, reminding the reader of the problems that the project initially raised. In what areas does your research support the general view, and in what areas does it not? When there are discrepancies, what are some of the possible explanations? This discussion should provide readers with a sense of what has been learned and what remains problematic.

The **generalizability** of the findings to other contexts should be explored. This refers to the extent that the findings may be extrapolated from the present study to other groups in general. It is commonly referred to as **external validity.**

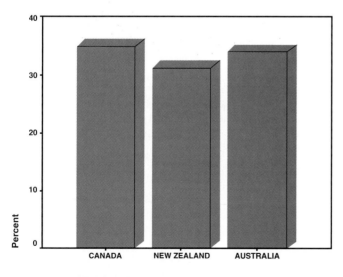

NAME OF COUNTRY

Figure 19.3   Sample bar graph. Percent with suicidal thoughts by country of origin.

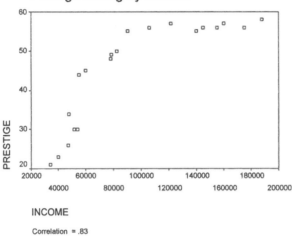

Prestige Rating by Income

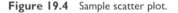

To perform this analysis using SPSS, use GRAPHS/SCATTER.

Figure 19.4 Sample scatter plot.

The impact of threats to external and internal validity on results should be discussed in this section (see Chapters 4 and 12). In so doing, the researcher communicates to readers an awareness of the limitations of the study and discusses their impact on the interpretation of the study findings.

The **implications** of the study findings are explored in the discussion section. The author highlights the importance of the study in terms of its potential contributions to practice, education, theory, and research, as appropriate. This component is particularly critical if the results are to be used by research consumers to inform practice or to identify new and challenging research questions. Recommendations emerging from the study should be clearly articulated in ten-

tative terms so they may be tested in subsequent investigations.

7. Conclusion

The final section should try to briefly state what the central problem was and what conclusions have been identified. This section may also include suggestions for how the current project may have been improved and what other issues the researcher identifies as worthy of further exploration.

8. Final Checklist

Table 19.8 contains a checklist of items that authors of quantitative reports may wish to use to provide some guidance for when a paper is ready to submit.

Table 19.8   Checklist for Determining When Your Paper Is Ready for Submission

Section	Description
Title	Short, informative title should be selected
Abstract	If needed, keep to one half a page
Introduction	Excite interest of reader; indicate why the topic is of interest. Normally the Introduction is short; keep literature references to a minimum.
Review of Literature	Include summary table if possible; it is generally best to organize the review around findings by variable not article summaries; should anticipate hypotheses (diagrams) to follow.
Statement of Hypotheses	Include causal model diagrams or formal statements of hypotheses to be tested. Diagrams force precision.
Methodology	Description of variables, measurement procedures, sampling, and analytical procedures identified
Results	Provide a description of sample studied; include summary tables for major hypotheses tested
Discussion	Link findings of study to the body of literature reviewed earlier. What questions remain? Which direction do you see as the most productive for researchers to pursue?
Conclusions	Summarize the major findings of the study. Keep this section short.
References	Are in-text references consistent? Are all in-text references included in the References Cited section at the end of the paper? Have you consistently used the APA referencing format?
Spell Check	Run the paper through a spell checker to catch any errors.
Format	Examine the paper to be certain you are not breaking tables in the middle; use different sized fonts for subtitles.
View Document	Use word processor's "view document" to check on page layout.
Print	Print your paper!
Proofread	A final check before you submit it.

C. ORGANIZATION OF QUALITATIVE REPORTS

Although some content discussed in the previous section is appropriate for some qualitative investigations, it would be unwise to expect qualitative reports to conform to the established format of a conventional quantitative study. Qualitative research emanates from a different worldview (see Chapter 1), and reporting formats must respect this difference. Qualitative researchers are concerned with capturing the essence of phenomena of concern to nurses and communicating the meaning of human experiences, with a level of detail that makes the experience come alive for the reader. The researcher creates "scenes" or vivid descriptive accounts of his or her experience over time with the participants rather than reporting facts and figures. Each tradition of qualitative research elects to do this using a different narrative structure. In preparing to write a qualitative report, one should obtain a high-quality model of a report using that particular tradition. This proves extremely helpful in guiding the researcher with the final report. One can learn a great deal about the proper structure and style for writing qualitative reports by a careful study of relevant phenomenological, ethnographic, grounded theory, or historical studies.

1. Guidelines for Qualitative Reports

In searching for models of qualitative studies, you will notice that there is no shortage of styles or formats in the literature. From this rich diversity of approaches, Miles and Huberman (1994, p. 304) have identified a set of minimum guidelines to assist beginning researchers in drafting a qualitative report. These include:

1. The report should tell us the essence of the study.
2. It should describe the social and historical context of the setting (or settings) where data were collected.
3. It should describe the natural history of the inquiry, including what was done and by whom and how. This is similar to the methods section of a quantitative account. It should convey how key concepts emerged over time, which variables appeared and disappeared, and which codes led to important insights.
4. It should communicate raw data in the form of vignettes, quotations, photographs, and so on, so that the reader can draw conclusions in parallel with the researcher. Drawing conclusions unsubstantiated by data is the antithesis of research.
5. Finally, in the discussion or conclusion section, researchers should articulate their conclusions and the impact on the nursing world.

Many qualitative investigators agree that it would be unwise to develop a set of canons for reporting qualitative findings. It appears at this juncture in our research history that the field of nursing agrees. Most researchers believe the study's questions, context, and audience should drive the design of the qualitative report. A balance between interpretation and description is important.

A major difference in reporting qualitative studies compared with quantitative ones is that whereas the latter deals with numbers, the former, coming from a different paradigm, reports themes or processes. Editors are becoming more sensitive to the differences in report styles and are less likely to force a qualitative investigator to conform to the reporting style adopted by quantitative researchers.

2. Sample Outlines of Qualitative Reports

Parsons (1997) used the phenomenological method to investigate the male experience of caregiving for a family member with Alzheimer's disease. She interviewed eight men—five spouses and three sons—to determine what their experiences were like. From the analysis of the interview data, nine themes emerged. The themes were interrelated to form a whole that captured the experience of caregiving for the male caregivers (the essence). Below is an outline of the report:

1. Abstract
2. Introduction and statement of topic and purpose
3. Review of literature
4. Methodology
   • Participants
   • Procedure
   • Data analysis
5. Findings
   • Enduring
   • Vigilance
   • A sense of loss
   • Aloneness and loneliness
   • Taking away
   • Searching to discover
   • The need for assistance
   • Reciprocity
   • Overstepping the normal boundaries
   • The essence
6. Discussion

If you consult the original source, you will notice that the terms *abstract* and *introduction* do not appear in the article. We have included them in our outline, however, because clearly they are evident in the structure of the report. Journal articles often omit any heading at the beginning of an article and consider all the material before the methodology section as an introduction. The introduction of this report identifies the research topic, the statement of purpose, the review of the literature, and the significance of the problem for nursing.

The methods section is divided into subsections and identifies the design (phenomenology), the sample selection process (participants), and the procedure for data collection and analysis. In qualitative reports, a great amount of detail is expected in the data collection and analysis section because so much of the findings depend on the researcher's interpretation of the data. Because of this, it is important to describe any procedures taken to protect and evaluate the quality of the data.

The results section is called "Findings" and is organized according to the nine themes that emerged and the description of the essence of the experience. This is typical of the style of reporting found in a phenomenological study. Quotations are used to illustrate important points. The themes are summarized and descriptive data are integrated into the materials. The discussion section discusses the importance of the findings to nursing.

You will notice that although there are similarities in the overall structure of this phenomenological report and some quantitative reports, there are significant differences in the organizational sections and the content within the sections differs.

To further explore the similarities and differences in quantitative and qualitative reports, let's look at the organizational structure of a grounded theory study. Stetz and Brown (1997) provide an in-depth description of *Taking Care,* one of the phases of a grounded theory of caregiving for families experiencing life-threatening illnesses such as cancer or AIDS. In-depth interviews

were conducted with 26 family caregivers of persons with cancer or AIDS during a 4-month period. Data were analyzed in terms of the strategies, consequences, and interactions involved in the caregiving experience. The researchers structured their report according to the following outline:

1. Abstract
2. Introduction
3. Theoretical framework
4. Purpose
5. Methods
   - Procedure
   - Sample
   - Instrument
   - Data analysis
6. Findings
   - Strategies for taking care
   - Consequences of taking care
   - Interactions and taking care
7. Limitations
8. Practice recommendations

This outline follows a logical step-by-step approach to the challenging but exciting task of writing up qualitative research results. In most qualitative outlines such as this one, you will notice that the findings section, in particular, usually portrays a range of subheadings unique to the specific study. The subheadings reflect the key ideas or concepts that emerge from the analysis of the qualitative data. This section quickly provides the reader of the report with a rich description of the critical findings of the report. For example, in their findings section, Stetz and Brown use the subheadings of "Strategies," "Consequences," and "Interactions" involved in the caregiving experience. These findings vividly portray the family caregivers' experiences in caring for ill family members. In other ways, the outlines of quantitative and qualitative reports are similar because both use the general headings of "Title," "Abstract," "Introduction," "Method," "Results," "Discussion," and "Conclusion."

It is important to remember that a research project is not complete until the final report is written and disseminated to appropriate audiences. The "perfect" research project is of little value if the results are not communicated to others. It is the researcher's professional accountability to make certain that results are published as soon as possible upon completion of the project.

E X E R C I S E S

1. Select a nursing research journal that publishes both quantitative and qualitative studies. Review an issue of it and determine if the quantitative articles within it adhere to the organizational headings provided in this chapter. Compare and contrast the organizational structure used by the quantitative and qualitative researchers to write their reports.

2. Select one article containing tables or graphs (or both). Assess them against the guidelines provided in the chapter. Select a second article that does not contain tables and create a table based on the data presented in the "Results" section.

3. Read the introductory section of a nursing research study. Carefully edit that section for redundant words, phrases, and sentences. Did you significantly shorten the section as a result of your editing? Did you sacrifice clarity for brevity?

4. Visit your nursing library and review the following types of research publications:
   - Scientific nursing journal
   - Professional journal that publishes research related articles
   - Nursing student thesis
   - Popular literature report of a research study

   Compare and contrast the structure of each report. Who was the intended audience? Did the author do a reasonable job of communicating the study to the intended audience? What suggestions, if any, would you make to improve the style of the presentations?

RECOMMENDED READINGS

American Psychological Association (1998). *Publication Manual of the American Psychological Association,* Washington D.C.: American Psychological Association.

Bell, L. (1995). *Effective Writing: A Guide for Health Professionals.* Toronto: Copp Clarke. An excellent resource for those interested in writing for publication, either for health-care professionals or the general public. Special sections on health research, health care, and health promotion are included.

Creswell, J.W. (1998). *Qualitative Inquiry and Research Design.* Thousand Oaks, CA: Sage. A good description of the different narrative styles used in each qualitative tradition.

Hodges, J.C., Whitten, M.E., Brown, J., and Flick, J. (1994). *Harbrace College Handbook:*

The purpose of this chapter is to provide beginning researchers with a set of skills for critically appraising research efforts. This is an essential skill for all nurses who wish to engage in evidence-based practice, use research findings to contribute to improved client care, or be responsible consumers of research. Unless nurses can correctly assess the merits of a research report, they are at a loss in terms of using research to guide practice and will be unable to contribute to extending the field of nursing's research knowledge base. This chapter discusses what a research critique is and outlines the process for evaluating the quality of research studies. Guidelines are provided for conducting critiques of quantitative and qualitative research reports. Samples of research report critiques are provided.

A. UNDERSTANDING THE CRITIQUING PROCESS

1. What Is a Research Critique?

A **research critique** is a critical appraisal of a piece of completed research. It involves a high level of critical thinking and analysis of each component of the research study. Critiques may be conducted on research reports, manuscripts, or published articles based on research studies or they may be done on research proposals. A critique provides constructive criticism of a specific piece of work for the purpose of promoting excellence in research. Through specific commentary, a critique can identify both the strengths and limitations of a study and assist the nurse in deciding how best to apply the study findings in practice. Critiques are usually three to four pages long and address the major aspects of the research process. **Critical appraisal** involves judging whether or not a research study is described clearly and comprehensively enough to decide if the findings and implications are logical and believable and

should be considered seriously in your practice. The outcome of a critique should influence future research and knowledge development in nursing.

2. What Is the Role of the Critic?

The major role of a **research critic** is to provide an objective evaluation of a study's merits. To do this, a critic must read a report comprehensively and offer constructive comments on all aspects of the report, as well as on the specific strengths and limitations of the study. Comments should be offered in a spirit that promotes mutual respect and collegiality among the researchers and the reviewer. The intent of a critique is to contribute positively to a research program. Although the areas needing improvement should be communicated clearly by the critic, tactfulness is needed so that researchers are not offended or discouraged in their attempts to advance nursing knowledge.

3. What Are the Stages of the Critique Process?

A critique of a research report involves a review of the report in its totality, as well as a microscopic examination of each component of the study. The critic appraises the merit of a research project in four stages. These include:

Stage 1. Clearly understanding the meaning of the purpose and problem statement of a study and determining if the research design and methodology are consistent with the study purpose.

Stage 2. Studying the manner in which the study was conducted and determining if the methodology was applied properly.

Stage 3. Studying the findings of a study and assessing if the outcomes and conclusions are believable and supported by the findings (NHS, 1998).

Stage 4. Summarizing the overall quality of the study, identifying the strengths and limitations of the study, evaluating the contribution of the study to nursing, and identifying suggestions for improving the work. This is usually the last paragraph or two of a critique.

Each of the stages evaluates critical components of the research report unique to that stage of the critiquing process. Box 20.1 identifies the components of a quantitative research report that are evaluated at each stage.

B. CRITICALLY APPRAISING RESEARCH REPORTS

Some researchers suggest that critical appraisal of a research study is based on the match between the study purpose and the other elements of the study (Knafl and Howard, 1984; Cobb and Hagemaster, 1987; Forchuk and Roberts, 1993). Because research that evolves from various paradigms (i.e., positivist–empiricist or naturalistic–inductive worldviews) differs considerably in its purpose and underlying nature, it is important to discuss guidelines for evaluating studies that emanate from different paradigms separately. The critique of studies from the positivist–empiricist paradigm, which uses quantitative research methods, is discussed first, followed by a discussion of the critique process for qualitative studies.

I. Criteria for Critically Appraising Quantitative Research Reports

A number of nursing scholars have written comprehensive lists of guidelines and accompanying questions that are helpful in critically appraising *quantitative* research reports (Field, 1983; Fain, 1999, Parhoo, 1997; LoBionda-Wood and Haber, 1998). The authors of this text provide a set of criteria and a series of related questions based on ideas gleaned from the literature and their own research experience. The guidelines and questions should be applied with flexibility and in various combinations when evaluating quantitative nursing studies.

The criteria for evaluating quantitative research studies are presented first, followed by questions appropriate to each of the four stages of the critiquing process.

BOX 20.1 *Stages of the Critiquing Process and Components of a Quantitative Research Report*

Stage 1: Purpose, Problem Statement, and Congruency with Design and Methodology

- Study purpose
- Problem statement
- Theoretical framework
- Literature review
- Hypotheses or research questions
- Research design
- Sampling procedures
- Data collection procedures
- Instruments
- Data analysis

Stage 2: Conduct of the Research

- Protection of participants' rights
- Ethics of research
- Consistency and integrity of procedures

Stage 3: Outcomes of the Research Process

- Statistical significance of results
- Clinical significance of results
- Discussion of findings
- Implications for practice, education, and research

Stage 4: Overall Quality of Study

- Conclusions

Regardless of whether you are doing the critique of a research study or reading a critique published by someone else, the criteria and questions you pose are the same. The following criteria are suggested for evaluating quantitative research studies:

1. Relevant and clearly articulated statement of purpose
2. Consistency between explicitly stated purpose and problem statement or question or hypothesis
3. Comprehensive literature review identifies gaps in the research area and logically leads to the research questions under study
4. Theoretical framework provides a rationale for the study
5. Congruent match between the purpose, design, and method
6. Appropriate sample and sample selection procedures
7. Statistical procedures appropriate to the type of data collected and research questions posed
8. Adequate reliability and validity to accept findings and generalize to appropriate populations
9. Significance of study for nursing is apparent

The suggested questions in Box 20.2 are listed for your consideration when conducting each stage of the critique. It is helpful if you use the following steps to move through the stages of the critiquing process:

Step 1. Answer the questions in Box 20.2 by providing content from the study to show how the researcher specifically addresses or fails to address the essence of each item. Avoid answering questions with a simple "yes" or "no." This will do little to enhance the researcher's ability to improve the study.
Step 2. In situations in which you must answer "no" to an item, make a memo to yourself so that in the "Limitations"

section of the critique, you can suggest improvements to the researcher for strengthening the study in the future.
Step 3. As you go through the list of questions and respond positively to each item, make a note of what you consider the real strengths of the study. These can then be summarized in the strengths and "Limitations" section of the critique. It is important, however, not to unfairly criticize the researcher for something that was never a part of the original purpose (Wilson, 1993).
Step 4. As you apply the list of questions to your critique, you are advised to review the chapters in the text that relate to the particular design used in the study, as well as chapters on the various components of the research process. For your convenience, these are noted in parentheses after each heading.

2. Criteria for Critically Appraising Qualitative Research Reports

As more nurses engage in *qualitative* investigations, it is important to know how to evaluate their contributions to nursing pracice. What general standards exist for critically appraising the quality of a qualitative investigation? Qualitative studies emerge from the naturalistic–inductive paradigm and as such are based on a different set of assumptions and a different worldview and have a different purpose than quantitative studies. These differences make it difficult to evaluate qualitative studies using the same criteria as quantitative investigations. Qualitative research hopes to promote "understanding" of phenomena—that is, that deep structure of knowledge that comes from prolonged engagement and persistent observation in the field, from visiting personally with participants, and probing to obtain detailed meanings (Creswell, 1998). Because a critique of a study is based on the

BOX 20.2 *Stage 1: Key Questions for Critiquing Quantitative Designs*

Stage 1 Questions: Critical Appraisal of Purpose, Problem Statement, and Congruence with Design and Methodology

Purpose or Problem Statement (see Chapter 3)

- Is the study problem and purpose statement clearly articulated?
- Are the reasons for conducting the study stated?
- Is the study's potential contribution to nursing knowledge stated?
- Are the research objectives or research questions or hypotheses stated clearly and researchable (answerable through the collection of empirical data)?
- Are terms defined conceptually and operationally?

Literature Review (Chapter 3)

- Does the literature review or theoretical framework provide evidence that the researcher has synthesized the classic and current literature and placed the research question in the proper context?
- Does the literature review identify gaps in knowledge, suggest how the current study extends the knowledge base in this area, and point out contradictions in the current knowledge base?
- Does the researcher summarize the literature review, provide a rationale for the current study, and show how this study will extend previous research?

Design (see Chapters 4 to 8)

- Is the study design specified, including its advantages and limitations for the research problem?
- Is there evidence that a pilot study had been conducted and the findings were used to enhance the design?
- Is the design (overall plan of research) appropriate to the research purpose and capable of answering the research question?
- How does the design control for extraneous variables?

Sample (see Chapter 15)

- Was probability or nonprobability sampling used and the reason for the choice specified?

- Is the population to whom results will be generalized described?
- Are precautions taken to avoid collecting a biased sample (see Chapter 9) that would limit generalizability of findings?
- Are the demographic characteristics of the sample described?
- Is the sample representative of the population?
- Are inclusion and exclusion criteria identified?
- Is the sample size appropriate to meet assumptions of statistical tests?

Data Collection (see Chapters 13 and 14)

- Are data collection methods appropriate to meet the study purpose and answer the questions or hypotheses?
- What evidence is provided that data collection procedures are valid and reliable?
- Are adaptations to data collection tools described?
- Are data collection instruments described in sufficient detail to enable readers to ascertain method of scoring and range of values and what a particular score means?

Data Analysis (see Chapters 11, 12, and 16 to 18)

- Are data analysis procedures described?
- Are the statistical techniques appropriate for the study methodology (i.e., the type of data collected and analysis)?
- Do the statistical tests answer the research questions and specify the level of significance?
- If results are nonsignificant, is a power analysis conducted to explore nonsignificant findings (see Chapter 15)?

Stage 2 Questions: Critical Appraisal of the Conduct of Research

Human Rights (see Chapter 10)

- How are rights of research participants protected?
- Are ethical issues anticipated and handled appropriately?

Procedures

- Are techniques used to ensure that there is consistency in the data collection process?
- What procedures were used to keep research conditions the same for all participants?

continued on next page

BOX 20.2 *Stage I: Key Questions for Critiquing Quantitative Designs (Continued)*

- Are there strategies to limit errors in data collection, recording, and analysis?
- Did any unplanned circumstances influence the results?
- In experimental designs, is there evidence of manipulation of independent variables, randomization in selection of sample and assignment to experimental and control groups, and control of extraneous variables (Wilson, 1993)?

Stage 3 Questions: Critical Appraisal of Research Outcomes

Findings (see Chapters 9 and 19)

- Are the findings presented clearly and correctly and are they related to the theoretical framework?
- Is there a clear statement of whether or not the data support the hypotheses or answer each research question?
- Are tables and graphs clearly labeled, easy to comprehend, and congruent with results presented in text form (see Chapter 19 for table construction)?
- Are findings presented in an unbiased manner (see Chapter 9)?

Discussion (see Chapter 19)

- Are alternative explanations offered for the findings?

- Does the researcher discuss both clinical and statistical significance of findings?
- Does the researcher overgeneralize the findings beyond the appropriate population?
- Are limitations of the study such as sample size, inadequate instruments, sources of bias, and so on identified and their implications discussed?

Implications and Conclusions (see Chapter 19)

- Does the researcher identify important implications of the study for practice, education, or research (if appropriate)?
- How do the findings of the study advance nursing knowledge?
- Do new research questions emerge from the study?

Stage 4 Questions: Critical Appraisal of the Overall Quality of the Study

Overall Quality

- What are the major strengths of the study?
- What are the major limitations of the study?
- Was the study described in sufficient detail to facilitate a replication study?
- What are the major contributions of this study to knowledge development in nursing?
- What suggestions might enhance the study and correct the limitations?

---

match between its purpose and other elements of the study, it makes sense that qualitative studies that have a different purpose from quantitative investigations should have a different set of criteria for appraising their merit. As noted in Chapters 6 to 8, qualitative research includes a wide array of methods and designs, each reflecting a different tradition and perspective. Criteria used to evaluate qualitative research must take this into account. In critiquing a qualitative study, the critic asks, "Did the investigators get it right?" That is, did they publish an accurate and authentic account of the research phenomenon that is recognized easily by those who experienced it?

As with quantitative research, a number of authors have proposed guidelines for critiquing qualitative studies; however, they are not as numerous. Box 20.3 contains examples of criteria for critiquing qualitative studies. Before applying any of these criteria, you should first read the report of the study in its entirety to get a feel for the essence of the study and its contribution to nursing. After this, you should read the report, again paying attention to each stage of the critiquing process. Creswell (1998) notes there is a "gulf of distance" among the authors discussing criteria and standards for evaluating qualitative studies. The criteria must be general enough to be applied across the different qualitative traditions (i.e., grounded theory, phenomenology, ethnography, historical research). Considerable diversity and richness are evident in the criteria represented in Box 20.3.

Having examined the criteria present in Box 20.3, you are now ready to respond to specific questions for each stage of the critiquing process of qualitative reports (Box 20.4). The stages of the process do not differ greatly from those used in quantitative critiques, but the questions forming the content of each stage address concerns of qualitative studies. The questions in Box 20.4 are intended as guidelines to help you apply the criteria to qualitative investigations and provide a framework from which to analyze research reports. You are advised to consult Chapters 6 to 8 for applicable aspects of qualitative research designs as you respond to questions in this section.

In the final analysis, when one critiques a qualitative study, the central question that must be addressed is: "How do we know that the qualitative study is believable,

---

BOX 20.3 *Criteria for Critiquing Qualitative Research Reports*

Leininger's Criteria (1990)

- Credibility: The truth value or believability of the findings to the participants
- Confirmability: Direct evidence from the informants, including mutual agreement
- Meaning in context: Interpretations fit within broader understandings of the experience
- Recurrent patterning: Themes recur in sequence or regular patterns
- Saturation: New data are redundant; no new themes emerge when additional information is collected
- Transferability: Consistency or generalizability across settings

Lincoln (1995)

- Positionality: The text should reflect authenticity and honesty about its own stance and the position of the author
- Community rubric: Research should be addressed to and serve the purposes of the community it takes place in
- Voice: Research should give voice to participants, and multiple voices should be heard in the text
- Critical subjectivity: The researcher shows evidence of developing heightened self-awareness that enables one to understand his or her psychological and emotional states before, during, and after the research experience

- Reciprocity: Evidence that an intense sharing, trust, and mutuality exists
- Sacredness of relationships: The researcher respects the collaborative and egalitarian aspects of research and makes room for the lifeways of others
- Sharing of the privileges: The researcher shares rewards (e.g., royalties or publication rights) with the participants whose lives he or she portrays

Forchuk and Roberts (1993)

- The research domain, topic, or question is specified and the appropriate design selected
- All research procedures are in keeping with the stated purpose
- The research method is described and the rationale is provided for its selection
- Appropriate review of the literature is recorded and referred to when it is relevant to the research
- Participants, informants, context, and researcher are described in relevant detail
- Data gathering and analysis are described in detail and the researcher should discuss how these are appropriate for the method selected
- The researcher's interpretations and conclusions must be consistent with the data and the importance and relevance of the research for nursing are clearly addressed

BOX 20.4 *Key Questions for Critiquing Qualitative Designs*

Stage 1 Questions: Critical Appraisal of Purpose, Statement of Research Phenomenon, and Congruence with Design and Methodology

Purpose or Statement of the Phenomenon of Interest

- Is the research phenomenon of interest clearly stated?
- Is rationale provided for approaching the study in an inductive, qualitative manner?
- Is the philosophy of the research tradition described?
- Is a statement of self-understanding included?
- Is there a single broad research question? Are their subquestions?
- Does the initial question become more focused as data are collected and analyzed?
- Is the study purpose clearly stated (e.g., discovery, description, theory building, and so on)?

Literature Review

- Does the qualitative method used call for a literature review before data collection?
- Does the review indicate that the researcher has expertise in the chosen area, know where gaps exist, and show how this study will eliminate such gaps?
- If a review is appropriate only after data collection, is there evidence that this is done?
- Is a framework appropriate? If so, is it presented clearly?

Design

- Is the design (i.e., overall plan for the research) appropriate to the research purpose?
- Is there congruency between the methodology and the research question?
- Is the context for the study adequately described?
- Is the researcher–participant relationship understood?

Sample

- Is purposive sampling used?
- Are informants capable of informing the study?
- Is the selection of participants appropriate to allow for saturation of data?

Data Collection

- Is data collection congruent with the study purpose, research question, and qualitative tradition selected?
- Are prolonged engagement and persistent observation in the field used to build trust with participants and ensure validity of data collection?
- Are data collection strategies and procedures described in sufficient detail?

Data Analysis

- Are data analysis procedures clearly described and appropriate to the research tradition?
- What evidence is provided that data collection and analysis are concurrent and ongoing?
- Is there evidence of decision rules for analyzing data, and does the researcher remain true to the rules?
- What evidence is there of narrowing the coding as categories are systematically discarded when they are unsupported by the data and the researcher becomes more focused on data collection and analysis?
- Is there evidence of "theoretical saturation?"

Stage 2 Questions: Critical Appraisal of the Conduct of the Research

Human Rights

- How are the rights of research participants protected?
- Are ethical issues anticipated and handled appropriately?

Procedures

- What evidence is provided that research meets the criteria of rigor (credibility: findings must be understood and viewed as credible by the informants; trustworthiness: one can believe the findings are true; and usefulness: findings shed light on an important phenomenon)?
- Creswell (1998) identifies eight procedures for testing the truth value (appropriate representation of multiple realities) and notes that researchers should use at least two of these in any given study. The critic should ask which of these the researcher uses.

continued on next page

BOX 20.4 Key Questions for Critiquing Qualitative Designs (Continued)

1. Prolonged engagement and persistent observation in the field to build trust with participants, learn about the culture and context, and correct distortions introduced by the researcher's presence
2. Triangulation for purpose of corroborating evidence from different sources to shed light on a theme or perspective
3. Peer review as an external check of the research process; this person asks hard questions about the method, meanings, and interpretations and keeps the researcher honest
4. Negative case analysis, in which the researcher reworks the hypothesis until all cases fit it
5. The researcher articulates researcher bias so that the reader knows what prejudices, biases, or past experiences have shaped the researcher's approach to the study
6. Member checks to solicit informants' opinions of the accuracy and credibility of the findings and conclusions. Some methods, however, such as hermeneutic analysis, do not always conduct member checks because their emphasis is on the interpretation of meaning by the research team of the experience of the participants in the research project.
7. External audits in which a consultant examines both the process and product of the qualitative study to assess accuracy and determine if the findings, interpretations, and conclusions are supported by the data
8. Rich, in-depth descriptions of participants and setting are provided so that the reader can make decisions regarding transferability of findings to other settings

Stage 3 Questions: Critical Appraisal of the Research Outcomes

Findings

- Are the findings contextualized (i.e., presented within the context of the circumstances that influence their interpretation)?
- Do readers of the report recognize the phenomenon or vicariously experience it?
- Are the findings true to the data?
- Do the themes, categories, or theoretical statements present a comprehensive, plausible, and meaningful picture of the phenomenon?
- If models, diagrams, or figures are used, are they effective?
- Are the findings compatible with the field of nursing's knowledge base?
- Are reasons for incompatible findings explored by the researcher?

Discussion, Implications, and Conclusions

- Does the researcher identify implications of the study for nursing (i.e., in practice, theory building, instrument development, education, and research)?
- Is a context provided in which to use the findings?
- Do the implications and conclusions follow logically from the findings?
- Do new research questions emerge from the findings?

Stage 4 Questions: Critical Appraisal of the Overall Quality of the Study

- What are the major strengths of the study?
- What are the major limitations of the study?
- What are the major contributions of this study to knowledge development in the field of nursing?
- What suggestions might enhance the study and correct the limitations?

accurate, and 'right'?" (Creswell, 1998, p. 193). Application to the qualitative report of the criteria and questions provided in Boxes 20.3 and 20.4 should help the critic to answer this question. Although it is not possible within the scope of this text to describe specific critiquing details for all of the different qualitative approaches, we have summarized general standards for judging the quality of a qualitative study and pointed out significant differences where appropriate.

C. EXAMPLES OF RESEARCH CRITIQUES

Reading systematic reviews of nursing research studies is an excellent means for developing skill in carrying out a critical appraisal of a project as well as learning about an area of nursing practice. Resources are available to beginning researchers and nurses interested in locating critical appraisals of research studies applicable to nursing. Several sources of critical appraisals of nursing research studies include:

1. *The Western Journal of Nursing Research* regularly publishes critiques and commentaries of published research articles after the main study report. This mechanism provides a rich source of feedback to the author on the original study and gives the opportunity for the researcher to respond to the critique.
2. *Scholarly Inquiry for Nursing Practice: An International Journal* also publishes original research studies followed by critical responses to research studies by experts in the field. Both of these journals are highly recommended as quality examples of critiques for anyone interested in learning more about the skill of critiquing.
3. Many research texts provide critiques of nursing studies in their chapters on the critique process. Examples include Fain (1999), Brockopp and Hastings-Tolsma (1995), and LoBionda-Wood and Haber (1998).
4. Other resources available include experts in the field such as directors of nursing research units, research consultants with professional associations, and individuals designated to give advice on clinical effectiveness in health care institutions.

1. Example of a Critique of a Quantitative Study

The research critique requires a systematic analysis of each section of the quantitative report. The following is a critique of a research study by Asch (1996) titled *The Role of Critical Care Nurses in Euthanasia and Assisted Suicide.* Excerpts from the original study are provided in italics to give the reader the essence of each component of the research study. This is followed by the critique of that aspect of the report. Interested readers may wish to refer to a published critique of this report by Mawdsley (1997). Both the research report and Mawdsley's critique may be read in their entirety by consulting the references in the recommended readings for the original source.

a. Stage 1: Purpose, Problem Statement, and Congruence with Design

(i) Purpose

. . . Evidence from the literature suggests that nurses outside the U.S.A. may be as willing as physicians to engage in euthanasia. The purpose of this study was to examine the role of U.S. critical care nurses in acts of euthanasia and assisted suicide.

Critique. The purpose of the study is clearly and explicitly stated. It is consistent with the background information presented. The purpose is important because critical care nurses are in key positions related to end-of-life and life-saving care.

(ii) Problem Statement

Little is known about the actual experiences and practices of critical care nurses when end-of-life decisions are imminent. In a survey of 943 Australian nurses, 218 reported being asked by a physician to engage in euthanasia; of these, 85% reported complying with the request. Moreover, 16 nurses reported complying with a patient's request for euthanasia without having been asked to do so by a physician. In a survey of 278 Australian nurses, 52 (19%) reported taking active steps to bring about the death of a patient, often without being asked to do so by the patient or the patient's family . . .

Critical care nurses frequently care for patients who wish to die, and these nurses are often in a position to hasten their deaths. And, like physicians they may also be in a position to engage in such activities outside the practice setting, on behalf of friends or relatives who wish to die.

. . . for purposes of this study euthanasia and assisted suicide are defined as events in which someone performs an act with the specific intent of causing or hastening a patient's death, but excluded are those acts that reflect the withholding or withdrawing of life-sustaining treatment. By this definition, we include such acts as providing an intentional overdose of narcotics or potassium chloride or providing explicit advice to patients about how to commit suicide but exclude such acts as withdrawing a mechanical ventilator, even though all these acts might result in the patient's death.

Critique. The problem statement is clearly articulated and identifies the need to explore the role of nurses in euthanasia and assisted suicide. This is an important area to consider because nurses are often in a position to understand and act on patients' wishes. The research question is not specifically stated but rather implied in the statement of purpose and problem. The problem is researchable and the terms are defined conceptually.

(iii) Literature Review

Euthanasia and assisted suicide have received considerable attention recently in the medical literature, pub-

lic discussion, and proposed legislation. Almost all the discussion in this area has focused on the role of physicians . . . In surveys of British and Australian physicians, 7 to 29% admit having performed euthanasia. In a recent survey, 218 of 828 physicians in Washington State reported receiving requests for assisted suicide or euthanasia. These physicians satisfied 38 of the 156 requests for assisted suicide and 14 of 58 requests for euthanasia . . . In one study of 1210 oncology nurses in the United States, 47% indicated that they would vote to legalize physician-assisted death, and 16% indicated that they would under a physician's order, administer a lethal injection to a competent, terminally ill patient who requested such assistance . . .

Critique. The literature review in this study is limited. It focuses on the role of health professionals in euthanasia and assisted suicide. Most of the literature in this area has focused on the role of physicians; hence, this gap in the literature is presented as the rationale for conducting this study. References suggest that nurses may be an important group to study because of their unique position in understanding the wishes of patients. The researcher cites current studies conducted in this area and notes that little is known about the actual experiences of nurses, particularly critical care nurses. The researcher provides no summary of the literature.

(v) Methods: Design

A survey was mailed to 1600 critical care nurses in the United States, asking them to describe anonymously any requests from patients, family members or others acting for patients, or physicians to perform euthanasia or assisted suicide, as well as their own practices.

Critique. The study used a descriptive survey design. The design was not explicitly stated; rather, it was implied by the mailed survey instrument sent to U.S. nurses. This design is appropriate to the research purpose and is capable of answering the research question. A strength of the survey is its ability to tap many variables, include many cases, and measure attitudes and perceptions of respondents. The researcher failed to identify both the advantages and limitations of the survey design to this study.

(vi) Methods: Sample

The subjects in this study were nurses practicing in the United States in intensive care units for adults. A random sample of 1600 subscribers to Nursing magazine who practiced in critical care settings was selected in order to represent a broad spectrum of attitudes and experiences. Nursing is the largest nursing journal in the world, with a circulation of nearly 500,000. Forty surveys were returned as undeliverable and 1139 completed surveys were returned by the cutoff date, a response rate of 71%. Subjects were excluded if they were not critical care nurses or did not practice in clinical care settings (165 subjects), or if they practiced in pediatric intensive care (46 subjects) or emergency departments (9 subjects). A sample of 852 nurses who practiced exclusively in critical care units for adults remained. Table 1 (p. 1375 of the article) shows selected demographic characteristics of the sample (age, gender, clinical experience, and practice site).

Critique. Significant concerns center on the procedure for randomly selecting the sample, the definition of critical care unit used as part of the inclusion criteria, and the representativeness of the sample to the population of practicing critical care nurses. Although *Nursing* magazine is a popular journal containing articles for generic as well as critical care nurses, there are many critical care journals from which a more representative sample of critical care nurses could have been selected. Furthermore, the definition of critical care unit used by the researcher to select the 1600 nurses was not specified. This resulted in eliminating more than 200 questionnaires because nurses did not work exclusively in adult critical care settings (Mawdsley, 2000). A clear definition of critical care unit is required because it may mean different settings to different nurses. For example, some may include coronary care, step-down units, post-anesthetic units, and so on. The type or size of critical care unit in which the nurses practiced was not specified. This is a serious omission because previous research has shown a relationship between withdrawing life support and the size of unit and the type of patient (Mawdsley, 1997). The sample size and the response rate were adequate.

(vii) Methods: Data Collection

Data were collected by means of an eight-page survey instrument that required 10 minutes to complete. The terms euthanasia and assisted suicide were defined for participants (see problem statement). To address the subjects' experience with requests that they perform euthanasia or assist in a suicide, they were asked: Have you ever been asked by a patient, family member, or other surrogate to administer a medicine to a patient or perform some other act with the intent of causing that patient's death—other than withholding or withdrawing life-sustaining treatment? To address the subjects' actual practice, they were asked: While a critical care nurse, have you ever administered a medicine to a patient or performed some other act with the intent of causing or hastening that person's death—other than withholding or withdrawing life-sustaining treatment? Most of the questions asked subjects to quantify their experiences during their careers and during the previous 12 months. They were asked whether their actions were undertaken at the request of patients, patients' families, other nurses, or physicians or with the advanced knowledge of these persons.

The initial surveys were mailed during January and February 1995, and two additional mailings of the same instrument to the same respondents followed at one-month intervals. As part of a related study of survey techniques, potential subjects were randomly assigned to one of two groups. One group received a coded postcard with the survey instrument, to be returned separately with the questionnaire. This minimized the mailing of new copies of the instrument to nurses who had already responded, while keeping specific responses anonymous. The second group of nurses did not receive postcards, so each subject in this group received three complete, identical packets. All mailings included stamped, addressed envelopes for return of the instruments with instructions not to return more than one completed questionnaire.

Critique. There is no validity or reliability information provided about the study instrument. This makes it difficult to determine if the instrument really does measure the nurse's role in euthanasia and assisted suicide. The researcher did provide definitions of euthanasia and assisted suicide, but no critical care case examples differentiating between euthanasia and withdrawing life support were provided, nor was the concept of *specific intent* defined. This is a serious omission because such information is essential to "understanding what is meant by *euthanasia* and *assisted suicide* and differentiating between euthanasia and withdrawing life support" (Mawdsley, 1997). The researcher further confuses these terms by referring to the withdrawal of ventilation as an example of withdrawing life support, but the administration of large doses of opioids to clients is defined as euthanasia. This is disturbing

because common practice in many critical care settings is to withdraw ventilation while providing opioids and sedatives to make the patient comfortable (Ignatavicus et al., 1999). The study participants were not given any validation of this common practice. Such lack of clarity in terms undermines the validity of the data collection instrument and the strength of the results.

(viii) Methods: Data Analysis
Critique. The researcher does not provide a description of the data analysis procedures. From the "Results" section, one assumes that descriptive statistics and measures of central tendency and dispersion were used to describe the data. Sufficient information is not provided on the analysis of qualitative data to determine how the handwritten comments and explanations from the respondents were treated. The quantitative measures appear appropriate given the type of data collected and the research purpose.

b. Stage 2: Conduct of the Research

(i) Human Rights
The completed surveys were anonymous. No identifying information was placed on the instruments or return envelopes. The protocol was approved by the human subjects committees of the University of Pennsylvania and the Philadelphia Veterans Affairs Medical Center. The study was reviewed by an independent board selected by a major professional nursing society and by two experts in the areas of bioethics and nursing.

Critique. The researcher clearly addresses the rights of participants and protects their anonymity and confidentiality. The study received ethical approval from an appropriate body.

(ii) Procedures
Refer to the "Methods: Data Collection" section.

Critique. No details are provided by the researcher on strategies to limit errors in data collection, recording, or analysis. Research conditions were not the same for all participants because one group received a coded postcard and the other group received three complete identical packets of questionnaires. However, all respondents did receive the same questionnaire by mail. The researcher does verify that the characteristics of the respondents and their responses did not differ between the two groups.

c. Stage 3: Research Outcomes

(i) Findings

Of the 1139 nurses who responded (71 percent), 852 said they practiced exclusively in intensive care units for adults in the United States. Of these 852 nurses, 141 (17 percent) reported that they had received requests from patients or family members to perform euthanasia or assisted suicide; 129 (16 percent of those for whom data were available) reported that they had engaged in such practices; and an additional 35 (4 percent) reported hastening a patient's death by pretending to provide life-sustaining treatment ordered by a physician. Some nurses engaged in these practices without the request or advance knowledge of physicians or others. The method most frequently used for euthanasia was the administration of a large dose of an opiate to a terminally ill patient.

Critique. Findings were accurately presented. Tables were easy to read and clearly presented but were only briefly discussed in the text. Textual discussion of the handwritten comments of respondents was brief and weak. A more detailed discussion of the nurses' description of their activities would have enhanced the reader's understanding of the nurse's role in euthanasia and assisted suicide.

(ii) Discussion

As public debate continues over the social, moral, and professional issues surrounding euthanasia and assisted suicide, 19% of the nurses in this study reported engaging in these practices. Some reported doing so on several occasions, and some without the knowledge of physicians, patients, or surrogates and without their request.

If these practices had been sporadic, they might be attributed to a few lone practitioners, operating beyond the margins of their profession. Although the moral appropriateness of an action is not measured by its pervasiveness, some will find it hard to accept the conclusion that so many nurses in this sample were acting inappropriately. We need to find another explanation.

One possible explanation is that although these activities may have been undertaken with the intent to hasten death, they may nevertheless reflect a continuum of moral acceptability and professional practice. At one end of the continuum, perhaps, are nurses who report hastening death in hidden ways— for example, deliberately giving lethal overdoses of medications. Others practiced at the limits of their authority—for example, titrating intravenous drips within prescribed ranges but beyond required doses. Some nurses appealed fully or in part to the doctrine of double effect, arguing either that their intent was only to relieve suffering or that their intent was both to relieve suffering and to hasten death. Finally, some nurses reported hastening death by administering high doses of opiates while withdrawing patients from mechanical ventilation. In these cases the death was imminent and was an accepted goal.

Because so many different kinds of activities are reflected in the responses of nurses it is difficult to ascribe a single meaning to the results or to take a single moral stance toward them. Further-

more, a weakness of the study was the failure to distinguish between euthanasia and assisted suicide in the questionnaire. In either case, however, the intent to cause death was explicit . . .

The results are subject to nonrespondent bias . . . as nurses most upset by the survey might be those least likely to engage in such practices and least likely to respond. The high response rate suggests that such a bias could not have altered the findings much. Finally, the results of the study are based on self-reports. Some respondents may have underreported or overreported activities and some may have misunderstood the questions. These limitations call for caution in interpreting the point estimates provided by the study.

Critique. The discussion is well done. Alternative explanations are offered for the research findings. The researcher is thorough in the discussion, mentioning important limitations such as the questionable representativeness of the sample, potential sample bias, and the lack of clarity in definition of terms. However, the researcher fails to discuss the limitations created by the lack of establishing the validity or reliability of the data collection instrument. Furthermore, the researcher failed to ask some key questions such as:

- Under what conditions were large amounts of opiates administered by nurses?
- Why was there no differentiation between the administration of opioids during euthanasia and the withdrawal of life support?
- Why did the researcher not acknowledge the common practice of withdrawing mechanical ventilation in the presence of large amounts of opioids and sedatives and fit these actions into the definitions of euthanasia and assisted suicide? Doing so would have eliminated confusion for the respondents.

These are questions to keep in mind when a researcher reports that nurses engage in euthanasia without the consent of patients and families (Mawdsley, 1997).

(iii) Implications and Conclusions

The issues surrounding euthanasia and assisted suicide are complex. In some cases the practice can appear to be a genuine response to human suffering. Permitting health professionals to carry out these activities may seem appropriate when the decision clearly fosters the patient's autonomy. From this perspective distinctions made between euthanasia and the withholding or withdrawing of life-sustaining treatment appear artificial and hard to sustain. In most cases, the aims and consequences of the actions are the same. On the other hand should euthanasia be sanctioned, it might become too easy an option. Maintaining legal and professional prohibitions against euthanasia or assisted suicide may limit such tragedies better than any procedural safeguards . . . The results of this study should prompt nurses, physicians, and other health care professionals to examine their practices more openly and collaboratively, with the aim of understanding and reducing disagreement over goals and plans . . . Regardless of the policy implications of this study it is clear that nurses in this study practice, often with little support, in extraordinarily difficult situations. In these complex environments, professional, moral, personal, and religious values frequently collide.

Critique. Conclusions are well explored and implications of the study findings for practice and future research are clearly stated. The study challenges nurses to ponder why a small number of critical care nurses reported hastening death without the consent of patients, families, or physicians. It also raises the question of whether nurses can clearly differentiate between euthanasia and withdrawing of life support. "The study highlights the necessity for clear terminology regarding end-of-life decisions so that when one member of the health-care team proposes withdrawing life support, everyone is clear regarding the meaning of the term." (Mawdsley, 1997, p. 11).

d. Stage 4: Overall Quality of Study

(i) Major Strengths
The major strengths of this study include its ability to challenge readers to face the ethical dilemmas encountered everyday in clinical practice, the clear identification of the limitations of the study by the researcher, and the indications for the direction of future research.

(ii) Major Limitations
The major limitations of the study include the lack of reporting on the validity and reliability of the study instrument, the lack of clarity regarding terms, and the questionable representativeness of the sample to the population of practicing critical care nurses in the United States.

(iii) Suggestions for Improvement
Much of the confusion for study participants in completing the instrument could have been eliminated if the researcher had acknowledged the common practice of withdrawing ventilation in the presence of large amounts of opioids and sedatives and had incorporated these actions into the definitions of euthanasia and assisted suicide. In conclusion, the study addresses an important area of practice that is underinvestigated in the nursing literature and brings to the forefront an important dilemma for nurses and other health-care professionals.

2. Example of a Critique of a Qualitative Study

The following is a critique of the report *Phenomenological Study of Nurses Caring*

for Dying Patients (Rittman et al., 1997). Excerpts from the original study are provided in italics to give the reader the essence of each component of the research study. This is followed by the critique of that aspect of the report. The research report may be read in its entirety by consulting the reference in the recommended readings for the original source. The questions provided in Box 20.4 provide a framework to analyze the report using the four stages of the critiquing process.

a. Stage 1: Purpose, Statement of Research Phenomenon, and Congruence with Design and Methodology

(i) Purpose or Statement of Research Phenomenon
Little is known about how nurses experience caring for dying patients. Yet, entering the patient's world often involves dealing with death and dying and is a major challenge to oncology nurses. The purpose of this study is to explore the experiences of nurses engaged in relationships with patients who were dying in order to describe skills and shared practices of oncology nurses. Three questions guided the study: (a) What skills do nurses use in providing care to dying patients and their families? (b) What do nurses experience while caring for dying patients? (c) What meanings sustain nurses while working with dying patients?

Critique. The purpose of the study and the research phenomenon are clearly stated. The researcher refers to the lack of knowledge about nurses' experience of caring as a rationale for conducting a qualitative investigation in this area. A single broad question was used to address the study purpose. Nurses were asked to describe an experience of caring for a dying patient. In addition, three subquestions guided the study. No reference is made to the philosophical stance on which the phenomenological approach is based. Because the philosophical framework directs the questions that are asked and influences the collection and interpretation of data in qualitative studies, it would be helpful for the researcher to outline the philosophical orientation of the approach.

(ii) Literature Review

No section titled "Literature Review" is found in this report; rather, a section called "Background" is presented by the researcher. The following excerpt is from the "Background" section.

> These findings expand earlier work on how nurses care for dying patients in oncology nursing. Previous findings have been reported on the meaning of oncology nursing practice, description of critical behavior in caring for dying patients, and coping strategies used when caring for dying patients and their families. Saunders and Valente described bereavement tasks of nurses after a patient dies. Findings from our study indicate that many bereavement tasks described by Saunders and Valente occur in the daily practice of oncology nurses and are used from admission throughout the dying process to achieve a good death . . . This study also expands current understanding of reciprocity in relationships between nurses and patients. Findings revealed that nurses and patients experienced a mutually beneficial process during their relationships. Being engaged with patients who are dying provided an opportunity for nurses to deal with their own mortality and to develop a certain comfort with death. Nurses often spoke of death not as an enemy but as a friend.

Critique. With the phenomenological approach, the review of the literature is not usually conducted until data analysis is complete (see Chapter 6). The rationale for delaying the review of the literature until this time is to limit the introduction of bias into the study process. The researcher is aiming for a pure description of the phenomenon. In this study, the researcher appropriately conducted a literature review after data analysis, to place the study findings in the context of what is already known about the topic of nurses caring for dying patients. The researcher does a thorough job of relating current findings to earlier work on the topic.

(iii) Method: Design

> The hermeneutic method was used to uncover meaning embedded in nurses' stories or narratives about caring for dying patients. The purpose of a hermeneutic analysis is to achieve an understanding of the phenomenon being studied.

Critique. The research design is clearly articulated and appropriate to the research purpose. Hermeneutic phenomenology is a special kind of phenomenology designed to reveal concealed meanings in phenomena. It bridges the gap between the familiar and unfamiliar in our worlds.

(iv) Method: Sample

> Data consisted of six narratives written by experienced oncology nurses working on an oncology unit who are considered by their peers and head nurse to have a high degree of expertise. All of the nurses had at least five years of oncology nursing experience. They also reported that they had personally experienced the death of a family member or a close friend.

Critique. It is implied that purposive sampling was used to select nurses who had experience caring for dying patients. The researcher reports the number of nurses in the study but does not describe how the six were selected from among other nurses on the oncology unit meeting the inclusion criteria.

(v) Method: Data Collection

Nurses were asked to describe an experience of caring for a patient who was dying. They were asked to select an experience that was important to them because it taught them something about what it means to care for a dying patient. Stories included as much detail as possible about the nurses' thoughts and feelings in the situation.

Critique. The data collection method was clearly identified and congruent with the study purpose, the research question, and the qualitative tradition. The three guide questions used to facilitate the writing of the nurses' narratives were previously identified. There is insufficient detail, however, related to the length of the data collection period, the context and setting in which the narratives were written, and the length of the narratives. Also, there is no information on whether the data were *saturated* (see Chapter 6). A more detailed discussion of data collection procedures is required to enable replication of the study.

(vi) Method: Data Analysis

A research team was used for data analysis purposes. The team included the principal investigator, two experienced oncology staff nurses, the head nurse of the oncology unit, and a nurse administrator responsible for supervising the oncology service but not directly involved with the direct care. The method of data analysis was adapted from the process described by Dikelmann et al. (1989). The team first read each narrative as a whole to gain an understanding of the text. Members then wrote descriptions of the meanings evoked by the data. The team shared interpretations and began identifying possible themes in the data. The principal investigator wrote in-depth interpretations of each narrative. These interpretations were validated by the participants to find out if the interpreta-

tions fit with their lived experience of oncology nursing practice. During discussions and further analysis of all data, the themes cutting across all narratives were identified.

Critique. The use of a research team for analyzing and interpreting data in a hermeneutic study is a desirable way to proceed because different perspectives provide for a rich interpretation of the data. In this case, the team has a good cross-section of nurses with varied and related experiences. This is a valuable asset in the analysis process. The researcher refers to the data analysis process used by Dikelmann et al. but does not give any detail about what the process was except to say that themes that cut across all narratives were identified by the research team after discussion of their shared interpretations. What differences of opinion existed, and how were differences in interpretation handled by the research team? Mention is not made of decision rules for analyzing the data, nor is reference made to *saturation* of data. It would be helpful to have the researcher provide a more in-depth discussion of the process for identifying themes. For example, what steps were taken to organize and categorize the data? How were the data collapsed into four main themes? The researcher failed to summarize the literature at this point, which would have facilitated the readers' understanding of how pattern categories and themes were recognized and accepted. This is usually when the literature review is conducted in a phenomenological study. However, it can be implied from the background section of the report that the literature was used effectively to inform the analysis.

b. Stage 2: Conduct of the Research

(i) Human Rights
Critique. There is no mention of protection of human subjects by the researcher.

It is not known what the procedure for informed consent was or if anonymity was guaranteed. It can be inferred that the writing of the narratives by the nurses who told their stories was considered consent to participate, but we do not know the extent to which the consent was free, informed, and noncoercive. It would be helpful to know if approval was received from an ethics review board.

(ii) Procedure
Critique. Three criteria are used by qualitative researchers to assess the truth value of their findings—credibility, trustworthiness, and usefulness. Although the researcher does not explicitly address the procedures for assessing this, it can be inferred from the description of the data analysis. The use of the research team provides an opportunity for shared responsibility for the interpretations made by the members. The team approach helps to keep the principal investigator honest about the method, meanings, and interpretations of the data. The interpretations of the team members were shared with the participants to determine if the interpretations fit with their lived experience of oncology nursing practice. This use of member checks is a very valuable way to check the accuracy and credibility of the findings and conclusions. No mention is made of researcher bias. It would be helpful for the researcher to identify the prejudices, biases, and past experiences of the research team that shaped the approach to the study. Also, the relationship between the research team and the participants should be clarified. This information is useful in qualitative investigations because the researcher–participant relationship influences the sharing of the experience in phenomenological investigations. Although the researcher briefly described the participants, little attention was given to providing in-depth descriptions of the research setting or the partic-

ipants. This would have made it easier to judge the usefulness of the findings.

c. Stage 3: Research Outcomes

(i) Findings
The shared experiences of nurses caring for dying patients was represented in the data that clustered around four themes: knowing the patient, preserving hope, easing the struggle, and providing for privacy.

Critique. The presentation of results is consistent with a phenomenological study. The findings are presented in the context of the group that was studied: oncology nurses who cared for dying patients. When reading this report, readers are able to recognize what the experience is like for nurses caring for dying patients. Rich descriptions of the themes enable readers to vicariously experience the meanings associated with oncology nursing practice. The four themes present a meaningful and comprehensive picture of the experience of caring for dying patients. The findings include a balance between the researcher's interpretation of the meanings and the participants' quotations from their narratives. The findings appear true to the data.

(ii) Discussion, Implications, and Conclusions
The four themes contribute to knowledge development about how nurses enter into and experience caring for dying patients. The themes expand our understanding of the nurses' experience in oncology nursing practice. Nurses who have expertise in caring for dying patients establish different levels of involvement in different situations. Ranging from intense and meaningful closeness to engagement with less intensity. The ability to develop different levels of intensity in relationships helped nurses manage the emotional demands in their practice. Whatever the level of involve-

Chapter 21

Research Utilization in Nursing

CHAPTER OUTLINE

KEY TERMS

Change agent

Conceptual utilization

Instrumental utilization

Evidence-based practice

Planned change

Research–practice gap

Research utilization

It is not enough for nurses to conduct high-quality, relevant research; the research must also be used in practice to improve client care and benefit society. The purpose of this chapter is to discuss the nature and value of research utilization in nursing. Steps in the research utilization process are outlined and popular utilization models and projects are briefly described. Barriers to and strategies for using research findings in practice are discussed. An example of a research utilization project that is guided by the theory of planned change is presented. The chapter concludes with a discussion of what the future holds for research utilization in nursing.

A. UNDERSTANDING RESEARCH UTILIZATION

Research utilization is a complex process that includes critically analyzing the literature, selecting appropriate interventions, implementing them, and evaluating the outcome (Goode et al., 1996).

I. What Is Research Utilization?

In the field of nursing, **research utilization** may be defined simply as the use of research findings in practice to improve care. It occurs at two levels: instrumental and conceptual. **Conceptual utilization** refers to the use of findings to enhance one's understanding of a problem or issue in nursing. Through conceptual utilization, you use the knowledge gained from research to cognitively restructure the way you think about a situation, problem, or phenomenon in nursing. It enables you to see different alternatives and possibilities in nursing situations. **Instrumental utilization** is the direct, explicit application of knowledge gained from research to change practice. It includes (but is not limited to) the adoption of nursing interventions, new procedures, clinical protocols, and guidelines.

A number of research utilization models are available to guide you in promoting quality care. Examples include the Western Interstate Commission for Higher Education (WICHE), Conduct and Utilization of Research in Nursing (CURN) model, Nursing Child Assessment Satellite Training (NCAST) project, Stetler Model, Dracup-Breu Model, Iowa Model of Research in Practice, and Horne Model. The models have many features in common. Box 21.1 illustrates the major components of each model. Because of space limitations, only the Iowa Model is featured in the research utilization example provided at the end of the chapter.

2. Why Is Research Utilization Important in Nursing?

The ultimate value of research utilization is twofold: (1) to facilitate an innovative change that will lead to improved client outcomes and (2) to validate existing nursing procedures and interventions. In today's environment of fiscal restraint and professional accountability, it is critical that nurses are able to demonstrate that the services they provide are relevant, cost effective, based on evidence, and lead to improved client outcomes. The use of research to direct client care is one way to engage in **evidence-based practice**. Such practice challenges nurses to critically examine traditional practices, procedures, and nursing rituals and question those that are not substantiated by research or other evidence. The use of empirical evidence to inform nursing practice ensures effective use of scarce nursing resources.

Research utilization is important at all levels of nursing. It is crucial to the nurse at the bedside as well as to nurses at the broader levels in the health-care organization and the profession at large. Box 21.2 highlights the value of research utilization to each level.

BOX 21.1 *Research Utilization Models*

The **Iowa Model** focuses on change in practice based on research findings applied by the skilled practitioner and emphasizes an organizational focus with administrative support as an essential component. The six main concepts of the model are:

- Identification of knowledge or problem-focused triggers
- Primary goal is change in practice
- Uses a process of planned change
- Administrative support is essential
- Application of findings at the practitioner level
- Evaluation of change by those who implemented it

The **Western Interstate Commission for Higher Education (WICHE)** was the first federally funded nursing research utilization project in the United States. The five components of this model include:

- Definition of nursing care problem
- Retrieval of relevant research
- Critical review of the research
- Development of research-based plan of care
- Evaluation of the effects of change

The **Conduct and Utilization of Research in Nursing (CURN)** was a federally funded project carried out by the Michigan Nurses Association with the purpose of developing research-based protocols for clinical practice. The components of the project include:

- Identification of research studies and establishment of a research base
- Transformation of findings into research-based protocols
- Transformation of protocols into specific nursing interventions
- Clinical trials in the practice setting
- Evaluation of the research-based practice

The **Nursing Child Assessment Satellite Training (NCAST)** focused on teaching nurses new health assessment techniques for children. It was directed at individual nurses. It used Roger's diffusion of innovation theory. Nurses across the United States were taught specific assessment techniques using several communication techniques. An evaluation process was used to determine the most effective mode. The following components composed the dissemination of new knowledge in this model:

- Recruitment of appropriate learners
- Translation of research into clinical terminology
- Dissemination via various satellite modes
- Evaluation of outcomes

The **Stetler Model** (1994) is a prescriptive model designed to guide individual nurses in the implementation of research findings. The components of this model include:

- Preparation to specify the reason for the research review
- Validation is the critical appraisal of research
- Decision making related to application or nonapplication of results
- Translation involves identifying the practice implications from the research
- Evaluation of outcomes and dissemination of findings

The **Dracup-Breu Model** focuses on using research to solve specific problems in the clinical setting. The six steps of this model include:

- Identify the problem
- Select appropriate research
- Establish project objectives
- Analyze the setting and devise the plan
- Implement the plan
- Evaluate outcomes

The **Horne Model** focuses on research utilization at the organizational level rather than at the individual level of the practitioner. The four components of the model are:

- Organizational commitment identified in goal statements and in the commitment of resources to research utilization
- Change agents whose primary responsibility is to create change in practice that is research based
- The process of planned change is used to prepare the organization
- The outcomes of research-based practice include new policies, procedures, and protocols based on research evidence.

SOURCE: Compiled using data from Goode, C., Butcher, L., Cipperley, J., et al. (1996). *Research Utilization: A Study Guide* (2nd ed). Ida Grove, IA: Horn Video Productions.

BOX 21.2 *Value of Research Utilization*

Value of research utilization

- Promotes critical thinking and reflective practice
- Enhances professional self-concept
- Ensures provision of safe and effective care
- Practice is based on current, scientifically sound knowledge
- Self-confidence of the nurse is enhanced

Value to the researcher

- Validates the efforts of the researcher
- Motivates scholars to continue to discover new knowledge
- Reinforces professional accountability
- Helps uncover new clinical problems for investigation

Value to the health-care agency

- Cost-effective nursing care
- High-quality care
- Improved client outcomes
- Retention and recruitment tool
- Professionally satisfied and stimulated nursing staff

Value to the profession

- Enhanced autonomy of practice
- Positive professional image
- Strengthen professional status
- Expand the field of nursing's scientific knowledge base

Research utilization is also important to clients. You will recall from Chapter 1 that nursing research's goal is the improvement of client care. With this goal in mind, research utilization in nursing takes on a different level of significance than in other disciplines in which the purpose of research may be the discovery of knowledge itself for its own value. In nursing, research utilization should result in the improvement of practice and enhanced client care.

Despite the many advantages that are articulated by a variety of experts in the field, there remains a significant *gap* between what we know in nursing as a result of research and the actual application of this knowledge in practice. This is referred to as the **research–practice gap.** Recent literature suggests there is a 10- to 15-year gap between the discovery of potential innovations and the implementation of these innovations in practice (Bostrom and Wise, 1994). All nurses share responsibility to reduce this gap by appropriately implementing empirical findings in practice. This chapter can help you to develop the basic skills to do so.

3. What Are the Steps in the Research Utilization Process?

The research utilization process is different from but complimentary to the research process (see Chapter 1). Although the research process is essential to enable the use of findings in practice, by itself it is not enough. It would be naive to think that if you conduct a scientifically sound study and disseminate the results in a usable and understandable format to those who can use the knowledge, then your findings will be implemented. Unfortunately, the task of narrowing the research–practice gap is complicated by a number of political, organizational, social, and personal factors, some of which are beyond the control of nurse researchers or practitioners. Let us consider the steps that nurses can take to narrow the research–practice gap through research utilization.

Step 1. The first task in narrowing the research–practice gap is to select a relevant problem area that requires empirical evidence to bring about a positive change in practice. Consensus on the problem area should be reached among those responsible for the research utilization. Open discussion at team conferences or unit meetings is one way to identify topics and reach a shared vision about the problem to be addressed. There are two types of triggers that help nurses to identify potential practice problems that can be improved through research: problem-focused triggers and knowledge-focused triggers (Oates, 1997).

Problem-focused triggers are usually evident to nurses in the practice setting. They represent clinical problems such as the increased incidence of urinary tract infections in settings where nurses have been replaced by less skilled workers or insomnia in clients receiving intermittent intravenous therapy.

Knowledge-focused triggers emerge from the use of journal clubs in practice when research articles are discussed by nursing members at regular club meetings, the attendance of nurses at professional and academic conferences where scientific papers are presented, the reading of research literature, and the reflection on standards and guidelines for care. A knowledge-focused trigger may be a report in a nursing journal about the use of a new injection technique for administering insulin to juvenile diabetics.

Step 2. Review the literature to determine what is known about the problem and related topic areas (see Chapter 3). After the literature sources have been identified and retrieved, they should be carefully critiqued using the guidelines provided in Chapter 20 to determine if the research is sufficient in quantity and quality to merit implementation of the findings in practice. A helpful way to synthesize the literature and summarize the research findings is to create a grid that concisely displays the findings. You may need to review the format for setting up such a grid (see Table 3.1). The research utilization team may wish to divide the literature sources among members to critique the studies and then come together to discuss their findings and synthesize the results.

Step 3. Determine if the findings from the literature are appropriate to apply in your practice setting. Is there a significant research base to enable adoption of the innovation in practice? You should look for a preponderance of evidence that supports the use of the findings in your practice setting. The research base should be substantial in both quantity and quality to support implementation of the findings. Look for integrative reviews of the literature, meta-analyses of research studies dealing with your clinical problem, and replication studies that yield similar findings. It would be unwise to suggest a change in practice based on only one study. A number of authors have suggested guidelines for evaluating implementation of research findings. Before making a decision to adopt an innovation in practice, the following criteria should be considered by those responsible for research utilization:

- **Utility to nursing practice:** Does nursing have control over the intervention, procedure, or problem?
- **Applicability to practice:** Is the study sample, setting, context, and clinical problem applicable to your situation?
- **Replication:** Have the findings been replicated by others? If so, under what conditions?
- **Scientific merit:** Is the methodology rigorous, yielding valid and reliable results and scientifically sound conclusions?
- **Client safety:** What risks and benefits are available to the client if the innovation is adopted or not adopted?
- **Feasibility:** Are there adequate resources (i.e., time, money, people, expertise) available to implement the findings?

Step 4. After a decision is taken by the utilization team to implement the findings, a plan must be developed in writing to communicate the research-based intervention or protocol. This will ensure consistency in approach and substantiate the research base for the innovation. Such written research-based protocols and procedures should be included in the policy and procedure manuals of agencies and institutions (LoBionda-Wood and Haber, 1998).

Step 5. Implementation of the planned innovation follows. This involves carefully detailing and executing strategies for change. Usually new attitudes and new behaviors must be established and old attitudes and behaviors discouraged. All staff involved with the innovation must be part of the change process. Strategies for implementing the change are varied and may include involvement of stakeholders in the change process; education of all staff on the nature, merits and feasibility of the innovation; and feedback on the change process and the effects of the innovation. A number of models are available to guide the implementation of innovation based on research evidence (Lewin, 1951; Rogers, 1995; and Healthcare Quest, 1997). Figure 21.1 illustrates the steps for carrying out a planned change in practice. The change process is elaborated on later in the chapter.

Step 6. Evaluation of the success of the innovation is the final step in the research utilization process. Have the intended outcomes been achieved as a result of the introduction of the innovation? What changes, if any, are required to continue with the innovation? If the innovation did not produce the desired outcomes, the utilization team must assess what went wrong and make suggestions for future practice. In addition to outcomes of the utilization project, the process component of research-based practice should also be evaluated. This involves information on how the innovation is being implemented, barriers to implementation, and factors that enhance the implementation process.

Step 7. Dissemination of the findings of the research utilization process is the final step. The results of the evaluation of the innovation implementation and the evaluation of the process component of research-based practice need to be communicated to others in the nursing community. By publishing the results of the research utilization project in professional journals, in clinically based journals, in scholarly papers, and at scientific and nursing practice conferences, the nursing community accumulates evidence that can be used to support or challenge original research and direct future research utilization projects.

B. BARRIERS TO RESEARCH UTILIZATION

In the 1980s, nursing, medical, and scientific journals and conferences were the only available sources of reliable research data of relevance to practice. Now, however, a preponderance of readily accessible sources for research data are available to nurses. Such sources include:

1. The Cochrane Database of Systematic Reviews, which is a subset of the Cochrane Library. The Cochrane Collaboration movement was founded in 1993 by individuals from nine countries and is a major force in the British Commonwealth countries. Although it focuses primarily on medicine, it has recently influenced the field of nursing to engage in evidence-based practice (Estabrooks, 1999).
2. The Agency for Health Care Policy and Research (AHCPR) in the United States, which is a major depository of research evidence in nursing
3. The new Canadian Institute for Health Research, which is shaping the agenda for health research in Canada
4. *The Annual Review of Nursing Research,*

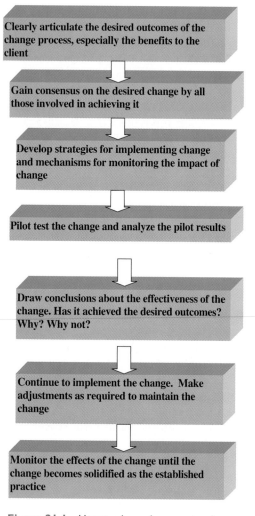

Figure 21.1   How to plan and carry out a change in practice.

which focuses on integrative research reviews of nursing studies

5. An array of nursing research journals that publish the latest in research findings such as *Nursing Research,* the *Western Journal of Nursing Research, Applied Nursing Research,* and *Clinical Nursing Research,* to name a few.

Despite these sources of research-based knowledge, the reality of nursing practice is that much of what we do as nurses is not based on scientific research. Similar to other professions, the field of

nursing has had difficulty enticing its members to respond to research evidence by changing their practice. Many "sacred cows" persist in nursing and go unquestioned even in the face of new evidence that has potential to improve client outcomes. Why is this the case? A discussion of factors that act as barriers to research utilization may help in understanding the gap that exists between the discovery of new knowledge and its implementation in practice. Barriers may be classified according to the following headings: characteristics of the nurse, characteristics of the setting, characteristics of the research, and characteristics of the innovation.

1. Characteristics of the Nurse

Knowledge, attitudes, and beliefs are three factors to consider in assessing characteristics of the nurse that may influence research utilization. Nurses require two kinds of knowledge to utilize research in practice. Nurses must be knowledgeable about the specific research studies that relate to their practice setting; this means they must read widely in the research literature. A study by Estabrooks (1999) suggests that there is a huge gap between publishing for scientific credit and publishing for consumption by clinicians. She notes that in a random sample of 1500 staff nurses, 38.7 percent read professional nursing journals rather than traditional scientific journals, in which most research studies are reported. Hence, many nurses are not exposed to research findings in the literature they read. Nurses must also be knowledgeable about the critiquing process so they can critically evaluate findings and be responsible consumers of research. Although most baccalaureate programs introduce nurses to skills in reading, interpreting, and evaluating research studies, there remains a strong need to build on this knowledge through continuing education sessions, conferences, and in-service sessions. Many nurses who are prepared at the diploma or associate degree level do not have the necessary skills or knowledge to critically evaluate research studies.

In addition to knowledge, nurses must develop positive attitudes and belief systems toward research utilization. A healthy attitude toward research is positively correlated with research utilization. In her work with nurses conducting research in clinical settings, Morrison (1998) uncovered a number of beliefs held by staff nurses that create unnecessary obstacles and limit research efforts. A number of erroneous beliefs of staff nurses about research were identified. These fallacies and other erroneous beliefs are listed in Table 21.1. The articulation of negative beliefs is a starting point in changing attitudes and in developing respect for use of research among clinical nurses.

Table 21.1   Fallacies About Research Held by Staff Nurses

Fallacies	Facts
The best design is experimental or quasi-experimental.	Nurses have a choice of many designs. The current trend is to use designs that capture the context even if there is less control.
A researcher must control all variables.	In addition to controlling variables in the study, they can be controlled statistically. In some designs, control is not the goal.
The best measurement is physiological.	False. The best measurement is holistic (i.e., a combination of bio, psycho, social).
The literature is searched for the exact study using the same sample and equipment.	Search for conceptual similarities, even if the studies were conducted on a different sample and a slightly different topic.
Clinical expertise is a prerequisite.	Research expertise and commitment are important qualifications.
Research is conducted only by academics who know little about practice.	Academics and practitioners work together as members of a research team.
Research is easy and can be conducted quickly by anyone.	Everyone should not conduct research, it requires time, and is not easy.
Ask for help when problems arise.	Seek help during the planning stages so that problems can be prevented and practice influenced positively.
Power and prestige accompany research funding.	Real prestige comes from publication of results.
Hire someone to collect and analyze data.	You learn best by completing your own data collection and analysis.
It is not important to inform others.	Professional ethics requires informing others and seeking appropriate permission.
It is not necessary to clarify ownership of work.	These issues should be openly discussed prior to conducting the study.
If a study is not funded, it has no value.	The merit of a study is judged by the quality of its design and execution.
Oral presentations are better than poster presentations.	It depends on the audience, both have their place.

Source: Adapted from Morrison (1998). Erroneous beliefs about research held by staff nurses. *The Journal of Continuing Education in Nursing, 29*(5), 196–203.

Lack of time is a barrier often cited by nurses. Many nurses do not have time while on duty to read and critically evaluate research. Given the recent cuts to health care and the downsizing of the nursing workforce, more and more demands are being placed on nurses' time. Pringle (1999) notes that it is unrealistic to expect staff nurses who do not feel valued, who are overworked and underpaid, and who feel their opinions do not count because they are rarely asked, to engage in research utilization on their own time. Nurse researchers, administrators, and educators must support the work life issues that staff nurses have so that their circumstances can be improved. Only by working together can we expect staff nurses to engage with researchers to identify clinical problems, test interventions, and apply new knowledge in practice for better client outcomes (Pringle, 1999).

2. Characteristics of the Setting

Health-care organizations have factors operating that both promote and oppose innovation. For a research culture to exist in an organization, five characteristics must exist (Crookes and Davies, 1998):

1. An ethos of *openness to new ideas* and a willingness to question the status quo with an eye toward continual quality improvement. Health-care organizations and those in positions of power often have a vested interest in maintaining the status quo. They fail to initiate change and to reflect on new and innovative answers to problems.
2. *Interpersonal and information linkages* are essential for new research ideas to be communicated openly and receive support. In bureaucratic structures, communication flow may be slowed or unidirectional from the top down. This impedes the cascading of information and limits upward movement of feedback or ideas. The formation of quality circles or research dissemination groups may improve the channels of communication.
3. *Freedom from organizational constraints,* which implies that subordinates will assume responsibility for accountable practice and managers will encourage and reward innovative practice. Often health-care organizations value tradition and discourage change and change agents from engaging in innovative practice. They fail to reward nurses for change actions and prefer to maintain the status quo, which they believe to be in keeping with their vision of the institution.
4. *Supportive leadership* requires a commitment to change and innovation. Leaders are either change agents themselves, opinion leaders, or supporters of others on their team who demonstrate skill in directing change and innovation. Traditionally, leaders in health care have often operated with an authoritative management style, which is opposed to change.
5. *Trust* must be present to risk the failures that come at times with change and innovation. If the environment is one in which collegiality and mutual trust exist, it is likely the staff will work to achieve common goals. However, if trust does not exist, then politics and personal interests will predominate and set the stage for failure of innovation.

3. Characteristics of the Research

The best research studies are of little value if they are incomprehensible to those who apply knowledge in practice or if they are published in sources that are foreign to typical staff nurses. Nurse clinicians must be able to read and understand research results if they are to apply the findings in practice. This places the burden on the researcher to communicate results clearly and comprehensively and to overtly identify the relevance of their findings for nursing practice. Researchers need to publish widely in journals that are user friendly to nurses who are in direct care positions.

Nurses need to focus on the type of research questions asked and ensure that they are studying problems of importance to nursing practice. This is best accomplished by working together with staff nurses to identify clinical problems that require a solution. Staff nurses can become part of the research team. This helps to improve the research skills of the staff nurse as well as enhance the relevance of clinical research programs.

Replication of research studies is warranted. In the past, a lack of replicated research acted as a barrier to the utilization of findings. Nurses did not appear to value the merit of replication studies. Today we realize that studies need to be replicated in different settings and with different populations so that a sound body of evidence may become increasingly available to staff nurses who are interested in evidence-based practice.

4. Characteristics of the Innovation

The attributes of a particular innovation can be a barrier to successful implementation. Rogers and Shoemaker (1971) identified five characteristics that predominate in successful attempts at innovation. If any of these five are missing, the implementation may be impeded:

1. The innovation must offer a *relative advantage* over the status quo. If the innovation is not perceived to improve the current situation, then implementation is unlikely.
2. *Compatibility* of the innovation with the current practice enhances the likelihood of successful adoption. If the innovation is quite different from existing

norms and practices, then innovation is difficult. In such situations, it may be better to settle for small changes and work gradually toward the bigger picture.
3. The *complexity* of the innovation is inversely related to its successful adoption.
4. The *trialability* or pilot testing of an innovation is less threatening than totally endorsing a major change in practice. If it is not possible to introduce the innovation in stages, it will be more difficult to convince others to take the risk of total implementation.
5. *Observability* refers to how visible the benefits and limitations of the innovation are to participants and observers. In other words, "seeing is believing," so the more obvious the drawbacks, the more difficult the implementation. Conversely, the more obvious the advantages, the easier the implementation.

Based on the attributes of the nurse, the setting, the research, and the innovation, a number of challenges are continuously presented to nurses who are hoping to implement an innovation in practice. Let us now consider some strategies one can use to overcome such barriers and successfully implement research findings in practice.

C. STRATEGIES TO FACILITATE RESEARCH-BASED PRACTICE

The implementation of research findings is a daunting challenge for individual nurses. The presence of a change agent is required on the unit. Vaughan and Pillmoor, cited in Crookes and Davies (1998), define a **change agent** as a person or group of people who can take an idea for change from the "drawing board," carry it through all the stages of its implementation, and evaluate its success or failure. Change agents must be able to respond to the barriers in

go a long way in promoting use of research findings to improve client care.

- Scholars should incorporate research findings into their textbooks and scholarly publications when appropriate. They also need to create theories to help explain research findings and work with researchers to test theory through research.
- Administrators should set institutional goals that include the use of research findings to promote excellence in practice. Management can support the efforts of practitioners to work to accomplish such goals by rewarding research utilization efforts in tangible ways such as extra days off, financial stipends, employment honor rolls, and special dinners and other celebrations to recognize staff efforts. Financial and human resources need to be designated for research utilization efforts.

D. EXAMPLE OF RESEARCH UTILIZATION

The process of research utilization is a complex one requiring critical thought, planned action, and deliberate choices by nurses committed to excellence in practice. This chapter equips you with some basic skills to help you overcome barriers to research utilization and proceed logically with a plan of action. This section presents an example of a research utilization project that was guided by the Iowa Model for Research-Based Practice (Fig. 21.2) and the Theory of Planned Change (Havelock, 1972, 1995).

I. Background to the Project

The placement of an intravascular catheter is a common treatment for children who require antibiotics, chemotherapy, total parenteral nutrition, or fluid therapy. Infection of central lines in ill children is a serious problem that negatively impacts client outcomes.

A large children's hospital in Philadelphia used a needleless valve device to maintain the intravascular catheter. The device provided staff nurses with a route to administer medication and draw blood samples. A potential problem of this system was the risk of infection caused by the increasing frequency with which needleless systems had stagnant blood around the valved device. Hence, a clinical nurse specialist organized a multidisciplinary team to discuss the problem and decide how to provide better care to children on the unit with intravascular devices.

2. Research Utilization Model

The Iowa Model for Research-Based Practice (see Fig. 21.2) provided an algorithm (i.e., a set of steps) for the research utilization team to follow in addressing the problem. The model is initiated by identification of a problem trigger or a knowledge focus trigger. In this situation, both triggers were present. The multidisciplinary research utilization team identified the *problem trigger* as contamination of the needleless device. The intermittent nature in which intravascular catheters are entered contributed to the team's finding many valves that contained stagnant blood. When blood is stagnant for long periods of time, the potential for microorganism growth exists; this is a serious problem in a pediatric population with compromised immune systems. The team believed that the valve should be removed until more data could be obtained. The *knowledge trigger* emerged from the Bloodborne Pathogen Standard and the guidelines produced by the Centers for Disease Control and Prevention to protect health-care workers from injury and to provide protection to clients.

Applying the Iowa Model, the next step was to identify relevant research literature on the topic. In the autumn of 1995, the clin-

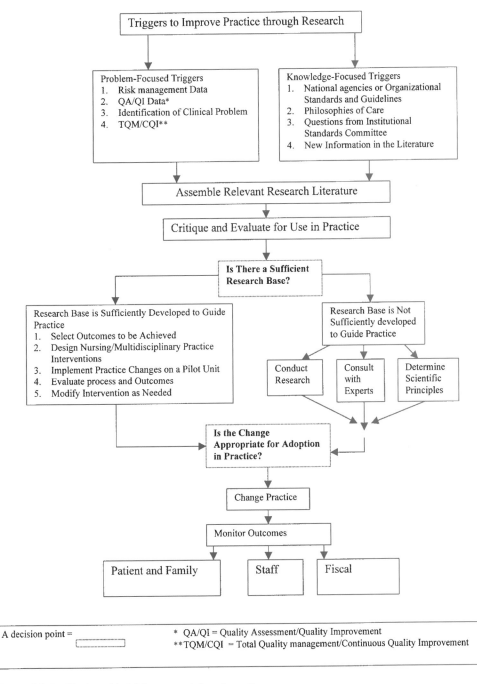

Figure 21.2 The Iowa Model for research-based practice.

ical nurse specialist and staff educator for pediatrics and the pediatric intensive care unit (PICU) completed a critical review of the literature and conducted interviews with equipment vendors. The consensus was that there was sufficient evidence to support conducting an evaluation of a new product: a nonvalved needleless system. A

3-month trial period of the new product was granted to the pediatric setting and the PICU.

To prepare for the trial, communication was established with the nurses through the unit-based council, with physicians through individual meetings, and with vendors through the clinical nurse specialist (CNS). The CNS conducted an in-service with 100 percent of the staff on all shifts. Throughout the trial period, vendors were available and nurses considered to be expert users of the new system supported other staff members on all shifts. The research utilization team maintained a visible presence during the trial, providing information as needed to staff members. An evaluation survey was conducted midway through the trial and again in the summer of 1996. The results from both surveys were positive. Results were shared with the nursing directors of pediatrics and PICU, the physician group, the purchasing department, and the hospital's product eval-uation committee. The CNS presented a summary of the trial to pediatric nurses, physicians, and the product evaluation committee and recommended that the product be used in the pediatric department. As a result, the product was accepted for use with modifications.

3. Planned Change

Many factors must be considered in initiating a planned change. Someone (i.e., a change agent) must be mandated to help plan and manage change, and a problem must be identified. In this situation, the change agent was the CNS and the client system was the nursing staff and together they developed a well-thought-out plan to guide the change process and implement a new procedure for maintenance of intravascular catheters. Havelock's Theory of Planned Change guided the project (Box 21.3).

BOX 21.3 *Nurse Researchers at Work*

APPLICATION OF HAVELOCK'S THEORY OF PLANNED CHANGE

A needleless system was chosen and approved for trial in the general inpatient and PICU. The product representatives, along with their clinical nurse, in-serviced the staff on the needleless system.

Unfreezing Phase

All staff members were involved in in-services on the product in an interactive, hands-on format. The problems of stagnant blood or fluid were identified with the present needleless device. The product representatives and the CNS were identified as resources.

Moving Phase

A plan to introduce the system into the unit for trial was presented at each unit-based council meeting. The staff members gained acceptance after information was given and the product was in-serviced. At this stage, "super users" were identified as clinical resources for the staff on a 24-hour basis. Phone numbers of the CNS, staff educator, and product representatives were available at each nursing station to address questions or concerns with the product.

Refreezing Phase

After the trial, survey results were shared with the nursing and physician staff. Finally, a decision was made to approve the product and integrate it into the system. The final stage of refreezing was the gradual withdrawal of the CNS to allow the bedside practitioner to function autonomously.

SOURCE: Oates, K. (1997). Models of planned change and research utilization applied to product evaluation. *Clinical Nurse Specialist, 11*(6), 270–273. Cited with permission.

4. Evaluation of the Change

The evaluation of the change was conducted during and at the end of the trial to determine appropriateness of the change. It is necessary to continue to monitor outcomes after successful implementation. The Iowa Model divides outcomes into three categories: patient and family, staff, and fiscal. Outcomes are monitored through quarterly quality improvement tools, infection control data, monthly product cost, and satisfaction of the staff and patients (and patients' parents). Staff must continue to provide feedback to the CNS on the change. In this example, as the change was consolidated in the system, the change agent (i.e., the CNS) was gradually removed, leaving the client system (i.e., the staff) to monitor and maintain the change. Individuals within the client system that could maintain the change must be identified. When the client system had embraced the change and acted as the change agent, the change process was terminated.

E. THE FUTURE OF RESEARCH UTILIZATION

What does the future hold for research utilization? Given today's increasing emphasis on quality, evidence-based practice, accountability, and fiscal responsibility in health care, it is likely that research utilization will be a major focus of all health professionals in the future. Having reached the last chapter in this book, you have obviously made the commitment to learn the skills required to be a responsible consumer of research and now have sufficient knowledge to engage in research-based practice at a beginning level. The utilization of research is a complex process requiring an informed consumer who has sufficient knowledge to be able to:

1. Sort through published results and decide which findings are credible and which are not.
2. See patterns, inconsistencies, and contradictions in findings from several studies on the same topic.
3. Decide whether a summary of evidence compiled by someone else is credible (Brown, 1999, p. 188).

In the past, the field of nursing missed opportunities to shape practice through nursing research. Today, however, nurses are better educated and better prepared than ever before to engage critically in evidence-based practice and to value it as an important part of professionalism.

The future of nursing research utilization will require commitment from individual nurses, hospital and community-based nursing units, the health-care delivery system, and the education system. We must all do our share to ensure that the many fine examples of nursing and interdisciplinary health research are used by practitioners to shape and improve nursing practice and health care for our clients. If research-based practice is to become part of the culture of nursing, then the following should occur:

- Practitioners must seek out continuing education opportunities that are research-based.
- Organizations must provide nurses with the computer and library resources to do literature searches and the time for practitioners to read research and implement findings in practice.
- Job descriptions of nurses should reflect the necessity of using research findings in practice.
- Organizations should hold practitioners accountable for using research findings appropriately in their practice.
- Nursing education must incorporate research findings into course content.
- Research skills should be presented to students as fundamental skills essential to understanding the nursing liter-

ature and to being a responsible consumer of research findings.

- Textbooks should be selected for their
  inclusion of research-based knowledge
  and citations of empirical studies.
- The discipline must communicate
  clearly to its members and students the
  importance of being informed consumers of researched-based knowledge
  (Brown, 1999).

If these activities are consistently
adopted, the field of nursing will be successful in communicating the high value
it places on research-based practice.

The future will see nurses engaged in
networking extensively across a global
village to bring the latest research findings to their nursing practice areas.
Through the use of the Internet and journals such as the *Online Journal of Knowledge Synthesis for Nursing,* nurses will
have access to evidence they can use to
shape future practice. Clinical settings
will support nurses in promoting comprehensive research activity. Indeed, the
future for research utilization looks
bright in nursing. In this era of innovation
and health-care reform, everyone must
share in the responsibility to see practice
improved through appropriate application of research findings.

A word of caution, however—research
utilization will not always be easy. Many
nurses may question why it is important
to do research. Some will say that research dollars are better spent in direct
care at patients' bedsides. This caution-
ary note is included not to discourage
you but rather to prepare you for con-
frontation, skepticism, and doubt you
may face, and the fact that you will raise
more questions than you answer. Improvements in practice will only occur
when you can demonstrate that new
knowledge leads to better health outcomes. Research is necessary to create
this new knowledge. Be persistent and
have faith in your ability to create positive change through research. Even the
most die hard cynics must agree with
change in the face of powerful evidence.

As you conclude reading this text, we
hope it is just the beginning of your research career in nursing. We encourage
you to re-read sections of this text as you
engage in research-based practice. As
you progress to more advanced levels of
nursing practice, you will come to realize
that you can make a difference through
research. You now have the attitude,
knowledge, and skills to do so. What remains is the desire, motivation, and commitment to make it happen. Remember
that the ultimate value of research is the
extent to which it is used in practice.

E X E R C I S E S

1. Select a problem from the practice setting that is of concern to the field of
   nursing. Do a review of the literature to
   determine the quantity and quality of
   research available on the problem
   topic. Summarize the critique of the literature. Make a determination as to
   whether or not there is sufficient evidence to proceed with a research utilization project. Justify your decision.

2. Using a theory of planned change,
   identify the steps one would engage in
   to implement a research utilization
   project to deal with the problem you
   identified in exercise 1. How would you
   evaluate the success or failure of the
   plan? Why is consolidation of the innovation in practice important to a research utilization project?

3. You are attending a clinical conference on your nursing unit and a comment is made that the ongoing nursing research utilization project is taking too much staff time and shouldn't be part of staff nurses' jobs. How would you respond to such a comment? Whose responsibility is research utilization? Provide a rationale for your answer.

4. As a practicing nurse, how would you increase research use in nursing?

5. What strategies would you suggest for dealing with the following barriers to research utilization?
  • Lack of time

  • Authoritative management style

  • Negative staff attitude toward research

  • Limited research critiquing skills

  • Limited replication studies on the topic

6. Select a nursing procedure from the procedure manual at your clinical agency or your nursing skills text. Do a literature search to determine what, if any, research evidence is available to support the steps in the procedure.

RECOMMENDED READINGS

Bostrom, J., and Wise, L. (1994). Closing the gap between research and practice. *Journal of Nursing Administration, 24*(5), 22–27. Comprehensive descriptions tell how a group of nurses improved the quality of nursing care by facilitating the transfer of research knowledge to current practice.

Crookes, P., and Davies, S. (1998). *Research into Practice.* London: Bailliere Tindall. This is an excellent guide to critically evaluating, synthesizing, and utilizing research-based literature in professional practice.

Goode, C., Butcher, L., Cipperley, J., et al. (1996). *Research Utilization: A Study Guide.* Ida Grove, IA: Horne Video Productions. This helpful guide takes readers step by step through the process and activities involved in research utilization.

National Health Services (1998). *Changing Clinical Practice.* London: Department of Health. A brief review of the process involved in changing clinical practice.

Nilson, K., Nordstrom, G., Krusebrant, A., and Bjorvell, H. (2000). Perceptions of research utilization: Comparisons between health care professionals, nursing students, and a reference group of nurse clinicians. *Journal of Advanced Nursing, 31*(1), 99–109. A good discussion of barriers to and facilitators of nurses' use of research findings in practice from various perspectives.

Oates, K. (1997). Models of planned change and research utilization applied to product evaluation. *Clinical Nurse Specialist, 11*(6), 270–273. A good example of both the research utilization process and the change process applied to a clinical practice problem.

Parahoo, K. (2000). Barriers to and facilitators of research utilization among nurses in Northern Ireland. *Journal of Advanced Nursing, 31*(1), 89–98. A survey of nurses' perceptions of barriers to—and facilitators of—research utilization.

Part 8

APPENDICES

A ppendix A contains an introduction to analyzing data, creating new variables, and working with output using SPSS for Windows (version 10.0). Appendix B contains a sample questionnaire. This questionnaire will serve as an illustration of formatting and also be used in the sample data set and exercises contained in the instructor's manual for this text.

Appendix **A**

Using SPSS for Windows*

APPENDIX OUTLINE

If you are just starting to work with SPSS, it would be a good idea to review the materials in Chapter 16 because it includes an introduction to the Statistical Package for the Social Sciences (SPSS) and reviews the procedures for logging onto the computer and accessing an SPSS system file. This Appendix provides guidelines for the basic procedures most likely to be used by the nursing researcher. Sample output is annotated to assist you in using SPSS.

In addition to the instructions on how to begin an SPSS session included in Chapter 16, you may wish to review Chapter 18, which discusses four key multivariate procedures. Also, a number of manuals available from SPSS present many additional features and options for the various procedures. Some of these manuals are listed at the end of Appendix A; you may wish to consult them as you develop your facility in working with SPSS.

*SPSS is a trademark of SPSS, Inc. of Chicago, Illinois, for its proprietary computer software.

A. METHODS OF ISSUING SPSS COMMANDS

SPSS procedures may be run using either a **point-and-click** method or by entering **syntax** commands. Many users find that both techniques are useful. Beginning users typically find the point-and-click method easiest. We primarily focus on this method here.

After each procedure is completed, the results are sent to the **Output Viewer** that is automatically displayed on your monitor; you can save, edit, and print your output from the Output Viewer. You can also directly copy the output to a word processor file from the Output Viewer. We will begin by examining the fundamentals of submitting commands to SPSS and then discuss how to work with output followed by a presentation of the basic procedures that have been covered in this text.

1. Point-and-Click Commands

The toolbar across the top of the SPSS Data Editor screen provides the starting point for issuing analysis commands to SPSS. One can draw samples, select cases, sort cases, add or delete variables, and initiate a vast range of statistical procedures by clicking on the appropriate toolbar item. The main statistical procedures are listed below. To access each of them, the user simply clicks an item on the toolbar and follows the sequence to identify the desired procedure. The ones we focus on here are as follows:

- **ANOVA:** Analyze/General Linear Model/Univariate
- **COMPUTE:** Transform/Compute
- **CORRELATE:** Analyze/Correlate/Bivariate
- **CROSSTABS:** Analyze/Descriptive Statistics/Crosstabs
- **DESCRIPTIVES:** Analyze/Descriptive Statistics/Descriptives
- **DISCRIMINANT:** Analyze/Classify/Discriminant

- **FACTOR:** Analyze/Data Reduction/Factor
- **FREQUENCIES:** Analyze/Descriptive Statistics/Frequencies
- **GRAPHS:** Graphs/Scatter/Define
- **IF:** File/New/Syntax (enter IF commands on screen)
- **LIST:** File/New/Syntax (enter LIST commands on screen)
- **MEANS:** Analyze/Compare Means/means
- **PARTIAL CORRELATION:** Analyze/Correlate/Partial
- **RECODE:** Tansform/Recode/Into Different Variables
- **REGRESSION:** Analyze/Regression/Linear (Method=Backward)
- **RELIABILITY:** Analyze/Scale/Reliability (Model=Alpha)
- **SPEARMAN CORRELATION:** Analyze/Correlate/Bivariate/Spearman
- **t-TEST GROUPS:** Analyze/Compare Means/Independent-Samples t Test
- **t-TEST PAIRS:** Analyze/Compare Means/Paired-Samples t Test
- **Z SCORE:** Analyze/Descriptive Statistics/Descriptives/(Save Standardized values as variables)

After a procedure has been selected, an SPSS procedure screen appears and the user simply uses the mouse to select variables and move them into the appropriate analysis boxes shown on the Window. A few general tips in using the method are listed below:

- To illustrate an SPSS procedure window, the crosstabs one is shown in Figure A1.
- To select one variable, simply click on it.
- To select multiple variables from a list, hold down the Control button and click on the variables.
- To select several variables in a sequence, click on the first one in the sequence, move the mouse to the last one, hold the Shift key down, and click on that item; all the variables between the two clicked on will then be high-

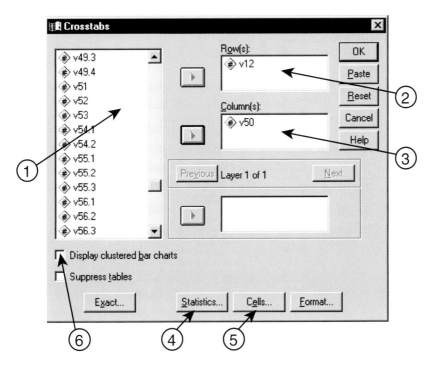

Notes:
1.   The variables in the file are listed in this pane.
2.   Move the dependent variable(s) to the **Row(s)** analysis pane
      by highlighting the variable(s) and then clicking it over by

      by clicking on the ▶ button.
3.   Move the independent variable(s) to the **Column(s)** pane by

      highlighting the variable(s) and then click on the ▶ to move it
      over.
4.   Click on **Statistics** to select the Statistics you want (probably
      Chi-Square)
5.   Click on **Cells** to indicate how you want percentages run
      (choose column)
6.   Click on **Display clustered bar charts** if you wish to have a
      bar chart of the data

Figure Al   Crosstab Screen

lighted and may then be moved to an analysis box by clicking the ▶ key.

• To move quickly through a variables list, click and hold down the scroll bar button (to the right of the variables list) and slowly drag down the scroll bar button.

• Click on the various Options and Sta-

tistics boxes to see the additional procedures that are available within each procedure.

2. Syntax Commands

To enter syntax commands, the user brings up a Syntax Editor screen, types commands into the screen, and then submits the commands to SPSS for processing. To bring up a Syntax Editor screen, click on File/New/Syntax on the toolbar. An SPSS Syntax box appears at the bottom of the screen; if you click on it, the Syntax Editor screen appears. You then type in SPSS commands into the screen and, when ready to submit, point and click on Run on the window's toolbar. See Figure A2 for a copy of the Syntax window.

It is a good idea to retain a copy of the syntax commands used when running an analysis. When you exit from SPSS, you will be asked if you wish to keep a copy of the syntax file. If you respond yes, then you will be prompted for a name for the file. These files use a file extension of .sps.

Another use of syntax files is that when using the point-and-click method, you can also click on Paste before you click on OK when running procedures; this pastes into a Syntax Editor file the syntax commands for the procedure you have just invoked. These syntax files are worth retaining because if you discover errors in your data, you can fix them and then quickly re-run the analysis by simply resubmitting the commands contained in the syntax file.

If you wish to list several variables for the first 25 cases, it may be done using the LIST command in a syntax file. This procedure is available only as a syntax command and is useful when confirming that various RECODE, IF, or RECODE commands are working properly (see LIST procedure).

3. Working with Output Viewer

The results of each analysis are sent to the Output Viewer. You can edit, print, and save output from the Viewer. Figure A3 shows output as it appears in the Output Viewer for an analysis of suicide thoughts by gender. The Output Viewer provides two panes: (1) the outline pane, on the left, lists items in the output and you can click on these to move, save, or delete them; and (2) the contents pane, on the right side, shows the output from the analysis.

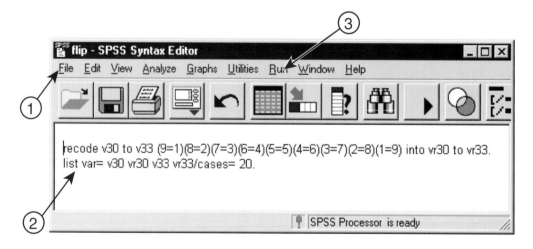

Notes:
1.   To get Syntax Editor Screen click: **File/New/Syntax.**
2.   Enter SPSS procedure commands in screen.
3.   When ready to submit, click on Run on the toolbar.

Figure A2   Syntax Editor Screen

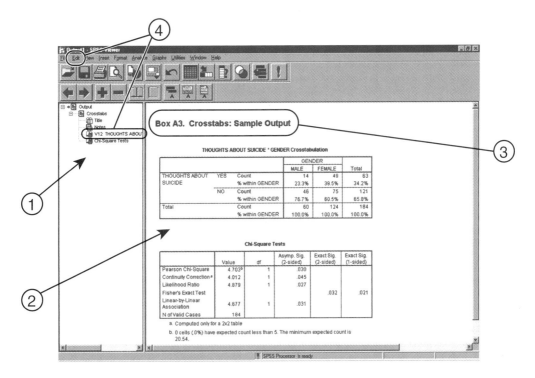

Notes:

1. The left pane indicates elements; click on an element to have it highlighted.
2. The pane on the right displays the results of the analysis; to edit the results (changing width of columns etc. click anywhere on output and then double click on it; now you can change widths of columns etc.).
3. To add your table title click on title and then double click; type in new title.
4. To copy to another file; on left pane click on element(s) you wish to copy, and then on toolbar click **Edit/Copy Objects**; switch to file you wish to copy the material into and do a **Copy/Paste**.

Figure A3   Output Viewer Screen

Some tips for using the Output Viewer are:

- To go directly to a section of the output, simply click on the name of the section on the outline pane (the screen on the left side).
- To delete a section of output, simply click on the item on the left screen and press the Delete button. You will generally want to get rid of the "case processing summary."
- To print one or more sections, click on the items on the left pane and then print the results (you can preview what will be printed by clicking on the Preview icon).
- You can move objects around by clicking and dragging to new locations on your output.
- You have various templates available to choose the format of your output; to see options available, double Click on the table (this activates the Pivot

Table), click on Format, and click on Tablelooks

A number of optional formats will be presented and you can choose from among them.

- You can highlight a section (or sections) on the left pane, Edit/Copy the material into the clipboard, and then bring up your word processing program and Edit/Paste the material into the new file.
- If you wish to attach your name as a header for your output, go to File/Page Setup/Options when you are in the Output Viewer and type in what you want in the header panel. Click on Make Default and the header will appear on all your subsequent outputs.
- On lengthy outputs, you may find that not all the output shows. Double click inside the box containing the output, move the cursor to the bottom of the output, and drag down the bottom margin. When you do this, the remainder of the output will show on the screen.
- If you find that there are unwanted page breaks in the output, double click inside the output (a thick border should be showing). The little square box marks page breaks; you can delete these using the Delete or Backspace key. Recheck your preview to ensure that the unwanted page breaks are gone before you print.
- When you get errors using the Syntax procedure, it is a good idea to read the error carefully and then highlight and delete the error message before you resubmit the job. Note that you can run point-and-click procedures without returning to the Data Editor because the analysis toolbar is at the top of the Output Viewer screen.
- When you exit SPSS, you will be asked if you wish to save your output viewer file. This file will have a .spo file extension.

B. BASIC SPSS PROCEDURES

There are two basic procedures for examining *individual* variables. When you want a count of the number of cases that fall into each category of a nominal or ordinal variable, use the FREQUENCIES procedure described later. If you have a ratio level variable and you wish to calculate the mean and standard deviation, use the DESCRIPTIVES procedure described later.

When analyzing the relationship *between* variables, there are many procedures that may be used. Beginning researchers are advised, however, to apply the 3M approach (model, measurement, method) to determine which procedure is appropriate given the relationship being examined and the level of measurement involved in the measures (see Chapter 16).

The following sections present the basic procedures of SPSS. Each procedure is illustrated with annotations on the sample output that should help the researcher understand and interpret the results of the analysis. The procedures are listed alphabetically to make them easier to find.

I. ANOVA: Analysis of Variance

Experimental researchers use analysis of variance (ANOVA) when their design has more than one independent variable or has more than two treatment levels. (t tests are typically used in studies with fewer than 30 cases in each of the two groups and when there is one treatment level and one independent variable.) The inclusion of additional complexity is relatively simple and provides an opportunity to explore the interaction of treatment variables (when effects change for different combinations of treatment variables) in influencing the dependent variable.

Although regression analysis is appropriate in many situations, there are several situations in which analysis of variance (ANOVA or MANOVA [multivariate analysis of variance]) would be more appropriate than regression analysis. For example, if you had predictor variables that have qualitative differences (e.g., three different drugs); or if rather than having a ratio variable measuring the amount of time spent in the hospital, we have a variable that indicates whether the person was hospitalized or treated as an outpatient, we again would probably opt for analysis of variance. In short, if an independent variable is made up of values that differ in *kind* rather than in *quantity*, we would opt for analysis of variance.

A second situation that is better handled with analysis of variance is one in which the relationship between the independent and the dependent variable changes over the continuum. Perhaps the relationship is nonlinear; once again, analysis of variance should be considered as an alternative to regression.

Typically, analysis of variance techniques should used when:

- An experimental design is being used.
- The dependent variable (or variables) is measured at the ratio level.
- One or more of the treatment variables are measured at the ratio level and others at the nominal or ordinal levels.
- You have multiple dependent measures that you wish to examine simultaneously (i.e., in MANOVA).
- Ratio level independent variables may be identified as *covariates.*
- In nonexperimental designs, you wish to examine whether there are significant interactions among independent variables.

a. Point-and-Click Method

- Analyze
- General Linear Model
- Univariate or Simple Factorial

Move the dependent variable and then the variables for the various factors and any *covariates* by clicking on them and then clicking them to their appropriate screens by using the arrow keys; you will be prompted to identify the lowest and highest values of treatment values such as 0, 2; in this case, the implied values include 0, 1, and 2. ANOVA assumes that there are no blank categories, so you will have to RECODE values if there are no values in one of the categories implied by the range indicated. Click OK when you are ready to process the data.

b. Sample Output: ANOVA

Note that the variations that are compared in an analysis of variance are composed of two elements: random error and possible treatment effects. The test that is done compares the ratio in the following way:

$$F = \frac{\text{Random error} + \text{possible treatment effects}}{\text{Random error}}$$

The interpretation of the results of an ANOVA test is split between a concern for:

- The main effect of treatment variable A (Box A1 indicates that COUNTRY has a statistically significant main effect on egalitarianism).
- The main effect of treatment variable B (Box A1 indicates that v50 [gender] does not have a statistically significant main effect on egalitarianism).
- An interaction of the treatment variables $(A \times B)$ (the interaction between COUNTRY and GENDER is not statistically significant).
- An error term (within groups). This is the "residual source of variation."

2. COMPUTE: Creating New Variables

COMPUTE allows researchers to create new variables by performing mathematical operations on variables.

BOX A1 ANALYSIS OF VARIANCE: Sample Output

Between-Subjects Factors

		Value Label	N
NAME OF COUNTRY	0	CANADA	65
	1	NEW ZEALAND	57
	2	AUSTRALIA	60
GENDER	1	MALE	59
	2	FEMALE	123

Tests of Between-Subjects Effects

Dependent Variable: EGALITARIANISM

Source	Type III Sum of Squares	df	Mean Square	F	Sig.
Corrected Model	1575.426[a]	5	315.085	4.531	.001
Intercept	139602.183	1	139602.183	2007.419	.000
COUNTRY	1194.586	2	597.293	8.589	.000
V50	33.219	1	33.219	.478	.490
COUNTRY * V50	125.990	2	62.995	.906	.406
Error	12239.591	176	69.543		
Total	186677.000	182			
Corrected Total	13815.016	181			

[a.] R Squared = .114 (Adjusted R Squared = .089)

Notes

1. Degrees of freedom column.
2. F test of significance value.
3. Test of significance results: needs to be 0.05 or less to be statistically significant.

a. Point-and-Click Method

- Transform
- Compute

As illustrated in Figure A4, enter the name of the new variable you wish to create in the Target Variable window (you will now see a window that allows you to place a variable label on the new variable); then move the cursor to the Numeric Expression window and type in the computational formula you wish to use. Enter OK, and the new variable will be created.

Figure A4 shows the screen illustrating

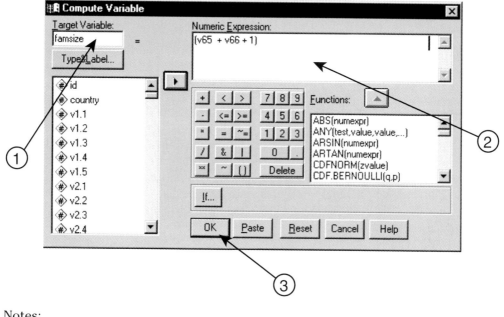

Notes:
1. Name new variable here
2. Type in numerical expression here
3. Click OK when done

Figure A4   Compute Screen

---

the creation of a new variable, *famsize*, representing the addition of values in two variables (i.e., number of brothers plus number of sisters plus 1 added to the total). Computations within parentheses are performed first and are used to control the order of the mathematical operations. Make certain that there are an equal number of open and closed parentheses. SPSS uses the following symbols to indicate basic functions:

- + Addition
- − Subtraction
- * Multiplication
- / Division
- ** Exponentiation

Many other functions are available to the researcher in SPSS; three commonly used ones include:

- RND(var) = rounds to whole number

- SUM(var list) = sums values in variable list
- MEAN(var list) = mean of values

3. CORRELATIONS: Correlational Analysis

When variables are measured at the ratio level, then various correlational techniques are appropriate. As discussed in Chapter 11, a correlation, or r, measures the strength of an association between two variables. The values can range from +1.00 to −1.00. Typically, they are reported to two decimal places, as in 0.56. Explained variance is the square of the correlation coefficient or r^2.

a. Point-and-Click Method

- Analyze

- Correlate
- Bivariate

The correlation screen will appear. Click on and move variables to the Variable window. For ratio variables, you should use Pearson correlations; however, if you are using ordinal variables, you should use Spearman correlations; click on the appropriate box. You may also specify one- or two-tailed tests; click OK when everything is set appropriately.

Box A2 includes a summary table of correlations. The CORRELATIONS procedure may also be used along with the PARTIAL CORRELATION procedure to test for intervening variables and for sources of spuriousness variables. See the PARTIAL

CORRELATION section to see how that type of correlation is run.

4. CROSSTABS: Crosstabular Analysis

CROSSTABS is a procedure used to examine the association between a nominal or ordinal dependent variable and a nominal, ordinal, or ratio independent variable. To have sufficient cases in each of the table cells when there are several categories in the independent variable, they would be recoded (i.e., a new variable would be created regrouping the categories into two or three *meaningful* categories) before the analysis is run.

BOX A2 CORRELATIONS: Sample Output

Correlations ①

		Government Increase Foreign Aid	More Money Should be Given to Welfare	Homo-Sexuality Okay	Abortion Woman's Personal Choice ③
GOVERNMENT INCREASE FOREIGN AID	Pearson Correlation	1.000	.323**	.029	−.023
	Sig. (1-tailed)	.	.000	.347	.379
	N	184	183	182	183
MORE MONEY SHOULD BE GIVEN TO WELFARE	Pearson Correlation	.323**	1.000	.272**	.234**
	Sig. (1-tailed)	.000	.	.000	.001
	N	183	184	183	184
HOMOSEXUALITY OKAY	Pearson Correlation	.029	.272**	1.000	.435**
	Sig. (1-tailed)	.347	.000	.	.000
	N	182	183	183	183
ABORTION WOMAN'S PERSONAL CHOICE	Pearson Correlation	−.023	.234**	.435**	1.000
	Sig. (1-tailed)	.379	.001	.000	.
	N	183	184	183	184

**. Correlation is significant at the 0.01 level (1-tailed). ②

Notes

1. Pearson correlation is the r value.

2. One-tailed test requested (** indicates significance at the 0.01 level).

3. N = number of cases.

a. Point-and-Click Method

- Analyze
- Summarize
- Crosstabs

The CROSSTABS screen will now appear.

- Place the dependent variable (or variables) in the Row(s) window.
- Place the independent variable (or variables) in the Column(s) window.
- Click on Statistics, on Chi-Square, and then on Continue.
- Click on Cells and click on Column Percentages. Then click Continue.
- Click OK.

b. Sample Output and Notes

Box A3 presents the results from a simple CROSSTABS analysis. Note where the chi-square value is printed and the probability is identified. Usually CROSSTABS results are reformatted when prepared for presentation in a paper. See Table A1 for suggestions on how to reformat a CROSSTABS table for presentation in a paper.

Table A1 presents the relationship between gender and suicidal thoughts. Because we are attempting to assess the impact of the independent variable on the dependent one, we are interested in the percent of respondents who have thoughts of suicide. Thus, we might describe the findings as indicating that while 23.3 percent of the male respondents report having had thoughts of suicide, this was true for 39.5 percent of the female respondents. In short, we compare percentages in each column. Usually it is sufficient to use one row (in this case, just the row for those reporting having had thoughts of suicide).

For analyses involving three or more variables simultaneously, the procedures are the same, with the control variable identified in the Layer 1 of 1 window (Box A4 provides a sample output).

When control variables are used, it is necessary to minimize the number of categories in the independent and in the control variables. Generally, there should be no more than two or three categories within these variables. There are two major reasons for this limitation: (1) the number of cases in each cell will become too small if there are many categories in either the independent or the control variable, and (2) the interpretation of the table is very difficult if simplicity is not maintained.

Chapter 17 discusses interpretations of three-variable cross-tabular tables. Remember that to apply *Jackson's rule of thirds,* it is necessary to compare the original difference in the percentages between the categories of the independent variable and re-run the relationship, controlling for the intervening (or source of spuriousness) variable. Only if the original difference is reduced by more than one-third *in each category of the control variable* do we have any evidence consistent with the proposed model.

5. DESCRIPTIVES: Computing the Mean and Standard Deviation

The DESCRIPTIVES procedure computes means and standard deviations and is appropriately used for ratio level variables. The output provides the mean, standard deviation, and the minimum and maximum values for the variable (or variables) identified on the variable list. In addition, the number of valid (nonmissing) cases is reported (Box A5 provides a sample output.)

a. Point-and-Click Method

- Analyze
- Descriptive Statistics
- Descriptives

The DESCRIPTIVES screen will now appear. Identify the variables for which you

BOX A3 CROSSTABS: Sample Output

②

THOUGHTS ABOUT SUICIDE * GENDER Crosstabulation

			GENDER		Total
			MALE	**FEMALE**	
THOUGHTS ABOUT SUICIDE	YES	Count % within GENDER	14 (23.3%)	(49) (39.5%)	63 34.2%
	NO	Count % within GENDER	46 76.7%	75 60.5%	121 65.8%
Total		Count % within GENDER	60 100.0%	124 100.0%	184 100.0%

① →

③ ← 49

④ ← 121

⑤

Chi-Square Tests

	Value	df	Asymp. Sig. (2-sided)	Exact Sig. (2-sided)	Exact Sig. (1-sided)
Pearson Chi-Square	4.703[b]	1	.030		
Continuity Correction[a]	(4.012)	1	.045		
Likelihood Ratio	4.879	1	.027		
Fisher's Exact Test				(.032)	.021
Linear-by-Linear Association	4.677	1	.031		
N of Valid Cases	184				

⑥

⑦⑧

[a.] Computed only for a 2×2 table
[b.] 0 cells (.0%) have expected count less than 5. The minimum expected count is 20.54.

Notes

1. The dependent variable is suicidal thoughts.
2. The independent variable is gender.
3. Number of females who have thought about suicide.
4. Compare these percentages when discussing results.
5. df = degrees of freedom.
6. With 2 × 2 tables, use this value as the chi-square value; if not a 2 × 2 table, use the Pearson chi-square value.
7. Use this value to test null hypothesis (no relationship between suicide thoughts and gender).
8. Because the value is < 0.05, the decision is to reject the null hypothesis; there is a statistically significant relationship between suicidal thoughts and gender

want DESCRIPTIVES by moving desired variables to the Variable window. Click OK when ready.

If Optional Statistics are desired, click on Options. If a standardized (Z score) version of the variable (or variables) is desired, click Save Standardized. SPSS will create a standardized version of the variable and will add a Z to the beginning of the variable name (e.g., v24 will become zv24). The new variable is immediately available for use.

Table AI   Suicide Thoughts by Gender

| | GENDER | | | | | |
| | Male | | Female | | Total | |
Thoughts About Suicide	N	%	N	%	N	%
Yes	14	23.3	49	39.5	63	34.2
No	46	76.7	75	60.5	121	65.8
Total	60	100.0	124	100.0	184	100.0

Chi-square 4.012 (corrected for continuity); degrees of freedom = 1; Sig. = .032 (2 tailed test)

BOX A4 CROSSTABS: Sample Output Showing a Control Variable

THOUGHTS ABOUT SUICIDE * GENDER * NAME OF COUNTRY Crosstabulation

| | | | | GENDER | | |
NAME OF COUNTRY				MALE	FEMALE	Total
CANADA	THOUGHTS ABOUT SUICIDE	YES	Count	8	14	22
			% within GENDER	26.7%	40.0%	33.8%
		NO	Count	22	21	43
			% within GENDER	73.3%	60.0%	66.2%
	Total		Count	30	35	65
			% within GENDER	22.2%	40.0%	34.5%
NEW ZEALAND	THOUGHTS ABOUT SUICIDE	YES	Count	4	16	20
			% within GENDER	22.2%	40.0%	34.5%
		NO	Count	14	24	38
			% within GENDER	77.8%	60.0%	65.5%
	Total		Count	18	40	58
			% within GENDER	100.0%	100.0%	100.0%
AUSTRALIA	THOUGHTS ABOUT SUICIDE	YES	Count	2	19	21
			% within GENDER	16.7%	38.8%	34.4%
		NO	Count	10	30	40
			% within GENDER	83.3%	61.2%	65.6%
	Total		Count	12	49	61
			% within GENDER	100.0%	100.0%	100.0%

①

Notes

1. Categories of the control variable (country).
2. To test if country of origin is spuriously influencing relationship between gender and suicidal thoughts, compare the percentage difference in suicide thoughts between males and females in each country. Have the differences (compared with those shown in Box A3) increased, stayed the same, decreased or disappeared, or are they mixed? See Chapter 17 for details about interpreting this output

BOX A5 DESCRIPTIVES: Sample Output, Including Z Score Values

Descriptive Statistics

	N	Minimum	Maximum	Mean	Std. Deviation
EGALITARIANISM	182	10.00	54.00	30.8187	8.7365
Zscore: EGALITARIANISM	182	−2.38296	2.65339	−2.9e-16	1.0000000
Valid N (listwise)	182				

① ② ③

Notes

1. Shows the mean value for an egalitarianism index score.
2. The standard deviation is shown.
3. The −2.9E-16 indicates the mean of the scores when converted to Z scores; the value is −0.0000000000000002.9, which is very close to zero!

b. Sample Output: DESCRIPTIVES

Box A5 shows the output you can expect from a DESCRIPTIVES analysis. See Chapter 19 for suggestions about how to compress the reporting of means and standard deviations for a number of variables.

6. DISCRIMINANT: Doing Discriminant Function Analysis

Discriminant function analysis is a procedure for examining the relationship between a nominal dependent variable and ratio independent variables. The basic idea behind discriminant function analysis is to correctly classify into which category of the dependent variable each case will fall. It can also be used to predict which category a case will fall into when measures of the dependent variable are missing. The statistics *Lambda* was discussed in Chapter 11. Readers should recall that this statistic measures the proportionate reduction in error that is achieved when a variable is added to an analysis. Lambda is used in discriminant function analysis to measure the success in correctly classifying cases. Similar to re-

gression analysis, standardized weightings are provided that permit the researcher to assess the relative impact of independent variables on the dependent one. Also, similar to regression analysis, it is possible to use *dummy* independent variables. See examples of how to construct these in the Regression Analysis section of this Appendix. For more details on discriminant analysis, see Chapter 18.

a. Point-and-Click Method

- Analyze
- Classify
- Discriminant

The Discriminant screen will now appear.

- Click on dependent variable and click ➤ to move to Grouping Variable window.
- Click on Define Range to specify minimum and maximum values for the dependent variable (hit the Tab key after each entry).
- Click on Continue.
- Click on Independent variables and click ➤ to move them to the Independent variables window.

- Click on Analyze and then click on Means.
- Click on Continue.
- Click on Classify and then click on Summary Table.
- Click on Continue.
- Click OK.
- Identify variables for which you want procedure run; click OK.

b. Sample Output and Notes

Box A6 presents sample output from a discriminant analysis of suicidal thoughts (v12) among respondents in an international survey. Selected for independent variables were FAMILY SES (socioeconomic status), v50 (gender, a dummy variable), v58 (size of home community), and EGAL (an index measuring egalitarianism).

The output shown in Box A6 shows how many cases were used in the analysis and the number of respondents who reported that they had thought about committing suicide ($n = 60$) and the number who reported that they had not had such thoughts ($n = 108$). The mean scores for each independent variable are then reported for each category of suicidal thoughts. Note that those with suicide thoughts had higher mean scores on egalitarianism, family SES, gender, and size of home community.

The last presentation on the output shows the percent of cases correctly classified. It is reported that 61.3 percent of the cases were correctly classified using the four independent variables. But how might we have fared if we had just randomly assigned cases to the suicidal thought or nonsuicidal thought categories? To compute the number of correct classifications we would have made using random assignment, the following steps may be taken:

- Compute the proportion of cases that fall into each category (in this case, 60 ÷ 168 = 0.36; 108 ÷ 168 = 0.64).

- Square the proportions and add them together and then multiply by 100 ($0.36^2 + 0.64^2$) × 100 = 53.9 %.
- Proportion of errors in random assignment ($1 - 0.54 = 0.46$).
- Proportion of errors using discriminant analysis based classifications ($1 - 0.61 = 0.39$).

The percent error reduction using the model compared with random assignment may be calculated by comparing the proportion of errors in model compared with random assignment divided by the proportion of errors using the model, multiplied by 100: $[(0.46 - 0.39) ÷ 0.46] × 100 = 15.2$ percent.

The results indicate that we were able to improve our classification of people into the thought-of-suicide category versus the have-not-thought-of-suicide category by 15.2 percent by using the information on the four independent variables. But how important were each of the independent variables?

There are two basic ways of estimating the relative importance of variables in correctly estimating into which category of the dependent variable that a case will fall:

1. Use the DISCRIMINANT procedure, including all variables on the first run. Then continue to repeat the analysis but exclude a different independent variable each time until you have an analysis excluding each independent variable. The contribution of each independent variable may then be judged by comparing the percentage of correct assignment using the variable with when it is not used, as in:

> Contribution = (% correct with variable included) − (% correct without variable included)

The variable that produces the greatest decrease in correct assignments when omitted is the most important factor, the one with the second greatest drop

BOX A6 DISCRIMINANT ANALYSIS: Sample Output

①

Group Statistics

THOUGHTS ABOUT SUICIDE		Mean	Std. Deviation	Valid N (listwise)	
				Unweighted	Weighted
YES	EGALITARIANISM	32.6833	8.9962	60	60.000
	FAMILY SES	68.4190	21.4355	60	60.000
	SIZE OF HOME COMMUNITY	5.2500	2.8560	60	60.000
	GENDER (Dummy)	.7667	.4265	60	60.000
NO	EGALITARIANISM	29.0926	8.5002	108	108.000
	FAMILY SES	63.3498	22.6049	108	108.000
	SIZE OF HOME COMMUNITY	5.0093	2.6102	108	108.000
	GENDER (Dummy)	.6204	.4876	108	108.000
Total	EGALITARIANISM	30.3750	8.8241	168	168.000
	FAMILY SES	65.1602	22.2634	168	168.000
	SIZE OF HOME COMMUNITY	5.0952	2.6945	168	168.000
	GENDER (Dummy)	.6726	.4707	168	168.000

Analysis 1: Summary of Canonical Discriminant Functions

Eigenvalues

Function	Eigenvalue	% of Variance	Cumulative %	Canonical Correlation
1	.091[a]	100.0	100.0	.289

[a]First 1 canonical discriminant functions were used in the analysis.

Wilks' Lambda

Test of Function(s)	Wilks' Lambda	Chi-square	df	Sig.
1	.916	14.307	4	.006

Standardized Canonical Discriminant Function Coefficients

	Function 1
EGALITARIANISM	.743
FAMILY SES	.528
SIZE OF HOME COMMUNITY	.146
GENDER (Dummy)	.591

②

continued on next page

Structure Matrix

	Function
	I
EGALITARIANISM	.660
GENDER (Dummy)	.500
FAMILY SES	.365
SIZE OF HOME COMMUNITY	.142

Pooled within-grouped correlations between discriminating variables and standardized canonical discriminant functions.
Variables ordered by absolute size of correlation within function.

Functions at Group Centroids

	Function
THOUGHTS ABOUT SUICIDE	I
YES	.403
NO	−.225

Unstandardized canonical discriminant functions evaluated at group means.

Classification Statistics

Prior Probalitities for Groups

		Cases Used in Analysis	
THOUGHTS ABOUT SUICIDE	Prior	Unweighted	Weighted
YES	.500	60	60.000
NO	.500	108	108.000
Total	1.000	168	168.000

Classification Results[a]

			Predicted Group Membership		
		THOUGHTS ABOUT SUICIDE	YES	NO	Total
Original	Count	YES	37	23	60
		NO	42	66	108
	%	YES	61.7	38.3	100.0
		NO	38.9	61.1	100.0

③

[a]61.3% of original grouped cases correctly classified.

Notes

1. The mean values for each independent variable is presented for both categories of the dependent variable

2. The relative importance of the independent variable in helping to classify the date into the suicide thoughts categories may be measured by the standardized values presented here. Hence the egalitarianism score of .743 is the most important item.

3. The 103 cases on this diagonal were correctly classified; the other diagonal contains 65 incorrectly classified cases.

is the second most important variable, and so forth.

2. Another method to assess the relative importance of factors may be derived by examining the *standardized discriminant function coefficients*. These coefficients are similar to the beta weights in regression analysis in that they are standardized (so that differences in the range and variability of values in a variable does not influence the coefficient; if it helps, think of these as Z scores in which each variable has a mean of 0 and a standard deviation of 1). The larger the coefficient, the more importance the variable has in predicting into which group the individual will fall. The relative importance of each variable is directly proportional to its coefficient and may be estimated in a manner similar to that suggested for the beta weights in regression analysis (see Regression section).

Box A6 should be examined. First, it should be noted that the total amount of the variation explained by the combination of variables can be determined by squaring the *canonical correlation*. In our example, the canonical correlation is 0.289, which mea that together the four independent va les are accounting for 8.4 percent of variance in suicidal thoughts (0.289   0.0835 × 100 = 8.4%).

The *eigenvalue* (0.091) represents the ratio of the between-groups variance to the within-groups variance. The higher this value, the greater the ability of the independent variables to discriminate between categories of the dependent variable.

The *Lambda* value varies from 0 to 1.0 and is a direct measure of the discriminating power of the model being tested—that is, the higher the value, the higher the discriminating ability of the model to distinguish between categories of the dependent variable. In this case, the Lambda is 0.916.

A *chi-square* value is reported along with the degrees of freedom (df) and the prob-

ability of the difference occurring on a chance basis (Sig.). In our illustration, the significance level is 0.006, which means that because of chance factors in sampling, that much of a difference could only be observed six times in a thousand samples.

The number of functions that the DISCRIMINANT procedure will calculate is one fewer than the number of categories in the dependent variable. Thus, as is the case in the example we are using, when there are two categories in the dependent variable, one function will be computed; if we had three categories, two functions would be calculated.

As in regression analysis, if there is a high correlation among the independent variables (e.g., above 0.70), then it is a good idea to either drop one of the highly correlated variables or multiply them together to provide a composite measure of the two variables.

7. FACTOR: Doing Factor Analysis

Factor analysis is a procedure used to explore communalities among a number of variables (see Chapter for a comparison to regression analysis). The typical uses in nursing include instrument development, instrument validation, and data reduction. Simply stated, factor analysis is a tool used to identify groups of variables that cluster together within a data set. For example, if a researcher had 20 Likert items measuring nurses' job satisfaction, factor analysis might be used to see if the various indicators fall into three or four groupings. One factor might be "job autonomy," another might be "feeling a part of the team," and so forth. To do a factor analysis in SPSS, access the procedure as follows:

a. Point-and-Click Method

- Analyze
- Data Reduction
- Factor

The Factor Analysis screen will now appear.

Some of the terms that need to be understood in reading factor analysis output include the following key terms:

- An **eigenvalue** is the sum of the squared factor loadings for any one factor. Thus, the eigenvalue is a measure of how much of the total variance is explained by a given factor. The higher the eigenvalue relative to other ones, the greater the variance explained by that factor.
- A **correlation matrix** is said to be factorable if there are reasonably robust correlations among the items. Ordinarily, one would expect the interitem correlations to average above 0.25 to consider the variables to be worthy of factor analysis. If it is any lower than that, and you may not find that any factors would be extracted.
- A **marker variable** is one that produces the highest correlation with the underlying factor that is identified in the analysis. The marker variable is useful to the researcher in attempting to label the underlying factor.

In determining the second factor, a rotation is required, either (1) an orthogonal (varimax is the most common version of orthogonal rotations) forces a 90 degree rotation, producing an entirely independent solution or (2) an oblique rotation that selects the second best solution but does not insist on the 90 degree rotation.

There are two main ways in which factors are extracted:

1. The **principal components method,** which includes an analysis of all the variance in the observed variables, not just the shared variance among the variables.
2. The **principal factors method** (known in SPSS as the *Principal Axis Factoring method*). This approach relies on the shared variances of the variables included in the analysis and appears to be the most commonly used approach.

Box A7 illustrates some of the output that results from a factor analysis. In this case, two significant factors were extracted from the communalities among the eight variables purporting to measure liberalism. By examining these factors, we note that factor 1 seems to include those items related to public policy issues, so we labeled the factor "Public Policy Liberalism." The second factor included two items with heavy loadings ("abortion is a woman's personal choice" and "homosexuality is okay"). This factor we identified as "Individual Rights Liberalism."

It is interesting to compare the results with a RELIABILITY analysis of the same items. The results are the same and the researcher would end up creating two indexes, one for the public policy liberalism and one for the individual rights liberalism.

8. FREQUENCIES: How Many Cases in Each Category?

Nominal and ordinal variables are examined using the FREQUENCIES procedure. This procedure provides a count of the number of cases falling into each category. This procedure is also used to check the distribution of a variable before recoding it. FREQUENCIES can also produce bar charts and histograms. Click on Options to select whether you want bar charts, pie charts, histograms, or none (the default). Various statistics are available on request. By double clicking on the output, various changes may be made to the various charts (Box A8 provides a sample output.)

a. Point-and-Click Method

- Analyze
- Descriptive Statistics
- Frequencies

The Frequencies screen will now appear. Click on the variables for which you want frequencies run and move them to the Variables window by clicking on the ➢ button on the menu. When you have the variables you want listed, click OK. The

BOX A7 *Factor Analysis of Liberalism Measures: Sample Output*

Total Variance Explained

Factor	Initial Eigenvalues			Extraction Sums of Squared Loadings			Rotation Sums of Squared Loadings		
	Total	% of Variance	Cumulative %	Total	% of Variance	Cumulative %	Total	% of Variance	Cumulative %
1	2.471	35.295	35.295	1.842	26.320	26.320	1.622	23.165	23.165
2	1.405	20.075	55.370	.839	11.993	38.313	1.060	15.148	38.313
3	.801	11.449	66.819						
4	.650	9.283	76.102						
5	.642	9.167	85.269						
6	.549	7.841	93.109						
7	.482	6.891	100.000						

Extraction Method: Principal Axis Factoring.

Factor Matrix[a]

Factor 1: Public Policy Liberalism	Factor 1	Factor 2
GOVERNMENT INCREASE FOREIGN AID	.546	−.360
INCREASE OF VISIBLE MINORITIES IN JOBS	.535	−.179
VISIBLE MINORITY NOT GIVEN EQ EDUCATION	.550	−4.76E-02
IMMIGRATION POLICIES TOO STRICT	.513	−.243
ABORTION WOMAN'S PERSONAL CHOICE	.310	.610
HOMOSEXUALITY OKAY	.438	.490
MORE MONEY SHOULD BE GIVEN TO WELFARE	.636	6.161E-02

Extraction Method: Principal Axis Factoring.
[a]2 factors extracted. 16 iterations required.

continued on next page

BOX A7 *Factor Analysis of Liberalism Measures: Sample Output (Continued)*

Rotated Factor Matrix[a]

Factor 2: Individualism Rights Liberalism	Factor	
	I	2
GOVERNMENT INCREASE FOREIGN AID	.651	26.20E-02
INCREASE OF VISIBLE MINORITIES IN JOBS	.556	9.243E-02
VISIBLE MINORITY NOT GIVEN EQ EDUCATION	.508	.216
IMMIGRATION POLICIES TOO STRICT	.567	2.612E-02
ABORTION WOMAN'S PERSONAL CHOICE	−1.20E-02	.684
HOMOSEXUALITY OKAY	.157	.639
MORE MONEY SHOULD BE GIVEN TO WELFARE	.533	.353

Extraction Method: Principal Axis Factoring.
Rotation Method: Varimax with Kaiser Normalization.
[a]Rotation converged in 3 iterations.

③

Notes

1. Two significant factors are identified in the analysis of the eight variables.

2. The loadings on factor I indicate that all but two of the items have factor loadings above 0.5.
3. On factor 2, two items predominate: abortion should be a woman's personal choice and homosexuality is okay.

output will be sent to the Output Viewer and displayed on your monitor.

b. Sample Output: FREQUENCIES

It is often preferable to present nominal or ordinal data in summary tables. Table 19.3 illustrates such a table for nominal or ordinal data, which is based on information generated using the FREQUENCIES procedure. In summary tables, it is useful to report both the numbers and the percentages.

Box A8 shows a sample output from a FREQUENCIES procedure. The circled

items draw attention to key points on the output.

9. GRAPH: Graphing Results

There are a variety of graphing procedures available in SPSS, including bar charts, line charts, pie charts, scatterplots, and histograms, among others (see Figure A9). The SCATTER procedure enables the researcher to produce a scatterplot of the relationship between two variables. The researcher may also designate various labels to be placed on the output as well as specify the scale for each dimension of the plot.

Box A8. Frequencies: Sample Output

MOTHER'S EDUCATIONAL BACKGROUND

		Frequency	Percent ①	Valid Percent ②	Cumulative Percent ③
Valid	NO EDUCATION	3	1.6	1.7	1.7
	1-3YRS	7	3.8	3.9	5.6
	4-8YRS	26	14.0	14.6	20.2
	9-12YRS	70	37.6	39.3	59.6
	13-15YRS	31	16.7	17.4	77.0
	16+YRS	41	22.0	23.0	100.0
	Total	178	95.7	100.0	
Missing	9	8	4.3		
Total		186	100.0		

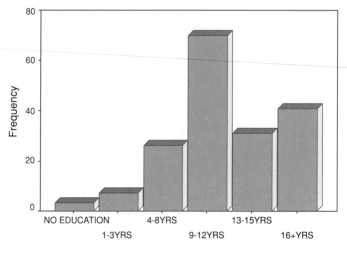

MOTHER'S EDUCATIONAL BACKGROUND

MOTHER'S EDUCATIONAL BACKGROUND

Notes:
1.   Percentage calculated including the missing cases.
2.   Percentages calculated excluding the missing cases.
3.   Cumulative percentage: this column is useful for determining cut-points when recoding ordinal variables.
This barchart was produced by clicking on the Graphics icon on the toolbar and then selecting Bar.

Box A9.
Scatterplot: Mother's Occupation & Family Socioeconomic Status

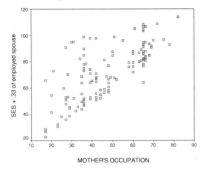

MOTHER'S OCCUPATION

Bar Chart: Father's Education

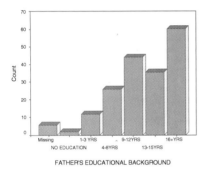

FATHER'S EDUCATIONAL BACKGROUND

Pie Chart: Father's Education

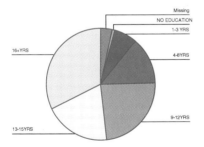

a. Point-and-Click Method

- Graphs
- Bar/Line/Area/Pie/High-Low/Scatter/ Histogram
- Define

Identify the variable (or variables) as ap-propriate for the type of graph you are creating. Then click OK.

b. Sample Output and Notes

The sample output shows the results of a scatterplot of the relationship between two variables, with the dependent variable on the vertical axis. Various options are available to permit researchers to control the intervals printed along the two dimensions and to print various statistics. By double clicking on the output in the Output Viewer, a nurse researcher can alter various settings on the charts, including such things as the size of the units used for scaling, colors, the format of bars, and so forth. Consult an SPSS manual for other graphics options.

10. IF: Creating New Variables

A third way new variables can be created is through IF statements. The simple form of the command (using Syntax editor) is as follows:

- COMPUTE newvar = 0.
- IF (v15 LT 25) newvar = 1. (See footnote to Box A10 for a list of abbreviations used.)

Here the new variable is initially set to 0. Then whenever v15 has a value less than 25, NEWVAR is set to 1.

More complex uses of the IF statement are illustrated in the following example. Suppose we are studying poverty in a community and we have survey data on 300 people over the age of 18 years. We wish to create a variable identifying different types of poverty, taking into account the variables known as age and income. The following represents one way of creating the new variable:

COMPUTE poortype = 0
IF (age LT 25 AND income LT 20000)
poortype = 1

BOX A10 Creating an Occupational Prestige Index Using IF Statements

The following syntax commands were used to create a family socioeconomic index using: (1) the higher of the mother's and father's occupational prestige score plus (2) one third of the lower spouse's score. In cases of a "housewife" or "house husband," the score is based on the employed person's occupational prestige. The original data used 99 as a missing value and 98 for housewife or house husband. The comments on the right side explain the commands.

Syntax Commands	Comments
des var= v63 v64.	V63 = father's occupation
missing values v63 v64().	V64 = mother's occupation
des var= v63 v64.	removes missing values; checks
if (v64 ge v63 and v64 lt 98) ses = v64.	values before and after removal
if (v63 ge v64 and v63 lt 98) ses = v63.	uses mother's score if higher
if (v64 ge 98 and v63 lt 98) ses = v63.	than father's, etc.
if (v63 ge 98 and v64 lt 98) ses = 64.	if one spouse not in work force
list var= id v63 v64 ses/cases = 25.	other spouse's score is used;
des var = v63 v64 ses.	ses score computed
compute ses1 = ses.	to add 1/3 of lower person's
var labels ses1 "SES + .33 of employed spouse".	score the following is used:
if (v64 ge v63 and v64 lt 98) ses1 = (ses1 + (v63 * .33)).	adds 1/3 of father's score
if (v63 gt v64 and v63 lt 98) ses1 = (ses1 + (v64 * .33)).	adds 1/3 of mother's score
missing values v63,v64(98,99).	puts missing values back on
des var= v63 v64 ses ses1.	computes new means lists 25
list var= v63 v64 ses ses1/cases= 25.	cases to confirm data

SPSS Abbreviations

- gt = greater than
- ge = greater than or equal to
- lt = less than
- le = less than or equal to

- eq = equal to
- ne = not equal to
- and = both conditions must be met
- or = either condition must be met

IF (age GE 25 AND age LT 65 AND income LT 25000) poortype = 2
IF (age GE 65 AND income LT 20000) poortype = 3
VARIABLE LABELS poortype "Type of Poor."
VALUE LABELS poortype 0 "all ages, nonpoor."
1 "under 25 under $20 K"
2 "25–64, under $25 K"
3 "over 64, under $20 K"

The above set combines age and income levels to create a new variable called POORTYPE, which identifies the nonpoor (those with incomes more than $20,000 for the young and old and those with more than $25,000 for the middle-aged respondents) and three categories of the poor (young respondents with incomes under $20,000; middle-aged respondents with incomes under $25,000; and senior respondents with incomes under $20,000).

Another illustration of the IF statement is the creation of an SES index that identifies for each respondent the higher of the mother's or father's occupational prestige rating. On the assumption that information has been collected on both the mother's and father's occupations and that the prestige scores for the occupations have been entered into the computer, our task is to develop a new variable that will use the higher of the mother's or father's occupational prestige rating to reflect the SES level of the family unit. The challenge here is to have SPSS compute the index. Box A10 shows how the new variable could be created using SPSS.

Examine Box A10 carefully. Because "housewife" (coded as 98) and those who did not answer the question (coded as 99) were both identified as missing values, it was necessary to remove the missing values identifiers before the index could be created. Through the use of IF statements, SPSS was then instructed to use the higher of the mother's or father's occupational prestige score to determine the value for the new variable (i.e., SES). In this index, we have combined several elements:

- Selected the higher of the mother's and father's occupational prestige score
- If either is not in the labor force, the score for the one who is is used to indicate the occupational prestige
- If both are in the labor force, the higher occupational prestige score is used and then one third of the other person's occupational prestige is added in to derive the "Family SES" score

It is crucial in creating more complex variables to list a number of cases to be certain that the values are being properly assigned to the new variable. After the IF statements have been completed, it is necessary to have SPSS do some procedure before the missing values for v63 and v64 (the two occupational prestige scores) are reassigned. The syntax commands are illustrated in boldface in Box A10.

11. LIST: Listing Variables

After any computation creating or modifying a variable is completed it is a good idea to list some of the cases out so that you can confirm that the changes have

been properly executed. LIST is available through a syntax command, as follows:

- File
- New
- Syntax

The blank syntax screen should now appear on your monitor. Use the following command format to initate a listing of cases for each specified variable:

list var = id v1 v1r/cases = 30

On the toolbar click on Run and click on either All or Selection (if you have highlighted the LIST command line). SPSS will then list the values for the specified variables (id, v1, v1r) for the first 30 cases in the file. The researcher can then check to see that the changes made in v1r are correct. If the "cases" specification is omitted, all the cases will be listed for the variables identified on the variable list.

12. MEANS: Comparing Means

The MEANS procedure is used to compare the mean values of a dependent variable across categories on an independent variable. The test of significance associated with the test is a one-way analysis of variance.

a. Point-and-Click Method

- Analyze
- Compare Means
- Means

Identify the dependent variables for which you want MEANS procedure run. Click them over to the Dependent List window by pressing the ≻ button. Identify the independent variable list and click those over to the Independent List window. Check the Options window to select any statistics you want; click them over to the Cell Statistics. When done, click Continue and then OK.

b. Sample Output and Notes

Box A11 presents the results resulting from the use of the MEANS procedure. Note that the average values for all respondents on the egalitarianism index are presented for each country.

When you have a dependent variable measured at the ratio level and either a nominal or ordinal independent variable, then it is appropriate to compute the mean values of the dependent variable for each category of the independent variable. Table A2 presents the kind of data that would be appropriate for this kind of analysis. Note that the dependent variable (income) is ratio level one and the independent variable is nominal (gender).

The categories of the table should be carefully labeled. The means and standard deviations of the dependent variable along with the number of cases are normally reported in columns across the table (Table A2 provides an example).

BOX A11 MEANS ANALYSIS: Sample Output

Report

EGALITARIANISM

COUNTRY	Mean	N	Std. Deviation
Canada, New Zealand	32.4000	125	8.4204
Australia	27.3509	57	8.4779
Total	30.8187	182	8.7365

ANOVA Table

	Sum of Squares	df	Mean Square	F	Sig.
EGALITARIANISM* Between Groups (Combined)	998.034	1	998.034	14.016 ①	.000 ②
Canada, New Zealand, Australia Within Groups	12816.982	180	71.205		
Total	13815.016	181			

Measures of Association

	Eta	Eta Squared
EGALITARIANISM* Canada, New Zealand, Australia	.269	.072

Notes

1. The F statistic here.
2. The significance value here; because it is less than 0.05, we reject the null hypothesis; there is a statistically significant difference between the countries in their level of egalitarianism.

Table A2   Mean Income by Gender

Gender	Mean Income, dollars	Standard Deviation	Cases, *n*
Male	37,052	14,707	142
Female	34,706	11,693	37
Combined mean	36,567	13,474	179

If appropriate, test of significance values entered here.

A summary table may be used to report the relationship between one dependent variable and a series of independent variables. A sample of such a table is presented in Figure 19.6.

In cases in which there are many categories in the independent variable, they will have to be regrouped into two or three before the analysis is run (click on the Transform/Recode/Into Different Variable procedure).

In interpreting the outcome of an analysis, compare the mean values for each category. In Table A2, for example, the average incomes of the men are compared with those of the women.

The MEANS procedure may be used to test for intervening variables or for sources of spuriousness models (Box A12).

Note that the test to see if the relationship between egalitarianism and country is spurious, caused by the number of each gender who happened to be in the sample, we first compare the original mean difference between the countries (32.4000 − 27.3509 = 5.0491). Second, we now see if the difference holds up when we control for the gender of the respondents: Box A12 indicates that among the male respondents, the difference is 3.1849 (31.7143 − 28.5294 = 3.1849). For the female respondents, the difference in egalitarian scores is 5.897 (32.7470 − 26.8500 = 5.897). Using Jackson's rule of thirds, we note that among the men, the difference decreased, but among the female respondents, the difference remained the same. The result is mixed and therefore does not support the spuriousness model.

13. PARTIAL CORRELATION: Testing for an Intervening Variable

The computations for testing for intervening or sources of spuriousness models when you have ratio level variables involve a combination of CORRELATIONS and PARTIAL CORRELATIONS. Box A13 shows how such models may be tested. Jackson's rule of thirds may be applied (see Chapter 17). And for each, the question is what happens to the original relationship when control variables are applied. Box A13 indicates that the correlation between v63 and v64 is 0.45; when "community size" is controlled, the correlation between v63 and v64 drops to 0.42. Because the partial correlation remains within one third of the value of the original relationship, it would lead us to argue that the control variable is not a source of spuriousness.

Testing for a source of spuriousness using CORRELATIONS and PARTIAL CORRELATION is identical to testing for an intervening variable. And if the results were to come out as shown in Box A13, we would reject the source of spuriousness model. Remember, to find support for the source of spuriousness model, the partial correlation would have to be less than 0.30, which would indicate that the original relationship had been reduced by more than one third ($0.45 \times 0.33 = 0.30$).

a. Point-and-Click Method

- Analyze
- Correlate
- Partial

BOX A12 *MEANS ANALYSIS: Sample Output with a Control Variable*

Report				
EGALITARIANISM				
Canada, New	**GENDER**	**Mean**	**N**	**Std. Deviation**
Canada, New Zealand	MALE	31.7143	42	9.8161
	FEMALE	32.7470	83	7.6602
	Total	32.4000	125	8.4204
Australia	MALE	28.5294	17	10.8519
	FEMALE	26.8500	40	7.3504
	Total	27.3509	57	8.4779
Total	MALE	30.7966	59	10.1349
	FEMALE	30.8293	123	8.0253
	Total	30.8187	182	8.7365

Notes

1. Is gender spuriously causing a false relationship between country and egalitarianism?
2. If gender is spuriously causing the relationship, then when we control for gender, the difference between the countries should disappear within both of the gender categories.
3. Original difference between countries was 5.0491 (32.4 − 27.3509).
4. Compare these values to get the difference scores.
5. Applying Jackson's rule of thirds: 5.0491 ÷ 3 = 1.68
   - Increased: 5.0491 + 1.68 = 6.7291 and over
   - Stayed the same: 5.0491 ± 1.68 = 3.37 to 6.7290

- Decreased or disappeared: < 3.37
- Mixed: different category for each cell of control

6. To find evidence consistent with a source of spuriousness (or an intervening variable), the results of the test must indicate that the difference falls into the decreased or disappeared category in both categories of the control variable. In the present case, the difference between both the males (in the different countries) and the females (in the different countries) would have to be less than 3.37.
7. Observed differences: males: 3.1849 (decreased or disappeared category); females: 5.897 (stayed the same category).
8. Conclusion: the relationship is not spuriously caused by gender differences.

Identify variables for which you want Partial Correlations run; click OK.

14. RECODE: Collapsing and Switching Categories

The RECODE procedure is used to temporarily change a variable during analysis or to create a new variable. The procedure is primarily used to regroup the values in a variable. Survey researchers, in particular, have many occasions to use this procedure. For example, you may have eight categories reflecting community size and you may wish to regroup the cases into three categories. The best way to proceed with an ordinal variable is to run a FREQUENCIES on the variable, noting on the "Cumulative Frequencies" column where cut-points of 33 percent and 66 percent are located. To do this sequentially, click on the toolbar.

BOX A13 PARTIAL CORRELATION: Sample Output

PARTIAL CORRELATION COEFFICIENTS

Controlling for.. V58 ⟵———————— ⑤   ②

	V63	V64
V63	1.0000	.4192 ⟵
	(0)	(122) ⟵ ③
	P= .	P= .000
V64	.4192	1.0000
	(122)	(0) ④
	P= .000	P= .

(Coefficient/(D.F.)/2-tailed Significance)

". " is printed if a coefficient cannot be computed

Notes

1. V63 = father's occupational prestige; V64 = mother's occupational prestige; V58 = community size.
2. The top number is the partial correlation coefficient.
3. The middle number refers to the number of cases in the analysis.
4. The last number is the test of significance (probability).
5. The control variable name (V58) is identified.

CORRELATIONS: Zero-Order Correlation: Sample Output

		Father's Occupation	Mother's Occupation
FATHER'S OCCUPATION	Pearson Correlation	1.000	.446** ⟵ ②
	Sig. (1-tailed)		.000
	N	179	131
MOTHER'S OCCUPATION	Pearson Correlation	.446**	1.000
	Sig. (1-tailed)	.000	
	N	131	133

**Correlation is significant at the 0.01 level (1-tailed).

Notes

1. Testing to see if size of community is spuriously influencing relation between mother's and father's occupational prestige.
2. Original zero-order correlation (shown above) is 0.45.
3. With control for community size (see PAR-

TIAL CORRELATION table), first-order partial is 0.42.

4. Conclusion: relationship is within one third of its original magnitude; therefore, community size is not spuriously accounting for relationship between mother's and father's occupational prestige.

a. Point-and-Click Method

- Transform
- Recode
- Into Different Variables

A second important use for the RECODE procedure involves reverse-scoring variables. Suppose we have three nine-point Likert-type items we wish to reverse score (i.e., change the 9's into 1's, 8's into 2's, etc.) In most cases, it is safest to create a new variable containing the new codes.

Hint: If you are frequently reverse scoring Likert items, consider doing it in the Syntax Editor (to get there, click on File/New/Syntax) to create a template file containing the following:

RECODE v33 (9 = 1)(8 = 2)(7 = 3)(6 = 4) (5 = 5)(4 = 6)(3 = 7)(2 = 8)(1 = 9) INTO V33R. VARIABLE LABELS V33R "Reversed V33".

Save the file with a name such as flip.sps. In the future when you wish to flip a nine-point scale, just access flip.sps, change the variable names to the ones you want, and run the job.

Note that the new variable names simply have an "R" appended to the original name. It is a good idea to maintain the original name in the new name so that the researcher will know that it is a recoded version of the original variable. Variable labels may be attached as indicated.

15. REGRESSION: Doing Multiple Regression Analysis

The REGRESSION procedure does various forms of multiple regression analysis. Regression analysis was one of the procedures featured in Chapter 18. Recall that this type of analysis allows the researcher to determine an equation to describe the relationship between a dependent variable and multiple independent variables as well as to indicate the amount of variation explained by each independent variable.

a. Point-and-Click Method

- Analyze
- Regression
- Linear

Identify the dependent variable, clicking it into the Dependent window. Next move the independent variables over to the Independent(s) window. On the Method window, switch to Backward; on the Statistics window, click on Estimates, Model fit, and Descriptives. Then click on Continue and then OK.

b. Sample Output and Notes

Box A14 presents a regression analysis examining the relationship between Family SES and three independent variables: mother's educational background, father's educational background, and size of home community. Given that we have requested the BACKWARD solution, note that all the independent variables are entered into the equation at step 1, then the variable that is not statistically significant is removed and the equations are recomputed and shown at step 2. If we had more nonsignificant variables, the process would have continued until only statistically significant variables remain. Note that the R^2 (explained variance) value, the b coefficients (labeled B), and beta weights are all reported on the output (see Model Summary) as well as the test of significant (labeled Sig.). The "model" numbers refer to the steps. In this case, SPSS went through three steps to arrive at the final solution. Only the father's educational level remained as a significant predictor of Family SES.

Table A3 presents an example of regression results' table. Note that along with the b coefficients and the beta weights, and the variance explained (R^2) by the models tested. In cases where a number of statistically significant predictors survive to the last model, one can use the following formula to compute the percent contribution of each of the independent variables (Jackson, 1999):

$$\% \text{ Variance explained by each variable} = \frac{\beta_1 \times R^2}{\Sigma \beta\text{'s}} \times 100$$

where β_1 is the beta weight for the variable; R^2 is the r^2 (explained variance) for the equation; and β's is the sum of the beta weights (ignoring $+$ and $-$ signs).

Table A4 shows how these calculations could be presented. Note that this is a rough estimate because the betas represent the particular variables in the equation and would change if other variables were included.

Pure researchers have particular interest in the beta weights because they provide a basis for directly comparing the impact of the different independent variables on the dependent one. Applied researchers are usually more concerned with b coefficients, especially those that

Descriptive Statistics

	Mean	Std. Deviation	N
① → FAMILY SES	65.4439	22.2776	165
MOTHER'S EDUCATIONAL BACKGROUND	4.39	1.17	165
FATHER'S EDUCATIONAL BACKGROUND	4.59	1.30	165
SIZE OF HOME COMMUNITY	5.13	2.72	165

Model Summary

Model	R	R Square	Adjusted R Square	Std. Error of the Estimate
1	.390[a]	.152	.136	20.7083
2	.389[b]	.152	.141	20.6460
3	.385[c]	(.148) ←	.143	20.6242 → ⑤

[a]Predictors: (Constant), SIZE OF HOME COMMUNITY, MOTHER'S EDUCATIONAL BACKGROUND, FATHER'S EDUCATIONAL BACKGROUND
[b]Predictors: (Constant), SIZE OF HOME COMMUNITY, FATHER'S EDUCATIONAL BACKGROUND
[c]Predictors: (Constant), FATHER'S EDUCATIONAL BACKGROUND

Notes

1. Dependent variable: family socioeconomic status (SES). Independent variables: mother's education, father's education, and size of home community. All variables were entered initially, then dropped one at a time, until only statistically significant variables remain.
2. SPSS recomputes the model each time a variable is dropped; only one statistically significant variable remains at the end of this analysis.
3. Final equation: Family SES = 35.1 + 6.6 (father's education).
4. Beta weights show the relative influence of variables.
5. R^2 is the total explained variance by the formula predicting "family SES."

Coefficients[a]

Model	Unstandardized Coefficients		Standardized Coefficients		
	B	Std. Error	Beta	t	Sig.
1 (Constant)	33.459	7.230		4.628	.000
MOTHER'S EDUCATIONAL BACKGROUND	−.313	1.899	−0.16	−.165	.869
FATHER'S EDUCATIONAL BACKGROUND	6.739	1.711	.392	3.939	.000
SIZE OF HOME COMMUNITY	.476	.597	.058	.798	.426
2 (Constant)	32.944	6.504		5.065	.000
FATHER'S EDUCATIONAL BACKGROUND	6.546	1.245	.381	5.257	.000
SIZE OF HOME COMMUNITY	.481	.594	.059	.810	.419
3 (Constant)	(35.118	5.918		5.934	.000
FATHER'S EDUCATIONAL BACKGROUND	6.610)	1.241	.385	5.324	.000

[a]Dependent Variable: Family SES

② → Model

④

Beta ← (④)

③

Table A3   Simplified Table Summarizing Results of Statistically Significant Variables in Predicting Variations in Prestige Rating, Fictional Data

Multiple Regression Analysis
Dependent variable = prestige rating
Multiple R = 0.91493
R^2 = 0.083709

	df	Sum of Squares	Mean Square
Regression	2	3036.73385	1518.36692
Residual	12	590.99949	49.24996
F = 30.82981			
Signif F = 0.0000			

Variables in the Equation

Variable	B	SE B	Beta	T	Sig T	Percent Contribution
ED	3.65645	1.45103	0.54434	2.520	0.0269	47.8
Income	4.573087E-04	2.42024E-04	0.40817	1.890	0.0832	35.9
(Constant)	−8.96285	11.81029		−0.759	0.4626	

Total variance explained = 83.7; variance unexplained = 16.3.

Variables in the Equation

Variable	Beta In	Partial	Min Toler	T	Sig T
EX	-0.06440	-0.11431	0.18567	-0.382	0.7100

can be changed through policy alterations. They provide the basis for understanding how much change in the dependent variable may be produced for each change in the independent variable. Variables can be grouped for presentation to illuminate the degree to which different variable types influence the dependent variable (e.g., how much of the variation in the dependent variable is caused by socioeconomic variables compared with the variety of experience variables).

A second method for estimating the relative importance of variables is to calculate a *part correlation coefficient.* This coefficient is calculated for each independent variable and represents the difference in the R^2 when the variable is included versus when it is not included. The variables may then be ordered in

Table A4   Calculating the Percentage Contribution of Each Independent Variable

Variable	Beta	Calculation	Percent Contribution
ED	0.54434	([0.54434 * 0.83709]/0.95251) * 100 =	47.8
Income	0.40817	([0.40817 * 0.83709)/0.95251) * 100 =	35.9

Total variance explained = 83.7; variance unexplained = 16.3.

terms of the unique contribution of each independent variable. To get Part Correlations in regression analysis, click on Statistics and then click on the PART and PARTIAL CORRELATIONS window.

In presenting the results of a regression analysis, most researchers present the final table after the nonsignificant variables had been dropped. But you will want to include the following:

- Note the names of the variables that remained.
- Note the names of the variables that were dropped.
- Point out total variation explained (R^2 value).
- Note the percentage contribution of each of the statistically significant variables.
- Discuss the implications of the findings.
- In addition, the formula describing the relationship may be presented. In the case presented here, the formula would be as follows: family SES = 35.1 + 6.6 (father's education)
- Note that the formula uses b coefficients and the a value is the constant (the general form of the equation is $Y = a + b_1 X_1 + b_2 X_2$)

c. Dummy Variable Analysis

There may be times when a researcher wishes to use a nominal variable within a regression analysis. Using dummy variables can do this. Suppose we had three religious categories, Protestant, Catholic, and Jewish. To submit religion as a variable, we would create two new variables (one less than the number of categories) and enter each of these into the regression analysis. These variables are coded as 1 for presence and 0 for absence. These are best created using the RECODE procedure, as in:

(i) Point and Click
- Transform

- Recode
- Into Different Variables . . .

Using this procedure, create one fewer new variable than categories in the original religious affiliation variable. Each of the new variables will be entered into the regression analysis as an independent variable. In the example of a three-category religious affiliation variable (Protestant, Catholic, and Jewish), one would make one variable PROT with a coding of 1 for Protestants and everyone else coded 0. A second variable, CATH, would be coded 1 for the Catholics and 0 for everyone else. The third religious category, Jewish, is taken into account in the residual category of the two previous categories. One has to be cautious in interpreting the results when dummy variables are used. These variables are at some disadvantage in explaining variance because they have only two values, 0 and 1. In short, we may somewhat underestimate the importance of the variable religion in such an analysis.

d. Some Cautions

Caution 1. Ensure variables are theoretically independent from one another. What this means is that one cannot use aspects of the dependent variable as independent variables. Include only meaningful potential causes of the dependent variable, not alternate measures of it.

Caution 2. Watch out for highly correlated independent variables. The weightings that will be attached to the variables will be unstable if the independent variables are strongly correlated with one another. The program prints out a warning if there is a problem in this area.

Caution 3. Interpret weightings with care. Understand that the weightings are for the particular combination of independent variables for a particular sample and that these weightings may not apply reliably to other samples.

Caution 4. Monitor the number of cases carefully. By default, SPSS deletes a case if it has a missing value in any of the variables in the equation. Thus, if there are several variables in an analysis, there is a danger of losing many cases. And as the number of cases drops closer to the number of variables, the R^2 increases dramatically. *To determine the number of cases used in the analysis, add 1 to the total degrees of freedom reported in the table.* If a large number of cases have been dropped, try running the analysis using PAIRWISE treatment of missing cases. If there are still many missing, try MEANS (this will substitute the mean of the variable for any missing cases).

An additional possibility, after an initial narrowing down of the variables has been done, is to resubmit the analysis, naming only the significant variables plus perhaps two or three that were dropped in the last few steps. This preserves the cases that were dropped because of missing values in variables that are not in the final equation.

16. RELIABILITY: Assessing Internal Consistency

Indexes combine two or more indicators to reflect complex variables such as SES, quality of life, health status, or an attitude toward a particular nursing issue. Frequently, a researcher constructs subindexes that may be treated alone or combined with other subindexes to form a composite measure. For example, a researcher measuring attitudes toward abortion may construct a subindex for "soft reasons" (e.g., economically inconvenient, preference for having a baby later) and "hard reasons" (e.g., pregnancy as a result of rape, severely handicapped). These subindexes might also be combined to form an overall index. In each case, however, the researcher has to ensure that appropriate items are included in each subindex.

Chapter 13 presents a discussion of item analysis and introduces the principles of index construction. The RELIABILITY procedure evaluates which items should go into an index. RELIABILITY examines the components of a proposed additive index providing a variety of diagnostics for each item. The procedure does not actually compute the index; rather, it provides an assessment of each item. The actual index would be constructed with a COMPUTE command. Of particular note for beginning nurse researchers is that RELIABILITY computes item means and standard deviations, interitem correlations, a series of item-total comparisons, and *Cronbach's alpha* for index reliability.

The RELIABILITY procedure in SPSS uses the internal consistency approach to reliability. The method that is used to calculate the *standardized* alpha involves the number of items going into the index and the average interitem correlation among the items, as in:

$$\text{Alpha} = \frac{n \text{ (average inter-item correlation)}}{1 + (\text{average inter-item correlation } (n - 1))}$$

Where n is the number of items proposed for the index being tested and the average interitem correlation is the average of the correlations between the items: this value is printed when the SUMMARY options MEANS is selected

The standardized alpha for the index evaluated in Box A15 would be as follows:

$$\text{Alpha} = \frac{5(0.3507)}{1 + [0.3507 (5 - 1)]}$$

$$\text{Alpha} = 1.7535 \div 2.4028$$

$$\text{Alpha} = 0.7298$$

Cronbach's alpha varies with the average interitem correlation, taking into account the number of items that make up the in-

BOX A15 *RELIABILITY ANALYSIS: Sample Output*

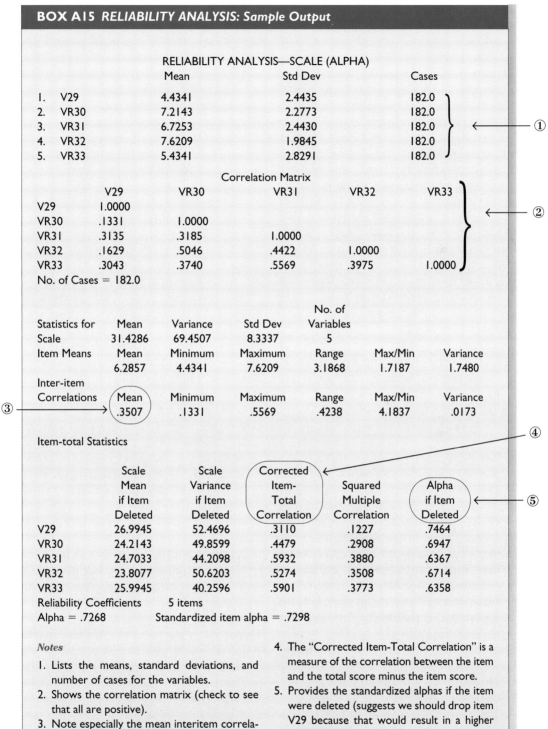

RELIABILITY ANALYSIS—SCALE (ALPHA)

		Mean	Std Dev	Cases
1.	V29	4.4341	2.4435	182.0
2.	VR30	7.2143	2.2773	182.0
3.	VR31	6.7253	2.4430	182.0
4.	VR32	7.6209	1.9845	182.0
5.	VR33	5.4341	2.8291	182.0

①

Correlation Matrix

	V29	VR30	VR31	VR32	VR33
V29	1.0000				
VR30	.1331	1.0000			
VR31	.3135	.3185	1.0000		
VR32	.1629	.5046	.4422	1.0000	
VR33	.3043	.3740	.5569	.3975	1.0000

②

No. of Cases = 182.0

Statistics for	Mean	Variance	Std Dev	No. of Variables		
Scale	31.4286	69.4507	8.3337	5		
Item Means	Mean	Minimum	Maximum	Range	Max/Min	Variance
	6.2857	4.4341	7.6209	3.1868	1.7187	1.7480
Inter-item Correlations	Mean	Minimum	Maximum	Range	Max/Min	Variance
	.3507	.1331	.5569	.4238	4.1837	.0173

③

Item-total Statistics

	Scale Mean if Item Deleted	Scale Variance if Item Deleted	Corrected Item-Total Correlation	Squared Multiple Correlation	Alpha if Item Deleted
V29	26.9945	52.4696	.3110	.1227	.7464
VR30	24.2143	49.8599	.4479	.2908	.6947
VR31	24.7033	44.2098	.5932	.3880	.6367
VR32	23.8077	50.6203	.5274	.3508	.6714
VR33	25.9945	40.2596	.5901	.3773	.6358

④ ⑤

Reliability Coefficients   5 items
Alpha = .7268   Standardized item alpha = .7298

Notes

1. Lists the means, standard deviations, and number of cases for the variables.
2. Shows the correlation matrix (check to see that all are positive).
3. Note especially the mean interitem correlation (should be above 0.25).
4. The "Corrected Item-Total Correlation" is a measure of the correlation between the item and the total score minus the item score.
5. Provides the standardized alphas if the item were deleted (suggests we should drop item V29 because that would result in a higher alpha).

dex. If there is an increase in either the interitem correlation or the number of items, alpha increases. For example, with two items and a 0.4 mean correlation, the alpha value would be 0.572; with eight items and a 0.4 mean interitem correlation, the alpha would be 0.842. With 0.6 interitem correlations, the alpha for two versus eight items would be 0.750 and 0.924, respectively. Table 13.4 summarizes the relationship between items and interitem correlations (see Chapter 13 for more details).

In examining Box A15, note that we are examining five nine-point Likert-type liberal gender attitude items, known as v29, v30, v31, v32, and v33. Note that v30 to v33 are inverse measures (the higher the score, the *less* liberal the attitude). Let us go through the steps to evaluate these items.

Step 1. Reverse score any items that are negative (in this case, v30 to v33) using the RECODE procedure.

Step 2. Point-and-Click Method
- Analyze
- Scale
- Reliability
  Identify variables for which you want procedure run (V29, V30R, V31R, V32R, and V33R). Click on Statistics and then click to place a checkmark on all items in the Descriptives pane. In the Summaries pane, check *Means* and *Correlations.* In the Interitem pane, check *Correlations.* In the ANOVA pane, check *None.* After this is done, click on *Continue.* At the Reliability Analysis window, check *OK.*

Step 3. Examine the results shown in Box A15.
  As a rule of thumb, you have an acceptable index if:
- The *correlation matrix* indicates that the correlations between the items are positive (in this case, all are positive because they vary from 0.13 to 0.56).
- The *mean interitem correlations* should

be above 0.25 (in the case we are examining, the value is 0.3507). Note here, however, that if you were using items based on Likert items with fewer than nine points, you might wish to accept a slightly lower mean interitem correlations, perhaps as low as 0.25.

- Examine the *item-total statistics.* This part of the analysis examines the individual items, comparing each with the total score for the index being evaluated. The *corrected item-total correlation* presents the correlation between the item and the total index score with the effects of the individual item removed. Generally, you would expect each of these items to be above 0.25.
- At the bottom of the table, two alphas are reported. Earlier the calculation for the standardized item alpha was demonstrated. We attempt to get as high an alpha as possible when constructing an index. The alpha reported in Box A15 is 0.7268.
- The *alpha if item deleted column* reports on what the alpha would be if the item were deleted. In Box A15, we note that if we dropped v29, the alpha would be 0.7464; for all other cases, the alpha would be lowered if the item were deleted. Our decision will be to drop v29 when the final index is calculated using the COMPUTE procedure.

Step 4. If two or more items are to be removed from the final index, it is necessary to resubmit another RELIABILITY job. If one or no items need to be eliminated, then one can go immediately to step 5.

Step 5. After deciding which items are to be included in the index, a new job should be run, adding together the items using a COMPUTE command. (Either point-and-click or syntax commands may be used.) The Syntax command would look like:

COMPUTE sexatt = v30r + v31r + v32r + v33r.
VARIABLE LABELS sexatt "Sex Role Attitude."

The system file should be updated, saving the new index scores with a **File/Save** command. There are many other options available within the RELIABILITY procedure. It is possible to compute split-half coefficients and various coefficients proposed by Louis Guttman. Consult the *SPSS User's Guide* for additional models and options.

17. SPEARMAN: Correlation for Ordinal Data

Spearman correlations are used when ordinal level measurement has been attained. They may be reported and interpreted in the same manner as Pearson correlations. Similar to Pearson correlations, they vary from -1.00 to $+1.00$ and measure the strength of an association.

a. Point-and-Click Method

- Analyze
- Correlations
- Bivariate
- Spearman

In the Bivariate Correlations box, click on **Spearman.** Identify the variables for which you want the procedure run. Then Click **OK.**

18. t-TEST: Comparing Means

The t-TEST procedure tests whether the difference in the means between two groups is statistically significant. For a between-subjects design, use the Independent Samples t-Test; for a within-subjects design, use the Paired Samples t-Test. (Recall that a between-subjects test involves the comparison of two groups of subjects. Typically one group is exposed to a treatment and the other group is not exposed to it. A within-subjects test is used when the same subject is exposed to the different treatments; these are also known as repeated measures designs.)

a. Point-and-Click Method

- Analyze
- Compare Means
- Independent Samples t-Test
  or
- Paired Samples t-Test

The following steps need to be taken to complete the analysis:

- For the between-subjects design (using the Independent Samples t-Test), move the test variable to the Test Variables window. Next place the Grouping Variables in its window. You will need to then enter the values for the Grouping (usually 1 and 2, or 0 and 1). Click OK.
- For the within-subjects design (using the Paired Samples T-Test), move the paired variables to the window and click OK.

b. Sample Output and Notes

Box A16 shows sample output from two t-TEST analyses. The first shows the command format and results from a between-subject design; the second shows how to set up a job to do a within-subjects analysis.

19. Z SCORE: Using Z Scores to Create an Index

Z scores are used to standardize variables so that each variable will have a mean of 0 and a standard deviation of 1. Suppose you wished to create an index that adds the mother's educational category to her occupational prestige, equally weighting the two elements. One way to proceed (dealing with the different range of variables involved) would be to standardize the scores (Z scores) and then add together the standardized scores. Z scores versions of variables are available in the DESCRIPTIVES procedure by simply naming the relevant variables and clicking on the box

BOX A16 T-TEST: Sample Outputs

(A) Within-Subjects Sample Output

Paired Samples Statistics

		Mean	N	Std. Deviation	Std. Error Mean
Pair	time 1 speed	13.260	10	.324	.102
1	time 2 speed	13.160	10	.267	8.459E-02

① (arrow to Mean)

Paired Samples Correlations

	N	Correlation	Sig.
Pair time 1 speed & time 2	10	.941	.000

② (arrow to Correlation)

Paired Samples Test

| | Paired Differences | | | | | | | |
| | | | | 95% Confidence Interval of the Difference | | | | |
	Mean	Std. Deviation	Std. Error Mean	Lower	Upper	t	df	Sig. (2-tailed)
Pair time 1 speed time 2 speed	1.000E-01	.115	3.651E-02	1.74OE-02	.183	2.739	9	.023

③ ④ ⑤

(B) Between-Subjects Sample Output

Group Statistics

	Type of Tire	N	Mean	Std. Deviation	Std. Error Mean
TIME	Standard	10	18.390	2.168	.685
	Experimental	10	18.060	2.447	.774

①

Independent Samples Test

| | | Levene's Test for Equality of Variances | | t-test for Equality of Means | | | | | 95% Confidence Interval of the Difference | |
		F	Sig.	t	df	Sig. (2-tailed)	Mean Difference	Std. Error Difference	Lower	Upper
TIME	Equal variances assumed	.524	.478	.319	18	.753	.330	1.034	−1.842	2.502
	Equal variances not assumed			.319	17.741	.753	.330	1.034	−1.844	2.504

② ③ ④

continued on next page

BOX A16 t-TEST: Sample Outputs (Continued)

Notes (Within-Subjects t-TEST)

1. The mean times at time 1 and time 2 shown here.
2. The correlation of the measures at the two times is 0.941.
3. The t-test value.
4. The degrees of freedom.
5. The two-tailed test of significance.
6. Conclusion: reject the null hypothesis; there is a statistically significant difference in the speeds at the two times.

Notes (Between-Subjects t-TEST)

1. The mean lap times for the "standard" and "experimental" tires shown here.
2. Computed t value.
3. Degrees of freedom.
4. Two-tailed test of significance.
5. Conclusion: accept the null hypothesis; there is no statistically significant difference between the lap times on the different tires.

---

called **Save Standardized Values as Variables.** A **Z** will be prefixed to the name of the variable. Next you would simply do a COMPUTE, adding together the new standardized variables. The COMPUTE could be done as follows:

COMPUTE newses = zv62.1 + zv64.

VARIABLE LABELS newses "SES Score: Education plus Prestige."

Incidentally, if you wished to weight the elements so that two thirds of the final scores were based on occupational prestige and one third on educational level, the COMPUTE command would be altered to:

COMPUTE newses = (zv62.1 * 0.33) + (zv64 * 0.67).

The previous section presented the basic commands for examining relationships.

The SPSS package contains a broad range of options, statistics, file management, and analysis procedures. The chances are that most analyses you wish to do are possible within SPSS. After you have mastered the basic procedures, you will be ready to begin exploring SPSS in greater detail.

C. SPSS MANUALS

There are many manuals currently available for SPSS for Windows version 10.0. The major ones of particular relevance to this text are listed in the Recommended Readings section. They are available in the United States from SPSS Inc., Publication Sales, 444 N. Michigan Ave., Chicago, Illinois 60611. In Canada, the distributor of SPSS publications is Prentice Hall Canada Inc., 1870 Birchmount Road, Scarborough, Ontario, M1P 2J7. In Canada, call 1-800-567-3800.

RECOMMENDED READINGS

SPSS. (1999). *SPSS Base 10.0 Applications Guide.* Chicago: SPSS Inc. This basic manual contains the basic procedures covered in *Doing Nursing Research.*

SPSS. (1999). *SPSS Advanced Models 10.0.* Chicago: SPSS Inc. This advanced techniques manual is of interest to those doing GLM repeated measures and loglinear and other advanced techniques.

SPSS. (1999). *SPSS 10.0 Syntax Reference Guide.* Chicago: SPSS Inc. For those who prefer to use syntax commands, this is the complete reference guide—some 1412 pages long!

A Student-designed Questionnaire

The following questionnaire is part of a study being conducted as a Nursing 300 project. To ensure the confidentiality of your responses, please do *not* write your name on the questionnaire. Thank you for your cooperation.

1. Gender: I am:

   Male————————1❏
   Female————————2❏

2. In what year were you born? 1 9 ___ ___

3. What program of study are you currently enrolled in?

   Bachelor of Arts ————————————————01 ❏
   Bachelor of Business Administration ————02 ❏
   Bachelor of Education ——————————————03 ❏
   Bachelor of Engineering ————————————04 ❏
   Bachelor of Music ——————————————————05 ❏
   Bachelor of Science in Nursing ——————————06 ❏
   Bachelor of Science in Human Nutrition ————07 ❏
   Bachelor of Science in Human Kinetics————08 ❏
   Bachelor of Science ——————————————————09 ❏
   Bachelor of Arts in Information Systems ————10 ❏
   Other ——————————————————————————————11 ❏
      If other, please specify_____

4. What year of study are you currently in?

   Freshman ————————————1 ❏
   Sophomore ————————————2 ❏
   Junior ————————————————3 ❏
   Senior ————————————————4 ❏
   Other ————————————————5 ❏
      If other, please specify_____

5. Approximately, what was the population of your hometown/or city before coming to the university?

Rural area under 1000 ——————1 ☐
1000–4,999 ———————————2 ☐
5000–9999 ———————————3 ☐
10,000–19,999 ——————————4 ☐
20,000–29,999 ——————————5 ☐
30,000–39,999 ——————————6 ☐
40,000–49,999 ——————————7 ☐
50,000 and over ————————8 ☐

6. What is your religious affiliation?

Roman Catholic ————01☐   Jewish ————————07☐
Anglican ——————02☐   Buddhist ————————08☐
United ——————————03☐   Muslim ——————————09☐
Baptist ————————04☐   None ——————————10☐
Presbyterian ————05☐   Other ————————11☐
Other Protestant ————06☐   Please specify_____

7. Currently, how often do you attend church services?

More than once a week————————————1 ☐
Once every week ————————————2 ☐
2–3 times a month ——————————3 ☐
Once a month ——————————————4 ☐
7–10 times a year ——————————5 ☐
2–6 times a year ——————————6 ☐
Once a year————————————————7 ☐
Never ——————————————————8 ☐

8. What is (or was) the main occupation of your father? (e.g., social worker, elementary school teacher)?

Job position_____

Brief job description_____

9. What is (or was) the main occupation of your mother? (e.g., high school teacher, homemaker, lawyer)?

Job position_____

Brief job description_____

10. Ann is 50 years old and is a cancer patient. She is in the last stage of the disease. It has been decided by her physician that no treatment options will serve any benefit to treat her cancer or reduce discomfort. She has left the hospital of her own free will and wishes to die. **The physician prescribes medication for Ann, knowing she intends to overdose on it.** In regards to the physician's actions, I . . .

Strongly Disagree   1   2   3   4   5   6   7   8   9   Strongly Agree

11. Ben is 30 years old and has been paralyzed from the neck down as a result of an accident some years ago. He will be bedridden for the rest of his life. He no longer has control over urine or bowel movements and needs to be fed and cared for. He finds a passive life in an institution unbearable. Ben wishes to die. **The physician prescribes medication for Ben and sets it up so that he will be able to take it in overdose amounts himself when he chooses.** In regards to the physician's actions, I . . .

Strongly Disagree   1   2   3   4   5   6   7   8   9   Strongly Agree

12. Margaret is a 90-year-old woman who lives by herself. She has weak vision and arthritis and can no longer do the things she enjoys. Margaret spends most of her day alone except for 1-hour visits from a home-care nurse. She is lonely and wishes to die. **The physician prescribes medication for Margaret, knowing she intends to overdose on it.** In regards to the physician's actions, I . . .

Strongly Disagree   1   2   3   4   5   6   7   8   9   Strongly Agree

13. Ann is 50 years old and is a cancer patient. She is in the last stage of the disease. It has been decided by her physician that no treatment options will serve any benefit to treat her cancer or reduce discomfort. She has left the hospital of her own free will and wishes to die. **She has asked her physician to inject a lethal drug into her to bring about her death and the physician has agreed to do it.** In regards to the physician's actions, I . . .

Strongly Disagree   1   2   3   4   5   6   7   8   9   Strongly Agree

14. Ben is 30 years old and has been paralyzed from the neck down as a result of an accident some years ago. He will be bedridden for the rest of his life. He no longer has control over urine or bowel movements and needs to be fed and cared for. He finds a passive life in an institution unbearable. Ben wishes to die. **He asks his physician to give him a lethal injection to end his life and the physician has agreed to do it.** In regards to the physician's actions, I . . .

Strongly Disagree   1   2   3   4   5   6   7   8   9   Strongly Agree

15. Margaret is a 90-year-old woman who lives by herself. She has weak sight and arthritis and can no longer do the things she enjoys. Margaret spends most of her day alone except for 1-hour visits from a home care nurse. She is lonely and wishes to die. **She has asked her physician to inject a lethal drug into her to bring about her death, and the physician has agreed to do it.** In regards to the physician's actions, I . . .

Strongly Disagree   1   2   3   4   5   6   7   8   9   Strongly Agree

16. I would help a friend fight for the right to die if that was his or her choice.

Strongly Disagree   1   2   3   4   5   6   7   8   9   Strongly Agree

17. I would refuse to provide a terminally ill person with a lethal dosage of a drug, if he or she requests it.

Strongly Disagree   1   2   3   4   5   6   7   8   9   Strongly Agree

18. I would rather die than live with a chronic, painful, nonterminal illness.

    Strongly Disagree   1   2   3   4   5   6   7   8   9   Strongly Agree

19. I would personally give a lethal injection to a terminally ill individual, if requested by the person.

    Strongly Disagree   1   2   3   4   5   6   7   8   9   Strongly Agree

20. I would provide emotional support to a terminally ill friend who wished to end his/her life.

    Strongly Disagree   1   2   3   4   5   6   7   8   9   Strongly Agree

21. People have the right to take their own lives if they are terminally ill.

    Strongly Disagree   1   2   3   4   5   6   7   8   9   Strongly Agree

22. People have the right to take their own lives if they have suffered a great financial loss.

    Strongly Disagree   1   2   3   4   5   6   7   8   9   Strongly Agree

23. Active euthanasia is defined as an action by a person with the intention of hastening the death of another person who is terminally ill or in such a condition that causes suffering. Active euthanasia is wrong under all circumstances.

    Strongly Disagree   1   2   3   4   5   6   7   8   9   Strongly Agree

24. Physician-assisted suicide is an action taken by the physician that assists a person in ending his or her own life. Physician-assisted suicide should be legalized.

    Strongly Disagree   1   2   3   4   5   6   7   8   9   Strongly Agree

25. I am in favor of active euthanasia.

    Strongly Disagree   1   2   3   4   5   6   7   8   9   Strongly Agree

26. I am in favor of physician-assisted suicide.

    Strongly Disagree   1   2   3   4   5   6   7   8   9   Strongly Agree

27. I feel depressed.

    Strongly Disagree   1   2   3   4   5   6   7   8   9   Strongly Agree

28. I worry about the way I look.

    Strongly Disagree   1   2   3   4   5   6   7   8   9   Strongly Agree

29. I feel lonely.

    Strongly Disagree   1   2   3   4   5   6   7   8   9   Strongly Agree

30. I worry about what others think.

    Strongly Disagree   1   2   3   4   5   6   7   8   9   Strongly Agree

31. I have a tendency to get involved in unhealthy relationships.

    Strongly Disagree   1   2   3   4   5   6   7   8   9   Strongly Agree

32. I usually avoid talking about my feelings.

    Strongly Disagree   1   2   3   4   5   6   7   8   9   Strongly Agree

33. I find that other people's moods influence my own mood.

    Strongly Disagree   1   2   3   4   5   6   7   8   9   Strongly Agree

34. I occasionally question whether my life is worth living.

    Strongly Disagree   1   2   3   4   5   6   7   8   9   Strongly Agree

35. My religious beliefs are strong.

    Strongly Disagree   1   2   3   4   5   6   7   8   9   Strongly Agree

36. I have been "at the bedside" of one who was dying:

    Yes————————1☐

    No—————————2☐

37. Indicate whether or not anyone from the following categories is currently suffering from a long-time illness or has died following a long period of suffering. (Check Yes or No for each item.)

	Yes	No
Close friend	___	___
Acquaintance	___	___
Immediate family member	___	___
Relative	___	___
Neighbor	___	___
Other	___	___

    If other, please specify_____

38. If yes for any part of question 37, **for the person you had the most contact with:** How much time did you spend with that person while he or she was sick?

    Lived with ———————————1☐
    Visited every day————————2☐
    Visited 2–3 times a week—————3☐
    Visited once a week—————————4☐
    Visited 2–3 times a month ————5☐

39. How long was this person ill?

  1–2 weeks ——————————1☐
  Less than a month ————2☐
  Less than 6 months ———3☐
  Less than 1 year ————4☐
  1 year or more ——————5☐

40. I would rather die than become dependent on my family to care for me.

   Strongly Disagree   1   2   3   4   5   6   7   8   9   Strongly Agree

41. I believe in a superior being with whom I have a relationship.

   Strongly Disagree   1   2   3   4   5   6   7   8   9   Strongly Agree

42. I would rather die than live in a nursing home.

   Strongly Disagree   1   2   3   4   5   6   7   8   9   Strongly Agree

43. If a family member had cancer and decided against having chemotherapy, I would question his or her decision.

   Strongly Disagree   1   2   3   4   5   6   7   8   9   Strongly Agree

44. God would not allow anyone to have more pain than they could handle.

   Strongly Disagree   1   2   3   4   5   6   7   8   9   Strongly Agree

45. I love to get up each day to live life to the fullest.

   Strongly Disagree   1   2   3   4   5   6   7   8   9   Strongly Agree

46. I believe that a "higher being" is there for those in times of anguish and suffering.

   Strongly Disagree   1   2   3   4   5   6   7   8   9   Strongly Agree

47. I often overcommit myself.

   Strongly Disagree   1   2   3   4   5   6   7   8   9   Strongly Agree

48. I love to be the center of attention.

   Strongly Disagree   1   2   3   4   5   6   7   8   9   Strongly Agree

49. When children are young, a mother's place is in the home.

   Strongly Disagree   1   2   3   4   5   6   7   8   9   Strongly Agree

50. I worry about dating and relationship problems.

   Strongly Disagree   1   2   3   4   5   6   7   8   9   Strongly Agree

fore the introduction of the treatment variable.

Baseline measure: A measure taken after stability has been achieved in the dependent variable at the beginning of a set of observations.

Baseline stability: Several measures are taken; the treatment variable is not introduced until the measures achieve stability.

Beneficence: The duty to promote or do good.

Beta: The probability of making a type II error.

Beta weight: Associated with regression analysis, the beta weight is a standardized measure of the relative influence of an independent variable (compared with other independent variables) on the dependent one.

Between-subjects design: Study design in which each group of experimental subjects is exposed to either the control group treatment or to the experimental group treatment.

Bias: A preference or predisposition to favor a particular conclusion.

Biased sample: A sample that is not representative of the population it is intended to reflect.

Bimodal distribution: A distribution with two peaks.

Blocked design: Experiments in which subjects have been grouped together on a particular variable that needs to be controlled; subjects are then randomly assigned to treatment and control conditions.

Bracketing: A cognitive process used by researchers to set aside one's biases and personal perspectives about a research topic. Its purpose is to make known what the researcher believes about the research topic so he or she can then approach the topic with less bias.

Candidate variable model: A model that proposes several independent variables as possible causes of variation in a dependent variable.

Causal explanation: When an event or sequence of events is explained by making reference to preceding, influencing events.

Causal model: A diagram showing the causal connections between variables.

Change agent: A person or group of people who can take an idea for change from the "drawing board," carry it through all the stages of its implementation, and then evaluate its success or failure. Change agents must be able to respond to the barriers that mitigate against research utilization.

Chi-square test: A test of statistical significance associated with contingency table analysis, in which the dependent variable is a nominal one.

Classic experimental design: A between-subjects design involves a *control* and an *experimental* group. Measures are taken from members in both groups before treatment and repeated after the treatment has been experienced.

Cleaning the data: The systematic search for errors in a data set so that they can be corrected before data analysis begins.

Clinically significant: Findings that must have meaning for patient care in the presence or absence of statistical significance; this requires the nurse to interpret the findings in terms of their value to nursing.

Closed-ended questions: Precoded, single-choice questionnaire items.

Cluster sample: Sample with population divided into groups (or *clusters*). The first units or clusters to be sampled are the largest, followed by smaller and smaller units selected at random (see also Multistage area sample).

Coefficient of reliability: A measure of agreement between the coders on the categorization of the items being analyzed. The proportion of times there is agreement is reflected in the coefficient.

Comparative studies: Studies that typically involve cross-cultural or historical analyses of social behavior.

Componential analysis: Analysis that looks for all the contrasts among the cultural categories in the domains. It is the systematic search for the *attributes* (components of meaning) associated with cultural categories.

Concept: A general idea referring to a characteristic of an individual, group, or nation.

Conceptual framework: Does not contain a specific theory that explains the expected relationship between variables but rather synthesizes relevant literature about the proposed hypotheses.

Conceptual hypothesis: A statement of the relationship between two or more conceptual variables.

Conceptual level of research: Entails the definition of variables that are to be used.

Conceptual map: A diagram of the concepts and relationships expressed in a theoretical framework. A conceptual map is often a more efficient way to communicate what is known about a phenomenon than is a verbal description.

Conceptual utilization: The use of findings to enhance one's understanding of a problem or issue in nursing. Through conceptual utilization, a nurse uses the knowledge gained from research to cognitively restructure the way one thinks about a situation, problem, or phenomenon in nursing.

Conceptual variable: An idea that has a dimension that can vary.

Concurrent validity: When two different tests are given and the scores correlate highly with each other.

Conditional variable: A variable that accounts for a change in the relationship between an independent variable and a dependent variable when the general conditions change.

Confidentiality: Based on the ethical principal of respect for persons. Most surveys, interviews, experiments, and field studies are completed on the understanding that individual responses, or information that would permit the identification of the individual, will never be released.

Conflict theory or perspective: Argues that society is fundamentally characterized by conflict between interest groups; owners of the means of production (e.g., factories, farms, businesses), the bourgeoisie, seek to exploit workers, the proletarians, whose labor is undervalued and underpaid.

Confirmability: The objectivity of the data. Meanings emerging from the data have to be tested for their plausibility, their sturdiness, their "confirmability," so that two independent researchers would agree about the meanings emerging from the data.

Confirmatory factor analysis: Usually conducted after an exploratory analysis has occurred or when the researcher has a hypothesis about the existing factor structure that is to be tested. It is usually based on theory.

Confounding variable One that may unintentionally obscure or enhance a relationship.

Consequentialist: This view of research ethics stresses that ethical judgments about a research project should be made in terms of its consequences for the subject, for the academic discipline, and for society.

Constant comparative method: Used when each piece of data is coded and compared with other pieces for similarities and differences in the lives of those interviewed.

Constructs: Concepts specified in such a way that they are observable in the real world. Making a concept potentially observable facilitates testing of the idea.

Construct validity: A situation in which a theoretically derived hypothesis turns out as predicted.

Contemporary applied research: The goal is to produce knowledge that can be used for the specific purpose of generating positive change. Unlike conventional research, which mainly contributes to knowledge development that may not necessarily be used in practice, the emphasis in contemporary applied research is to use the research to "inform the change."

Content analysis: A technique for making inferences by objectively and systematically coding information.

Content validity: The extent to which the measure reflects the dimension (or dimensions) implied by the concept.

Control by constancy: Within-subject designs in which the same subject experiences different levels of the treatment; hence, the subject acts as his or her own control.

Control group design: An experimental design the researcher uses randomized assignment to groups (or precision matching) to adjust for known and unknown variations between the two groups.

Controlled observations: Observations in which other confounding factors are minimized or taken into account.

Control variable: One that is taken into account in exploring the relationship between an independent and dependent variable. There are three basic types of control variables: the intervening variable, the conditional variable, and the source of spuriousness (or confounding) variable.

Convenience sample: A nonprobability sampling procedure that involves selection on the basis of ease or convenience.

Core variable: A variable that focuses the theory and accounts for most of the variation in a pattern of behavior that is both relevant and problematic for the participants involved.

Correlation analysis: A procedure for measuring how closely two ratio level variables co-vary together.

Correlation coefficient (r):   A measure of the strength of association between two variables; a correlation may vary from +1 to −1.

Correlation matrix: A table showing the correlation coefficients between all designated variables.

Counterbalancing: In experimental designs, counterbalancing involves introducing, changing, maintaining, and then returning to the first level of the experimental treatment to control for effects of learning on the subject's performance.

Covariates: Ratio level treatment variables.

Credibility: The accuracy of the description of the phenomenon under investigation. The portrayal of the reality must be faithfully represented and plausible to those who have experienced that reality.

Criterion validity: The extent to which a measure is able to predict accurately.

Critical appraisal: Involves judging whether or not a research study is described clearly and comprehensively enough to decide if the findings and implications are logical and believable and should be considered seriously in your practice.

Critical approach: Views human behavior as fundamentally characterized by different groups attempting to enhance their interests at the expense of less powerful groups. The fundamental goal of the critical approach is to bring about a truly egalitarian society—one in which there is an equality of opportunity *and* an equality of result.

Critical value: This value is determined by looking up the appropriate cell on a statistical table. In order for a null hypothesis to be rejected, the critical value must be equaled or exceeded by the computed test value. (When a computer program is used, these values are not necessary because the exact probabilities are provided on the computer output).

Cronbach's alpha: Used in assessing the internal consistency of an index. This test is based on the strength of the intercorrelations of all the items in the instrument as well as the number of items used. The alpha value ranges from 0 to 1, with 1 indicating perfect internal consistency and 0 indicating no internal consistency.

Crossover design: Assign subjects randomly to a specific sequencing of treatment conditions. For example, half of the subjects (group 1) receive treatment A (the nicotine patch) followed by treatment B (Zyban), and the other half (group 2) receive treatment B (Zyban) followed by treatment A (the nicotine patch).

Cross-sectional: Data collected at one point in time.

Cross-tabulation tables: Present information so that the relationship between a nominal level dependent variable can be related to an independent variable.

Cultural scene: An ethnographic term used to refer to a culture under study.

Cultural themes: Recurrent patterns in the data that are used to connect domains.

Culture: A way of life belonging to a designated group of people. It includes all the ways a group of people solve problems as reflected in their language, dress, food, traditions, and customs. It is a pattern of living that guides the group's thoughts, actions, and sentiments.

Curvilinear relationship: One in which the plot between the variables goes in one direction and then switches to another one.

Data collection: The process of gathering information from identified participants to answer a research question.

Data distribution: A listing of all the values for any one variable.

Data entry: The process of transferring the information collected in a study to a computing device.

Data massaging: The practice of playing with the data until the analysis producing the strongest association is identified and retained. In massaging the data, the bias will usually be to find evidence supporting expected or preferred outcomes.

Data reduction: The researcher may collect a large amount of data and then reduce the data through factor analysis. A single composite variable or several variables measuring different dimensions of a concept may be created out of a conglomerate of variables through factor analysis.

Debriefing: Researchers explaining studies to subjects after the data have been collected, noting any deception and why it was necessary and reassuring subjects that their participation was appreciated and helpful.

Declaration of Helsinki: This declaration differentiates between *therapeutic research* and *nontherapeutic research*. *Therapeutic research* is research that provides participants with an opportunity to benefit from an experimental treatment. *Nontherapeutic research* is research that generates new knowledge that will bring future benefits to society, but those acting as participants most likely will not benefit from their participation in the research.

Deductive explanation: When the phenomenon to be explained is a logically necessary consequence of the explanatory premises, as in if A = B and B = C, then A = C.

Deductive reasoning: A process by which a nurse reaches a conclusion by moving from the general to the specific. It is the approach used to test predictions and validate existing relationships through quantitative research methods.

Degrees of freedom: In cross-tabular tables, the number of cells in which the expected frequency would have to be computed before the remaining cells could be determined by subtraction, given that the total expected must equal the total observed.

Dehoaxing: The process of a researcher informing subjects in a study about what was really going on in an experiment, particularly informing them of any deception that was used.

Demand characteristic: A distortion introduced when people respond in terms of how they think they are expected to respond.

Deontological: A view of research ethics that proposes absolute moral structures that must never be violated.

Dependability: Both the stability and the trackability of changes in the data over time and conditions. The issue of dependability in qualitative investigations reflects the reality that situations constantly change and people's realities differ.

Dependent variable: A variable that is viewed as being influenced by other variables; it is the "effect" in a cause-and-effect relationship.

Descriptive research: Research that is about *what* and how many of *what.*

Descriptive statistics: Statistics that include various tools, conventions, and procedures for describing variables or the relationship between variables. Means, standard deviations, normal distributions, and Z scores are used to describe individual variables; cross-tabulations, means across categories, and correlations are some of the procedures used to describe relationships between variables.

Design: Similar to a blueprint for a study, it guides the investigator in planning and implementing a study. It provides a detailed plan for data collection and analysis and is the critical element linking the theoretical framework and questions with the resultant data.

Dialectic critique: Makes explicit, internal contradictions in the data rather than complimentary explanations. By exposing the contradictory nature of phenomena in the change situation, the researchers and participants come to a clearer understanding of the change process.

Discrepancy: The difference between the ways things are in practice and the way they should be, or between what one knows and what one needs to know to eliminate a problem

Discriminant function analysis: Used in situations in which the dependent variable is measured at the nominal or ordinal level and the researcher wishes to examine the impact of several independent variables simultaneously. This procedure provides weightings maximizing the likelihood of correctly predicting the category of the dependent variable each case will fall into.

Domain analysis: Moving from observing a *social situation* (a set of behaviors carried out by people in a social situation) to discovering a *cultural scene.*

Double blind: In experimental designs, those in which neither experimenters nor subjects are aware of the experimental condition that is being applied to the subject.

Double standard: In research, using different means of measuring identical behaviors, attitudes, or situations for each gender, for example.

Dummy variable: One that is coded 1 for presence and 0 for absence of a characteristic and represents one category of an independent variable. Dummy variables are used in multiple regression and in discriminant analysis to enable the researcher to incorporate nominal variables.

Effect size: Concerned with the strength of the relationship among study variables. It is a measure of how false the null hypothesis is, or in other words, how strong the effect of the independent variable is on the dependent variable.

Eigenvalue: The sum of the squared factor loadings for any one factor in factor analysis.

Elite bias: A danger because informants are more likely to be drawn from the more articulate, high-status elements in a society. Hence, unless care is taken, there is a tendency to overrepresent the views of the elite in one's research.

Emic: An insider's or native's point of view and how they derive meaning from their experiences.

Empathetic explanation: One in which the experience of coming to see and coming to understand are stressed.

Empirical knowledge: Knowledge of the experienced or empirical world. This knowledge is generated through scientific methods and is usually organized into laws and theories that help to describe, predict, and explain phenomena.

Epistemology: The study of the nature of knowledge. It seeks to determine how we know what we know. A number of authors have studied ways of knowing in nursing.

Equivalence: The degree of agreement among two or more different observers using the same measurement tool or the agreement between two or more alternate forms of an instrument.

Error checking: A process to locate and correct errors in the data before data analysis.

Ethical knowing: Focuses on obligation on what ought or should be done. This pattern of knowing in nursing requires an understanding of different philosophical positions regarding what is good, what is right, and what is desired.

Ethics: The study of moral principles.

Ethics review board (ERB): Committee that is used to approve research involving humans. The purpose of the review is to ensure that ethical principles are appropriately applied to research involving human subjects. Most ERBs reviewing biomedical research operate under the guidelines of the Declaration of Helsinki.

Ethnography: A qualitative research method that attempts to understand human behavior in the cultural context in which it is embedded.

Ethnomethodology: Typically involves a detailed examination of a single event or case; associated with the interpretive approach.

Ethnonursing: The study and analysis of the local people's viewpoints, beliefs, and practices about nursing care.

Etic: The view of the researcher or an outsider.

Evaluation case study: In-depth explorations of phenomena, usually over an extended period of time, using diverse data collection procedures to collect detailed information about an individual, group, organization, program, or social phenomenon.

Evaluation research: A systematic appraisal using the methods of social research for the purpose of generating knowledge and understanding that can be used for decision making. It is an applied form of research that provides utilitarian answers to practical questions for decision makers.

Evidence-based practice: Nursing practice that is informed and modified in light of systematic research that evaluates the effectiveness of alternative interventions.

Expectancy: An anticipation of particular research results; this may lead to a distortion of results in the direction of expectations.

Experiment: A scientific investigation that tests cause-and-effect relationships while controlling for the influence of other factors.

Experimental group: The group that is exposed to the treatment intervention.

Experimenter effect: A tendency to produce findings that are consistent with the experimenter's expectations.

Expert sampling: A type of purposive sampling used with the Delphi technique.

Explanatory research: Seeks to provide answers to "why?" questions.

Exploratory factor analysis: Used when a researcher does not *a priori* identify the factor structure of the variables in the data set. It is similar to stepwise regression analysis in that the variance of the first factor identified is partialed out before analysis of the second factor proceeds.

External validity: The extent to which results may be extrapolated from a particular study to other groups in general.

Extinction: The cessation of a behavior that was once displayed.

***F* distribution:** Used to test whether there is a significant difference in the means of various categories.

Face validity: An evaluation of an indicator that, on inspection, appears to reflect the concept you wish to measure.

Factor analysis: A multivariate procedure used primarily to determine the structure of a set of variables—that is, to show how variables cluster together to form unidimensional constructs. It determines the structure of a set of variables by analyzing the intercorrelations among them. It sorts the variables into categories according to how closely related they are to other variables. Variables that are highly correlated are grouped together into a factor.

Factorable: A correlation matrix is said to be factorable if there are reasonably robust correlations among the items. Ordinarily one would expect the interitem correlations to average above 0.25 to consider the variables to be worthy of factor analysis; if it is any lower than that, you may not find that any factors would be extracted.

Factor extraction: The analyst seeks to determine the number of factors that need to be extracted in order to capture or explain the variation in the data set. To proceed, the analyst then selects a method for how additional factors will be identified through a process of factor rotation.

Factor loadings: The b weights (similar to the bs in regression analysis) in the factor analysis equation. Factor loadings may be combined to yield a *factor score,* which measures the extent that factor scores are similar, thus reflecting the underlying common factor (or factors).

False dilemma: Occurs when a researcher argues that something is caused by either A or by B. Then, having provided some evidence that B is not responsible, the researcher falsely concludes that A must be the cause.

Familism: A special case of gender insensitivity that involves treating the family as the unit of analysis when, in fact, it is individuals within the family unit that engage in a particular activity or hold a certain attitude. Familism is also a problem when we assume that a particular phenomenon has an equal impact on all members of the family when, in fact, it may affect different family members in different ways.

Feminist theory: The basic premise is that one cannot adequately understand human societies without paying attention to the universal role of patriarchy, which refers to a domination of the social groups by men, who have greater power and privilege than women and children.

Field experiment: When a researcher's intervention occurs in a natural setting rather than in a laboratory and is usually simple, limited, and quickly completed.

Field notes: Attempt to capture the essence of the group being studied. Included are descriptions of events and people as well as the interpretations of the researcher and the participants.

Field studies: Include investigations in which a researcher observes and records the behavior of individuals or groups in their natural settings.

File: The name for a data set, or the text of a report, entered into a computer.

Focus group: Typically consists of 6 to 12 individuals who are asked to discuss topics suggested by a facilitator. The idea is for the researcher to observe the interactions among focus group members detecting their attitudes, opinions, and solutions to problems posed by the facilitator.

Folk wisdom: An important source of ideas for the researcher are those passed down from generation to generation; such ideas should not, however, be accepted as true until tested in a rigorous scientific fashion.

Formative evaluation: A form of inquiry that focuses on how well a new service or ongoing program or activity is meeting its objectives. The thrust of formative evaluation research is to identify what is and what is not working currently, so that remedial action can be taken to improve the situation at hand.

Formal theory: Includes properties, propositions stating the relationships between them, and the propositions forming a deductive system.

Four-variable causal models: A testable model containing four variables.

Frequency distribution table: A systematic listing of all the values on a variable from the lowest to the highest with the number of times (frequency) each value was observed.

Functional explanation: One in which the presence of a particular phenomenon is explained in terms of the role it plays in maintaining a particular system.

Gamma: A measure of the strength of association between ordinal level variables.

Gatekeeper: An individual with special group status who can lead the researcher to other *key informants.*

Gender insensitivity: A disregard of the differential impacts of research conclusions or of social policy on men and women.

Generalizability: The extent that the findings may be extrapolated from the present study to other groups in general.

Generalization: A statement that attempts to describe a pattern of behavior or of relationship that is, on average, correct.

Grand theories (or **conceptual models**): These embody the beliefs, traditions, goals, and values of the discipline. They take into account the phenomena of central concern to nursing: person, health, nursing, and environment. They broadly define these concepts and link them together through relationship statements reflective of the theorist's view of the discipline. They explain universal relationships that describe what the discipline of nursing is all about and remain broad, abstract representations of reality.

Grounded theory: The idea that the conclusions of a qualitative study should be grounded in the data—that is, based on direct and careful observations of everyday life within the group.

Halo effect: A carry-over effect, in which a researcher's first rating may influence the second and subsequent ratings.

Hawthorne effect: Any variability in a dependent variable that is not the direct result of variations in the treatment variable (see also Source of spuriousness variable and Confounding variable).

Health promotion research: The systematic investigation into the processes and substance of health promotion action. It encompasses a broad range of studies, including much of the research in health policy, lifestyle, and socio-epidemiology.

Hierarchical regression: The researcher determines the order of entry, or hierarchy, of the variables put into a regression equation. This technique is used in testing path models.

History: In the context of experimental design, history refers to concurrent events that, along with the experimental manipulation, may be influencing variation in the dependent variable.

Holistic ethnography: Defines culture as a way of life and studies it as an integrated whole.

Hypotheses: Statements of predicted relationship between two or more variables.

Illegitimate appeal to authority: To argue that something is bad (e.g., euthanasia) by citing the opinion of a person who is not an expert in the particular field but who is well known for accomplishments in another field.

Implications: The author highlights the importance of the study in terms of its potential contributions to practice, education, theory, and research, as appropriate.

Independent variable: A "cause" in a cause-and-effect relationship. It is a variable that has been selected as a possible influence on variations in a dependent variable.

In-depth interviews: Personal interviews in which probing is used to explore issues in detail.

Index: A combined score based on two or more indicators.

Index system: Through a compilation of items, enables the researcher to create and manipulate concepts and emerging ideas.

Individually delivered questionnaires: Questionnaires handed to the respondents by a researcher.

Inductive reasoning: Moves from the specific to the general; specific situations are observed and then combined into a larger, more general statement that can be tested through qualitative or quantitative research methods.

Inferential statistics: Deal with making extrapolations from a sample to the population from which it was drawn; they also deal with tests of statistical significance.

Informant: Participant in an ethnographic investigation.

Informed consent: The right of a potential respondent to be informed as to the nature of the study, the kinds of issues will be explored, how the respondent was selected, and who is sponsoring the research. When studies are done involving children, infirm patients, or incompetent adults, the organization or individual responsible for the prospective respondent should provide consent in writing.

Informed opinion: An opinion based on evidence that has been collected under controlled circumstances.

Institutional review board: See Ethics review board.

Instrument decay: A deterioration in the measurement instrument over the course of measurements in a study.

Instrument development: A process involving application of specific rules to create a tool to measure some research phenomenon. It is a major use of factor analysis. Usually instrument development proceeds with a large number of items used to represent the research phenomenon later reduced to fewer items.

Instrument validation: Factor analysis is an important tool for validating new research instruments. In nursing research, it is used most frequently for this reason. Factor analysis offers an empirical method of identifying the underlying factors that compose a construct.

Instrumental utilization: The direct, explicit application of knowledge gained from research to change practice. It includes but is not limited to the adoption of nursing interventions, new procedures, clinical protocols and guidelines, and so on.

Internal consistency approach to reliability: Involves comparing an individual item's correlation to the total index score. If an item is consistent with the total score, it will correlate with it.

Internal validity: A researcher has demonstrated that the treatment does, in fact, produce the changes in the dependent variable.

Interpretive perspective: Relies mainly on field studies, with an emphasis on participant observation studies (joining a group and participating in it), in-depth interviews with people, and on ethnomethodology (typically a detailed examination of a single event or case). Each of these studies typically involves a few cases that are described in detail. A key question for these researchers is, "Does the explanation offered make sense to the people whose behavior is being explained?" Communication of the results of such studies usually emphasizes verbal descriptions rather than numerical analyses.

Interquartile range: A measure of how far apart the values are in the middle 50 percent of a distribution.

Intersubjectivity: Describes how subjective awareness and understanding can be reached in a common world.

Intervening variable: A variable that links an independent variable to a dependent one. An intervening variable represents an explanation of how the independent variable influences the dependent variable.

Interview panels: Groups in which at least one follow-up interview is conducted with them.

Interview schedules: Outline of the major questions that are to be raised. The interviewer has autonomy in exploring questions in detail.

Jackson's rule of thirds: In interpreting three-variable relationships, if the original difference between the categories increases by one third or more, it should be interpreted as an *increase,* or a strengthening, of the original relationship. If the difference remains within one third of the original, it should be interpreted as an indication that the relationship has *remained the same.* If the difference decreases by more than one third, it should be interpreted as a *decrease or disappearance* of the relationship. Finally, if the relationship is markedly different when different control categories are compared with one another (e.g., it disappears in one category but stays the same in the other), the result is *mixed.*

Justice: The idea that all participants must be treated fairly. The protection of participants from incompetence and the right to receive research treatments are expectations of the justice principle.

Key character files: Files established on key players in the organization or group being observed. Here items that provide clues as to the personality and manner of operation of each individual are drawn from the master file.

Key informants: Group members who are most knowledgeable about the study phenomenon.

Kuder-Richardson coefficient: A method for testing internal consistency in an index.

Lambda: A statistic measuring the *proportionate reduction in error* that occurs in estimating a dependent variable given knowledge of the independent variable.

Leptokurtic distribution: Has little variability—a small standard deviation relative to the magnitude of the values—and is sharply peaked.

Likert-based index: An index or instrument based on a combination of statements that use a numeric scale after each statement for response.

Likert items: Asking respondents to categorize a statement by indicating whether they strongly disagree, disagree, are undecided or neutral, agree, or strongly agree with the statement.

Linear regression equation: A relationship between a number of independent variables and a dependent variable and which provides for the best linear (additive) weightings of the independent variables and a constant calculated so as to maximize the prediction of the dependent variable.

Literature review: A critical step in focusing the research problem and statement of purpose. It is a process of reviewing the current knowledge about the research problem, describing the characteristics of previous studies in the area, noting the similarities and differences in research results, evaluating the strengths and limitations of previous studies, and identifying gaps in knowledge relevant to the research problem.

Lived experiences: The everyday human experiences that are real to the individuals who experience them.

Longitudinal studies: Studies that involve data collection from the same group at different points in time.

Looking glass self: The idea that our perception of self is reflected in how others see us and that we come to see ourselves as others see us.

Macrovariables: Properties or characteristics of societies, as opposed to qualities of individuals.

Magnitude estimation procedures: Procedures that are useful when comparative judgments are required. In this type of procedure, a respondent estimates the magnitude of a series of stimuli compared with a fixed standard.

Marker variable: A variable that produces the highest correlation with the underlying factor that is identified in the factor analysis procedure. A marker variable is useful to researchers attempting to label the underlying factor.

Master field file: Made up of the complete journal of field notes.

Master table: Records all collected information so that required tables can be derived from it without going back to tally sheets.

Matched pairs: The researcher predetermines significant characteristics in the sample that might influence the dependent variable and matches the sample according to those characteristics. For example, if a researcher is interested in measuring the impact of a health promotion program on participants, the researcher would try to "match" each program participant with another person with a similar predetermined characteristics at the outset of the program.

Maturation: Any changes that occur in an individual subject over the course of an experiment which may, along with the experimental manipulation, influence the outcome of the experiment.

Maxi ethnography: A large, comprehensive study of general and particular features of a designated culture.

Mean: More formally known as the *arithmetic mean* and less formally known as the *average,* it is computed by summing the values of a variable and dividing the result by the total number of cases.

Measurement: The process of reflecting abstract concepts with empirical indicants or numbers.

Measurement error: The extent to which indicants fail to reflect the true underlying values of variables.

Measures of central tendency: Use one number to typify a set of values.

Measures of dispersion: The extent of the variability, or dispersion, of values in a distribution.

Mechanistic model: Model that asserts that a particular behavior is completely controlled by one or more external actions or events.

Median: The midpoint of a distribution.

Meta-analysis: The statistical analysis of a large collection of results from individual studies for the purpose of integrating findings.

Methodological triangulation: The application of diverse methods to generate and collect data about one phenomenon.

Microvariables: Properties or characteristics of individuals as opposed to properties of a society.

Middle-range theories: Located on the theory continuum midway between the most abstract ideas (grand theory) and the most concrete ideas (practice theory). They deal with limited aspects of nursing phenomena and are more testable and generalizable than grand theories. They contain well-defined concepts and propositions.

Mini ethnography: A small-scale ethnography focused on a narrow area of inquiry.

Missing evidence: The idea that evidence necessary for an argument to be true may be missing.

Missing value code: A value assigned to a variable for cases in which the information is absent or not applicable.

Mode: The most frequently occurring response to a nominal variable.

Mortality: Subjects selecting themselves out of a study.

Multicolinearity: The extent of the correlation among the independent variables.

Multiple regression analysis: An equation to predict variations in a dependent variable from two or more independent variables.

Multistage area sample: When sampling involves an attempt to reflect a large unit such as a state, province, or country and no list of the population is available, then one develops a sample by stages. At each stage of the sampling process, every individual (or unit) must have a known chance of being selected.

Multivariate analysis of variance (MANOVA): Used in examining relationships between a ratio level dependent variable and independent variables measured at any level. MANOVA techniques also permit the researcher to examine multiple dependent variables simultaneously.

Multivariate models: Models that involve numerous variables.

Mutually exclusive categories: Situations in which category boundaries are established so that no category overlaps another one.

Natural setting experiments: Experiments in which everyday situations can be manipulated, allowing for the researcher to observe reactions of people to the intervention.

Naturalistic observational studies: When the researcher records observations without the subjects being aware that they are being observed.

Needs assessment: A form of inquiry that assesses the needs, problems, concerns, or conditions of a group, community, or organization that should be addressed in future planning activities.

Nodes: Qualitative data containers for thoughts about a project. The nodes store the index categories developed by the qualitative researcher.

Nominal measurement: A quantitative measure in which the numbers are arbitrarily assigned to categories of the variable.

Nonmaleficence: The duty to not inflict harm, either emotional or physical.

Nonparallel constructions: Particularly problematic if used in gender references. They may lead to confusion or misrepresentation by violating the principle that parts of a sentence that are parallel in meaning should be parallel in structure.

Nonprobability sampling techniques: Techniques that do not provide potential respondents with a known chance of being asked to participate in a study. Convenience, quota, and referral (snowball) samples are examples of nonprobability sampling techniques.

Normal distribution: Approximates a bell-shaped curve, in which there are few cases on the extremes with most clustered at the mean of the distribution.

Normative bias: Value judgments are made by the investigator regarding normalcy and the appropriateness of phenomenon-related feelings and behaviors based on current conceptual models, theories, and available empirical data.

NUD*IST: A software program developed specifically for qualitative data analysis. It stands for non-numerical unstructured data indexing searching and theorizing.

Null hypothesis: States that there will be no relationship between the variables.

Nuremberg code: Formulated as a result of unethical medical research experiments conducted by Nazi scientists predominantly on inmates of concentration camps before and during World War II. The code addresses issues of informed consent, protection of subjects from risk or harm, the right of participants to withdraw from experimentation, and adequate qualifications of those conducting research.

Objective: Observations that are free from bias.

Observational measurement: Frequently conducted in nursing research to determine how participants respond in specific situations. It is a data collection method that is particularly well suited to phenomena that are best viewed from a holistic rather than a reductionistic perspective. For example, direct observation of a child's separation anxiety behavior would most likely yield better data than what would be achieved through a survey.

One-tailed test: Situations in which we are predicting which particular tail of the normal distribution the result will fall into if the null hypothesis is to be rejected.

One-way analysis of variance: Provides a test of significance for the effect of one independent variable on a dependent variable.

Open-ended question: Asks a respondent to answer a question or to offer a suggestion or opinion but to do so without any preset categories provided for the answer.

Operant conditioning theory: The process by which behavior is modified by the rewards and punishments that result from the behavior being displayed.

Operationalization: The selection of indicators (measures) to reflect conceptual variables used in the implementation of a research project.

Operational level: Consists of the measurement of variables as well as the collection and analysis of data.

Ordinal measurement: Consists of a measure in which there is an order in the values assigned but in which the intervals between the values are not equal.

Overgeneralization: A statement that claims to refer to all people but is based on evidence that does not represent all people.

Overspecificity: Involves situations in which single gender terms are used when members of both genders are involved (e.g., "the doctor . . . he").

Panel studies: Studies that monitor specific organizations or individuals over time.

Partial correlation: Measures the strength of association between two ratio level variables while simultaneously controlling for the effects of one or more additional variables.

Partial theory: Explains an assumed or known relationship by specifying a testable causal model.

Participant: Used to refer to the individuals who inform the study in qualitative investigations. These individuals are viewed as active participants in the research process and as equal partners with the investigator.

Participant observation studies: Those in which the researcher is involved in the daily lives of the study group, observing and recording as much as possible about their lives.

Participatory action research: Uses critical social theory methods; it is research for the purpose of taking action and creating change.

Path model: A graphic representation of a complex set of proposed interrelationships among variables.

Patriarchy: The domination of the social groups by men, who have greater power and privilege than women and children.

Percentage: Represents a proportion multiplied by 100; thus, a percentage represents *how many* for every 100 of something.

Personal knowledge: The interpersonal interactions and relationships between a nurse and a client. It is concerned with the knowing and encountering of the individual self.

Phenomenological approach: A qualitative research method that describes the meaning of a lived experience from the perspective of the participant. Lived experiences are the everyday human experiences that are real to the individuals who experience them. Phenomenology seeks to achieve a deep understanding of the phenomenon being studied through a rigorous, systematic examination of it. Its purpose is to describe the essences of lived experiences.

Phone survey: Survey that relies on information reported by the respondent over the telephone.

Pilot study: In survey research, a study that involves having a small sample of respondents complete a questionnaire or undergo an interview. Pilot studies are used to determine items to be included in indexes and to determine, from open-ended questions, the categories that should be used in a fixed choice format.

Plagiarism: The unacknowledged borrowing of other authors' ideas or words.

Planned change: An intentional process that involves a change agent who works to bring about a demonstrable improvement in the status quo.

Platykurtic distribution: Has a great deal of variability that tends to be flat and wide.

Population: A collection of individuals, communities, or nations about which one wishes to make a general statement.

Positivist approach: The approach used in the physical sciences. It emerged from a branch of philosophy known as logical positivism, which operates on strict rules of logic, truth, axioms (general principles), and predictions.

Power analysis: A procedure used to determine the power of a statistical test; in other words, to determine the probability that an inferential statistical test will detect a significant difference that is real or correctly reject a null hypothesis.

Practice theories: Theories that are narrower in scope and more specific than middle-range theories. Concepts are specifically and narrowly defined and readily measured. Practice theory propositions produce clear directives for application in practice. Much of what nurses follow today in hospital procedure manuals is actually practice theory that has been developed inductively by expert nurses who have observed and described ways of practicing based on trial and error.

Precise communication: Unambiguous information.

Precision matching: A method of achieving equivalence between control and experimental groups by ensuring that the groups are matched on certain key variables.

Precoded, single-choice questions: Questions that ask a respondent to indicate which category applies to him or to her.

Prediction: In regression analysis, the extent to which variation in a dependent variable can be accurately estimated with knowledge of the independent variables.

Predictive research: Moves beyond explanation to the prediction of precise relationships between dimensions or characteristics of a phenomenon or differences between groups. Predictive research typically engages the empirical method of experimentation.

Predictive validity: If you were attempting to develop a measure to predict success in nurse registration examinations, you could assess the validity of your measure by correlating it with success rates on RN examinations. A high correlation would indicate high predictive validity.

Pre-experimental design: A design that does not permit clear causal inferences about the impact of a treatment on the dependent variable.

Presence–absence questions: Questions that request respondents to check off which items in a list do or do not apply to them.

Primary sampling units: May be census tract areas, or other similar units, normally several hundred of them; these units are numbered and, using an equal probability technique, a selection of at least 30 units is made from them.

Principal components method: Includes an analysis of all the variance in the observed variables, not just the shared variance among the variables in factor analysis.

Principal factors method: Known in the Statistical Package for the Social Sciences (SPSS) as the principal axis factoring method, this approach relies on the shared variances of the variables included in the analysis and appears to be the most commonly used factor analysis approach.

Probabilistic explanation: Involves arguing that a particular case will be similar to others in the same general category.

Probability levels: The test statistic computes the chance that a result is caused by sampling fluctuations. This is reported in various ways, normally labeled as the *p* value or significance value.

Probability sampling procedures: Involve techniques for selecting sampling units so that each has a known chance of being included.

Problem statement: A narrative that elaborates on the research problem and identifies the specific area of concern. It provides direction for the entire study and guides the study toward a quantitative or a qualitative design.

Process consent: The researcher renegotiates the consent with the participants as unforeseen circumstances arise. This allows the participants to be part of the decision-making process as the study unfolds.

Pronoun problem: Encourages stereotypic thinking by referring to doctors and managers as *he* and nurses as *she.*

Proportion: Represents the part of one that is represented by a category (e.g., how many females there are in a population compared with the total population). Proportions always begin with a decimal point.

Proportionate reduction in error: Associated with the statistic *Lambda,* which measures the reduction in error in estimating variation in a dependent variable, given knowledge of an independent variable. If two variables are strongly associated, then errors in predicting variations in the dependent variable will be considerably reduced if information on the independent variable is taken into account.

Propositions: Statements of proposed relationships between two or more concepts in a theory. Propositions link concepts of a theory together so that something can be described, explained, or predicted. Propositions may also be referred to as axioms or theorems.

Prospective: Reference to data that are collected from the present to a future point in time.

Provincialism: The tendency to see things as one's culture sees them.

Proxemics: The study of the norms surrounding personal space and the conditions under which such space will or will not be violated.

Pure research: Research that focuses on understanding phenomena of interest.

Purposive sampling: Selecting and interviewing or observing participants who have had experience with the phenomena of interest.

Qualitative research: Research that uses concepts, classifications, and attempts to interpret human behavior that reflects not only the analyst's views but the views of the people whose behavior is being described; the emphasis is on verbal descriptions as opposed to numerical ones.

Quality control monitoring system: Procedures to ensure that interviewers are following established procedures for selecting respondents, asking questions, and entering data.

Quantitative research: Seeks to quantify, or reflect with numbers, observations about human behavior.

Quasi-experimental design: Design in which it has not been possible to do any or all of the following: (1) randomly assign subjects to a treatment or control group or (2) control the timing or nature of the treatment. The quasi-experiment design comes as close as possible to the experimental design in order to measure the impact of a treatment.

Questionnaire: Made up of a series of set questions that either provide a space for an answer or offer a number of fixed alternatives from which the respondent makes a choice.

Quota sample: Respondents are selected on the basis of meeting certain criteria. The first respondent to meet the requirement (or requirements) is asked to participate and sampling continues until all the categories have been filled—until the quota for each has been reached.

r^2:   A measure of the amount of variation in the dependent variable is explained by an independent variable.

R^2:   A measure of the amount of variation in the dependent variable that is explained by the combination of independent variables (regression analysis).

Random error: Inconsistencies that enter into the coding process but that have no pattern in the errors.

Random variable: Varies without control but is taken into account by the way groups are set up in an experiment.

Random sample: Provides each unit (usually a person) in the population with an equal chance of being selected for participation in a study.

Randomization: A process of assigning subjects to a treatment or a control group so that each subject has an equal chance of being assigned to either group.

Randomized clinical trial: Uses one or more control groups and experimental groups, depending on the number of interventions. Subjects are randomly allocated to the groups.

Range: Indicates the gap between the lowest and highest value in a distribution.

Rank-ordering questions: Questions in which a respondent is asked to indicate an ordering of response items, usually from most preferred to least preferred.

Rate: The frequency of a phenomenon for a standard sized unit (such as incidence per 1000 or per 100,000).

Ratio measurement: Quantitative measurement in which intervals are equal and there is a true zero point.

Ratios: Used to compare rates or other measures across categories.

Reflexive critique: A process that enables participants and researchers to make explicit, alternative explanations for events or experiences. It facilitates discussion between the researchers and participants and leads to greater insights and acceptance of multiple explanations for events.

Regression analysis: A method for analyzing the relationship between a ratio level dependent variable and independent variables. This form of analysis provides weightings that may be used in an equation to describe the relationship. Standardized weightings provide a means for estimating the relative impact of independent variables on the dependent one.

Regression line: A straight line describing the relationship between an independent and dependent variable drawn so that the vertical deviations of the points above the line equal the vertical deviations below the line.

Reliability: The extent to which, on repeated measures, an indicator yields similar readings.

Reliable knowledge: Knowledge you can count on; knowledge that allows you to predict outcomes.

Repeated measures analysis of variance: To test for differences among the mean scores of the treatment conditions when the researcher has exposed the *same* subject to two or more treatment conditions.

Replacement of terms: Replacing general theoretical concepts by specific instances of these concepts.

Research: The systematic inquiry into a subject to discover new knowledge or to validate or refine existing knowledge.

Research bias: Defined as systematic distortions in research outcomes.

Research critic: The role is to provide an objective evaluation of the study's merits. To do this, the critic must read the report comprehensively and offer constructive comments on all aspects of the report, as well as on the specific strengths and limitations of the study.

Research critique: A critical appraisal of a piece of completed research. It involves a high level of critical thinking and analysis of each component of the research study. Critiques may be conducted on research reports, manuscripts, or published articles based on research studies, or they may be done on research proposals. A critique provides constructive criticism of a specific piece of work for the purpose of promoting excellence in research.

Research design: Similar to a blueprint for a study, it guides an investigator in planning and implementing a study. It provides a detailed plan for data collection and analysis and is the critical element linking the theoretical framework and questions with the resultant data.

Researcher affect: Reference is made to a process whereby the researcher, having "fallen in love" with a particular explanation for a particular relationship or view of the world, may inadvertently engage in procedures that lead to conclusions supporting the preferred explanation.

Research hypothesis: The statement of relationship between variables.

Research–practice gap: The gap between what we know in the field of nursing as a result of research and the actual application of this knowledge in practice.

Research problem: A situation or circumstance that requires a solution to be described, explained, or predicted.

Research process: The research process is simply a series of actions taken by the researcher to discover new knowledge or validate or refine existing knowledge.

Research question: The research problem stated in the interrogative form. It is stated in the present tense. The advantage to stating the problem in the interrogative form is that a question invites an answer.

Research report: A comprehensive description of key aspects of the project that includes a minimum of four major sections: "Introduction," "Methods," "Results," and "Discussion."

Research topic: The broad general area you wish to investigate.

Research utilization: A complex process that includes critically analyzing the literature, selecting appropriate interventions, implementing them, and evaluating the outcome.

Response bias: Exhibited if respondents who want to appear consistent give the same responses as they did the first time; others might want to help the researchers and, suspecting the study is to demonstrate how good something is, respond by being more positive after the experimental stimulus has been given.

Response rate: The percentage of delivered questionnaires that are completed and returned.

Response set: A situation in which a respondent tends to answer similarly to all items.

Retrospective: Reference to data collection about behavior that occurred in the past.

Review of the literature: A section of a paper that tries to provide an overview of the "state of scientific knowledge" on the topic being researched.

Role modeling: Emulating someone else's attitudes and behaviors.

Salience: The degree of interest in the topic of the research by the respondent; the greater the salience of the topic to respondents, the greater the response rate.

Sample: Selected from a population and interpreted to represent that population.

Sampling error: The difference between the values emerging from the sample and those emerging from the population on a particular phenomenon.

Sampling fraction: The sample size in relation to the population.

Sampling frame: The list from which a sample is drawn.

Sample interval: See Skip interval.

Saturation: Used in qualitative investigations, situation in data collection in which the participants' descriptions become repetitive and confirm previously collected data.

Secondary data: Information collected by persons other than the researcher.

Scalable items: Items in which there is a hierarchy among them. This means that when items are arranged from low intensity to high intensity, if a person responds positively to an item at the high end, they are expected to respond positively to all lower intensity items.

Scale: A complex combination of indicators in which the pattern of the responses is taken into account.

Scientific method: Viewed in Western cultures as the most sophisticated method of acquiring knowledge, it combines the process of logical reasoning with systematic planned investigation, data collection, analysis, and evaluation.

Selected evidence: Evidence that results when one chooses to report only the studies that support a particular point of view, ignoring the evidence that runs counter to what the researcher is attempting to demonstrate.

Selection: Subjects selecting themselves into a study.

Semantic differential: Items are used to study subjective feelings toward objects or persons.

Sexism: Discrimination on the basis of gender.

Sexist language: Problems that include the pronoun problem, the man problem, and the nonparallel construction problem.

Sexual dichotomism: Treating the genders as discrete social, as well as biological, cohorts rather than two cohorts with shared characteristics.

Significant others: Help define the world for individuals by serving as models for attitudes and behavior.

Simple random sample: Provides each unit (usually a person) in the population with an equal chance of being selected for participation in a study.

Simultaneity paradigm: Reality is characterized by a mutual process of human—environment interaction. Persons exist in open participation with the universe and are more than and different from the summed parts studied in the totality paradigm. The wholeness or unitary nature of the human being is primary in this paradigm.

Single blind: Study in which the subjects are not aware of the type of intervention that will be administered.

Situation-specific theory: Answers a set of coherent questions about situations that are limited in scope and focus.

Skip interval: Determined by dividing the total sample requirement into the total number of units in the population being surveyed; this number should then be rounded to the nearest, but lower, whole number.

Snowball sampling: A name for a referral sampling procedure. As a researcher completes one interview, he or she asks if there is anyone else known to the respondent who might be appropriate for the study.

Source of spuriousness variable: A variable that is viewed as possibly influencing both the independent and the dependent variable in such a way that it accounts for the relationship between them.

Spearman correlation: Statistic used to measure the strength of association between two ordinal level variables.

Split-half method: A method for testing reliability involves randomly splitting index items into two groups, computing the indexes, and then correlating the resulting scores. Internal reliability would be indicated by a high correlation between the two indexes.

SPSS (Statistical Package for the Social Sciences):   A collection of procedures for processing social science and nursing data.

Stability: Concerned with the consistency of the results with repeated measures.

Standard deviation: The average amount of deviation from the mean value of the variable.

Standard error of the means: A measure of variability in the means of repeated samples.

Statement of purpose: Flows from the problem statement and is included in it. One research problem statement may be the basis for several research purposes. The research purpose is usually a single declarative statement that focuses the study and clearly identifies what the researcher intends to do.

Statistical regression: Demonstrated when a sample is selected on the basis of extreme scores and retesting shows a tendency toward less extreme scores.

Stratified sample: A sample that gives individuals within designated categories an equal chance of selection.

Structural equation modeling: An advanced statistical method designed to test theories.

Structured interviews: Face-to-face interviews in which questions are read to the respondents. Such interviews ordinarily do not provide for in-depth probes on some of the questions.

Summary tables: Tables that compress the results of many analyses into one table.

Summated rating indexes: Indexes in which the scores for each item are summed, or summed and averaged, to yield each individual's score.

Summative evaluation: Conducted to determine the effectiveness, value, and worth of an innovation. For many evaluation projects, it includes evaluation of the costs as well as the effectiveness of the program or intervention.

Surveys: A method for collecting information by having respondents complete a questionnaire.

Symbolic interactionist theory: Pays attention particularly to how one's self-concept is formed. People develop a sense of self that is influenced by how others see them and by how others react to them.

Systematic errors: Errors that distort the data in one particular direction.

Systematic sample: Provides each unit (usually a person) in the population an equal chance of being selected for participation in a study by choosing every *n*th unit, starting randomly.

t Test: A test of significance usually used with small samples.

Tally sheets: Used to record information during the data collection phase of observational studies.

Taxonomy: A set of categories organized on the basis of a single semantic relationship.

Test of significance: Reports the probability that an observed association or difference is the result of sampling fluctuations and not reflective of a "real" difference in the population from which the sample has been taken.

Testing: When questions are repeated, some respondents may want to appear consistent and, therefore, give the same responses in both tests.

Themes: Recurrent ideas or patterns that emerge in the data representing common threads of meaning in the narrative of participants.

Theoretical frameworks: Brief descriptions or explanations of a theory or portions of a theory to be tested in a research project. A theoretical framework describes the basic structure of ideas (theories, concepts, propositions) within which the study is to be conducted and the results interpreted. It is a verbal description of existing theory relevant to the phenomena under investigation based on a review of the literature.

Theoretical memos: The ideas a researcher holds about codes and the relationships as they strike him or her during analysis.

Theoretical level: The most abstract, general conceptualization of the research problem.

Theoretical substruction: A process of discovery in which a researcher begins with observations and tries to make sense of them and to identify the concepts the data seem to reflect. As observations are made, the concepts are continuously identified and refined.

Theoretical triangulation: A strategy for theory testing that involves the testing of two competing or alternative theories within one study.

Theory: A systematic vision of reality that describes, explains, or predicts something.

Theory development: Factor analysis is used to identify structures of variables or constructs that can be interpreted meaningfully by the researcher. The researcher explains why variables that have been defined mathematically are clustered together the way that they have emerged. It can also lead to the conceptualization of research phenomena and their underlying dimensions and show important intercorrelations and relationships among constructs. These are important steps in theory development.

3M approach: A method used to identify which SPSS procedure to use; the Model/Measurement/Method.

Totality paradigm: Reality exists independent of the knower, humans are viewed as the sum of their parts, persons adapt to an external environment through cause-and-effect relationships, and health is viewed along a continuum from illness to wellness.

Transferability: Concerned with the *generalizability* or *fittingness* of study findings to other settings, populations, and contexts. In assessing transferability of findings, the research consumer hopes to show that the results are not context bound.

Treatment level: The number of different categories of a variable that will be exposed to the subject in an experiment. A study, for example, that when using three treatment levels, might compare the effects of seeing a short, medium, or long film.

Treatment variable: Variable whose effect on some dependent variable is being assessed in an experiment.

Triangulation: Using a variety of techniques to test research questions.

True value: The underlying exact quantity of a variable at any given time.

Trustworthiness: The process of establishing the validity and reliability of qualitative research.

Two-tailed test: Situations in which the researcher has not predicted into which particular tail of the normal distribution the result will fall into if the null hypothesis is to be rejected.

Two-way analysis of variance: A multifactor analysis of variance, when the design has two or more independent variables.

Type I error: Results when a researcher rejects a null hypothesis that should be accepted.

Type II error: Results when a researcher accepts a null hypothesis that should be rejected.

Unilineal model: A model in which the same patterns of development are followed by all societies.

Unit of analysis: The basic type of object under investigation. Usually researchers define the unit and deal with only one unit at a time; it may be a speech, it may be a paragraph from the speech, or it may be a number of individuals or a number of groups. The information collected describes the unit under investigation.

Unwarranted conclusion: An error in reasoning; confusing correlation and cause is an example of this type of error.

Utilitarian perspective: Ethical judgments about a research project should be made by evaluating its consequences for the participants, for society, and for the academic discipline. This view entails the belief that the good of a research project is defined by the consequences of the results.

Validity of a measurement: The extent that a measure reflects the concept, reflecting nothing more or nothing less than that implied by the conceptual definition.

Variables: Characteristics of research concepts that are directly measurable and that vary.

Variance: The average amount of deviation from the mean value of the variable; it is the standard deviation squared.

Verifiable: Information that could be confirmed by tests conducted by others.

Verstehen: A German word meaning the empathetic understanding of behavior.

Visual analog scale: Measures the intensity of participants' sensations and feelings about the strength of their attitudes, beliefs, and opinions about specific stimuli such as pain, fatigue, nausea, quality of life, health status, appetite, self-care ability, and so on.

Within-subject design: Study design that exposes one subject to the different experimental treatments; because the subject is the same person, background characteristics, attitudes, and intelligence are all perfectly controlled.

Z score: Expresses an observation's location relative to the mean (in standard deviation units) within a normal distribution.

Bibliography

Aamodt, A.M. (1991). Ethnography and epistemology: Generating nursing knowledge. In J.M. Morse, (Ed.), *Qualitative Nursing Research* (pp. 40–53). Newbury Park, CA: Sage.

Abrahamson, M. (1983). *Social Research Methods.* Englewood Cliffs, N.J.: Prentice-Hall.

Aish, A.E. & Isenberg, M. (1996). Effects of Orem-based nursing interventions on nutritional self-care myocardial infarction patients. *International Journal of Nursing Studies, 33*(3), 259–270.

Alcock, D., Lawrence, J., Goodman, J., & Ellis, J. (1993). Formative evaluation: Implementation of primary nursing. *Canadian Journal of Nursing Research, 25*(3), 15–27.

Alliex, S. (1998). *Hurdling: The process of nurse-patient interaction in the presence of technology.* Qualitative Health Research Conference, Hotel Vancouver, Vancouver, BC. February, 1998.

Alpers, R. (1998). The changing self-concept of pregnant and parenting teens. *Journal of Professional Nursing, 14*(2), 111–119.

American Nurses Association (1995). *Code for nurses with interpretive statements.* Washington, DC: American Nurses Association.

American Nurses Association (1989). *Commission on nursing research: Education for preparation in nursing research.* Kansas City, MO: Author.

American Nurses Association (1985). *Human Rights Guidelines for Nurses in Clinical and Other Research.* Kansas City, MO: Author.

American Nurses' Association (1976). *Preparation for Nurses for Participation in Research.* Kansas City, MO: Author.

American Psychological Association (1998). *Publication Manual of the American Psychological Association* (5th ed.). Washington D.C.: American Psychological Association.

American Psychological Association (1994). *Publication Manual of the American Psychological Association* (4th ed.). Washington, D.C.

Anderson, N. (1961). *The Hobo.* Chicago: Phoenix Edition, [1923].

Anderson, N.L. (1996). Decisions about substance abuse among adolescents in juvenile detention. *Image: Journal of Nursing Scholarship, 28*(1), 65–70.

Arathuzik, D., & Aber, C. (1998). Factors associated with national council licensure examination: Registered nurse success. *Journal of Professional Nursing, 14*(2), 119–126.

Asch, D.A. (1996). The role of critical care nurses in euthanasia and assisted suicide. *The New England Journal of Medicine,* May 23, 1374–1379.

Atkinson, P., & Hammersley, M. (1994). Ethnography and participant observation. In N.K. Denzin & Y.S. Lincoln, (Eds.), *Handbook of Qualitative Research* (pp. 248–261). Thousand Oaks, CA: Sage.

Azen, I. (1985). From intentions to action: A theory of planned behavior. In J. Kuhl & J. Beckman (Eds.), *Action Control: From Cognition to Behavior* (pp. 11–39). New York: Springer.

Azen, I. (1991). The theory of planned behavior. *Organizational Behavior and Human Decision Processes, 50,* 179–211.

Babbie, E. (1992). *The Practice of Social Research,* (6th ed.). Belmont: Wadsworth.

Bailey, P., Maciejewski, J., & Karen, I. (1993). Combined mother and baby care: Does it meet the needs of families? *Canadian Journal of Nursing Research, 25*(3), 29–39.

Baker, C. (1996). Subjective experience of symptoms in schizophrenia. *Canadian Journal of Nursing Research, 28*(2), 19–37.

Banik, B.J. (1993). Applying triangulation in

nursing research. *Applied Nursing Research, 6*(1), 47–52.

Banks-Wallace, J. (1998). Emancipatory potential of storytelling in a group. *Image: Journal of Nursing Scholarship, 30*(1), 17–21.

Barnsley, J., & Ellis, D. (1992). *Research for change. Participatory action research for community group.* Vancouver, BC: Women's Research Center, 101-2245 West Broadway.

Baron, S.W. (1989). The Canadian West Coast punk subculture: A field study, *Canadian Journal of Sociology, 14*(3), 289–316.

Barragan, L. (1998). Nursing practice draws upon several different ways of knowing. *Journal of Clinical Nursing, 7,* 209–217.

Beal, J. (2000). A nurse practitioner model of practice. *The American Journal of Maternal Child Nursing, 25*(1), 18–24.

Beauchamp, T.L., & Childrens, J.F. (1989). *Principles of Premedical Ethics* (3rd ed.). Oxford: Oxford University Press.

Beck, C.T. (1996). Grounded theory: Overview and application in pediatric nursing. *Issues in Comprehensive Pediatric Nursing, 19,* 1–15.

Beck, C.T. (1994). Reliability and validity issues in phenomenological research. *Western Journal of Nursing Research, 16*(3), 254–267.

Beck, C.T. (1993). Qualitative research: The evaluation of its credibility, fittingness, and auditability. *Western Journal of Nursing Research, 15*(2), 263–265.

Becker, H.S., Blanche, G., Hughes, E.C., & Strauss, A.L. (1961). *Boys in White.* Chicago: The University of Chicago Press.

Beecher, H.K. (1966). Ethics and clinical research. *New England Journal of Medicine, 274*(24), 1354–1360.

Begley, S. (1993). The meaning of junk, *Newsweek* (March 23), 62–64.

Bell, L. (1995). *Effective Writing: A Guide for Health Professionals.* Toronto: Copp Clarke.

Bellack, J.P., Graber, D.R., O'Neil, E.H., Musham, C., & Lancaster, C. (1999). Curriculum trends in nurse practitioner programs: Current and ideal. *Journal of Professional Nursing, 15*(1), 15–28.

Benner, P. (1984). *From Novice to Expert.* Menlo Park, CA: Addison-Wesley.

Bennett, J.A. (1997). A case for theory triangulation. *Nursing Science Quarterly, 10*(2), 97–102.

Berg, B.L. (1995). *Qualitative Research Methods for the Social Sciences.* Boston: Allyn and Bacon.

Berland, A., Whyte, N.B., & Maxwell, L. (1995). Hospital nurses and health promotion.

Canadian Journal of Nursing Research, 27(4), 13–33.

Berman, H., McKenna, K., Arnold, C., & MacQuarrie, B. (2000). Sexual harassment: Everyday violence in the lives of girls and women. *Advances in Nursing Science, 22*(4), 32–46.

Bertrand, L.D., & Abernathy, T.J. (1993). Predicting cigarette smoking among adolescents using cross-sectional and longitudinal approaches. *Journal of School Health, 63*(2), 98–103.

Betz, C.L., & Beal, J. (1996). Use of nursing models in pediatric nursing research: A decade of review. *Issues in Comprehensive Pediatric Nursing, 19,* 153–167.

Blalock, H.M., Jr. (1964). *Causal Inference in Nonexperimental Research.* Chapel Hill: The University of North Carolina Press.

Blalock, H.M., Jr. (1979). *Social Statistics.* Toronto: McGraw-Hill.

Blishen, B.R., & McRoberts, H. (1976). A revised socioeconomic index for occupations in Canada, *Canadian Review of Sociology and Anthropology, 13*(1), 71–79.

Blumer, H. (1969). *Symbolic Interactionism: Perspective and Method.* In W. Chenitz and J. Swanson, *From Practice to Grounded Theory: Qualitative Research in Nursing.* Menlo Park, CA: Addison-Wesley.

Borenstein, M., & Cohen, J. (1988). *Statistical Power Analysis: A Computer Program.* Hillsdale, NJ: Erlbaum Associates.

Bostrom, J., & Wise, L. (1994). Closing the gap between research and practice. *Journal of Nursing Administration, 24*(5), 22–27.

Bottomore, T.B., & Maximilien, R. (1988). *Karl Marx: Selected Writings in Sociology and Social Philosophy.* London: Penguin Books.

Boutlier, M., Mason, R., & Rootman, I. (1997). Community action and reflective practice in health promotion research. *Health Promotion International, 12*(1), 69–78.

Bradburn, N.M. & Sudman, S. (1980). *Improving Interview Method and Questionnaire Design.* San Francisco: Jossey-Bass.

Bramwell, L., & Hykawy, E. (1999). The Delphi technique: A possible tool for predicting future events in nursing education. *The Canadian Journal of Nursing Research, 30*(4), 47–59.

Brandt, A.M. (1978). Racism and research: The case of the Tuskegee syphillis study. *Hastings Center Report, 8*(6), 21–29.

Brent, E. E., Scott, J. K., & Spencer, J.C. (1988). *Ex-Sample* ™: *An Expert System to Assist in Designing Sampling Plans. User's Guide and*

Reference Manual, Version 2.0. The Idea Works Inc., 100 West Briarwood, Columbia: MI, 65203.

Brentro, M., & Hegge, M. (2000). Nursing faculty: One generation away from extinction? *Journal of Professional Nursing, 16*(2), 97–103.

Brink, P., & Wood, M. (1998). *Advanced Design in Nursing Research* (2nd ed.). Thousand Oaks CA: Sage.

Brockopp, D.Y., & Hastings-Tolsma, M.T. (1995). *Fundamentals of Nursing Research* (2nd ed.). Boston, MS: Jones & Bartlett.

Brown, M.N., & Keeley, S.M. (1990). *Asking the Right Questions: A Guide to Critical Thinking.* Englewood Cliffs, NJ: Prentice Hall.

Brown, S.J. (1999). *Knowledge for Health Care Practice: A Guide to Using Research Evidence.* Philadelphia, PA: W.B. Saunders.

Brundt, J.H., Lindsey, E., & Hopkinson, J. (1997). Health promotion in the Hutterite community and the ethnocentricity of empowerment. *Canadian Journal of Nursing Research, 26*(1), 17–29.

Bunkers, S.S., Petardi, L.A., Pilkington, F.B., & Walls, P. (1996). Challenging the myths surrounding qualitative research in nursing. *Nursing Science Quarterly, 9*(1),33–37.

Bunn, H., & O'Connor, A. (1996). Validation of client decision making instruments in the context of psychiatry. *Canadian Journal of Nursing Research, 28*(3), 13–29.

Bunting, S. M., & Campbell, J.C. (1994). Through a feminist lens: A model to guide nursing research. In. Chinn, P. (Ed.). *Advances in Methods of Inquiring for Nursing.* Gaithersburg, Maryland: Aspen Publications.

Bunton, R., & MacDonald, G. (1992). *Health Promotion: Discipline and Diversity.* London: Rortledge Press.

Burns, N., & Grove, S.K. (1999). *Understanding Nursing Research* (2nd ed.), Philadelphia: Saunders.

Burns, N., & Grove, S.K. (1997). *The Practice of Nursing Research: Conduct, Critique & Utilization.* Philadelphia: W.B. Saunders.

Butler, L. (1995). Valuing research in clinical practice. *Canadian Journal of Nursing Research, 27*(4), 33–49.

Butler, L., & Ginn, D. (1998). Canadian nurses' views on assignment of publication credit for scholarly and scientific work. *Canadian Journal of Nursing Research, 30*(1), 171–185.

Campbell, D.T., & Stanley, J.C. (1966). *Experimental and Quasi-Experimental Designs for Research.* Chicago: Rand McNally.

Canadian Nurses Association (1994). *Ethical Guidelines for Nurses in Research Involving Human Participants.* Ottawa: Author.

Canadian Nurses Association (1997). *Code of Ethics for Registered Nurses,* Ontario: CNA.

Caplan, A.L., Edgar, H., King, P.A., & Jones, J.H. (1992). Twenty years after—The legacy of the Tuskegee syphilis study. *Hastings Center Report, 22*(6), November–December.

Carmines, E.G., & Zeller, R.A. (1979). *Reliability and Validity Assessment.* Beverly Hills: Sage.

Carper, B.A. (1978). Fundamental patterns of knowing in nursing. *Advances in Nursing Science, 1*(1), 13–23.

Carper, D.A. (1992). Response to perspectives on knowing: A model of nursing knowledge (pp. 297–299) In Leslie H. Nicoll (Ed.) *Perspectives on Nursing Theory* (2nd ed). Philadelphia: Lippincott.

Carruth, A.K. (1996). Development and testing of the caregiver reciprocity scale. *Nursing Research, 45*(2), 92–97.

Centers for Disease Control and Prevention (CDCP) (1999). *HIV/AIDS Surveillance Report, 10*(1), 1–39.

Chalmers, K., Bramadat, I., & Sloan, J. (1997). Development and testing of the primary health care questionnaire (PHCQ). *Canadian Journal of Nursing Research, 29*(1), 79–96.

Chenitz, W.C., & Swanson, J. (1986). *From Practice to Grounded Theory: Qualitative Research in Nursing.* Menlo Park, CA: Addison Wesley.

Cherry, B., & Jacob, S. (1999). *Contemporary Nursing: Issues Trends and Management.* Philadelphia: Mosby.

Cheyn, E. (1972). The effect of spatial and interpersonal variables on the invasion of group controlled territories, *Sociometry,* 477–488.

Chinn, P.L., & Kramer, M. (1991). *Theory and Nursing: A Systematic Approach* (3rd ed.). St. Louis, MI: Mosby.

Chinn, P.L., & Kramer, M. (1995). *Theory and Nursing: A Systematic Approach,* (4th ed.). St. Louis, MI: Mosby.

Chow, J.D. (1999). Interruption to research design: Substance driven research. *Advances in Nursing Science, 22*(2), 39–47.

Clarke, E.G., & Danbolt, N. (1955). The Oslow study of the natural history of untreated syphilis. *Journal of Chronis Diseases, 2,* 311–344.

Clark, D., Clark, P., Day, D., & Shea, D. (2000). The relationship between health care reform and nurses' interest in union representation: The role of workplace climate. *Journal of Professional Nursing, 16*(2) 92–96.

Ciliska, D. (1998). Evaluation of two nursing interventions for obese women. *Western Journal of Nursing Research, 20*(1), 119–135.

Clairmont, D.H., & Jackson, W. (1980). *Segmentation and the Low Income Blue Collar Worker: A Canadian Test of Segmentation Theory,* Halifax: Institute of Public Affairs, Dalhousie University.

Cobb, G.W. (1999). *Introduction to Design and Analysis of Experiments.* New York: Springer.

Cobb, A.K., & Hagemaster, J. (1987). Ten criteria for evaluating qualitative research proposals. *Journal of Nursing Education, 26*(4), 138–143.

Coffey, A., & Atkinson, P. (1996). *Making Sense of Qualitative Data.* Thousand Oaks, CA: Sage.

Cohen, J. (1977). *Statistical Power Analysis for the Behavioral Sciences.* New York: Academic Press.

Colaizzi, P.F. (1978). Psychological research as the phenomenologist views it. In R.Valle & M. King (Eds.), *Existential Phenomenological Alternative for Psychology.* New York: Oxford University Press.

Connelly, L., Bott, M., Goffart, N., & Taunton, R. (1997). Methodological triangulation in a study of nurse retention. *Nursing Research, 46*(5), 299–302.

Cook, A.C. (1997). Investigator bias in bereavement research: Ethical and methodological implications. *Canadian Journal of Nursing Research, 29*(4), 87–93.

Corbin, J., & Strauss, A. (1990). Grounded theory research: Procedures, canons, and evaluative criteria, *Qualitative Sociology, 13*(1), 3–21.

Cormack, F.S. (1996). *The Research Process in Nursing* (3rd ed.). London: Blackwell Scientific Publications.

Creswell, J. (1994). *Research Design: Qualitative and Qualitative Approaches.* Thousand Oaks, CA: Sage.

Creswell, J.W. (1998). *Qualitative Inquiry and Research Design: Choosing Among Five Traditions.* London: Sage.

Crookes, P., & Davies, S. (1998). *Research into Practice.* Edinburgh: Billire Tindall.

Davidoff, H. (1953). *A World Treasury of Proverbs.* London: Cassell & Company.

Davis, D.L., & Joakinsen, L. M. (1997). Nerves as status, and nerves as stigma. *Qualitative Health Research, 7*(3), 370–391.

Dawes, M., Davies, P., Gray, A., Mont, J., Seers, K., & Snowball, R. (1999). *Evidence-based Practice: A Primer for Health Professionals.* London: Churchill-Livingston.

Deagle, G., & McWilliam, C. (1992). *Developing Healthy and Supportive Community Environments: A Strategy for Action.* Presented at Prevention Congress V. London, Ontario, 27 April.

Declaration of Helsinki (1986). In R.J. Levive (Ed.), *Ethics and Regulations of Clinical Research* (2nd ed., pp. 427–429). Baltemore-Munide Urban & Schwarzenberg.

Deets, C. (1990). Nursing's paradigm and a search for its methodology. In N. Chaska (Ed.) *The Nursing Profession: Turning Points,* St. Louis, MO: Mosby.

Deets, C. (1998). Nursing—A maturing discipline? *Journal of Professional Nursing, 14*(2), 65.

Deloughery, G.L. (1995). *Issues and Trends in Nursing* (2nd ed.). St. Louis, MI: Mosby.

Denzin, N., & Lincoln, Y. (1994). *Handbook of Qualitative Research.* London: Sage.

Department of Health, Education and Welfare (1973). *Final Report of the Tuskegie Syphilis Study Ad Hoc Advisory Panel.* Washington, D.C.

Deutscher, I. (1966). Words and deeds: Social action and social policy, *Social Problems, 13,* 235–254.

Dickoff, J., James, P., & Weednbach, E. (1968). Theory in a practice discipline: Practice oriented theory (Part 1). *Nursing Research, 17,* 415–435.

Dickson, G. (2000). Aboriginal grandmothers' experience with health promotion and participatory action research. *Qualitative Health Research, 10*(2), 188–213.

Diekleman, N., Allen, D., & Tanner, C. (1989). *The National League for Nursing Criteria for Appraisal for Baccalaureate Programs: A Critical Hermeneutic Analysis.* Publ. No. 15-2253. New York: NLN Press.

Diers, D. (1979). *Research in Nursing Practice.* Philadelphia: J.B. Lippincott.

Dillman, D.A. (1999). *Mail and Electronic Surveys: The Tailored Design Method.* New York: John Wiley & Sons.

Dillman, D.A. (1978). *Mail and Telephone Surveys: The Total Design Method.* New York: John Wiley & Sons.

Dillon, J.T. (1990). *The Practice of Questioning.* New York: Routledge.

Downie, R.S., & Calman, K.C. (1987). *Healthy Respect: Ethics in Health Care.* London: Faber & Faler.

Downs, F. (1984). Elements of a research critique. In Downs, F., & Newman, M. (Eds). *A Sourcebook of Nursing Research* (2nd ed.). Philadelphia: F.A. Davis.

Duffy, M. (1986). Primary prevention behaviors: The female-headed, one-parent family. *Research in Nursing and Health, 9,* 115–122.

Dulock, H. L., & Holzemer, W. L. (1991). Substruction: Improving the linkage from theory and method. *Nursing Science Quarterly, 4*(2), 83–87.

Edwards, M. (1998). *The Internet for Nurses and Allied Health Professionals.* New York: Springer-Verlag.

Edwards, N., Sims-Jones, M., & Breithaupt, K. (1998). Maternal smoking/non-smoking and feeding choice. *Canadian Journal of Nursing Research, 30*(3), 83–99.

Eichler, M. (1988). *Nonsexist Research Methods.* Boston: Allen & Unwin.

Eichner, K., & Habermehl, W. (1981). Predicting response rates to mailed questionnaires, *American Sociological Review, 46,* 361–363.

Emami, A., Torres, S., Lipson, J.G., & Ekman, S. (2000). An ethnographic study of a day care center for Iranian immigrant seniors. *Western Journal of Nursing Research, 22*(2), 169–188.

Erdos, P. L. (1983). *Professional Mail Surveys.* Malabar, Florida: Robert E. Krieger Publishing.

Estabrooks, C.A. (1998). Will evidence-based nursing practice make practice perfect? *Canadian Journal of Nursing Research, 30*(4), 273–295.

Fain, J.A. (1999). *Reading Understanding and Applying Nursing Research: A Text and Workbook.* Philadelphia: F.A. Davis.

Fawcett, J., & Downs, F. (1986). *The Relationship of Theory and Research.* Norwalk, CT: Appleton-Century Crofts.

Fawcett, J. (1999). *The Relationship of Theory and Research.* Philadelphia: F.A. Davis.

Fay, B. (1987). *Critical Social Science: Liberation and Its Limits.* Ithaca, N.Y.: Cornell University Press.

Featherman, D.L., & Stevens, G. (1982). A revised index of occupational status: Application in analysis of sex differences in attainment. In *Social Structure and Behavior: Essays in Honor of William Hamilton Sewell.* New York: Academic Press.

Ferketich, S., & Muller, M. (1990). Factor analysis revisited. *Nursing Research, 39*(1), 59–62.

Festinger, L., Reiken, H.W., & Schachter, S. (1956). *When Prophecy Fails.* New York: Harper & Row.

Feurstein, M. (1988). Finding the methods to fit the people: Training for participatory evaluation. *Community Development Journal, 23,* 16–25.

Field, W.E. (1983). Clinical nursing research: A proposal of standards. *Nursing Leadership,* December 6, 117–120.

Finfgeld, D. (1998). Courage in middle-aged adults with long-term health concerns. *Canadian Journal of Nursing Research, 30*(1), 153–169.

Fisher, D. (1993). Fed up with too many questions, Canadians are hanging up on pollsters, *Montreal Gazette,* (September 24, A8).

Fitzpatrick, J., & Whall, A.L. (1996). *Conceptual Models of Nursing: Analysis and Application.* (3rd ed.), Stamford, CT: Appleton & Lange.

Flaskerud, J., & Nyamathi, A. (2000). Attaining gender and ethnic diversity in health intervention research: Cultural responsiveness versus resource provision. *Advances in Nursing Science, 22*(4), 1–15.

Flynn (1992). The development of the healthy cities project in the US. In J. Ashton (Ed.), *Healthy Cities* (pp. 43–48). Buckingham: Open University Press.

Forcese, D.P., & Richer, S. (1973). *Social Research Methods.* Englewood Cliffs, N.J.: Prentice-Hall.

Forchuk, C. (1994). The orientation phase of the nurse-client relationship: Testing Peplau's theory. *Journal of Advanced Nursing, 20,* 532–537.

Forchuk, C., & Roberts, J. (1993). How to critique qualitative research articles. *Canadian Journal of Nursing Research, 25*(4), 47–57.

Ford-Gilboe, M., & Campbell, J. (1996). The mother headed single parent family: A feminist critique of the nursing literature. *Nursing Outlook, 44,* 173–183.

Fougere, A. (1992). Effects of eating breakfast on grade performance, Antigonish: St. Francis Xavier University, Research Methods Paper, Sociology 300.

Fowler, F.J. (1993). *Survey Research Methods* (2nd ed). Newbury Park, CA: Sage.

Frank-Stromberg, M., & Olsen, S. (1997. *Measurement in Nursing Research* (2nd ed.). Boston, MA: Jones & Bartlett.

Gale, A., Gardner, L., Greer, C., Jackson, N., Jasper, M., Rolfe, G., & Sherwood-Rogers, S. (1998). *An Action Research Project to Develop the Role of the Generic Health Care Support Worker.* 4th Qualitative Health Research Conference, Vancouver, B.C., February 19–21, 1998.

Gates, K.M. (2000). The experience of caring for a loved one: A phenomenological study. *Nursing Science Quarterly, 13*(1), 54–59.

Gates, M.F., & Lackey, N.R. (1998). Youngsters caring for adults with cancer. *Image: Journal of Nursing Scholarship, 30*(1), 11–16.

George, D., & Mallery, P. (2000). *SPSS for Windows Step by Step: A Simple Guide and Reference 9.0 Update* (2nd ed.). Boston: Allyn & Bacon.

George, J.B. (1995). *Nursing Theories: The Base for Professional Nursing Practice* (4th ed.). Norwalk, CT: Appleton & Lange.

Georgi, A. (1985). *Phenomenology and Psychological Research.* Pittsburgh: Duquesne University Press.

Gillis, A.J. (1990). Nurses' knowledge of growth and development principles in meeting the psychosocial needs of hospitalized children. *Journal of Pediatric Nursing, 5*(2), 78–87.

Gillis, A.J., MacLellan, M., & Perry, A. (1998). Competencies of liberal education in post RN baccalaureate students. *Journal of Nursing Education, 37*(9), 408–412.

Gillis, A.J. (1998). *The trends and variations in smoking.* Course paper for Nursing 300, St. Francis Xavier University.

Gillis, A.J. (1993). *The relationship of definition of health, perceived health status, self-efficacy, parental health promoting lifestyle, and selected demographics to health-promoting lifestyle in adduces out females.* Doctoral Dissertation, University of Texas at Austin.

Gillis, A.J. (1994). Determinants of health-promoting lifestyle in adolescent girls. *Canadian Journal of Nursing Research, 26*(2), 13–29.

Gillis, A.J. (1997). The adolescent lifestyle questionnaire: Development and psychometric testing. *Canadian Journal of Nursing Research, 29,*(1), 29–47.

Gillon, R. (1986). *Philosophical Medical Ethics.* Chichester: Wiley.

Glaser, B., & Strauss, A. (1967). *The Discovery of Grounded Theory.* Chicago: Aldine.

Glaser, B. (1978). *Theoretical Sensitivity.* Niel Valley, CA: Sociology Press.

Goffman, E. (1962). *Asylums.* Chicago: Aldine.

Gold, D. (1958). Comment on 'A Critique of Tests of Significance,' *American Sociological Review, 23* (February), 85–86.

Goode, C., Butcher, L., Cipperley, J., Ekstrom, J., Hayes, J., Lovett, M., & Wellendorf, S. (1996). *Research utilization: A study guide.* Ida Grove, Iowa: Horne Video Productions.

Gooding, B.A., Sloan, M., & Gagnon, L. (1993). Important nurse caring behaviors: Perceptions of oncology patients and nurses. *Canadian Journal of Nursing Research, 25*(3), 65–77.

Gott, M., & O'Brien, M. (1990). *The Role of the Nurse in Health Promotion: Policies, Perspectives & Practice.* Milton Keynes, England: Crown Copyright.

Goyder, J., & McKenzie-Leiper, J. (1985c). The decline in survey response: A social values interpretation, *Sociology, 19*(1), 55–71.

Goyder, J.C. (1982). Further evidence on factors affecting response rates to mailed questionnaires, *American Sociological Review, 47,* 550–553.

Goyder, J.C. (1985a). Nonresponse on surveys: A Canada-United States comparison, *Canadian Journal of Sociology, 10,* 231–251.

Goyder, J.C. (1985b). Face-to-face interviews and mailed questionnaires: The net difference in response rate, *Public Opinion Quarterly, 49,* 234–25.

Gray, M., & Smith, L. (1999). The professional socialization of diploma of higher education nursing students (Project 2000): A longitudinal qualitative study. *Journal of Advanced Nursing, 29*(3), 639–647.

Greenberg, M. (1998). *Therapeutic playing: A grounded theory of the utilization of humor within the nurse-client relationship in an acute care setting.* Qualitative Health Research Conference. Hotel Vancouver, Vancouver, BC. February, 1998.

Grunburg, Martha. (1998). *Therapeutic playing: A grounded theory of the Welzation of Humor within the nurse-client relationship in an acute care setting.* 4th QHRC-UBC School of Nursing, Vancouver, BC. Feb 19–21.

Hahn, E.J., Bryant, R., Peden, A., Robinson, K., & Williams, C.A. (1998). Entry into community based nursing practice: Perceptions of prospective employers. *Journal of Professional Nursing, 14*(5), 305–314.

Hall, J.M., & Stevens, P.E. (1991). Rigor in feminist research. *Advances in Nursing Science, 13*(3), 16–29.

Halldórsdótter, S., & Hamrin, E. (1997). Caring and uncaring encounters within nursing and health care from the cancer patient's perspective. *Cancer Nursing, 20*(2), 120–128.

Hamblin, R.L. (1971). Ratio measurement for the social sciences, *Social Forces, 50,* 191–206.

Hammersley, M., & Atkinson, P. (1995). *Ethnography: Principles in Practice* (2nd ed). New York: Routledge.

Hanna, B. (1997). From raw data to chapters via the support of NUD*IST. *Health Infomatics Journal, 3,* 61–65.

Hanson, M.J. (1997). The theory of planned behavior applied to cigarette smoking in African-American, Puerto Rican, and Non-

Hispanic, white teenage females. *Nursing Research, 46*(3), 155–162.

Harding, S. (1987). Is there a feminist method? In Harding S. (Ed.). *Feminism and Methodology.* Bloomington, IN: Indiana University Press.

Harding, S. (1991). *Whose Knowledge? Whose Science? Thinking from Women's Lives.* Ithica, NY: Cornell University Press.

Hart, E., & Bond, M. (1998). *Action Research for Health and Social Care.* Philadelphia: Open University Press.

Harton, H.C., & Latane, B. (1997). Social influence and adolescent lifestyle attitudes. *Journal of Research on Adolescence, 7*(2), 197–220.

Hartrick, G.A. (1997). Women who are mothers: The experience of defining self. *Health Care for Women International, 18,* 263–277.

Havelock, R., & Zlotolow, S. (1995). *The Change Agent's Guide to Innovation in Education* (2nd ed.) Englewood Cliffs, NJ: Educational Technology Publications.

Havelock, R. (1972). *Bibliography on knowledge Utilization and Dissemination.* Ann Arlor, MI: Institute for Social Research.

Healthcare Quest. (1997). *Getting Audit Ready to Benefit Patients.* Romsey.

Heberlein, T.A., & Baumgartner, R. (1978). Factors Affecting Response Rates to Mailed Questionnaires. *American Sociological Review, 43.*

Hinds, P., Vogel, R., & Clarke-Sleffen, L. (1997). The possibilities and pitfalls of doing a secondary analysis of a qualitative data set. *Qualitative Health Research, 7*(3), 408–425.

Hilton, B., Thompson, R., & Moore-Dempsey, L. (2000). Evaluation of the AIDS Prevention Street Nurse Program: One step at a time. *Canadian Journal of Nursing Research, 32* (1), 17–38.

Hochschild, A.R. (1983). *The Managed Heart: Commercialization of Human Feeling.* Berkeley: University of California Press.

Hodges, J.C., Whitten, M.E., Brown, J., & Flick, J. (1994). *Harbrace College Handbook: for Canadian Writers,* (4th ed.). Toronto: Harcourt Brace, Canada.

Holden, C. (1979). Ethics in social science research, *Science, 206* (November), 537–540.

Hollingshead, A. B. (1975). *Four Factor Index of Social Status.* Unpublished manuscript. Yale Station, New Haven, CT. 06520.

Holroyd, E., Katie, F., Chun, L., & Wai Ha, S. (1997). Doing the month: An exploration of postpartum practices in Chinese women. *Health Care for Women International, 18,* 301–313.

Homans, G.C. (1964). Bringing men back in. *American Sociological Review, 29,* 809–818.

Horne Video Productions (1996). *Research utilization: A study guide* (2nd ed.). Ida Grove, Iowa: Author.

Hoskins, C.N. (1988). *The Partner Relationships Inventory.* Palo Alto, CA: Consulting Psychologists Press.

Howell, D.C. (1997). *Statistical Methods for Psychology* (4th ed.). Belmont, CA: Duxbury Press, Wadsworth Publishing.

Huber, P.W. (1991). *Galileo's Revenge: Junkyard Science in the Courtroom.* New York: Basic Books.

Hughes, D. (1998). *The invisible burden: Women's lives with fibromyalgia.* Qualitative Health research Conference, Hotel Vancouver, Vancouver, BC, February, 1998.

Humenick, S., Hill, P., Thompson, J., & Hart, A.M. (1998). Breast-milk sodium as a predictor of breastfeeding patterns. *Canadian Journal of Nursing Research, 30*(3), 67–83.

Humphreys, L. (1970). *Tearoom Trade.* Chicago: Aldine Press.

Humphris, D. (1999). Types of evidence. In S. Hamer & G. Collinson (Eds.), *Achieving Evidence-based Practice: A Handbook for Practitioners.* Edinburgh: Harcourt.

Hyman, H. (1955). *Survey Design and Analysis.* New York: Free Press.

Ibbotson,T. (1999). *An Ethnographic Study of the Diffusion Process of Telemedicine in Scotland.* Middlesex: Brunel University.

Im, E. (2000). A feminist critique of research on women's work and health. *Health Care for Women International, 21,* 105–119.

Im, E., & Meleis, A. (1999). Situation-specific theories: Philosophical routes, properties, and approach. *Advances in Nursing Science, 22*(2) 11–24.

Iowa Model for Research-Based Practice to Promote Quality Care (1994). The University of Iowa.

Israel, G.A. & Shurman, S.U. (1990). Social support, control, and the stress process. In K. Glanz, F. Lewis, & B. Rimer (Eds.) *Health Behavior and Health Education.* San Franciso, CA: Jossey-Bass.

Iversen, G.R., & Norpoth, H. (1976). *Analysis of Variance.* Beverly Hills: Sage.

Jackson, W. (1973). *University Preferences and Perceptions of Pictou County Students.* Antigonish: St Francis Xavier University.

Jackson, W., & Poushinsky, N.W. (1971). *Migration to Northern Mining Communities: Structural and Social Psychological Dimen-*

sions. Winnipeg: Center for Settlement Studies, University of Manitoba.

Jackson, W. (1999). *Methods: Doing Social Research* (2nd ed). Scarborough, Ont.: Prentice Hall (Canada).

Janke, J. (1999). The effects of relaxation therapy on preterm labor outcomes. *Journal of Obstetric, Gynecologic, and Neonatal Nursing, 28,* 255–263.

Janson-Bjerklie, S., Carrieri, V., & Hudes, D. (1986). The sensation of pulmonary dyspnea. *Nursing Research, 35*(3), 154–159.

Jeans, M.E. (1992). Editorial: Clinical significance of research: A growing concern. *Canadian Journal of Nursing Research, 24*(1), 1–2.

Jeans, M.E. (1990). Editorial: Research dollars: Who's passing the buck? *Canadian Journal of Nursing Research, 22*(3), 1–2.

Kachigan, S.K. (1986). *Statistical Analysis: An Interdisciplinary Introduction to Univariate & Multivariate Methods.* New York: Radius Press.

Kalisch, B.J., Kalisch, P.A., & Belcher, B. (1985). Forecasting for nursing policy: A news-based image approach. *Nursing Research, 34*(1), 44–49.

Kalischuk, R. (1998). *Family healing following adolescent suicide.* Qualitative Health Research Conference, Hotel Vancouver, Vancouver, BC, February, 1998.

Kang, D., Coe, C., Karaszewski, J., & McCarthy, D. (1998). Relationship of social support to stress responses and immune function in healthy and asthmatic adolescents. *Research in Nursing and Health, 21,* 117–128.

Kaviani, N., & Stillwell, Y. (2000). An evaluative study of clinical preceptorship. *Nurse Education Today, 20,* 218–226.

Kerlinger, F.N. (1973). *Foundations of Behavioral Research.* New York: Holt, Rinehart & Winston.

Kerlinger, F.N. (1986). Foundations of behavioral research (3rd ed.). New York: Holt, Rinehart, and Wilson.

Kerr, J., & MacPhail, J. (1996). *Canadian Nursing: Issues and Perspectives* (3rd ed.). St. Louis: Mosby.

Kidd, P., & Parshall, M. (2000). Getting the focus and the group: Enhancing analytical rigor in focus group research. *Qualitative Health Research, 10*(3), 293–308.

Kikchi, J., Polivka, B., & Stevenson, J. (1991). Triangulation: Operational definitions. *Nursing Research, 40,* 364–366.

Killien, M.G. (1998). Postpartum mothers' return to work: Mothering stress, anxiety, and gratification. *Canadian Journal of Nursing Research, 30*(3), 53–67.

Kimchi, J., & Simmons, H. (1994). *Developing a Philosophy of Nursing.* Lincoln: Sage.

Kinnear, P., & Gray, C. (1999). *SPSS for Windows Made Simple* (3rd ed.). East Sussex, UK: Psychology Press.

Kinzel, C. (1992). *The Alberta Survey 1992: Sampling Report.* The University of Alberta: Population Research Laboratory.

Kish, L. (1965). *Survey Sampling.* New York: Wiley.

Klein, R.D. (1983). How to do what we want to do: Thoughts about feminist methodology. In Bowles, G., & Klein, R.D. (Eds.) *Theories of Women's Studies* (pp. 88–104). London: RKP.

Klostermann, B., Perry, C., & Britto, M. (2000). Quality improvement in a school health program. *Evaluation and the Health Professions, 23*(1), 91–106.

Knafl, K., & Howard, M. (1984). Interpreting and reporting qualitative research. *Research in Nursing and Health, 7,* 17–24.

Konrad, T. R., & DeFriese, G. (1990). On the subject of sampling. *American Journal of Health Promotion, 5*(2), 147–153.

Krahn, H. (1991). Sociological methods of research. In L. Tepperman and R. Jack Richardson (Eds.), *The Social World: An Introduction to Sociology.* Toronto: McGraw-Hill Ryerson, pp. 34–66.

Kulig, J., & Thorpe, K. (1996). Teaching and learning needs of culturally diverse post RN students. *Canadian Journal of Nursing Research, 28*(2), 119–125.

LaPiere, R.T. (1934). Attitudes vs. actions, *Social Forces, 13,* 230–237.

Larson, P. (1981). Oncology patients and professional nurses' perception of important caring behaviors. (Doctoral dissertation, University of California, San Francisco, 1981). *Dissertation Abstracts International, 42,* 568B.

Larson, P. (1984). Important nurse caring behaviors perceived by patients with cancer. *Oncology Nurses Forum, 11,* 46–50.

Lastrucci, C.L. (1967). *The Scientific Approach.* Cambridge, MA: Schenkman Publishing.

Lather, P. (1993). Fertile obsession: Validity after post structuralism. *Sociological Quarterly, 34,* 673–693.

LeCompte, M.D., & Goetz, J.P. (1982). Problems of reliability and validity in ethnographic research. *Review of Educational Research, 52*(1), 31–60.

Lederman, R., & Miller, D. (1998). Adaptation to pregnancy in three different ethnic groups: Latin American, African-American, & Anglo-American. *Canadian Journal of Nursing Research, 30*(3), 37–53.

Lee, K.H. (1997). Korean urban women's experience of menopause: New life. *Health Care for Women International, 18,* 139–148.

Lee, M. (1992). *Smoking Behaviours.,* Antigonish: St. Francis Xavier University (Research methods paper).

Leenerts, M., & Magilvy, J. (2000). Investing is self-care: A midrange theory of self-care grounded in the lived experience of low-income HIV-positive white women. *Advances in Nursing Science, 22*(3), 58–75.

Leininger, M. (1970). *Nursing and Anthropology: Two Worlds to Blend.* New York: John Wiley & Sons.

Leininger, M. (1978). *Transcultural Nursing: Concepts Theories and Practices.* New York: John Wiley & Sons.

Leininger, M. (1985). *Qualitative Research Methods in Nursing.* Orlando, FL: Freene & Atratton.

Leininger, M. (1991). *Culture Care Diversity and Universality: A Theory of Nursing.* New York, NY: National League for Nursing Press.

Leininger, M. (1990). Ethnomethods: The philosophic and epistemic bases to explicate transcultural nursing knowledge. *Journal of Transculteral Nursing, 1,* 40–51.

Lenz, E.R., Pugh, L.C., Milligan, R.A., Gift, A., & Suppe, F. (1995). Collaborative development of middle-range nursing theories: Toward a theory of unpleasant symptoms. *Advances in Nursing Science, 17,* 1–13.

Lenz, E.R., Pugh, L.C., Milligan, R.A., Gift, A., & Suppe, F. (1997). The middle range theory of unpleasant symptoms: An update. *Advances in Nursing Science, 19,* 14–27.

Levin, J., & Fox, J.A. (1991). *Elementary Statistics in Social Research,* (5th ed.). New York: HarperCollins.

Lewin, K. (1951). *Field Theory in Social Sciences.* New York: Harper & Row.

Likert, R. (1931). A technique for the measurement of attitudes. *Archives of Psychology.* New York: Columbia University Press.

Lincoln, Y., & Guba, E.G. (1994). Competing paradigms in Qualitative Research. In N.K. Denzin & Y.S. Lincoln (Eds.), *Handbook of Qualitative Research* (pp. 105–117). Thousand Oaks, CA: Sage.

Lincoln, Y., & Guba, E.G. (1985). *Naturalistic Inquiry.* Beverly Hills, CA: Sage.

Lincoln, Y.S., & Guba, E.G. (1981). *Effective Evaluation: Improving the Effectiveness of Evaluation Results Through Responsive and Naturalistic Approaches.* San Francisco: Josey-Bass.

Lincoln, Y.S. (1995). Emerging criteria for quality in qualitative and interpretive research. *Qualitative Inquiry, 1,* 275–289.

Lindeman, C.A. (1975). Priorities in clinical nursing research. *Nursing Outlook, 23,* 693–698.

Lindsey, E., & Stafduhar, K. (1998). From rhetoric to action: Establishing community participation in AIDS-related research. *Canadian Journal of Nursing Research, 30*(1), 137–153.

LoBiondo-Wood, G., & Haber, J. (1998). *Nursing Research: Methods Critical Appraisal and Utilization* (4th ed). St. Louis: Mosby.

Lodge, M. (1981). *Magnitude Scaling: Quantitative Measurement of Opinions.* Beverly Hills: Sage.

Long, E.R., Suppe, F., Gift, A., Pugh, L.C., & Milligan, R.A. (1995). Collaborative development of middle-range nursing theories: Toward a theory of unpleasant symptoms. *Advances in Nursing Science, 17,* 1–13.

MacDonald, L. (1991). Attitudes toward the elderly (Research Methods Paper). Antigonish: St. Francis Xavier University.

MacKinnon, M. (1997). What a difference a nurse makes—Then and now. *Western Journal of Nursing Research, 19*(6), 795–801.

MacLeod, C.J., & Hockey, L. (1989). *Further Research for Nursing.* London: Scutari-Press

Malinozwski, B. (1925). *Magic, Science and Religion.* New York: Doubleday.

Manson-Singer, S. (1994). The Canadian health communities' project: Creating a social movement. In A. Pederson, M. O'Neil & I. Rootman (Eds.), *Health Promotion in Canada,* Toronto: WB Saunders.

Marshall, C., & Rossman, G.B. (1995). *Designing Qualitative Research* (2nd ed.). Thousand Oaks, CA: Sage.

Martof, E. (2000). Personal communication with authors.

Martin, D. W. (1991). *Doing Psychology Experiments* (3rd ed.). Pacific Grove: Brooks/Cole Publishing Company.

Massey, V.H. (1995). *Nursing Research* (2nd ed.). Springhouse, PA: Springhouse.

Mason, C., Orr, J., Harrisson, S., & Moore, R. (1999). Health professionals perspective on service delivery in two Northern Ireland communities. *Journal of Advanced Nursing, 30*(4), 827–834.

Masterson, A. (1996). *Clarifying Theory for Practice: Study Guide. Distance Learning.* London: Royal College of Nursing.

Mawdsley, C. (1997). Study says critical care nurses quick to aid in death of terminally ill: A research critique. *CACCN, 8*(2), 8–11.

Maynard-Tucker, G. (2000). Conducting focus groups in developing countries: Skill training for local bilingual facilitators. *Qualitative Health Research, 10*(3), 396–410.

McDonald & Daly cited in Parahoo. (1997).

McEwen, M. (1993). The health motivation assessment and inventory. *Western Journal Nursing Research, 15*(6), 770–776.

McKay, L., & Diem, L. (1995). Health concerns of adolescent girls. *Journal of Pediatric Nursing, 10*(1), 19–27.

McQueen, D. (1994). *Health Promotion Research in Canada: A European/British Perspective.* In A. Pederson, M. O'Neill, & I. Rootman (Eds.). *Health Promotion in Canada.* Toronto: W.B. Saunders.

Mead, G.H. (1934). *Mind, Self, and Society.* Chicago: University of Chicago Press.

Mead, M. (1935). *Sex and Temperament in Three Primitive Societies.* New York: Morrow.

Meehan, T.C. (1998). Therapeutic touch as a nursing intervention. *Journal of Advanced Nursing, 28*(1), 117–125.

Meerabeau, L. (1992). Tacit nursing knowledge: An untapped resource or a methodological headache? *Journal of Advanced Nursing, 17,* 108–112.

Meleis, A. (1991). *Theoretical Nursing: Developments and Progress* (2nd ed.). Philadelphia: Lippincott.

Meleis, A. (1997). *Theoretical Nursing: Development and Progress* (3rd ed.). Philadelphia: Lippincott.

Meyer, J.E. (1993). New paradigm research in practice: The trials and tribulations of action research. *Journal of Advanced Nursing, 18,* 1066–1072.

Miles, M., & Huberman, M. (1994). *Qualitative Data Analysis.* Thousand Oaks, CA: Sage.

Mill, J.S. (1925). *A System of Logic* (8th ed.). London: Lognmans, Green and Co.

Miller, D. C. (1977). *Handbook of Research Design and Social Measurement* (3rd ed). New York: Longman.

Mishel, M., & Murdaugh, C. (1987). Family adjustment to heart transplantation: Redesigning the dream. *Nursing Research, 36*(6), 332–338.

Mitchell, G. (1994). Intuitive knowing: Exposing a myth in theory development. *Nursing Science Quarterly, 7*(1), 2–3.

Mitchell, M., & Jolley, J. (2000). *Research Design Explained* (4th ed.). Orlando: Harcourt Brace Jovanovitch College Publishers.

Monette, D.R., Sullivan, T.J., & DeJong, C.R. (1990). *Applied Social Research: Tool for the Human Services* (2nd ed.). Fort Worth: Holt, Rinehart and Winston.

Montgomery, K. (2000). Getting organized: Qualitative data collection. *Applied Nursing Research, 13*(2), 103–104.

Moody, L. E., Wilson, M. E., Smyth, K., Tittle, M., & Vancott, M. L. (1988). Analysis of a decade of nursing practice research: 1977–1986. *Nursing Research, 37,* 374–379.

Moore, P.A. (1995). The utilization of research in practice. *Professional Nurse, 10,* 536–537.

Morris, R. (1996). The culture of female circumcision. *Advances in Nursing Science, 19*(2), 43–53.

Morris, J., Penrod, J., & Hupcey, J. (2000). Qualitative outcome analysis: Evaluating nursing interventions for complex clinical phenomena. *Journal of Nursing Scholarship, 32* (2), 125–130.

Morrison, E.F. (1998). Enormous beliefs about research held by staff nurses. *The Journal of Continuing Education in Nursing, 29*(5), 196–203.

Morse, J. (1991). *Qualitative Nursing Research: A Contemporary Dialogue.* Newbury Park, CA: Sage.

Morse, J. (1992). The power of induction. *Qualitative Health Research, 2*(1), 3–6.

Morse, J. (1998). *Qualitative Methods: The State of the Art.* Keynote address presented at the 4th Qualitative Health Research Conference, Vancouver, British Columbia, February 19– 21, 1998.

Morse, J. M., & Field, P.A. (1995). *Qualitative Research Methods for Health Professionals.* Thousand Oaks: Sage.

Morris, J., Penrod, J., & Hupcey, J. (2000). Qualitative outcome analysis: Evaluating nursing interventions for complex clinical phenomena. *Journal of Nursing Scholarship, 32* (2), 125–130.

Morton, J. (1994). The clinical usefulness of breast milk sodium in the assessment of lactogenesis. *Pediatrics, 93,* 802–886.

Moustaka, C. (1994). *Phenomenological Research Methods.* Thousand Oaks, CA: Sage.

Mueller, C. (2000). Personal communication to authors.

Munhall, P.L., & Boyd, C.O. (1993). *Nursing Research. A Qualitative Perspective.* New York: National League for Nursing Press.

Munhall, P.L. (1988). Ethical considerations in qualitative research. *Western Journal of Nursing Research, 10*(2), 150–162.

Munhall, P.L., & Oiler, C.J. (1986). *Nursing Research: A Qualitative Perspective.* Norwalk, CT: Appleton-Century-Crofts.

Munro, B.H. (2001). *Statistical Methods for Health Care Research* (4th ed.). Philadelphia: Lippincott.

Munro, B., & Page, E. (1993). *Statistical Methods for Health Care Research*. Philadelphia: J.B. Lippincott.

Murray (1999). Unwanted intimacy in female university students (Research Methods Paper). Antigonish: St. Francis Xavier University.

Musial, C.M., Jones, S.L., & Warner, C.D. (1998). Structural equation modeling and its relationship to multiple regression and factor analysis. *Research in Nursing & Health, 21,* 271–281.

National Health Services (NHS) (1998). *Changing Clinical Practice*. Leeds, England: Department of Health.

National Health Services (NHS) (1998). *Achieving effective practice: A clinical effectiveness and research information pack for nurses, midwives and health visitors*. Leeds, England: Department of Health.

Nelms, T. (2000). The practices of mothering in caregiving an adult son with AIDS, *Advances in Nursing Science, 22*(3), 46–57.

Neter, J., Wasserman, W., & Kutner, M. (1985). *Applied Linear Statistical Models*. Homewood, IL: Irwin.

Neuberger, J. (1992*). Ethics and health care. The role of researcher ethics committees in the U.K.* London: Kings Fund Institute.

Nilson, K., Nordstrom, G., Krusebrant, A., & Bjorvell, H. (2000). Perceptions of research utilization: Comparisons between health care professionals, nursing students, and a reference group of nurse clinicians. *Journal of Advanced Nursing, 31*(1), 99–109.

Norbuck, J.S., Lindsay, A.M., & Carrieri, V.L. (1982). Further development of the norbrick social support questionnaire: Normative data and validity testing. *Nursing Research, 32*(1), 4–9.

Norwood, S.L. (2000). *Research Strategies for Advanced Practice Nurses*. Upper Saddle River, NJ: Prentice Hall Health.

Nunnally, J.C. (1978). *Psychometric Theory* (2nd ed). New York: McGraw-Hill.

Nuremburg Code (1949). In R.J. Levine (Ed.), (1986). *Ethics and Regulation of Clinical Research,* (2nd ed., pp 425–426). Baltimore, Munich: Urban & Schwarzenberg.

Oakley, A. (1989). Who's afraid of the randomized control trial? Some dilemmas of the scientific method and good research practice. *Women and Health, 15*(4), 25–59.

Oakley, A. (1981). Interviewing women: A contradiction in terms. In H. Roberts (Ed.), *Feminist Research Methods: Exemplary Readings in the Social Sciences* (pp. 44–62). San Francisco: West View Press.

Oates, K. (1997). Models of planned change and research to product evaluation. *Clinical Nurse Specialist, 1*(6), 270–273.

O'Connell, K. (2000). If you call me names, I'll call you numbers. *Journal of Professional Nursing, 16*(2), 74.

O'Connell, A. (2000). Sampling for Evaluation. *Evaluation & the Health Professions, 23*(2), 212–234.

Ogden-Burke, S., Kauffman, E., Costello, E., Wiskin, N., & Harrison, M. (1998). Stressors in families with a child with a chronic condition. *Canadian Journal of Nursing Research, 30*(1), 71–97.

Olesen, V. (1994). Feminism's and models of qualitative research. In NK. Denzin & Y.S. Lincoln (Eds.). *Handbook of Qualitative Research* (pp. 158–174). Thousand Oaks, CA: Sage.

Oliver, S., & Redfern, S. (1991). Interpersonal communication between nurses and elderly patients: Refinement of an observation schedule. *Journal of Advanced Nursing, 16,* 30–38.

Onyskiw, J. (1996). The meta-analytic approach to research integration. *Canadian Journal of Nursing Research, 28*(3), 69–85.

Omery, A. (1983). Phenomenology: A method for nursing research. *Advances in Nursing Science, 5*(2), 49–63.

Orem, D. (1995). *Nursing: Concepts of Practice* (5th ed.). St Louis: Mosby.

Orne, M. T. (1962). On the social psychology of the psychological experiment: With particular reference to demand characteristics and their implications. *American Psychologist, 17,* 76–83.

Orne, R., Fishman, S., Manka, M., & Pagnozzi, M. (2000). Living on the edge: A phenomenological study of medically uninsured working Americans. *Research in Nursing and Health, 23*(23), 204–212.

Osgood, C.E., Suci, G.J., & Tannenbaum, P.H. (1957). *The Measurement of Meaning*. Urbana: University of Illinois Press.

Pallikkathayil, L., Crighton, F., & Aaronson, L. (1998). Balancing ethical quandaries with scientific rigor: Part I. *Western Journal of Nursing Research, 20*(3), 388–393.

Palo-Bengtson, L., & Ekman, S. (1997). Social dancing in the care of persons with dementia in a nursing home setting: A phenomenological study. *Scholarly Inquiry for Nursing Practice: An International Journal, 11*(2), 101–118.

Paltiel, F., Ross, E., & Neill, M. (1998). Coming of

age in the metropolis: The Toronto experience. *The Canadian Nurse, 94*(10), 22–30.

Palys, T. (1992*). Research Decisions: Quantitative and Qualitative Perspectives.* Toronto: Harcourt Brace Jovanovitch Canada.

Parahoo, K. (1997). *Nursing Research: Principles, Process and Issues.* London: MacMillan Press.

Parahoo, K. (2000). Barriers to and facilitators of research utilization among nurses in Northern Ireland. *Journal of Advanced Nursing, 31*(1), 89–98.

Parse, R. (1987). *Nursing Science: Major Paradigms, Theories and Critiques.* Philadelphia, PA: Saunders.

Parse, R., Coyne, A.B., & Smith, M.J. (1985). *Nursing Research: Qualitative Methods.* Bowie, MD: Brady.

Parse, R.R. (1992). Human becoming: Parse's theory of nursing. *Nursing Science Quarterly, 5,* 35–42.

Parse, R.R. (1993). The experience of laughter: A phenomenological study. *Nursing Science Quarterly, 6*(1), 39–43.

Parse, R.R. (1994). Quality of life: Sciencing and living the art of human becoming. *Nursing Science Quarterly, 7,* 16–20.

Parsons, K. (1997). The male experience of caregiving for a family member with Alzheimer's disease. *Qualitative Health Research, 7*(3), 391–408.

Patterson, G., & Zderad, L.T. (1976). *Humanistic Nursing.* New York: John Wiley & Sons.

Pederson, A., O'Neill, M., & Rootman, I. (1994). *Health Promotion in Canada: Provincial, National and International Perspectives.* Philadelphia, PA: W.B. Saunders.

Pence, G.E. (1990). *Classic Cases in Medical Ethics.* London: McGraw-Hill.

Pender, N.J. (1987). *Health Promotion in Nursing Practice* (2nd ed.). Norwalk, CT: Appleton & Lange.

Pender, N.J. (1996). *Health Promotion in Nursing Practice* (3rd ed.). Stanford, CT: Appleton & Lange.

Peplau, H. (1988). *Interpersonal Relations in Nursing* (reissued). London: MacMillan Education.

Peplau, H.E. (1987). Psychiatric skills, tomorrow's world. *Nursing Times, 83,* 29–33.

Peplau, H.E. (1992). Interpersonal relations: A theoretical framework for application in nursing practice. *Nursing Science Quarterly, 5,* 13–18.

Piliavin, J.A., & Piliavin, I.M. (1972). Effect of blood on reactions to a victim, *Journal of Personality and Social Psychology, 23,* 353–361.

Pineo, P.C., & Porter, J. (1967). Occupational prestige in Canada. *Canadian Review of Sociology and Anthropology,* 24–40.

Polit, D. (1996). *Data Analysis and Statistics for Nursing Research.* Stanford, CT: Appleton-Lange.

Polit, D., & Hungler, B. (1999). *Nursing Research: Principles and Methods* (6th ed.) Philadelphia, PA: J. B. Lippincott.

Polit, D.F., & Sherman, R.E. (1990). Statistical power in nursing research. *Nursing Research, 39*(6), 365–369.

Porter, C., Oakley, D., Ronis, D., & Neal, W. (1996). Pathways of influence on fifth and eighth graders report about having had sexual intercourse. *Research in Nursing and Health, 19,* 193–204.

Pranulis, M. (1997). Nurses' roles in protecting human subjects. *Western Journal of Nursing Research, 19*(1), 130–136.

Pringle, D. (1999). Another twist on the double helix: Research and practice. *Canadian Journal of Nursing Research, 30*(4), 165–181.

Public Citizen (1997). 'Dangerously flawed' AIDS research criticized. *http://japan.cnn.com/HEALTH/9704122/AIDS.*

Punch, M. (1986). *The Politics and Ethics of Fieldwork.* Sage: London.

Punches, N. (1996). *QSR NUD*IST User Guide* (2nd ed.). Thousand Oaks, CA: Sage.

QSR NUD*IST User Guide (1997). Thousand Oaks, CA: Sage.

Querker, A. (1997). Longitudinal research using computerized clinical databases: Caveats and constraints. *Nursing Research, 46*(6), 353–355.

Ratner, P., Johnson, J., & Jeffery, B. (1998). Examining emotional, physical, social, and spiritual health as determinants of self-rated health status. *American Journal of Health Promotion, 12*(4), 275–282.

Reifsnider, E. (1998). Follow-up study of children with growth deficiency. *Western Journal of Nursing Research, 20*(1), 14–29.

Reinharz, S. (1992). *Feminist Methods in Social Research.* New York, NY: Oxford University Press.

Reynolds, P.D. (1982). *Ethics and Social Science Research.* Englewood Cliffs: Prentice-Hall.

Ribbens, J. (1989). Interviewing—An unnatural situation? *Women's Studies International Forum, 12*(6), 579–592.

Richards, T., & Richards, L. (1994). Using computers in qualitative analysis. In N. Denzin & Y. Lincoln (Eds.), *Handbook of Qualitative Research.* Thousand Oaks, CA: Sage.

Rittman, M., Page, P., Rivera, J., Stuphin, L., & Godown., I. (1997). Phenomenological study of nurses caring for dying patients. *Cancer Nursing, 20*(2), 115–119.

Ritzer, G. (1988). *Sociological Theory* (2nd ed.). New York: Alfred A. Knopf.

Roberts, C.A., & Burke, S.O. (1989). Nursing research: A quantitative and qualitative approach. Boston, MA: Jones & Bartlett.

Robinson, R.R. (1997). Issues in clinical nursing research: You & research = nursing practice program. *WJNR, 19*(2), 265–269.

Roethlisberger, F.J., & Dickson, W.J. (1939). *Management and the Worker.* Cambridge, MA: Harvard University Press.

Rogers, E.M., & Shoemaker, F.F. (1971). *Communication of Innovations: A Cross-Cultural Approach.* New York: The Free Press.

Rogers, E.M. (1995). *Diffusion Innovations* (4th ed.). New York: Free Press.

Rosenbaum, J., & Carty, L. (1996). The sub culture of adolescence: Beliefs about care health and individuation within Leininger's theory. *Journal of Advanced Nursing, 23,* 741–746.

Rosenthal, R. (1966). *Experimenter Effects in Behavioral Research.* New York: Century.

Rosenthal, R., & Fode, K.L. (1963). The effect of experimenter bias on the performance of the albino rat. *Behavioral Science, 8,* 183–189.

Rosenthal, R. (1984). *Meta-analytic Procedures for Social Research: Applied Social Research Methods.* London: Sage.

Rosenthal, R., & Rosnow, R.L. (1991). *Essentials of Behavioural Research: Methods and Data Analysis* (2nd ed.). New York: McGraw-Hill.

Rossman, G.B., & Wilson, B.L. (1985). Numbers and words: Combining quantitative and qualitative methods in a single large-scale evolution study. *Evaluation Review, 9*(5), 627–643.

Rothe, J.P. (1994). *Qualitative Research: A Practical Guide.* Heidelberg, Ontario: RCI Publications.

Rothman, D. J. (1982). Were Tuskegee and Willowbrook studies in nature? *Hastings Center Report, 12*(2), 5–7.

Sandelowski, M. (1986). The Problem of Rigor in Qualitative Research, *Advances in Nursing Science, 8*(3), 27–37.

Sandelowski, M., & Pollack, S. (1986). Qualitative analysis: What it is and how to begin. *Research in Nursing and Health, 18,* 371–375.

Sandelowski, M. (1993). Rigor or rigor mortis: The problem of rigor in qualitative research revisited. *Advances in Nursing Science, 16* (2), 1–8.

Sandelowski, M. (1995). On the aestehtics of qualitative research. *Image: Journal of Nrusing Scholarship, 27*(3), 205–209.

Sandelowski, M. (2000). Combing qualitative and quantitative sampling, data collection, and analysis techniques in mixed method studies. *Research in Nursing and Health, 23,* 246–255.

Savage, J. (2000). Participant observation: Standing in the shoes of others? *Qualitative Health Research, 10*(3), 324–339.

Sayre, J. (2000). The patient's diagnosis: Explanatory models of mental illness. *Qualitative Health Research, 10*(1), 71–83.

Schmitt, R. (1972). Phenomenology. In Paul Edwards (Ed.). *The Encyclopedia of Philosophy, 6,* (pp. 135–151). New York: Nacullian/Free Press.

Schwartz, H., & Jacobs, J. (1979). *Qualitative Sociology: A Method to the Madness.* New York: The Free Press.

Schwarz, M., Landis, S.E., Rowe, J.E., Janes, C.L., & Pullman, N. (2000). Using focus groups to assess primary care patient's satisfaction. *Evaluation & the Health Professions, 23*(1), 58–71.

Seaman, C. (1987). *Research Methods: Principles, Practice and Theory for Nursing.* Norwalk, CT: Appleton & Lange.

Sennott-Miller, L., & C. Miller (1986). Magnitude estimation: Issues and practical applications. *Western Journal of Nursing Research, 8,* 31–40.

Sheppard, R. (1993). Yes, no, undecided or just hangs up? *Globe and Mail, August 23,* p. A11.

Sherman, D.W. (1996). Nurses willingness to care for AIDS patients and spirituality, social support, and death anxiety. *Image, 28*(3), 205–213.

Sherrod, R. A. (1998). Infertility education in baccalaureate schools of nursing. *Journal of Nursing Education, 37*(9), 412–415.

Shields, S.A. (1988). Functionalism, Darwinism, and the psychology of women: A study in social myth. In Ludy T. Benjamin, Jr., (1988) *A History of Psychology.* New York: McGraw-Hill.

Silva, M. (1986). Research testing nursing theory: State of the art. *Advances in Nursing Science's, 90,* 1–11.

Silverman, D. (1993). *Interpreting Qualitative Data: Methods for Analysing Talk, Text, and Interaction.* London: Sage.

Silverman, D. (1997). *Qualitative Research: Theory, Method and Practice.* London: Sage.

Simon, J.L., & Burstein, P. (1885). *Basic Research Methods in Social Science* (3rd ed.). New York: Random House.

Smeenk, F. W., deWitte, L. P., vanHaastregt, J. C., Schipper, R. M., Biezemanus, H. P., & Crebolder, H. F. (1998). Transmural care of terminal cancer patients: Effects on the quality of life of direct caregivers. *Nursing Research, 47*(3), 129–136.

Smith, D. E. (1987). *The Everyday World as Problematic: A Feminist Sociology.* Toronto: University of Toronto Press.

Smith, P. (1997*). Research Mindedness for Practice: An Interactive Approach for Nursing and Health Care.* New York: Churchill Livingstone.

Smith. (1991). *Strategies of Social Research* (3rd ed.). St. Louis: Holt, Rivehart, & Winston.

Solchany, J.E. (1998). Anticipating the adopted child: Women's preadoptive experiences. *Canadian Journal of Nursing Research, 30*(3), 123–129.

Sparkes, S., & Rizzoloo, M. (1998). World wide web search tools. *Image: Journal of Nursing Scholarship, 30*(2), 167–171.

Spiegelberg, H. (1975). *The Phenomenological Movement.* The Hague, Netherlands: Martinus Nijhoff.

Spradley, J.P. (1979). *The Ethnographic Interview.* New York: Holt, Rinehart and Winston.

Spradley, J.P. (1980). *Participant Observation.* San Diego, CA: Harcourt Brace College Publishers.

SPSS. (1999). *SPSS Advanced Models 10.0.* Chicago: SPSS Inc.

SPSS. (1999). *SPSS Base 10.0 Applications Guide.* Chicago: SPSS Inc.

SPSS Inc. (1999). *SPSS Base 10.0 User's Guide.* Chicago: SPSS Inc.

SPSS. (1999). *SPSS 10.0 Syntax Reference Guide.* Chicago: SPSS Inc.

Statistical Abstract of the United States (1994). Washington, DC: US Government Printing Office.

Sterling, T.D. (1959). Publication decisions and their possible effects on inferences drawn from tests of significance—or vice versa. *Journal of the American Statistical Association, 54,* 30–34.

Sterling, T.D., Rosenbaum, W.L., & Weinkam, J.J. (1995). Publication decisions revisited: The effect of the outcome of statistical tests on the decision to publish and vice versa. *The American Statistician, 49,* 108–112.

Stern, P. (1998). Grounded theory workshop II. *Qualitative Health Research Conference,* Vancouver, British Columbia, February 19–21.

Stern, P.N. (1980). Grounded theory methodology: Its uses and process. *Image, 12*(1), 20–23.

Stetler, C. B. (1994). Refinement of the Stetler/Marram Model for application of research findings to practice. *Nursing Outlook, 42*(1), 18–20.

Stetz, K.M., & Brown, M.A. (1997). Taking care: Care giving to persons with cancer and AIDS. *Cancer Nursing, 20*(1), 12–22.

Stevens, B., Stockwell, M., Browne, G., Dent, P., Gafini, A., Martin, R., & Anderson, M. (1995). Evaluation of a home-based traction program for children. *Canadian Journal of Nursing Research, 27*(4), 133–151.

Stevens, B.J. (1984). *Nursing Theory: Analysis, Application and Evaluation* (2nd ed.). Boston: Little, Brown.

Stevens, P.E., & Hall, J.M. (1992). Applying critical theories to nursing in communities. *Public Health Nursing, 9(*1), 2–9.

Stevens, S.S. (1966a). A metric for the social consensus, *Science, 151,* 530–41.

Stevens, S.S. (1966b). Matching functions between loudness and ten other continua. *Perception and Psychophysics, 1,* 5–8.

Stevens, S.S. (1951). Mathematics, measurement, and psychophysics. In S.S. Stevens (ed.), *Handbook of Experimental Psychology.* New York: Wiley.

Stevenson, B., Mills, E. M., Welin, L., & Beal, K. (1998). Falls risk factors in an acute care setting: A retrospective study. *Canadian Journal of Nursing Research, 30*(1), 97–113.

Stewart, M.J., Gillis, A., Brosky, G., Johnson, G., Kirkland, S., Leigh, G., Persaud, V., Rootman, I., Jackson, S., & Pawliw-Fry, B.A. (1996). Smoking among disadvantaged women: Causes and cessation. *Canadian Journal of Nursing Research, 28,* 41–60.

Stewart. M.J., Doble, S., Hart, G., Langille, L., & MacPherson, K. (1998). Peer visitor support for family caregivers of seniors with stroke. *Canadian Journal of Nursing Research, 30*(2), 87–117.

Strauss, A., & Corbin, J. (1990). *Basics of Qualitative Research: Grounded Theory Procedures and Techniques.* Newbury Park, CA: Sage.

Strauss, A., & Corbin, J. (1997). *Grounded Theory in Practice.* Thousand Oaks, CA: Sage.

Streubert, H., & Carpenter, D. (1995). *Qualitative Research in Nursing: Advancing the Humanistic Imperative.* Philadelphia: J.B. Lippincott.

Streubert, H., & Carpenter, D. (1999). *Qualitative Research in Nursing: Advancing the Humanistic Imperative* (2nd ed.). Philadelphia: J. B. Lippincott.

Streubert, H.J. (1991). Phenomenological research as a theoretic initiative in community health nursing. *Public Health Nursing, 8*(2), 119–123.

Strunk, W., & White, E.B. (2000). *The Elements of Style.* Galt, Ontario: Brett-MacMillan.

Sudman, S. (1967). *Reducing the Cost of Surveys.* Chicago: Aldine Publishing.

Sudman, S. (1976). *Applied Sampling.* New York: Academic Press.

Sudman, S., & Bradburn, N. (1983). *Asking Questions.* San Francisco: Jossey-Bass.

Sussman, S., Burton, D., Dent, C.W., Stacy, A.W., & Flay, B.R. (1991). Use of focus groups in developing an adolescent tobacco use cessation program: Collection norm effects. *Journal of Applied Social Psychology, 21,* 1772–1782.

Sykes, G.M. (1968). *The Society of Captives.* New York: Atheneum.

Teevan, J. J. (2000). *Introduction to Sociology: A Canadian Focus,* (7th ed.). Scarborough: Prentice-Hall Canada.

Thibaut, J.W., & Kelley, H.H. (1959). *The Social Psychology of Groups.* New York: Wiley.

Thomas, S. (2000). *How to Write Health Sciences Papers, Dissertations and Theses.* New York: Harcourt.

Travelbee, J. (1971). *Interpersonal Aspects of Nursing* (2nd ed.). Philadelphia: F.A. Davis.

Travers, K. (1997). Reducing inequities through participatory research and community empowerement. *Health Education and Behavior 24*(3), 344–356.

Tri-Council (1998). TriCouncil Policy Statement: *Ethical Conduct for Research Involving Humans.* Ottawa: Author.

Trost, S., Pate, R., Saunders, R., Ward, D., Dowda, M., & Felton, G. (1997). A prospective study of the determinants of physical activity in rural fifth-grade children. *Preventive Medicine, 26,* 257–263.

Tuck, I., Harris, L., Renfro, T., & Lexvold, L. (1998). Care: A value expressed in philosophies of nursing services. *Journal of Professional Nursing, 14*(2), 92–97.

UKCC(1993). *Code of Professional Conduct for the Nurse, Midwife, and Health Visitor.* London: United Kingdom Central Council.

Unger, J., Kipe, M., Simon, T., Johnson, C., Montgomery, S., & Iverson, E. (1998). Stress, coping, and social support among homeless youth. *Journal of Adolescent Research, 13*(2), 154–157.

Van Kaam, A. (1959). A phenomenological analysis exemplified by the feeling of being really understood. *Individual Psychology, 15,* 66–72.

Van Manen, M. (1990). *Researching the Lived Experience: Human Science for an Action Sensitive Pedagogy.* Ontario, Canada: Atthouse.

Varcoe, C., & Hilton, A. (1995). Factors affecting acute care nurses use of research findings. *Canadian Journal of Nursing Research, 27*(4), 51–73.

Walker, L., Fleschler, R. G., Heaman, M. (1998). Determinants of a healthy lifestyle in new fathers. *Canadian Journal of Nursing Research, 30*(3), 21–37.

Walker, L. (1998). Weight related distress in the early months after childbirth. *Western Journal of Nursing Research 20*(1), 30–44.

Waltz, C., & Bausell, R.B. (1981). *Nursing Research: Design, Statistics and Computer Analysis.* Philadelphia: F.A. Davis.

Waltz, C., Strickland, O., & Lenz, E. (1991). *Measurement in Nursing Research* (2nd ed.). Philadelphia: FA Davis.

Warwick, D.P., & Osherson, S. (1973). *Comparative Research Methods.* Englewood Cliffs, N.J.: Prentice-Hall.

Waterman, A. Webb, L., & Williams, W. (1995). Parallels and contradictions in the theory and practice of action research in nursing. *Journal of Advanced Nursing, 22,* 779–784.

Webb, C. (1984). Feminist methodology in nursing research. *Journal of Advanced Nursing, 9,* 249–256.

Webb, C. (1993). Feminist research. Definitions, methodology, methods and evaluation. *Journal of Advanced Nursing, 18,* 416–423.

Weitz, R. (1990). Living with the stigma of AIDS, *Qualitative Sociology, 13*(1), 23–38.

Weitzman, E., & Miles, J. (1995). *Computer Programs for Qualitative Data Analysis.* Thousand Oaks, CA: Sage.

Whyte, W.F. (1955). *Street Corner Society: The Social Structure of an Italian Slum* (2nd ed.). Chicago: University of Chicago Press.

Whyte, W.F., Greenwood, D., & Lazes, P. (1991*). Participatory Action Research: Through Practice to Science in Social Research.* Newbury Park, CA: Sage.

Wilson, H. (1993). *Introducing Research in Nursing* (2nd ed.). Redwood City, CA: Addison-Wesley Nursing.

Wolf, Z.R., & Heinzer, M. M. (1999). Substruction: Illustrating the connections from research question to analysis. *Journal of Professional Nursing, 15*(1), 33–37.

Woods, N. F., & Catanzaro, M. (1988). *Nursing Research: Theory and Practice.* St. Louis, MI: C. V. Mosby.

Zerwekh, J. (2000). Caring on the ragged edge: Nursing persons who are disenfranchised. *Advances in Nursing Science, 22*(4), 47–61.

Index

Basic Procedures in SPSS (Version 10.0)
Starting with the menu bar, click the following to access the analysis window for each procedure

ANOVA: Analyze/General Linear Model/Univariate

CORRELATE: Analyze/Correlate/Bivariate

CROSSTABS: Analyze/Descriptive Statistics/Crosstabs

DESCRIPTIVES: Analyze/Descriptive Statistics/Descriptives

DISCRIMINANT: Analyze/Classify/Discriminant

FACTOR: Data Reduction/Factor

FREQUENCIES: Analyze/Descriptive Statistics/Frequencies

GRAPHS: Graphs/Scatter/Define

MANOVA: Analyze/General Linear Model/Multivariate

MEANS: Analyze/Compare Means/means

SPEARMAN CORR: Analyze/Correlation/Spearman

REGRESSION: Analyze/Regression/Linear (Method=Backward)

RELIABILITY: Analyze/Scale/Reliability (Model=Alpha)

t TEST PAIRS: Analyze/Compare Means/Paired-Samples t Test

t TEST GROUPS: Analyze/Compare Means/Independent-Samples t Test

Other basic procedures:

COMPUTE: Transform/Compute

IF: Transform/Compute

LIST: Use Syntax editor to issue command

RECODE: Transform/Recode/Into Different Variables

SORT CASES: Data/Sort Cases

SELECT CASES: Data/Select Cases

Research for Nurses: Methods and Interpretation takes the mystery out of research and in simple language illustrates the synergy and importance of research in nursing practice.

Whether you are learning to use research or embarking on a research project, this text provides:

♦ Guidelines for understanding each stage in evaluating and conducting research

♦ Easy-to-follow steps that guide you through a research project and help you to relate the findings to a practice setting

♦ Comprehensive coverage on both qualitative and quantitative approaches and a balanced view of the advantages, strengths, and limitations of each approach

♦ A statistics primer that is understandable to even the most numerically challenged student

♦ A chapter on bias in research

♦ "Nursing Researchers at Work" boxes that present case studies and sample projects to demonstrate key approaches, methods, and findings in research and relate them to the nursing practice

♦ Instructions on how to process data using the Statistical Package for the Social Sciences (SPSS)

♦ Website links to 160 sample questionnaires

Also available from F. A. Davis-
The Taber's Suite including:
- Taber's Cyclopedic Medical Dictionary, 19th edition
- Taber's Electronic Medical Dictionary CD-ROM, v.2.0
- Taber's Dictionary/CD-ROM Package
- Taber's Medical/Pharmaceutical Spell Checker
- Taber's Online (www.tabers.com), subscription-based web version of Taber's Electronic Medical Dictionary

Available at your health science bookstore or by calling 800.323.3555.
In Canada, call 800.665.1148.

Visit www.fadavis.com for additional information on all F. A. Davis products.

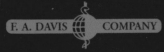

F. A. DAVIS COMPANY

The Taber's Publisher
www.fadavis.com
www.DrugGuide.com

ISBN 0-8036-0896-9

90000 >

EAN

9 780803 608962